T0251488

Experimental Models of Diabetes

Edited by

John H. McNeill, Ph.D.

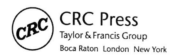

CRC Press
Taylor & Francis Group
Boca Raton London New York

CRC Press is an imprint of the
Taylor & Francis Group, an **informa** business

Library of Congress Cataloging-in-Publication Dat

Catalog record is available from the Library of Congress

Dedication

To my wife Sharon, the love of my life and my best friend,
who puts up with a lot and is always there for me.

Contents

The Editor

John H. McNeill, Ph.D., is Professor of Pharmacology and Toxicology and Dean of the Faculty of Pharmaceutical Sciences at The University of British Columbia in Vancouver, Canada.

Dr. McNeill graduated in 1960 from the University of Alberta with a B.Sc. (Pharm) degree. He obtained his M.Sc. from the same institution two years later and his Ph.D. in Pharmacology at the University of Michigan in 1967.

Dr. McNeill is a member of the Pharmacological Society of Canada, the American Society for Pharmacology and Experimental Therapeutics, the Western Pharmacology Society, the International Society for Heart Research, the Association of Faculties of Pharmacy, American Pharmaceutical Association, Sigma Xi, American Diabetes Association, Canadian Diabetes Association and Canadian Pharmaceutical Association. Dr. McNeill served on the Council and as President of the Pharmacological Society of Canada and the Western Pharmacology Society and on the Council of the North American Section and the international body of the International Society for Heart Research. He has served on and chaired many Canadian national research committees for the MRC, Canadian Heart and Stroke Foundation, Canadian Diabetes Association, and the PMAC-Health Research Foundation. He currently serves on the jury for the prestigious Prix Galien Award.

Dr. McNeill has received a number of awards for his research including the Upjohn Award (Pharmacological Society of Canada), McNeil Award (Association of Faculties of Pharmacy of Canada), and the Jacob Biely Award and Killam Award from The University of British Columbia. He has been an MRC Visiting Professor at a number of Canadian universities and at Montpellier University in France.

Dr. McNeill has presented numerous invited lectures in North America, Europe and Japan and has published over 350 manuscripts, reviews and book chapters. He is a founding editor of the *Journal of Pharmacological and Toxicological Methods*, has edited three books on methods used in evaluating biochemical and functional changes in the heart, and has edited or co-edited four books. His current major research interests are diabetes-induced cardiomyopathy, hyperinsulinemia and hypertension, investigational glucose-lowering agents, and mechanisms of action of insulin.

Contributors

Christopher R. Barnett   Diabetes Research Group, School of Biomedical Sciences, University of Ulster, Coleraine, County Londonderry, Northern Ireland, United Kingdom

Mary L. Battell   Division of Pharmacology and Toxicology, Faculty of Pharmaceutical Sciences, The University of British Columbia, Vancouver, British Columbia, Canada

Sharon Butler   Department of Agricultural, Food and Nutritional Science, University of Alberta, Edmonton, Alberta, Canada

Subrata Chakrabarti   Department of Pathology, University of Western Ontario, London, Ontario, Canada

Catherine J. Field   Department of Agricultural, Food and Nutritional Science, University of Alberta, Edmonton, Alberta, Canada

Peter R. Flatt   Diabetes Research Group, School of Biomedical Sciences, University of Ulster, Coleraine, Country Londonderry, Northern Ireland, United Kingdom

Jeffrey C. Flynn   Department of Medicine, University of Illinois at Chicago, Chicago, Illinois

Ivan C. Gerling   Department of Medicine, University of Tennessee, Memphis, Tennessee

Dong Cheol Han   Hyonam Kidney Laboratory, Soon Chun Hyang University, Seoul, Korea and Penn Center for Molecular Studies of Kidney Diseases, Renal — Electrolyte and Hypertension of Pennsylvania, School of Medicine, Philadelphia, Pennsylvania

Anthony R. Hebden   Heart and Stroke Foundation of British Columbia and Yukon, Vancouver, British Columbia, Canada

Costas Ioannides   Molecular Toxicology Group, School of Biological Sciences, University of Surrey, Guildford, Surrey, England, United Kingdom

Krista M. Kivilo   Department of Physiology and Biophysics, Case Western Reserve University, Cleveland, Ohio

Edward H. Leiter   The Jackson Laboratory, Bar Harbor, Maine

Gary D. Lopaschuk   Cardiovascular Research Group and Departments of Pediatrics and Pharmacology, University of Alberta, Edmonton, Alberta, Canada

Kathleen M. MacLeod   Division of Pharmacology and Toxicology, Faculty of Pharmaceutical Sciences, The University of British Columbia, Vancouver, British Columbia, Canada

Christopher H. S. McIntosh Department of Physiology, The University of British Columbia, Vancouver, British Columbia, Canada

John H. McNeill Division of Pharmacology and Toxicology, Faculty of Pharmaceutical Sciences, The University of British Columbia, Vancouver, British Columbia, Canada

Andras Mogyorosi Penn Center for Molecular Studies of Kidney Diseases, Renal-Electrolyte and Hypertension Division, Department of Medicine, University of Pennsylvania, School of Medicine, Philadelphia, Pennsylvania

Mahmood Mozaffari School of Dentistry, Oral Biology/Pharmacology, Medical College of Georgia, Augusta, Georgia

Raymond A. Pederson Department of Physiology, The University of British Columbia, Vancouver, British Columbia, Canada

Patrick Poucheret Laboratoire de Pharmacodynamie, Faculte de Pharmacie, Universite de Montpellier II, Montpellier, France

Brian Rodrigues Division of Pharmacology and Toxicology, Faculty of Pharmaceutical Sciences, The University of British Columbia, Vancouver, British Columbia, Canada

Stephen W. Schaffer Department of Pharmacology, School of Medicine, University of South Alabama, Mobile, Alabama

Kumar Sharma Division of Nephrology, Department of Medicine, Thomas Jefferson University, Philadelphia, Pennsylvania

William C. Stanley Department of Physiology and Biophysics, Case Western Reserve University, Cleveland, Ohio

Ramaswamy Subramanian Division of Pharmacology and Toxicology, Faculty of Pharmaceutical Sciences, The University of British Columbia, Vancouver, British Columbia, Canada

Subodh Verma Division of Cardiology, Faculty of Medicine, University of Calgary, Alberta, Canada

Violet G. Yuen Division of Pharmacology and Toxicology, Faculty of Pharmaceutical Sciences, The University of British Columbia, Vancouver, British Columbia, Canada

Fuad N. Ziyadeh Penn Center for Molecular Studies of Kidney Diseases, Renal-Electrolyte Division, Department of Medicine, University of Pennsylvania, School of Medicine, Philadelphia, Pennsylvania

Preface

The idea for publishing this book developed over a period of several years as my interest in studying diabetes increased. The need for a book that described the various animal models of diabetes and provided data on the effects of the diabetic state on the animals became apparent. Until fairly recently, most experimental studies of animal diabetes have been carried out in the early course of the disease. In addition, genetic models of Type 1 or Type 2 diabetes did not exist. Both of these situations have now changed and there is a considerable, but scattered, literature on these subjects. The book describes the models of both chemically induced (e.g., streptozotocin) and genetically occurring (e.g., BioBreeding Rat, Zucker Diabetic Fatty Rat) diabetes and provides data on the functional, biochemical, and pathological changes that occur over the course of the disease. Pharmacological information on experimental treatments of diabetes is also provided.

Having this information in one volume should be a great asset to those working in the field or contemplating the use of animal models in the study of diabetes. The relevance of each model to human disease is discussed in each section.

The authors are internationally known for their work in diabetes. The chapters have been peer-reviewed and edited and provide up-to-date, comprehensive, practical, and theoretical information on the topic.

I hope that the book will serve as a much-used reference and that the compiled information will save researchers precious time in building their knowledge background.

John H. McNeill, Ph.D.
Professor
Division of Pharmacology & Toxicology
Faculty of Pharmaceutical Sciences
The University of British Columbia
Vancouver, B.C.
Canada V6T 1Z3

Acknowledgments

I would like to thank my graduate students and colleagues for the discussions that led to the development of this book. In particular, Dr. Subodh Verma, then a student in my laboratory, was a significant factor early on in moving the project from an idea to a completed book. My secretary Sylvia Chan and my lab manager Mary Battell both contributed many extra hours of assistance in badgering authors, retyping manuscripts, and editing the proofs. My thanks to the authors for being on time (at least most of the time) and for putting up with my requests for revisions.

Section I

The Streptozotocin-Induced Diabetic Rat

1

Streptozotocin-Induced Diabetes: Induction, Mechanism(s), and Dose Dependency

Brian Rodrigues, Patrick Poucheret, Mary L. Battell, and John H. McNeill

CONTENTS

1.1 Introduction

1.1.1 Diabetes

The pancreas is an organ composed of exocrine (~98%) and endocrine (~2%) cells. The islets of Langerhans are clusters of endocrine tissue that are dispersed throughout the exocrine pancreas. There are four major cell types present within mammalian islets. These are β-cells (insulin producing), α-cells (glucagon producing), δ-cells (somatostatin

TABLE 1.1

Characteristic Features of Diabetes Subtypes

Characteristics	Type I (IDDM)	Type II (NIDDM)
Symptoms	Polyuria, polydipsia, fatigue, weight loss	Often asymptomatic in early years but may present with Type I symptoms especially in advanced stages
Age	<35 (common in youth)	>35 (frequent in adults)
Onset	Abrupt (days to weeks)	Weeks to months to years
Nutritional status	Undernourished	Majority are overweight
Ketosis	Prone	Resistant
Insulin	Mandatory	Required in <30%
Diet	Mandatory	Controls 30 to 50% cases
β-Cells	None (complete islet cell loss)	Varies
Islet cell antibodies	Yes	No
Family history	+ in 10%	+ in 30%
(Identical twins)	~50% concordance	~100% concordance

producing), and PP-cells (pancreatic polypeptide). The critical role of the pancreas in diabetes was not realized until it was discovered that complete removal of this organ resulted in hyperglycemia in dogs.[1] Subsequently, the Nobel prize was awarded to researchers who discovered that insulin from pancreatic extracts dramatically reduced hyperglycemia in pancreatectomized dogs.[2] Gepts[3] later demonstrated specific β-cell abnormalities and inflammmatory cells in the islets of Langerhans in patients with recently diagnosed insulin-dependent diabetes, and, using quantitative morphometry, it was found that Type I diabetes was associated with a specific and complete loss of pancreatic β-cells.[4]

Glucose stimulates the β-cells of the islets to release insulin, which then promotes glucose uptake and storage in various tissues. Considering these effects, hyperglycemia was believed to be due to insulin deficiency and hypoglycemia due to insulin excess. However, with the advent of insulin radioimmunoassays, it became apparent that the majority of patients with hyperglycemia were not completely insulin dependent and, in fact, had normal or even elevated concentrations of circulating insulin. Thus, diabetes mellitus is the name given to a multiple group of disorders with different etiologies. It is characterized by derangements in carbohydrate, protein, and fat metabolism caused by the complete or relative insufficiency of insulin secretion and/or insulin action. These aberrations account for the acute (fatigue, polyuria, polydipsia, etc.) as well as chronic (retinopathy, neuropathy, nephropathy, peripheral vascular disease, heart failure, etc.) complications of the disease.[5]

1.1.2 Classification of Diabetes

The classification of diabetes is based principally upon clinical symptoms and, when possible, on more specific etiologic characterization. Table 1.1 summarizes the two major types of diabetes: (1) diabetes associated with insulin-deficiency (Type I, insulin-dependent, IDDM; 5 to 10% of all cases) and (2) diabetes associated with insulin resistance (Type II, noninsulin-dependent, NIDDM; 90 to 95% of all cases). Other types of diabetes include gestational diabetes, impaired glucose tolerance, and diabetes resulting from other conditions or syndromes.[6]

1.1.2.1 Type I Diabetes

This disease is associated with a specific and complete loss of pancreatic β-cells, leaving islets composed of an increased number of α, δ, and PP cells. Thus, Type I diabetes can be thought of as a specific β-cytectomy, a phenomenon mimicked in animals with the use of chemical agents like alloxan or streptozotocin. Autoimmune destruction of pancreatic β-cells has been suggested to be the most common cause of IDDM. Although the factors that initiate this autoimmune response are not completely understood, it is more frequent in patients with certain human leukocyte antigen tissue types. Other initiating factors include viruses (i.e., Coxsackie B_4)[7] and chemical toxins. Less common causes of IDDM are conditions that result in a reduction in the mass of islet cell tissue, such as may occur with several types of pancreatitis, pancreatic carcinoma, and pancreatectomy.

1.1.2.2   Type II Diabetes

Patients with NIDDM represent 90 to 95% of the diabetic population. Between 60 and 90% of those having NIDDM are obese,[8] often exhibiting hyperinsulinemia and associated insulin resistance. Although the primary causes of the disease have not been identified at the molecular level, current research strongly suggests that this disease arises as a consequence of (1) failure of insulin action due to abnormalities at the cell surface (decreased affinity of the receptors for insulin) or within the cell (post-receptor defects) and (2) deficiency in insulin secretion or (3) a combination of these processes.[9] Although the majority of patients with NIDDM are insulin resistant, it is undecided whether the primary molecular defect lies within the insulin signal transduction pathway or in β-cell insulin secretion.[10,11]

1.2   Animal Models of Diabetes

Animal models featuring physiological and pathological changes characteristic of each diabetes subtype are important to understand this complex disease better and to propose potential treatments. For example, specific etiological factors and/or genetic backgrounds can be selected and combined to produce a particular type of experimental diabetes, allowing the researcher to explore particular biochemical or anatomical alterations. In this way, animal models can provide a means to study disturbances found in human diabetes.

1.2.1   NIDDM Animal Models

The genetic NIDDM models are produced through selective breeding, spontaneous mutations, or genetic engineering. Some examples include the db/db mouse, ob/ob mouse, KK mouse, NZO mouse, fa/fa Zucker rat, and fa/fa diabetic Zucker rat. Most of these models demonstrate various degrees of glycemia, insulinemia, and obesity. Chemically induced NIDDM is obtained through injection of agents that produce the desired pathology. The most commonly used agent is streptozotocin (STZ). A mild and stable form of diabetes, resembling Type II human diabetes, is produced by a single dose of STZ (90 mg/kg i.v.) in 2-day-old neonatal rats.[12] The induced β-cell injury is followed by limited regeneration, primarily as a result of ductal budding rather than mitosis of preexisting β-cells, creating a short-term normalization of glycemia. At 6 to 15 weeks of age, the rats have an impaired glucose disposal rate and significant β-cell secretory dysfunction. Surgical NIDDM can also be produced by removal of various amounts of pancreatic mass.

1.2.2 IDDM Animal Models

IDDM is caused by a marked reduction (>90%) in the number of pancreatic β-cells.[3] Genetic models of Type I diabetes include the NOD mouse and the BB diabetic rat. In these animals, diabetes occurs spontaneously with a total dependence on exogenous insulin for survival. Viral induction of IDDM allows for the identification of the role of environmental factors in the development of human diabetes. Chemically induced Type I diabetes is the most commonly used animal model of diabetes. Chemical agents that produce diabetes can be classified into three categories, and include agents that (1) specifically damage β-cells; (2) cause temporary inhibition of insulin production and/or secretion, and (3) diminish the metabolic efficacy of insulin in target tissues. In general, chemicals in the first category are of specific interest as they closely reproduce lesions that occur during β-cell destruction in IDDM. Moreover, these agents provide a relatively permanent diabetes that is suitable for long-term studies. Alloxan, a cyclic urea analog was the first agent in this category that was reported to produce a permanent diabetes in laboratory animals.[13] STZ[14] has replaced alloxan as the principal agent used to produce experimental diabetes. This is due to (1) the greater selectivity of β-cells for STZ;[15] (2) the lower mortality rate seen in STZ diabetic animals (effective diabetogenic dose of STZ is four to five times less than its lethal dose);[16] and (3) the longer half-life of STZ in the body (15 min).[17]

1.3   Streptozotocin Diabetes

STZ [2-deoxy-2-(3-methyl-3-nitrosourea) 1-D-glucopyranose] is a broad-spectrum antibiotic which is produced from *Streptomyces achromogenes*. The diabetogenic response to STZ was first detected by Upjohn Laboratories during testing of potential antibiotics from this organism. However, Rakieten et al.[14] were the first to describe that β-cell necrosis and the ensuing diabetic state could be produced after a single intravenous dose of STZ in rats and dogs.

1.3.1   Mechanism of the Diabetogenic Effect of STZ

The chemical structure of STZ comprises a glucose molecule with a highly reactive nitrosourea side chain that is thought to initiate its cytotoxic action. The glucose moiety directs this agent to the pancreatic β-cell,[18] where it binds to a membrane receptor to generate structural damage. A decrease in diabetes induction efficacy after substitution of glucose by other sugars supports the presence of a stereospecific membrane receptor or recognition site on the plasma membrane of the β-cell,[19-21] identified as probably being the glucose transporter GLUT2.[22] However, as no plasma membrane labeling was recorded with radioactive ^{14}C-STZ,[23] another explanation for β-cell plasma membrane damage is that it occurs secondary to other indirect actions of STZ.

At the intracellular level, three major phenomena are currently held responsible for β-cell death: (1) process of methylation, (2) free radical generation, and (3) nitric oxide (NO) production.

Methylation. The deleterious effect of STZ results from the generation of highly reactive carbonium ions (CH_3^+), formed from decomposition of the nitroso moiety. The CH_3^+ ions cause DNA breaks by alkylating DNA bases at various positions,[24] resulting in activation of the nuclear enzyme poly(ADP-ribose) synthetase as part of the cell repair mechanism.

As cellular pyridine nucleotides, particularly NAD^+ are utilized as substrates for the nuclear enzyme, a profound decline in NAD^+ occurs within 20 min. In effect, an abrupt and irreversible NAD^+ exhaustion leads to cessation of NAD^+-dependent energy and protein metabolism, ultimately leading to cell death. Inhibition of poly(ADP-ribose) synthetase by agents like 3-aminobenzamide and nicotinamide are known to protect β-cells from NAD^+ depletion and cell death after STZ exposure.[25]

Free Radicals. Free radical involvement in STZ effects have also been investigated. Hydrogen peroxide has been shown to be produced in pancreatic islets upon STZ exposure *in vivo* and *in vitro*.[26,27] Moreover, because superoxide dismutase, a free radical scavenger was demonstrated to provide some protection against the diabetogenic properties of STZ, it was concluded that oxidative stress could play a role in determining STZ toxicity.[28]

Nitric Oxide. Involvement of NO has also been proposed as a possible mechanism for mediating the diabetogenic effects of STZ.[29] The precise metabolic processes leading to NO generation from STZ are unclear,[30] but may involve the metabolism or spontaneous decay of STZ. Whatever the mechanism, STZ-generated NO seems to be significantly involved in the cytotoxicity toward β-cells.[31]

Recently, an integrated hypothesis was proposed to explain the mechanism of action of STZ. In this hypothesis, STZ, through production of superoxide, would generate peroxynitrite. The latter would dissociate into NO and hydroxyl radicals, thus leading to β-cell DNA damage and apoptosis.[32] Whatever the mechanism involved, nuclear and mitochondrial DNA are then repaired by the excision–repair process using nuclear poly(ADP-ribose) synthetase.[33,34] Indeed, the activity of this enzyme is significantly increased within 10 min after STZ injection.[35] The poly(ADP-ribose) synthetase uses NAD (whose concentration decreases within 20 min after STZ) as a substrate to produce the ADP-ribose units needed to repair DNA, thus depleting intracellular NAD levels. The decrease in intracellular NAD concentration could also be a consequence of a reduced uptake of its precursors and/or an impaired synthesis by the cell.[36] Indeed, one hypothesis suggests that alkylation and inhibition of intracellular enzymes involved in ATP production contribute to a decrease in NAD synthesis.[37]

In addition to the above effects of STZ on β-cells, this agent has also been used to induce diabetes with multiple low doses.[38] After multiple low-dose injection of STZ, islet degeneration due to direct STZ toxicity has been suggested to initiate an inflammatory response whereby mononuclear cells migrate from the bloodstream to the tissue, where they differentiate into macrophages.[39] These cells phagocytose the pancreatic β-cells, thereby releasing cytochemical mediators.[40] Subsequently, lymphocytic infiltration occurs.[41]

Several mechanisms have been postulated to explain why the fatal events described above occur selectively in β-cells. These include (1) a high affinity of STZ for the β-cell membrane, (2) unique SH groups that render the β-cell membrane especially sensitive to oxidative interactions, (3) a low capacity of β-cells to scavenge free radicals, and (4) a low NAD^+/DNA ratio in islets compared with other tissues.

1.4   Administration of STZ

1.4.1   Relationship of STZ Dose to Severity of Diabetes

Since its use to induce diabetes was first described in 1963 by Rakieten et al.,[14] STZ has been administered over a wide range of doses by several routes to rats and other animals.

Junod et al. [15] first described the triphasic pattern of changes in blood glucose and insulin in the 24-h period immediately following intravenous injection of 65 mg/kg STZ to male Wistar rats. An initial hyperglycemia that lasts for 1 h is followed by a critical period of marked hypoglycemia (lasting ~6 h), which is brought about by massive β-cell degranulation and an enormous release of pancreatic insulin. Stable hyperglycemia develops within 24 to 48 h and remains three to four times higher than normal in concert with an ~50% reduction in plasma insulin levels and a pancreatic insulin content less than 5% of control.[15] Although these animals are insulin deficient, they do not require insulin supplementation for survival and do not develop ketonuria. After a single injection, β-cell necrosis can be detected within 2 to 4 h on ultrastructural examination and within 24 h by light microscopy.[15] Then, 4 days following administration of STZ in adult rats, the remaining β-cells appear degranulated, with evidence of limited proliferation over several months, a probable consequence of preexisting precursor β-cells rather than a result of ductal or acinar cell transformation into β-cells.[42]

The report by Junod et al.[15] also established that a dose of 25 mg/kg resulted in no change in serum glucose and immunoreactive insulin or pancreatic insulin content up to 7 days after STZ. At the other end of the dose–response curve, 100 mg/kg STZ causes an intense β-cell necrosis. Disintegration and phagocytosis of necrotic cells is rapid, with practically no evidence of debris or inflammation visible after 3 days. In an identical rapid manner, there was a remarkable elevation of serum glucose within 24 h, a drop to about one half of the preinjection level of insulin, and the loss of 98% of the pancreatic insulin. In addition, this dose resulted in the appearance of ketonuria within the first 24 h, and death in most of the animals. That the deaths were due to the loss of insulin was established by administration of exogenous insulin. At doses between 25 and 100 mg/kg, there was a variation in the severity of the diabetes produced with increasing doses of STZ, as indicated by increasing levels of serum glucose and progressive decrease in the pancreatic insulin level at 24 h. The relative severity was also reflected in the changes in weight gain in the rats over a period of 5 weeks, with the rats that had received 55 and 65 mg/kg STZ failing to increase in body weight. This important paper provided several additional pieces of information. The authors reported that, at a dose of 35 mg/kg, about one quarter of the rats spontaneously recovered from the diabetes that had initially been exhibited. Moreover, there was a correlation between the pancreatic insulin content and the recovery from the diabetes. They also demonstrated that a second injection of STZ produced diabetes that was similar to that of a single dose of the total amount injected; i.e., two injections of 25 mg/kg resulted in a diabetes that was similar in severity to that produced by a single injection of about 50 mg/kg even though the rats exhibited no signs of diabetes following the first injection. Their results also documented a lack of correlation between the administered dose of STZ and the level of serum insulin at 24 h or at 7 days. This suggested that the pancreas compensated for the induced hyperglycemia by increasing the output of insulin from the remaining insulin-producing cells. These data indicated that pancreatic insulin content was a good measure of the severity of diabetes. The second valuable indicator of the severity of diabetes was the relative weight gain. This index has the obvious advantage of not requiring the sacrifice of the animals. Conversely, serum insulin level was not a good indicator of the severity of diabetes, and serum glucose was useful only up to that level where glucose starts to spill into the urine. An important point to note in the Junod et al. study[15] was that rats were fasted for 16 h prior to administration of STZ and rats that were sacrificed 10 h post-STZ continued to fast up to the time of death. This likely contributed to the deaths that occurred in the groups receiving the higher doses and may have resulted in an additional degree of severity of diabetes. This publication should be required reading for any scientist planning to work with STZ diabetic animals.

TABLE 1.2

Routes of Administration of STZ

Route	Dose (mg/)kg	Weight (g)	Strain (mmol/l)	Glucose	Ref.
i.v.	50	100–120	Sherman	16.5	14
i.v.	25–100	170–230	Wistar	Varied	15
i.v.	25–85	150–250	Sprague-Dawley	Varied	43
i.v.	30–70	250			
i.v.	30–100	150–200	Sprague-Dawley	Varied	45
i.p.	40–60	350–450	Wistar	Varied	46
i.p.	100	200	Sprague-Dawley	25.3	47
i.p.	35	260–270	Wistar	27.5	48
i.p.	100	180–220	Sprague-Dawley	>16.6	68
i.p.	70	140–160	Sprague-Dawley	23.9	69
i.p.	50	200–225	Sprague-Dawley	25.3	70
s.c.	40 twice	170–190	Sprague-Dawley	25	71
s.c.	40 twice				
i.c.	65	290–350	Sprague-Dawley	15.9	73
i.m.	20–120	100–300	Sprague-Dawley	Various	74

Note: i.v., intravenous (various veins were used; see individual publications); i.p., intraperitoneal; s.c., subcutaneous; i.c., intracardiac; i.m., intramuscular.

Junod's[15] finding of an STZ dose–response relationship was essentially confirmed by Bar-On et al.[43] in 1976 who administered 25 to 85 mg/kg STZ to Sprague-Dawley rats weighing 150 to 200 g. Doses of 25 or 35 mg/kg did not result in increased plasma glucose or triglyceride levels, whereas doses of 45 or 55 mg/kg did. These authors reported a mortality of one out of six in the 55-mg/kg dose group and rats in this group lost weight and appeared sick. Doses higher than 55 mg/kg were only administered to rats that received a high sucrose diet, and there was a 100% mortality in these animals.

The long-term stability of the diabetic condition was examined by Ar'Rajab and Ahrén.[44] Using 240- to 260-g male Sprague-Dawley rats, they were able to induce a state of diabetes that was long term only by using doses of 50 to 70 mg/kg STZ. The transient diabetes induced by doses of 30 and 40 mg/kg gave blood glucose levels that were elevated at day 1 to 7, but normalized by day 10. In these rats, the glucose-induced insulin release was absent at day 1 but normal at 3 months at which time the islet morphology also appeared normal. At doses of 50 to 70 mg/kg, the diabetes was stable. Insulin treatment for 1 week following injection of STZ normalized blood glucose in rats that received 55 mg/kg, but failed to provide a long-term normalization of plasma glucose in rats receiving 65 to 75 mg/kg. These studies reported no differences in the absolute plasma insulin levels between the groups in spite of the large differences in the plasma glucose levels.

While the above studies all report a dose dependency to the STZ effects, there is no agreement on the results of a particular dose. Junod et al.[15] used Wistar rats and fasted the rats prior to injection of the STZ, whereas Ar'Rajab and Ahrén[44] and Bar-On et al.[43] used Sprague-Dawley rats and did not fast prior to injection of STZ. Bar-On et al. reported at least one death (out of six) resulting from a 55-mg/kg dose while Ar'Rajab and Ahrén did not find deaths nor even weight loss up to 70 mg/kg. Results from other studies (summarized in Table 1.2) confirm that even when route of administration and dose of STZ are constant, there is wide variability in the severity of diabetes produced by various laboratories in different groups of rats.

Two additional important aspects of the relation between dose of STZ and severity of diabetes have been documented by Engle et al.[45] In this study, 150- to 200-g male Sprague-Dawley rats were injected with doses of 30 to 100 mg/kg STZ via the tail vein, and fasting serum glucose, blood urea nitrogen (BUN), urine output at 48 and 96 h, as well as decreases in weight gain were measured as an index of the severity of diabetes. Interestingly, the general pattern of changes in these groups with increasing dose of STZ was not seen in the group that received 100 mg/kg STZ. Instead, the 11 (out of 20) surviving animals in this group had values of serum glucose, BUN, urine output, and weight gain that indicated a severity of diabetes that was less than that of the group receiving 50 mg/kg. Evidently, the 11 surviving animals had been able to resist the effects of STZ. The second important point observed was when the animals were regrouped according to fasting serum glucose. When the data were sorted in this manner, fasting serum glucose appeared to be a good indicator of the severity of diabetes. Moreover, there was a wide variation in the severity of diabetes within a group of rats even when all the rats received the same dose of STZ.

1.4.2   Routes of Administration of STZ

All the studies described above used intravenous injection of STZ under ether or halothane anesthesia. However, other investigators have also used intraperitoneal injection of STZ to induce diabetes. Yogev et al.[46] studied rats made diabetic with an intraperitoneal injection of STZ with doses of 40, 50, and 60 mg/kg under ether anesthesia. This group used male Wistar rats weighing 350 to 400 g. All groups of rats receiving STZ had markedly elevated levels of plasma glucose and BUN, and lost weight over a 4-week period. The most severe changes were noted in the group receiving 50 mg/kg STZ. The authors did not comment on any deaths occurring in the group receiving 60 mg/kg, but the lower number of rats in that group suggested that mortality had occurred. If this is true, these results confirm the observations of Engle et al.[45] that the group of animals surviving the highest dose of STZ can be somewhat less diabetic than a group receiving (and surviving) a lower dose.

Giorgino et al.[47] induced diabetes (100 mg/kg STZ) in 200-g male Sprague-Dawley rats by the intraperitoneal route following an overnight fast. In these animals, fasting plasma glucose levels were markedly elevated, plasma insulin decreased to about 50% of control, and there was an approximately 20% decline in body weight within 5 days following STZ. Whiting et al.[48] also induced diabetes with an intraperitoneal injection of STZ in male Wistar rats of 260 to 270 g weight. Their dose of 35 mg/kg produced a marked degree of hyperglycemia 10 weeks after the injection of STZ, accompanied by weight loss. Additional routes of administration of STZ are described in Table 1.2.

1.4.3   STZ Diabetes in Female Rats

Rodrigues and McNeill[49] have examined cardiac function in male and female Wistar rats made diabetic with 55 mg/kg STZ. These authors reported a greater percent drop in body weight in the male rats compared with female rats even though there were no differences in serum glucose or insulin between the two diabetic groups. Diabetes did result in a greater depression in the rate of pressure development in an isolated working heart preparation from diabetic males compared with the pressure development in hearts from female rats. Other doses of STZ have also been used to induce diabetes in female rats (Table 1.3).

TABLE 1.3

Administration of STZ to Female Rats

Route	Dose (mg/kg)	Weight (g)	Strain	(mmol/l) Glucose	Ref.
i.v.	55	170–180	Wistar	35.3	49
i.v.	20, 40	234	Albino	7.1, 29.2	75
i.p.	75	175–200	Sprague-Dawley	24–25	76
i.p.	40, 80	200–250	Wistar	13, 21	77
i.p.	50	200	Sprague-Dawley	20.2	78

Note: i.v., intravenous; i.p., intraperitoneal.

1.4.4 Effect of Age on Diabetogenic Action of STZ

The age of the animals has some influence on the severity of diabetes produced by a given dose of STZ. As seen in Tables 1.1 and 1.2, rats of 100 to 400 g for males and 170 to 250 g for females have been used in many studies. The information listed in these tables is by no means exhaustive, and the range is likely greater. The study that has directly addressed the question of the effect of age on the diabetogenic effects of STZ has used smaller animals than those generally studied. Masiello et al.[50] used male Wistar rats of 50, 70, 90, 130, and 170 g body weight (age between 25 and 50 days) and doses of STZ from 40 up to 100 mg/kg i.v. Their data suggest that the smaller rats tolerate a higher dose of STZ, but since the experiments were only carried out to 48 h, the results are equivocal. Although Junod et al.,[15] using rats between 170 and 230 g, found that there were many deaths in rats receiving 100 mg/kg STZ i.v. as did Engle et al.[45] using rats in the 150 to 200 g body weight range, Dubuc[51] administered doses of 100 and 150 mg/kg STZ s.c. to Sprague-Dawley rats 20 to 24 days of age (about 50 g body weight) and apparently all the diabetic rats survived up to 15 weeks post-STZ. Yogev et al.[46] used rats of 350 to 450 g body weight and found persistent diabetes even at a dose of 40 mg/kg STZ i.p. Ramanadham et al.[52] used male Wistar rats to examine the effect of age/weight differences on the diabetes produced by STZ. The two weight ranges were 175 to 200 g (6 weeks of age) and 325 to 350 g (12 weeks of age). Examined 4 weeks following the induction of diabetes, the high-weight-range group had greater plasma levels of triglycerides, cholesterol, and phospholipid than the younger group. In addition, the low-weight group continued to gain weight while the high-weight group lost weight. The high-weight group did not show higher plasma glucose or a significantly greater reduction in plasma insulin, but, as stated above, these are not necessarily the best indexes of severity of diabetes. Newby et al.[53] induced diabetes in young, 140 to 220 g (6 to 8 week) male Wistar rats with 50 mg/kg STZ and in older, moderately obese, 450 to 500 g (6 to 8 month) rats with 30 mg/kg STZ. There was no difference in the serum glucose or insulin levels between these two groups of rats in spite of the different dosages of STZ used.

1.4.5 Preparation of STZ

The initial report on the diabetic action of STZ[14] reported that STZ is not stable in solution, requiring that solutions be made fresh daily. Furthermore, the compound is maximally stable at pH 4, and the stability decreases rapidly at higher or lower pH. As a consequence, most authors report that they prepare STZ in a citrate buffer with the pH adjusted to pH 4.5, or in acidified 0.9% saline at pH 4.5, and that the solution is injected within a short time (within 5 min).[43] The conventional requirement for pH 4.5 citrate buffer was brought into question by the study by Axler[54] who found an effective diabetogenic action in saline at pH 7.2 even when the solution was heated to 37°C for 30 min prior to being injected into female BALB/c mice. Povoski et al.[55] used solutions of STZ prepared and stored at 6°C for several days to induce diabetes in Syrian golden hamsters. They found no differences up to day 9 following injection of STZ using fresh STZ solutions compared with solutions stored at room temperature for up to 7 days. The dosage of STZ used was 50 mg/kg, and the procedure involved daily I.P. injections on 3 consecutive days. The plasma glucose levels 9 days after the final injection was 16.2 to 17.8 mmol/l. The authors concluded that it would be preferable to prepare the STZ solution, allow it to come to equilibrium, and store aliquots at 6°C.

Evan et al.[56] measured the half-life of STZ in plasma and determined that t½ was 6.9 min. Rakieten et al.[14] reported that the LD_{50} for STZ was about 130 mg/kg. STZ exists as two anomers at carbon-1. Rossini et al.[57] examined two lots of STZ, one 90% α, 10% β, and the other 75% β, 25% α, at doses from 10 to 60 mg/kg i.v. in Sprague-Dawley male rats. The α anomer produced slightly, but significantly greater levels of plasma glucose at 48 h after the injection at doses between 30 and 45 mg/kg but not at the higher or lower doses tested (10, 20, 50, 55, 60).

1.4.6 Susceptibility of Different Strains of Rats to STZ Diabetes

Two reports have examined the differences in induced diabetes in two closely related strains of rats: the Wistar and Wistar Kyoto (WKY) rat. Ramanadham et al.[52] used Wistar and WKY rats weighing between 175 and 200 g and administered doses of 55 and 65 mg/kg STZ i.v. Differences in the level of diabetes between the two strains were evident in the measurement of blood lipids. For example, WKY diabetic rats developed a much less severe hyperlipidemia than the corresponding Wistar diabetic rats. There was also less evidence of heart dysfunction in the diabetic WKY in contrast to the diabetic Wistar rat. Rodrigues et al.[58] confirmed and extended the findings of Ramanadham et al.[52] In this study, Wistar rats made diabetic with 55 mg/kg STZ had significantly higher fasting plasma glucose, significantly higher area under the glucose curve of an oral glucose tolerance test, and significantly lower pancreatic insulin content than WKY rats made diabetic with the same dose of STZ. At a higher dose of STZ (75 mg/kg), the difference in the plasma glucose (fasted or nonfasted) was not present, but the insulin output in response to an oral glucose challenge was significantly lower (as measured by area under the curve) and the pancreatic insulin content was less in the Wistar compared with the WKY diabetic rats. It is notable that even the higher dose of STZ failed to induce elevation in the plasma triglyceride levels in the WKY diabetic rats. The differences in the diabetogenic response to STZ between these two closely related strains of rats indicate that some differences should be expected between different strains of rats. Other strains of rats are even more sensitive to the effects of STZ. The spontaneously hypertensive rat has an elevated plasma glucose and triglyceride content following 35 mg/kg STZ while its parent strain, the WKY rat, fails to show such elevations.[59] Further, 3-month-old female spontaneously hypertensive rats receiving a dose of STZ as low as 10 mg/kg showed an increased plasma glucose level after administration of a 2-g/kg body weight load of glucose as compared with SHR rats that had not received STZ.[60]

1.5   Care of STZ Diabetic Rats

Because of the disease, some special care should be taken in dealing with diabetic rats. Clearly, all rats in a given experiment should be treated in an identical manner, so it will be necessary to provide the same care to all animals. The Canadian Council on Animal Care *Guide to the Use and Care of Experimental Animals* (Vols. 1 and 2) is an excellent source of information about correct care of rats in general.[61,62] Untreated STZ diabetic rats drink a large amount of fluid[63] and produce a correspondingly high urine volume.[45] A diabetic rat may drink up to its own weight in fluid each day. Care must therefore be taken that the housing is such that the animals can stay dry. If cages with bedding such as shavings are used, the bedding will need to be changed frequently, usually every day, and, in some circumstances, more than once per day. If the bedding is not changed, the rats get wet, and risk losing body heat. The diarrhea that frequently occurs in STZ diabetic rats[64] is an additional reason to see that bedding is always clean and dry. Generally, cages with bedding are preferred in experiments using STZ diabetic rats since wire-bottomed cages can lead to injuries to their feet, particularly in chronic experiments. Diabetic rats should always have sufficient water to drink and sufficient food. This holds true for all experimental animals at all times, but experimenters must be aware of the increased needs of diabetic animals. It may be necessary to fast rats overnight prior to various procedures. Provided that the rats are given sufficient time to regain weight between periods of fasting, this should not result in adverse effects on the rats. It is highly beneficial in chronic experiments to measure food and fluid intake and body weight gain in the rats since this can give valuable information about the health status of the rats. As with all experimental animals, the STZ diabetic rats should have sufficient space and not be crowded with many rats per cage. This may lead to competition for food and result in increased and unnecessary morbidity and mortality. In general, two to three STZ diabetic rats are housed per cage (21 cm high by 25.5 cm wide by 47 cm long). When inducing diabetes in spontaneously hypertensive rats, mortality over the course of 6 weeks can be reduced from 35% to about 15% by housing only two SHR STZ diabetic rats per cage.[65] Since rats are social animals, individual housing is not ideal and should only be used when required by the experiment.

1.6   Conclusion

In conclusion, numerous types of experimental diabetes are available to investigators to explore various physiological and biochemical defects observed during this disease. However, with the different animal models of diabetes, there will always be physiological, pathological, and morphological differences between models. Moreover, an unavoidable reality is that none of these animal models of diabetes are perfectly equivalent to the human disease state. Investigators working with STZ diabetic rats should give careful consideration to the dose of STZ used and ascertain the effect that is produced. It is not adequate to assume that the conditions stated by another investigator will produce rats with a similar degree of diabetes. At least one assessment of diabetic severity should be included in the experiment and reported in publications. The reliable indicators of the degree of severity of diabetes include relative weight gain, fasting plasma (or serum) glucose levels, area under the curve of an oral (or other route) glucose tolerance test, pancreatic insulin content at termination of the experiment, plasma lipid levels (particularly triglyceride levels), and fluid intake. Investigators may be doing studies where it is desired to produce a severe form of diabetes in rats which will be terminated within a short period of time, for example, 1 week,[66] or may be doing studies where the long-term survival of the rats without therapeutic intervention is critical, for example, more than 1 year.[67] The dose of STZ should be modified to be appropriate for the experiment. In addition, since diabetes may not be uniform among a group of animals, it is necessary to state a criterion for diabetes, for example, rats with 13 mM plasma glucose or greater. It is also valuable to state whether or not any mortality occurred among the diabetic animals and when the mortality occurred. Experiments involving more than one strain must be carefully considered but, provided the above points are considered, e.g., statement concerning criterion for successful diabetes induction, the data obtained can still provide valuable information leading to better understanding of this disease state.

Acknowledgments

The studies described in this chapter were supported by operating grants from Medical Research Council of Canada, the Heart & Stroke Foundation of B.C. and Yukon, and the Canadian Diabetes Association (J. H. McNeill) and the Canadian Diabetes Association (B. Rodrigues). The financial support of the Canadian Diabetes Association (scholarship to B. Rodrigues; fellowship to P. Poucheret) is gratefully acknowledged. We thank Sylvia Chan for her excellent secretarial assistance.

References

1. von Mering, J. and Minkowski, O., Diabetes mellitus nach Pankreasextirpation, *Arch. Exp. Pathol. Pharmakol.*, 26, 371, 1889.
2. Banting, F. G., Best, C. H., Collip, J. B., and Macleod, J. J. R., The preparation of pancreatic extracts containing insulin, *Trans. R. Soc. Canada*, Section V, 1922.
3. Gepts, W., Pathologic anatomy of the pancreas in juvenile diabetes mellitus, *Diabetes*, 14, 619, 1965.
4. Foulis, A. K. and Stewart, J. A, The pancreas in recent-onset Type I (insulin-dependent) diabetes mellitus: insulin content of islets, insulitis and associated changes in exocrine acinar tissue, *Diabetologia*, 26, 456, 1984.
5. Rubin, R. J., Altman, W. M., and Mendelson, D. N., Health care expenditures for people with diabetes mellitus — 1992, *J. Clincrinol. Endo. Metabol.*, 78, 809, 1994.
6. National Diabetes Data Group, Classification and diagnosis of diabetes mellitus and other categories of glucose intolerance, *Diabetes*, 28, 1039, 1979.
7. Yoon, J. W., Austin, M., and Orodera, T., Virus-induced diabetes mellitus: isolation of a virus from the pancreas of a child with diabetic ketoacidosis, *N. Engl. J. Med.*, 300, 1173, 1979.
8. Ekoe, J. M., Epidemiology of diabetes mellitus in Caucasian populations, in *Diabetes Mellitus and Its Long-Term Complications*, Elsevier, Amsterdam, 107, 1988.
9. Yli-Jarvinen, H., Role of insulin resistance in the pathogenesis of NIDDM, *Diabetologia*, 38, 1378, 1995.

10. Taylor, S. I., Accili, D., and Imai, Y., Insulin resistance or insulin deficiency, which is the primary cause of NIDDM? *Diabetes*, 43, 735, 1994.

11. Kahn, C. R., Insulin action, diabetogenes, and the cause of Type II diabetes, *Diabetes*, 43, 1066, 1994.

12. Bonnevie-Nielsen, V., Steffes, M. W., and Lernmark, A., A major loss in islet mass and β-cell function precedes hyperglycemia in mice given multiple low doses of streptozotocin, *Diabetes*, 30, 424, 1981.

13. Dunn, J. S., Sheehan, H. L., and McLetchie, N. G. B., Necrosis of islets of Langerhans produced experimentally, *Lancet*, 1, 484, 1943.

14. Rakieten, N., Rakieten, M. L., and Nadkarni, M. V., Studies on the diabetogenic action of streptozotocin (NSC 37919), *Cancer Chemother. Rep.*, 29, 91, 1963.

15. Junod, A., Lambert, A. E., Stauffacher, W., and Renold, A. E., Diabetogenic action of streptozotocin: relationship of dose to metabolic response, *J. Clin. Invest.*, 48, 2129, 1969.

16. Hoftiezer, V. and Carpenter, A. M., Comparison of streptozotocin-induced diabetes in the rat, including volumetric quantitation of the pancreatic islets, *Diabetologia*, 9, 178, 1973.

17. Agrawal, M. K., Streptozotocin mechanisms of action. Proceedings of a workshop held on 21 June 1980, Washington, D.C., *FEBS Lett.*, 120, 1, 1980.

18. Johansson, E. B. and Tjalve, H, Studies on the tissue-deposition and fate of [^{14}C]-streptozotocin with special reference to the pancreatic islets, *Acta Endocrinol.*, 89, 339, 1978.

19. Dulin, W. E. and Wyse, B. M., Studies on the ability of compounds to block the diabetogenic activity of streptozotocin, *Diabetes*, 18, 459, 1969.

20. Ganda, O. P., Rossini, A. A., and Like, A. A., Studies on streptozotocin diabetes, *Diabetes*, 25, 595, 1976.

21. Kawada, J., Okita, M., Nishida, M., Yoshimura, Y., Toyooka, K., and Kubota, S., Protective effect of 4,6-O-ethylidene glucose against the cytotoxicity of streptozotocin in pancreatic beta cells *in vivo*: indirect evidence for the presence of a glucose transporter in beta cells, *J. Endocrinol.*, 112, 375, 1987.

22. Schnedl, W. J., Ferber, S., Johnson, J. H., and Newgard, C. B., STZ transport and cytotoxicity, specific enhancement in GLUT2-expressing cells, *Diabetes*, 43, 1326, 1994.

23. Masiello, P., Karunanayake, E. H., Bergamini, E., Hearse, D. J., and Mellows, G., ^{14}C-streptozotocin: its distribution and interaction with nucleic acid and protein, *Biochem. Pharmacol.*, 30, 1907, 1981.

24. Uchigata, Y., Yamamoto, H., Kawamura, A., and Okamoto, H., Protection by superoxide dismutase, catalase and poly(ADP-ribose) synthetase inhibitors against alloxan- and streptozotocin-induced islet DNA strand breaks and against the inhibition of proinsulin synthesis, *J. Biol. Chem.*, 257, 6084, 1982.

25. Wilson, G. L., Patton, N. J., McCord, J. M., Mullins, D. W., and Mossman, B. T., Mechanisms of streptozotocin- and alloxan-induced damage in rat B cells, *Diabetologia*, 27, 587, 1984.

26. Gandy, S. E., Buse, M. G., and Crouch, R. K., Protective role of superoxide dismutase against diabetogenic drugs, *J. Clin. Invest.*, 70, 650, 1982.

27. Papaccio, G., Pisanti, F. A., and Frascatore, S., Acetyl-homocysteine-thiolactone-induced increase of superoxide dismutase counteracts the effect of subdiabetogenic doses of streptozotocin, *Diabetes*, 35, 470, 1986.

28. Robbins, M. J., Sharp, R. A., Slonim, A. E., and Burr, I.M., Protection against streptozotocin induced diabetes by superoxide dismutase, *Diabetologia*, 18, 55, 1980.

29. Kwon, N. S., Lee, S. H., Choi, C. S., Kho, T., and Lee, H. S., Nitric oxide generation from streptozotocin, *FASEB J.*, 8, 529, 1994.

30. Turk, J., Corbett, J. A., Ramanadham, S., Borher, A., and McDaniel, M. L., Biochemical evidence for nitric oxide formation from streptozotocin in isolated pancreatic islets, *Biochem. Biophys. Res. Commun.*, 197, 1468, 1993.

31. Tanaka, Y., Shimizu, H., Sato, N., Mori, M., and Shimomura, Y., Involvement of spontaneous nitric oxide production in the diabetogenic action of streptozotocin, *Pharmacology*, 50, 69, 1995.

32. Bedoya, F. J., Solano, F., and M. Lucas, M., N-Monomethyl-arginine and nicotinamide prevent streptozotocin induced double strand DNA break formation in pancreatic rat islets, *Experientia*, 52, 344, 1996.

33. Sandler, S. and Swenne, I., Streptozotocin, but not alloxan, induces DNA repair synthesis in mouse pancreatic islets *in vitro*, *Diabetologia*, 25, 444, 1983.
34. Pettepher, C. C., LeDoux, S. P., Bohr, V. A., and Wilson, G. L., Repair of alkali labile sites within the mitochondrial DNA of RINr38 cells after exposure to the nitrosourea streptozotocin, *J. Biol. Chem.*, 266, 3113, 1991.
35. Okamoto, H., Molecular basis of experimental diabetes: degeneration, oncogenesis and regeneration of pancreatic B-cells of islets of Langerhans, *Bioessays*, 2, 15, 1987.
36. Schein, P. S., Cooney, D. A., McMenamin, M. G., and Anderson, T., Streptozotocin diabetes further studies on the mechanism of depression of nicotinamide adenine dinucleotide concentrations in mouse pancreatic islets and liver, *Biochem. Pharmacol.*, 22, 2625, 1973.
37. Wilson, G. L., Hartig, P. C., Patton, N. J., and LeDoux, S. P., Mechanisms of nitrosourea-induced beta-cell damage: activation of poly(ADP-ribose) synthetase and cellular distribution, *Diabetes*, 37, 213, 1988.
38. Huang, S. W. and Taylor, G. E., Immune insulitis and antibodies to nucleic acids induced with streptozotocin in mice, *Clin. Exp. Immunol.*, 43, 425, 1981.
39. Bonnevie-Nielsen, V., Steffes, M. W., and Lernmark, A., A major loss in islet mass and beta cell function precedes hyperglycemia in mice given multiple low doses of streptozotocin, *Diabetes*, 30, 424, 1981.
40. Sandler, S. and Jansson, L., Vascular permeability of pancreatic islets after administration of streptozotocin, *Virchows Arch. Pathol. Anat.*, 407, 359, 1985.
41. Papaccio, G. and Esposito, V., Ultrastructural observations on cytotoxic effector cells infiltrating pancreatic islets of low dose streptozotocin treated mice, *Virchows Arch. Pathol. Anat.*, 420, 5, 1992.
42. Hamming, N. A. and Reynolds, W. A., DNA synthesis in pancreatic islet and acinar cells in rats with streptozotocin-induced diabetes, *Horm. Metab. Res.*, 9, 114, 1977.
43. Bar-On, H., Roheim, P. S., and Eder, H. E., Hyperlipoproteinemia in streptozotocin-treated rats, *Diabetes*, 25, 509, 1976.
44. Ar'Rajab, A. and Ahrén, B., Long-term diabetogenic effect of streptozotocin in rats, *Pancreas*, 8, 50, 1993.
45. Engle, M. J., Perelman, R. H., McMahon, K. E., Langan, S. M., and Farrell, P. M., Relationship between the severity of experimental diabetes and altered lung phospholipid metabolism, *Proc. Soc. Exp. Biol. Med.*, 176, 261, 1984.
46. Yogev, L., Yavetz, H., Gottreich, A., Oppenheim, D., Homonnai, Z. T., and Paz, G., Blood lutenizing hormone and prolactin concentrations in response to naltrexone challenge: studies on rats with diabetes induced by different doses of streptozotocin, *Life Sci.*, 54, 261, 1994.
47. Giorgino, F., Chen, J. H., and Smith, R. J., Changes in tyrosine phosphorylation of insulin receptors and a 170,000 molecular weight nonreceptor protein *in vivo* in skeletal muscle of streptozotocin-induced diabetic rats: effects of insulin and glucose, *Endocrinology*, 130, 1433, 1992.
48. Whiting, P. H., Bowley, M., Sturton, R. G., Pritchard, P. H., Brindley, D. N., and Hawthorne, J. N., The effect of chronic diabetes, induced by streptozotocin, on the activities of some enzymes of glycerolipid synthesis in rat liver, *Biochem. J.*, 168, 147, 1977.
49. Rodrigues, B. and McNeill, J. H., Comparison of cardiac function in male and female diabetic rats, *Gen. Pharmacol.*, 18, 421, 1987.
50. Masiello, P., De Paoli, A. A., and Bergamini, E., Influence of age on the sensitivity of the rat to streptozotocin, *Horm. Res.*, 11, 262, 1979.
51. Dubuc, P. U., Hormonal responses during development of streptozotocin diabetes in rats, *Endocrinol. Exp.*, 21, 275, 1987.
52. Ramanadham, S., Doroudian, A., and McNeill, J. H., Myocardial and metabolic abnormalities in streptozotocin-diabetic Wistar and Wistar-Kyoto rats, *Can. J. Cardiol.*, 6, 75, 1990.
53. Newby, F. D., Bayo, F., Thacker, S. V., Sykes, M., and DiGirolemo, M., Effects of streptozotocin-induced diabetes on glucose and lactate release by isolated fat cells from young, lean and older, moderately obese rats, *Diabetes*, 38, 237, 1989.
54. Axler, D. A., Stability of the diabetogenic activity of streptozotocin, *IRCS Med. Sci.*, 10, 157, 1982.

55. Povoski, S. P., McCullough, P. J., Zhou, W., and Bell, R. H., Jr., Induction of diabetes mellitus in Syrian golden hamsters using stored equilibrium solutions of streptozotocin,*Lab. Anim. Sci.*, 43, 310, 1993.

56. Evan, A. P., Mong, S. A., Gattone, V. H., Connors, B. A., Aronoff, G. R., and Luft, F. C., The effect of streptozotocin and streptozotocin-induced diabetes on the kidney,*Renal Physiol. Basel*, 7, 78, 1984.

57. Rossini, A. A., Like, A. A., Dulin, W. E., and Cahill, G. F., Jr., Pancreatic beta cell toxicity by streptozotocin anomers, *Diabetes*, 26, 1120, 1977.

58. Rodrigues, B., Cam, M. C., Kong, J., Goyal, R. K., and McNeill, J. H., Strain differences in susceptibility to streptozotocin-induced diabetes: effects on hypertriglyceridemia and cardiomyopathy, *Cardiovasc. Res.*, 534, 199, 1997.

59. Reaven, G. M. and Ho, H., Low-dose streptozotocin-induced diabetes in the spontaneously hypertensive rat, *Metabolism*, 40, 335, 1991.

60. Sato, T., Nara, Y., Kato, Y., and Yamori, Y., Hypertensive diabetic rats: different effects of streptozotocin treatment on blood pressure in adult SHR and in neonatal SHR,*Clin. Exp. Hyper. Theor. Pract.*, A13, 981, 1991.

61. Olfert, E. D., Cross, B. M., and McWilliam, A. A., Eds., *Guide to the Care and Use of Experimental Animals*, Vol. 1, 2nd ed., Canadian Council on Animal Care, Ottawa, 1993.

62. Canadian Council on Animal Care, *Guide to the Care and Use of Experimental Animals*, Vol. 2, Canadian Council on Animal Care, Ottawa, 1984.

63. Rodrigues, B., Cain, M. C., Jian, K., Lim, F., Sambandam, N., and Shepherd, G., Differential effects of streptozotocin-induced diabetes on cardiac lipoprotein lipase activity, *Diabetes*, 46, 1346, 1997.

64. Chang, E. B., Bergenstal, R. M., and Field, M., Diarrhea in streptozotocin-treated rats. Loss of adrenergic regulation of intestinal fluid and electrolyte transport,*J. Clin. Invest.*, 75, 1666, 1985.

65. Dai, S. and McNeill, J. H., Personal communication, 1994.

66. Shimoni, Y., Firek, L., Severson, D. L., and Giles, W., Short-term diabetes alters K⁺ currents in rat ventricular myocytes, *Circ. Res.*, 74, 620, 1994.

67. Dai, S., Thompson, K. H., and McNeill, J. H., One-year treatment of streptozotocin-induced diabetic rats with vanadyl sulfate, *Pharmacol. Toxicol.*, 74, 101, 1994.

68. Van Voorhis, K., Said, H. M., Abumrad, N., and Ghishan, F. K., Effect of chemically induced diabetes mellitus on glutamine transport in rat intestine, *Gastroenterology*, 98, 862, 1990.

69. Tanaka, Y., Konno, N., and Kako, K. J., Mitochondrial dysfunction observed *in situ* in cardiomyocytes of rats in experimental diabetes, *Cardiovasc. Res.*, 26, 409, 1992.

70. Chandrashekar, V., Steger, R. W., Bartke, A., Fadden, C. T., and Kienast, S. G., Influence of diabetes on the gonadotropin response to the negative feedback effect of testosterone and hypothalamic neurotransmitter turnover in adult male rats,*Neuroendocrinology*, 54, 30, 1991.

71. Domingo, J. L., Ortega, A., Llobet, J. M., and Keen, C. L., No improvement of glucose homeostasis in diabetic rats by vanadate treatment when given by gavage, *Trace Elem. Med.*, 8, 181, 1991.

72. Oster, M. H., Castonguay, T. W., Keen, C. L., and Stern, J. S., Circadian rhythm of corticosterone in diabetic rats, *Life Sci.*, 43, 1643, 1988.

73. Reinilä, A., Some advantages and disadvantages of streptozotocin from a morphologist's point of view, in *Streptozotocin: Fundamentals and Therapy*, Agarwal, M. K., Ed., Elsevier/North-Holland Biomedical Press, Amsterdam, 1981; chap. 4.

74. Nakhoda, A. and Wong, H. A., The induction of diabetes in rats by intramuscular administration of streptozotocin, *Experientia*, 35, 1679, 1979.

75. Akkan, A. G. and Malaisse, W. J., Iterative pulse administration of succinic acid monomethyl ester to streptozotocin diabetic rats, *Diabetes Res.*, 23, 55, 1993.

76. Géloën, A., Roy, P. E., and Bukowiecki, L. J., Regression of white adipose tissue in diabetic rats, *Am. J. Physiol.*, 257, E547, 1989.

77. Blades, R. A., Bryant, K. R., and Whitehead, S. A., Feedback effects of steroids and gonatrophin control in adult rats with streptozotocin induced diabetes mellitus, *Diabetologia*, 28, 348, 1985.

78. Kim, Y.-W., Kim, J.-Y., and Lee, S.-K., Effects of phlorizin and acipimox on insulin resistance in STZ diabetic rats, *J. Korean Med. Sci.*, 10, 24, 1995.

2

Alterations in Myocardial Energy Metabolism in Streptozotocin Diabetes

William C. Stanley, Gary D. Lopaschuk, and Krista M. Kivilo

CONTENTS

KEY WORDS: *cardiac, diabetes, fatty acids, glucose, glycolysis, heart, ischemia, lactate, myocardial metabolism, pyruvate dehydrogenase.*

2.1 Introduction

The aim of this chapter is to provide an overview of the abnormalities in myocardial energy substrate metabolism that accompany diabetes induced by streptozotocin (STZ). As described in Chapter 1 of this book, the administration of STZ damages pancreatic insulin-producing β-cells, leading to hypoinsulinemia, hyperglycemia, as well as elevated plasma free fatty acid and ketone body levels. Although diabetes affects a multitude of organs and tissues, for the sake of brevity and clarity, the heart was chosen as a model to describe the STZ-induced alterations of cellular energy metabolism. As a brief overview, this chapter is composed of six sections, with the significance of altered circulating hormone and substrate levels on the cellular energy metabolism being discussed first. The next four sections of the chapter elaborate on the alterations of carbohydrate, fatty acid, and ketone energy metabolism in the myocardium of STZ diabetic animals. The chapter concludes with an overview of the cross talk among carbohydrate, fatty acid, and ketone body energy metabolism.

Before launching into a description of the intricacies of the mechanisms regulating myocardial energy metabolism, it is important to address a few basic concepts concerning the experimental conditions used for studying cellular energy metabolism in STZ diabetic animals. First of all, diabetes-induced alterations in the rates of myocardial substrate utilization have largely been elucidated by studying isolated perfused rat hearts and cardiomyocytes. Defects inherent to the diabetic myocardium are difficult to isolate using *in vivo* animal models since relatively subtle alterations in circulating substrate levels lead to profound modifications in cellular metabolism. This complicates the differentiation of the effects of diabetes on circulating substrate levels from the effects of diabetes on the cardiac phenotype. Therefore, the design of studies investigating myocardial metabolism in diabetes must separate the direct influences of hyperglycemia, elevated plasma fatty acid, and ketone body levels from changes in cardiac gene expression or other cellular manifestations attributable to the diabetic heart. In consideration of the multitude of diabetes-induced changes at the cell, tissue, and whole organ level, studies are limited in experimental scope by the difficulty of matching the metabolic conditions in which the measurements are made.

While a myriad of studies have investigated heart metabolism in STZ diabetic rats, few have studied myocardial metabolism using large-animal models of diabetes. The development of an STZ diabetic pig model has provided a means to measure myocardial substrate metabolism *in vivo* under a variety of conditions.[20,32,59,109] The advantage of this model is a coronary anatomy, heart rate, and ventricular function similar to humans, as well as the ability to induce regional myocardial ischemia experimentally, and to take serial tissue and blood measurements. However, the primary drawbacks to this technique are the high cost and extensive labor requirements.

Another important consideration is the duration of STZ diabetes to which the animal is subjected. Many of the cardiovascular changes that occur in diabetes take several months to years to develop in experimental animals. Although many of the metabolic changes occur within the first 2 to 8 weeks following an injection of STZ, other alterations can take much longer (see Chapter 1 for specifics). The experimental data are incomplete regarding the time course of the metabolic changes induced by experimental diabetes. For the purpose of this review, the focus will be studies that use a longer duration of diabetes (>9 weeks).

Returning to the metabolic aspects of this chapter, the cellular energy currency, ATP, is regenerated from ADP and inorganic phosphate primarily via mitochondrial oxidative phosphorylation. Glycolysis and, to a far lesser extent, the tricarboxylic acid (TCA) (conversion of succinyl CoA to succinate yields a GTP) cycle also contribute to this process. However, in cardiomyocytes the majority of the reducing equivalents necessary for the operation of the electron transport chain are provided by the TCA cycle processing β-oxidized fatty acids. A nonsubstantial amount of NADH comes from glycolysis as well. More specifically, the TCA cycle is fueled by acetyl CoA derived from oxidation of fatty acids, ketone bodies, and pyruvate (Figure 2.1). Fatty acids metabolized by the heart are derived either from the plasma or the utilization of intracellular triacylglycerol stores, while ketones enter the TCA cycle via the acetoacetyl CoA intermediary. Pyruvate is synthesized in approximately equal parts from glucose and lactate. In the normal heart, 60 to 90% of acetyl CoA is derived from fatty acid β-oxidation,[53,71] while

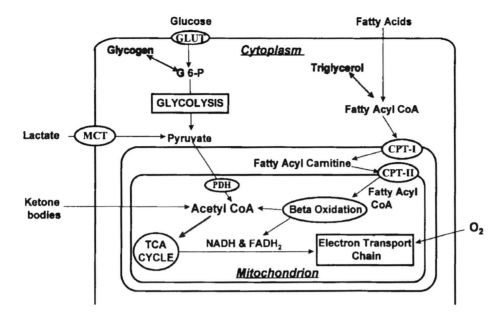

FIGURE 2.1
Overview of myocardial metabolism. See text for abbreviations.

pyruvate (originating from glucose or lactate) is the source of the remaining acetyl CoA.[71] In healthy, nondiabetic individuals ketone bodies are not a significant fuel for the heart due to very low circulating levels. Numerous studies in isolated buffer-perfused rat hearts have shown that experimental diabetes results in an increase in fatty acid oxidation,[74] as well as in a decrease in glucose transport,[36,63,95,96] glycolysis,[21,104] and glucose oxidation.[11,21,104] A detailed discussion of the exact energy metabolism mechanisms affected by STZ-induced diabetes is provided below.

2.2   Role of Circulating Hormone and Substrate Levels

As Chapter 1 has illustrated, an STZ injection induces diabetes in experimental animals by causing insulin levels to drop and therefore causing blood glucose levels to increase within a window of 24 to 48 h.[76] The resulting hyperglycemia is due to two main mechanisms. First, studies have shown that the sharp decrease in insulin results in inhibition of glucose uptake into peripheral tissues as a result of the presence of less GLUT 4 in the plasma membrane of muscle and adipose tissue. In addition there is less insulin stimulation of GLUT 4 expression,[70,106,114] glycogen synthesis,[14] and hexokinase activity[87] in peripheral tissues, where glucose metabolism is insulin driven. Concurrently, the insulin-dependent inhibition of lipolysis in adipocytes becomes impaired, thus causing plasma free fatty acid levels to increase and feedback to inhibit glucose and lactate uptake in muscle further.[66,101] In addition to altered insulin levels, an increase in glucagon, somatostatin, epinephrine, and norepinephrine levels has been shown and a decrease in thyroid hormone concentration has also been recorded.[76]

Fuel selection in the healthy heart is largely a function of the circulating substrate levels and the supply of fuels to the heart. The relative contribution of fatty acids to the rate of acetyl CoA production is a function of the arterial free fatty acid concentration.[41] Therefore, the rate of fatty acid uptake is increased when fatty acid levels are elevated (>0.8 mM) by fasting, catecholamine stress, hypoinsulinemia, acute myocardial infarction, or surgical stress.[65,72] Conversely, fatty acid uptake is decreased when fatty acid levels drop, such as after the ingestion of food. Similarly, the rate of lactate uptake by the heart increases linearly as a function of arterial concentration.[41] Thus, the rate of lactate uptake by the heart is increased during physical exercise, with lactate becoming the predominant source of pyruvate during more intense exercise with high arterial lactate concentration.[8,27,94,103] The rate of glucose uptake by the nondiabetic heart is increased when arterial glucose levels are elevated (10 to 15 mM) independent of fatty acid and insulin levels;[33,95,96,111] however, since the arterial glucose concentration does not vary much between 4 and 7 mM in people without diabetes, it does not appear to be a major regulator of normal myocardial glucose uptake.

Increased plasma triglyceride, fatty acid, and ketone body levels are several characteristics of STZ diabetic animals. Hypertriglyceridemia has been shown to be caused by the lack of insulin-dependent regulation of triglyceride-rich lipoprotein–triglyceride metabolism,[83,85] while the increase in free fatty acids is due to removal of insulin inhibition of lipolysis in adipocytes. The increase in hepatic fatty acid oxidation produces acetyl CoA that cannot enter the tricarboxylic acid cycle for the lack of carbohydrate-derived oxaloacetate. The excessive levels of acetyl CoA in hepatic mitochondria give rise to formation of ketone bodies (acetoacetate and β-hydroxybutyrate). Ketone bodies are readily taken up by the heart and converted back to acetyl CoA.

2.3 Carbohydrate Metabolism

2.3.1 Glucose Uptake

By 1912, Knowlton and Starling[46] had already shown that glucose uptake was depressed in hearts from depancreatized dogs. This phenomenon was further elucidated by the classic studies in the early 1960s by Morgan et al.,[63] which demonstrated a decrease in glucose uptake in perfused rat hearts from alloxan-induced diabetic animals, both in the presence and absence of insulin, as well as during anoxia. Since then, decreased rates of glucose transport in the heart have also been well documented in STZ diabetic models (Table 2.1). The main regulators of myocardial glucose uptake are the concentration of glucose transporters in the sarcolemma and the transmembrane glucose gradient. GLUT 1 and GLUT 4 isoforms of the GLUT glucose transporter family are expressed in cardiomyocytes, with GLUT 4 being predominant. Since the discovery of the family of glucose transporter proteins in the late 1980s, a number of studies have demonstrated that both the GLUT mRNA and protein content are downregulated in STZ diabetic rats[9,36,47,73] and swine[96] (Table 2.2). GLUT 1 and GLUT 4 proteins reside in the plasma membrane and in an intracellular microsomal pool. Insulin, hypoxia, or ischemia results in a translocation of GLUT 1 and GLUT 4 from the intracellular site into the plasma membrane, thus enabling myocardium to take up more glucose.[100,106,113] The diabetic rat heart has a decreased capacity to transport glucose into the cell due to less GLUT 4 protein present on the plasma membrane[25] (Figure 2.2); however, this can be normalized by daily treatment with subcutaneous insulin injections. Exercise training (in the form of treadmill running) in STZ diabetic rats can partially prevent the fall in GLUT 4 protein and mRNA, but not in

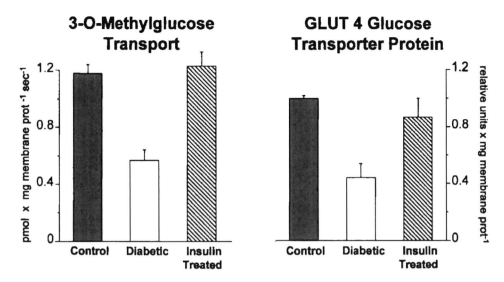

FIGURE 2.2
The rate of 3-O-methylglucose transport into sarcolemmal vesicles (left panel) and the concentration of GLUT 4 protein in isolated sarcolemmal membranes (right panel). (Adapted from data presented by Garvey et al.[25])

GLUT 1 protein.[73] The mechanism for this is unclear, but the effect may simply be due to the partial reduction in hyperglycemia induced by exercise training.[73,75]

The transmembrane glucose gradient is determined by the interstitial and intracellular free glucose concentrations. The interstitial glucose is a function of the arterial glucose concentration and blood flow.[33,34] Thus, in hyperglycemia, accompanying STZ induced diabetes, the interstitial glucose levels and transmembrane glucose gradient are increased, helping compensate for the decreased capacity for sarcolemmal glucose transport.[95] Hexokinase is also important in determining this transmembrane gradient by keeping the intracellular free glucose levels low by rapidly phosphorylating glucose into glucose-6-phosphate (G-6-P). This process not only renders glucose impermeable to the cell membrane, but it also maintains a high transmembrane glucose gradient. Hexokinase is activated by insulin, which increases the formation of G-6-P and the transmembrane glucose gradient, thereby increasing glucose uptake. Studies in isolated quiescent cultured cardiomyocytes suggest that glucose phosphorylation by hexokinase, rather than the transport across the sacrolemmal membrane, is the rate-limiting step in insulin-stimulated glucose utilization.[58] Thus, low insulin levels that are characteristic of the STZ diabetic animals could result in low hexokinase activity, leading to a decreased transmembrane glucose gradient and, therefore, resulting in decreased glucose transport in the STZ diabetic myocardium.

Glucose uptake is decreased in STZ diabetic dogs[3] and swine[37,95] under some conditions. When myocardial glucose uptake in nondiabetic normoglycemic swine or dogs is compared with STZ diabetic hyperglycemic animals, the rates of glucose uptake are not different either under normal aerobic conditions or when myocardial blood flow is reduced by 60%[3,96] (see Table 2.1). This occurs even though the diabetic animals have significantly reduced levels of GLUT 1 and GLUT 4 proteins. When nondiabetic swine are infused with somatostatin to prevent insulin release and are made acutely hyperglycemic to match the diabetic animals, they have a significantly greater rate of glucose uptake under both well-perfused and ischemic conditions when compared with hyperglycemic diabetic animals.[95] Therefore, it may be argued that hyperglycemia compensates for the decreased capacity for glucose transport across the sarcolemmal membrane in diabetic animals.[96]

TABLE 2.1

Effects of Streptoxotocin-Induced Diabetes on Glucose Uptake
and Oxidation, and Lactate Uptake

	Species	Effect of Diabetes % of Control	Ref.
Rate of Glucose Uptake			
1. Aerobic conditions	Rat (14d STZ)	56	1
	$+10^{-8}$ M ins	73	1
	Rat (28d STZ)	47	25
	Rat (7d STZ)	67	107
	Rat (5d alloxan)	28	48
	Rat (7d STZ)	32	62
	Pig (12w STZ)	24	95
	Pig (12w STZ)	43	37
	Dog (6w STZ)	46	3
2. Ischemia	Pig (12w STZ)	32	95
3. Anoxia	Rat (7d STZ)	22	62
4. Dobutamine	Pig (12w STZ)	79	37
Rate of Glycolysis			
1. Normal flow	Rat (6w STZ)	23	21
	Rat (6w STZ)	62	19
	Rat (6 w STZ)	54	6
	Rat (2w STZ)	70	5
	Rat (6w STZ)	68	55
2. Ischemia	Rat (6w STZ)	52	55
3. Reperfusion	Rat (6w STZ)	25	21
	Rat (6w STZ)	60	6
Rate of Glucose Oxidation			
1. Normal blood flow	Rat (4w STZ)	22–43	12
	Rat (6w STZ)	37	21
	Rat (6w STZ)	8	104
	Rat (6w STZ)	16	19
	Rat (7d STZ)	43	62
	Rat (3d STZ)	32	86
	Rat (6w STZ)	20	6
	Rat (STZ chronic)	15	81
	Rat (2w STZ)	39	5
	Rat (7d STZ)	21	84
3. Reperfusion	Rat (6w STZ)	10	21
	Rat (6w STZ)	58	6
Rate of Lactate Uptake			
1. Normal blood flow	Pig (12w STZ)	46	95
	Pig (12w STZ)	19	37
3. Dobutamine stimulation	Pig (12w STZ)	22	37
Rate of Lactate Output			
1. Normal blood flow	Pig (12w STZ)	500	95
	Pig (12w STZ)	333	37
	Rat (7d STZ)	43	62
	Rat (STZ)	112	81
2. Dobutamine	Pig (12w STZ)	581	37
3. Anoxia	Rat (7d STZ)	23	62

TABLE 2.1 (continued)

Effects of Streptoxotocin-Induced Diabetes on Glucose Uptake
and Oxidation, and Lactate Uptake

	Species	Effect of Diabetes % of Control	Ref.
Rate of FFA Uptake			
1. Normal blood flow	Pig (12w STZ)	73	95
	Pig (12w STZ)	57	37
	Rat (5d alloxan)	57	48
	Dog (6w STZ)	130	3
2. Ischemia	Pig (12w STZ)	57	95
3. Dobutamine	Pig (12w STZ)	33	37
Rate of Palmitate Oxidation			
1. Normal blood	Rat (4w STZ)	135	12
	Rat (6w STZ)	85	104
	Rat (7day STZ)	165	62
	Rat (2wk STZ)	100	5
Rate of Endogenous Triacylglycerol Metabolism			
	Rat (2d STZ)	100	90
Rate of β-Hydroxybutyrate Uptake			
1. Normal flow	Pig (12w STZ)	366	37
2. Dobutamine	Pig (12w STZ)	192	37
Glycogen Content	Rat (28d STZ)	460	107
Triacylglycerol Content	Rat (alloxan)	208–303	15,82
	Rat (2d STZ)	230–300	64,90
G-6-P Content	Rat (7d STZ)	438	16
	Rat (28d STZ)	3430	107

2.3.2 Glycogen Metabolism

Once in the cardiomyocyte, glucose can either proceed down the glycolytic pathway or be stored as glycogen. In addition to a decrease in glucose transporter concentration, diabetes results in a decreased activity of the G-6-P utilizing pathways. G-6-P is used for both glycogen synthesis and for glycolysis which forms pyruvate (see Figure 2.1). It has been demonstrated that the STZ diabetic rat myocardium has a higher glycogen content than the nondiabetic myocardium (see Table 2.1). In normal animals, the rate of glycogen synthesis is regulated by the concentration of G-6-P and the activity of glycogen synthase. Glycogenolysis results in the formation of G-6-P, and is regulated by the activity of glycogen phosphorylase. Studies in isolated rat hearts indicate that there is a high degree of simultaneous flux through glycogen synthetase and phosphorylase,[30,40] as suggested in earlier studies in humans.[110] The content of glycogen in the heart is highly dependent on diet, feeding state, and the metabolic flux of glycogen synthesis, while breakdown is dependent upon substrate availability and hormonal stimulation. Glycogen phosphorylase is activated when phosphorylated by phosphorylase kinase, which is activated by Ca^{2+}. The activity of phosphorylase kinase is regulated by protein kinase A, and thus is

TABLE 2.2

Effects of STZ-Induced Diabetes on Key Regulators of Myocardial Glucose Metabolism

	Species	Effect of Diabetes (% of control)	Ref.
Glucose Transporters			
GLUT-4 protein	Rat (28d STZ)	44	25
GLUT-4 mRNA	Rat (28d STZ)	57	25
GLUT-4 mRNA	Rat (7d STZ)	40	9
GLUT-4 protein	Rat (7d STZ)	79	9
GLUT-1 mRNA	Rat (7d STZ)	44	9
GLUT-4 mRNA	Rat (7d STZ)	70	4
GLUT-4 protein	Rat (7d STZ)	70	4
GLUT-1 protein	Rat (12w STZ)	81	36
GLUT-4 protein	Rat (12w STZ)	30	36
GLUT-1 protein	Pig (12w STZ)	34	37
GLUT-4 protein	Pig (12w szt)	50	37
Hexokinase Activity	Rat (12w STZ)	98	12
	Rat (7d STZ)	78	92,93
	Rabbit (alloxan)	103	38
Phosphofructokinase Activity	Rat (12w STZ)	98	12
	Rat (7d STZ)	79	93
Pyruvate Kinase	Rat (7d STZ)	43	93
Glyceraldehyde Phosphate Dehydrogenase Activity	Mice (genetic)	300	18
Pyruvate Dehydrogenase Activity			
Total PDH	Pig (12w STZ)	75	37
% Active PDH	Pig (12w STZ)	56	37
% Active PDH	Pig (12w STZ)	74	37
% Active PDH	Rat (2d alloxan)	22	60
% Active PDH	Rat (2d alloxan)	6	44
% Active PDH	Rat (2d alloxan)	15	108
Lactate Dehydrogenase Activity	Rat (2 d STZ)	100	99

activated by cAMP. Consequently, glycogen phosphorylase activity is controlled by both hormonal stimulation (e.g., β-adrenergic receptor stimulation leading to increased cAMP and Ca^{2+}) and metabolic feedback (AMP, Pi, and Ca^{2+}). Studies in diabetic rat hearts have shown no change in glycogen phophorylase activity from controls. There are two isoforms of glycogen synthase present in heart, G-6-P-dependent glycogen synthase and G-6-P-independent glycogen synthase; however, the effects of STZ diabetes have not been reported. Studies in rats have shown that high plasma fatty acid concentrations and a greater reliance on fatty acid and/or ketone body oxidation (such as occurs with diabetes, fasting, or during recovery from exhaustive exercise) will result in an inhibition of glycolysis, elevation of G-6-P, and an increase in myocardial glycogen levels.[8,52,98] All of these conditions result in inhibition of the glycolytic pathway and a redirecting of G-6-P to glycogen.

2.3.3   Glycolysis

STZ diabetic rat hearts have significantly lower rates of glycolysis, which cannot be simply explained by decrease in the capacity for glucose transport. The major regulator of arterial glucose uptake and oxidation in the heart *in vivo* is the arterial concentration of fatty acids. First described by Randle et al.[77-79] in the early 1960s, the glucose–fatty acid cycle (also known as the Randle cycle) involves the inhibition of glycolysis and pyruvate oxidation when there is a high rate of β-oxidation of fatty acids. In other words, when plasma fatty acid levels and the rate of fatty acid oxidation are high, the rates of glucose uptake and

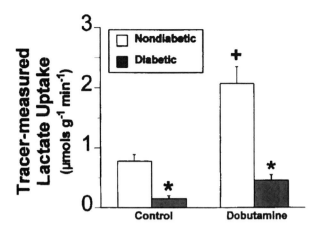

FIGURE 2.3
Myocardial lactate uptake measured with [U-¹³C] lactate tracer in normal and 12-week STZ (125 mg/kg) diabetic yucatan miniature swine under normal conditions and with dobutamine-induced work. ∗ Significantly different from the diabetic group; + different from the control period within the same group. (Adapted from data presented by Hall, et al., *Am. J. Physiol.*, 271, H2320–H2329, 1996.)

oxidation are subject to feedback inhibition. This effect is mediated by a variety of mechanisms. High levels of cytosolic citrate, which could occur when rates of fatty acid oxidation are high, can inhibit phosphofructokinase (PFK) activity, accumulation of G-6-P, and a decrease in the rate of glycolysis.[68] However, it is unclear if citrate regulates PFK activity *in vivo*. Rat heart mitochondria, unlike liver mitochondria, have a very low activity of the tricarboxylate carrier[10]; thus, the citrate concentration in the mitochondrial matrix may not correspond with cytosolic levels and, therefore, unlike the liver, may not be important in the regulation of heart PFK. Another possibility is a decrease in the transfer of glycolytically derived reducing equivalents from cytosolic NADH to the mitochondrial matrix due to an increase in the mitochondrial NADH/NAD+ ratio from increases in fatty acid and/or ketone body oxidation.[98]

2.3.4 Lactate Uptake

Lactate is a major source of pyruvate formation under well-perfused conditions *in vivo*, and under some conditions lactate uptake can exceed glycolysis as a source of pyruvate.[26,94,98] Studies with carbon-labeled lactate tracers in humans show that 80 to 100% of the lactate taken up by the healthy human heart is immediately released as labeled CO_2 into the coronary effluent,[26,27] suggesting that extracted lactate is rapidly oxidized by lactate dehydrogenase, decarboxylated by pyruvate dehydrogenase (PDH), and oxidized to CO_2 in the TCA acid cycle. The rate of lactate uptake is mainly a function of the transmembrane lactate gradient, the capacitance for transport across the plasma membrane, the rate of lactate oxidation to pyruvate, and the rate of pyruvate oxidation by PDH. Studies in anesthetized swine have demonstrated a decrease in lactate uptake in STZ diabetic animals under both normal conditions and when contractile work is increased with an infusion of dobutamine (Figure 2.3).[37] This impaired lactate uptake corresponded to a significant decrease in the activity of PDH, illustrating the importance of PDH activity in controlling lactate uptake in the diabetic heart.

Lactate transport across the sarcolemmal membrane is mediated by at least one inhibitable, stereoselective transport protein. A 45-kDa lactate transporter protein has recently been cloned, and is referred to as the monocarboxylate transporter-I (MCT-I).[24] Studies on isolated myocytes suggest that the rate of lactate efflux during hypoxia is limited by the capacity of the carrier.[105] At present, it is unclear if MCT-I is responsible for lactate efflux, influx, or both. The effects of diabetes on MCT-I have not been reported.

2.3.5   Pyruvate Dehydrogenase

Pyruvate decarboxylation is the key irreversible step in carbohydrate oxidation and is catalyzed by PDH. PDH is a large (~4600 kDa) multienzyme complex located in mitochondrial matrix. The rate of flux through PDH is regulated by the degree of phosphorylation of the enzyme as well as by substrate and product concentrations. It is inactivated by phosphorylation by PDH kinase, which is inhibited by pyruvate and ADP and activated by increases in acetyl CoA/free CoA and $NADH/NAD^+$.[61,77] Thus, an increase in substrates (pyruvate, CoA, and NAD^+) acts through a decrease in PDH kinase activity to keep the enzyme in the dephosphorylated active state, while, conversely, elevations in the products (acetyl CoA and NADH) stimulate PDH kinase and inactivate PDH. The activity of PDH can also be increased by dephosphorylation by PDH phosphatase, the activity of which is increased by Ca^{2+} and Mg^{2+}.[61,77] Pyruvate oxidation and the activity of PDH in the heart are decreased by elevated rates of fatty acid oxidation caused by increased plasma levels of fatty acids. Conversely, PDH activity is increased when fatty acid oxidation is decreased (i.e., due to a decrease in plasma fatty acid levels). Randle et al.[78,79] also showed that ketone bodies (β-hydroxybutyrate and acetoacetate) act to inhibit pyruvate oxidation by a similar mechanism.[78,79] β-hydroxybutyrate and acetoacetate are converted to acetyl CoA, which then inhibits flux through PDH, as described above. Clearly, this mechanism is not in operation in the normal healthy heart, where circulating ketone body levels are very low; however, it is of critical importance in diabetes when ketone body levels are elevated.

In addition to regulation of flux through PDH by phosphorylation of the enzyme, it is important to note that the rate of flux for any given phosphorylation state is largely a function of both the concentration of the products and substrates of PDH. Acetyl CoA produced from fatty acid oxidation in the mitochondrial matrix causes direct product inhibition of flux through PDH.[39] Thus, elevated rates of fatty acid and/or ketone body oxidation not only inhibit flux through PDH by elevating the concentrations of NADH and acetyl CoA, and stimulating PDH kinase and phosphorylating PDH, but also by inhibiting flux through PDH for any given PDH phosphorylation state. Flux through PDH is also dependent on the pyruvate concentration, which could be decreased in the diabetic heart because of a lower rate of glycolysis. However, it has not yet been unequivocally established that a decrease in pyruvate supply to PDH contributes to the low pyruvate oxidation in STZ diabetes.

Impaired pyruvate oxidation is a hallmark of the metabolic defects found in the diabetic heart. STZ diabetes results in both a decrease in the amount of enzyme found in the active dephosphorylated state, and in the maximal activity of PDH (measured by dephosphorylating the enzyme with the addition of purified PDH phosphatase) (see Table 2.2).[37,43,44] The metabolic significance of the decrease in PDH activity is a decrease in the rates of glucose and lactate oxidation. Studies in STZ diabetic swine show that there is a significant reduction in the rate of lactate uptake and in the activity of PDH, especially when the work of the heart is increased by infusing the β-adrenergic agonist dobutamine.[37] Studies in STZ diabetic rat hearts have shown that stimulation of PDH with dichloroacetate (DCA) results in an increase in myocardial glucose oxidation and contractile function in diabetic rat hearts perfused with fatty acids.[21] This suggests that the diabetes-induced inhibition of PDH contributes to the impaired contractile function observed in the diabetic heart. However, DCA stimulates glucose oxidation only twofold in diabetic hearts compared with

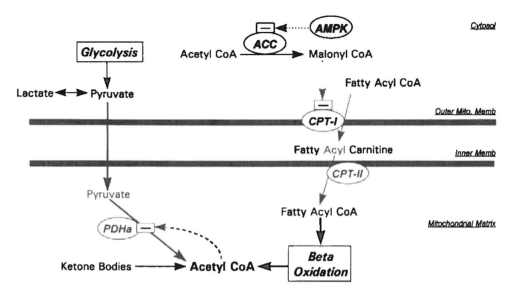

FIGURE 2.4
Schematic depiction of the interrelationship among pyruvate, fatty acid, and ketone body metabolism, with special emphasis on the role of malonyl CoA. See text for abbreviations.

fivefold in control hearts during aerobic perfusion,[21] which suggests that PDH activity in diabetic hearts is not as responsive to stimulation, possibly because of the increased use of free fatty acids resulting in higher intramitochondrial NADH/NAD⁺ and acetyl CoA/free CoA. Studies in alloxan diabetic rats suggest that the intrinsic ability of the enzyme to decarboxylate pyruvate is unaffected,[60] and that this decreased ability to activate PDH is due to a chronic increase in PDH kinase in the diabetic heart.[112] A similar upregulation of PDH kinase occurs in long-term starvation.[80]

2.4   Mitochondrial Energy Metabolism

The pathways for fatty acid, ketone body, and glucose and lactate oxidation merge at acetyl CoA (see Figure 2.1). Acetyl CoA combines with oxaloacetate to form citrate and enter the TCA cycle. The myocardial TCA cycle does not appear to be altered in diabetes. If total TCA cycle CO_2 production from glucose oxidation and both exogenous and endogenous fatty acid oxidation are measured, no differences in production are observed in diabetic vs. control rat hearts at the same rate of myocardial oxygen consumption.[21,90] Measurement of TCA cycle enzyme activities also do not differ in diabetic rats.[12,29,76] As a result, the primary alteration that occurs in diabetic hearts is not a change in TCA cycle activity, but rather in the source of acetyl CoA for the TCA cycle.

The next step in ATP production is the entry of NADH and $FADH_2$ into the electron transport chain, the extrusion of protons from the mitochondrial matrix, and the generation of H_2O and ATP by the ATP synthase. Biochemical evidence to date suggests that this process may be impaired in the diabetic heart. Isolated mitochondrial studies have demonstrated that state 3 respiration and oxidative phosphorylation rates are depressed in the diabetic heart.[51,76,91] How these relate to overall ATP production in the intact heart is still unclear. Although respiration has been shown to be depressed in diabetic heart mitochondria,

TABLE 2.3

Effects of STZ-Induced Diabetes on Key Regulators of Fatty Acid Metabolism

	Species	Effect of Diabetes (% of control)	Ref.
Fatty acid–binding protein	Rat (3w STZ)	133	29
Fatty acyl CoA synthase activity	Rat (3w STZ) liver	90	13
CPT I	Rat (STZ) liver	76	28
CPT II	Rat (STZ) liver	157	28
3-Hydroxyacyl CoA dehydrogenase	Rat (12w STZ)	150	12
	Mice (genetic)	100	50
	Rat (3w STZ)	103	29
β-Ketothiolases	Mice (genetic)	100	50
Acetoacyl CoA thiolase	Rat (8w STZ)	100	31

overall ATP production in the intact heart does not appear to be decreased.[43] The main difference in mitochondrial metabolism appears to be in a shift in the source of acetyl CoA for the TCA cycle, although one cannot rule out the potential negative effects of high rates of ketone body oxidation and the impaired rate of pyruvate carboxylation and anaplerosis, as recently noted in nondiabetic hearts.[42,88] Whether or not the capacity of mitochondria to produce adequate ATP is compromised at high workloads in diabetic hearts remains to be determined.

2.5   Fatty Acid Metabolism

2.5.1   Fatty Acid Supply

Fatty acids used by the heart are transported in the blood as either free fatty acids bound to albumin or as fatty esters complexed primarily to chylomicrons and very-low-density lipoproteins. All of these sources of fatty acids are elevated in the diabetic condition. The oxidation of chylomicron fatty acids is decreased in diabetic hearts,[29] which might be due to a diabetes-induced reduction in cardiac lipoprotein lipase activity and a decrease in heparin-releasable lipoprotein lipase activity. Therefore, in the diabetic heart it appears that the metabolism of fatty acids esterified to lipoproteins is decreased, whereas metabolism of nonesterified fatty acids is high. Concurrent with increases in nonesterified fatty acid metabolism, the diabetic heart appears to undergo a decrease in metabolism of fatty acids present in lipoproteins. However, the relationship between nonesterified fatty acid metabolism and lipoprotein fatty acid metabolism has not been clearly established.

The myocardium also experiences an increased content of triacylglycerol stores (see Table 2.1).[15] These triacylglycerols can be rapidly mobilized in diabetic rats depending on the presence or absence of high concentrations of exogenous fatty acids, resulting in the potential for a significant enhancement in lipolysis in the cardiac tissue.

2.5.2   Mitochondrial Fatty Acid Uptake

Esterified fatty acids are transferred across the mitochondrial membrane into the mitochondrial matrix by three carnitine dependent enzymes. The first one in the sequence, carnitine-palmitoyl transferase I (CPT I), catalyzes the formation of long-chain acylcarnitine from long-chain acyl CoA in the compartment between the inner and outer mitochondrial membrane (see Figure 2.4). The second enzyme, carnitine: acylcarnitine translocase, transports long-chain acylcarnitine across the inner mitochondrial membrane, whereas the last one in the sequence, carnitine palmitoyl transferase II (CPT II), regenerates long-chain acyl CoA in the mitochondrial matrix. Of the three enzymes involved in the transmitochondrial membrane transport, CPT I serves as the key regulatory enzyme. CPT I activity is inhibited by malonyl CoA, which is formed from carboxylation of acetyl CoA by acetyl CoA carboxylase (ACC) (see Figure 2.4). In STZ diabetic rat hearts, the authors have demonstrated that control of malonyl CoA production can be markedly repressed in diabetes. ACC expression and mRNA levels are not altered in STZ diabetic rat or swine hearts;[22,23,37] however, a significant depression of ACC activity has been observed.[54] This decrease occurs even in the presence of saturating concentrations of acetyl CoA. The above observation contrasts with data obtained from hepatic and adipose tissue measurements, in which a dramatic decrease in ACC expression occurs in STZ diabetes. ACC regulation is attributed to the cAMP-activated protein kinase and the 5′-AMP-activated protein kinase (AMPK). Phosphorylation of ACC inhibits its activity. In diabetes this regulation is induced by the increased activity in AMPK that, in turn, is activated by phosphorylation via a specific AMPK. ACC phosphorylation and inhibition lead to lower levels of malonyl CoA and removes the inhibition upon CPT I. These changes result in the enhancement of mitochondrial fatty acid uptake and oxidation in the diabetic heart. Such an increase in fatty acid oxidation is paralleled by a decrease in carbohydrate oxidation.

2.5.3　Fatty Acid β-Oxidation

Once in the mitochondrial matrix, long-chain acyl CoA passes through the β-oxidation enzyme system (or spiral) to produce acetyl CoA. Each successive cycle of the β-oxidation spiral results in a two-carbon shortening of the fatty acid (as acetyl CoA) and formation of one NADH and one $FADH_2$. The activity of β-hydroxyacyl-CoA dehydrogenase (a key enzyme of β-oxidation) has been shown to be normal[29,50] or high[12] in diabetic rat mitochondria (Table 2.3). Thus, in the diabetic heart the combination of high circulating levels of fatty acids and a normal or accelerated β-oxidative pathway results in the potential for a greater proportion of acetyl CoA for the TCA cycle to be derived from fatty acid oxidation.

2.6　Ketone Metabolism

Although ketosis is a classic symptom of poorly controlled diabetes, little attention has been given to subcellular regulation of acetoacetate and β-hydroxybutyrate metabolism, and their integration into carbohydrate and fatty acid metabolism. Studies in normal dogs[52] and isolated rat hearts[42,44,67,68,79,88] have demonstrated that increasing the concentration of acetoacetate and/or β-hydroxybutyrate in the perfusate increases the rate of their oxidation at the expense of glucose, lactate, and fatty acid oxidation. As discussed above, an increase in acetoacetate and/or β-hydroxybutyrate results in an increase in acetyl CoA and inhibition of PDH activity and the glycolytic pathway. The mechanism for ketone body inhibition of β-oxidation is unclear, although it is likely due to acetyl CoA inhibition of the terminal steps of the β-oxidation spiral.[42,88] Thus, the enhanced ability for the diabetic heart to oxidize fatty acids is paradoxically limited by competitive inhibition from ketone bodies under *in vivo* conditions.

2.7   Cross Talk Among Carbohydrate, Fatty Acid, and Ketone Metabolism

It is now well established how fatty acids and ketone bodies regulate glucose and lactate metabolism in the diabetic rat heart (see Sections 2.3 and 2.4). As the contribution of intramitochondrial acetyl CoA from fatty acid β-oxidation increases in diabetes, the contribution of glucose oxidation as a source of acetyl CoA decreases because of a decrease in PDH activity. What is less clear is how changes in glucose and lactate pyruvate metabolism regulate fatty acid oxidation in the diabetic heart. A decrease in acetyl CoA production from oxidation will result in a decrease in 3-ketoacyl CoA thiolase, the last enzyme of β-oxidation.[49] Whether or not this alters the mitochondrial uptake of fatty acids has not been established. A proposed mechanism by which glucose can alter fatty acid β-oxidation was proposed by Saddik et al.[89] and Stanley et al.,[97] who demonstrated in nondiabetic hearts that direct stimulation of PDH with DCA will markedly increase myocardial levels of acetyl CoA. These acetyl groups can be shuttled out of the mitochondria by a carnitine carrier, where the now cytoplasmic acetyl CoA can be converted to malonyl CoA by ACC. Increased malonyl CoA levels will decrease fatty acid oxidation rates, secondary to inhibition of CPT I.[2,35,56,89,97] In diabetic rat hearts, the opposite probably occurs, in which a decrease in glucose oxidation decreases cytoplasmic malonyl CoA and increases fatty acid oxidation rates. In support of this concept, Saddik et al.[89] have shown that decreasing glucose oxidation in nondiabetic hearts (by removing glucose from the perfusion medium) will result in a dramatic drop in malonyl CoA levels in the heart.[89]

Recent evidence also suggests that direct control of ACC by insulin may modify fatty acid oxidation in the diabetic heart. Gamble and Lopaschuk[22] and Makinde et al.[57] have recently demonstrated that insulin will activate ACC in the heart, secondary to an inhibition of AMPK. Furthermore, AMPK activity is increased in STZ diabetic rat hearts, which is accompanied by a decrease in ACC activity.[23] This suggests that the decrease in glucose metabolism in insulin-deficient diabetic rats is accompanied by an increase in fatty acid oxidation due to lack of insulin inhibition of malonyl CoA production by ACC.

As discussed, ketones can be readily oxidized by the heart, and can be a significant source of energy in the diabetic heart (Section 2.6). The formation of acetyl CoA from ketones will inhibit PDH and decrease glucose oxidation. How and if glucose and lactate metabolism alters ketone metabolism is not as clear, nor is how ketone oxidation and fatty acid oxidation interact. Inhibition of fatty acid oxidation by ketone oxidation[44,88] may be due to inhibition of thiolase activity by acetyl CoA. Whether or not ketone bodies alter malonyl CoA production by ACC has yet to be determined.

2.8   Benefits of Altering Energy Metabolism in the STZ Diabetic Rat Heart

It has been well established that STZ diabetes will result in the development of cardiomyopathies (see References 17, 45, and 102 for reviews). Although many underlying biochemical changes contribute to these diabetic cardiomyopathies, it is clear that alteration in energy metabolism in the heart is also an important contributing factor. This is supported by studies that have shown that acute and chronic manipulation of energy metabolism can benefit heart function in STZ diabetic rats. For instance, acute inhibition of fatty acid oxidation and stimulation of glucose oxidation[7,69,104] both improve heart function in diabetic rats. Chronic interventions that decrease fatty acid oxidation will also improve heart function in diabetic rats (see Reference 98 for a review). As a result, pharmacological modification of myocardial energy metabolism may be a promising approach to treating cardiomyopathies in patients with diabetes.

2.9 Summary

Conceptual understanding of the metabolic abnormalities in the diabetic heart comes largely from animals studies using the STZ model of diabetes. The hallmarks of diabetic cardiomyopathy are a decreased capacity for glucose transport and glycolysis, impaired pyruvate oxidation, and enhanced fatty acid and ketone body oxidation. These abnormalities persist during myocardial ischemia and reperfusion, and frequently correspond to greater contractile dysfunction. Correction of these metabolic abnormalities in animal models of STZ diabetes generally results in improved contractile recovery, thus suggesting that these metabolic lesions are the cause of the greater degree of histological and functional damage observed in the diabetic heart following ischemia. Understanding of these metabolic abnormalities is limited, especially in the interrelationships among fatty acid, ketone body, and carbohydrate metabolism.

References

1. Almira, E. C., R. G. Araceli, and B. R. Boshell, Insulin binding and glucose transport activity in cardiomyocytes of a diabetic rat, *Am. J. Physiol.*, 250, E402-E406, 1986.
2. Awan, M. M. and E. D. Saggerson, Malonyl-CoA metabolism in cardiac myocytes and its relevance to the control of fatty acid oxidation, *Biochem. J.*, 295, 61-66, 1993.
3. Barrett, E. J., R. G. Schwartz, L. H. Young, R. Jacob, and B. L. Zaret, Effect of chronic diabetes on myocardial fuel metabolism and insulin sensitivity, *Diabetes*, 37, 943-948, 1988.
4. Bourey, R. E., L. Koranyi, D. E. James, M. Mueckler, and M. A. Permutt, Effects of altered glucose homeostasis on glucose transporter expression in skeletal muscle of the rat, *J. Clin. Invest.*, 86, 542-547, 1990.
5. Broderick, T. L., G. Haloftis, and D. J. Paulson, L-propionylcarnitine Enhancement of substrate oxidation and mitochondrial respiration in the diabetic heart, *J. Mol. Cell. Cardiol.*, 28, 331-340, 1996.
6. Broderick, T. L., G. Panagakis, D. DiDomenico, J. Gamble, G. D. Lopaschuk, A. L. Shug, and D. J. Paulson, L-carnitine improvement of cardiac function is associated with a stimulation in glucose but not fatty acid metabolism in carnitine-deficient hearts, *Cardiovasc. Res.*, 30, 815-820, 1995.
7. Broderick, T. L., H. A. Quinney, and G. D. Lopaschuk, L-carnitine increases glucose metabolism and mechanical function following ischemia in diabetic rat heart, *Cardiovasc. Res.*, 29, 373-378, 1995.
8. Brooks, G. A. and G. A. Gaesser, End points of lactate and glucose metabolism after exhausting exercise, *J. Appl. Physiol.*, 49, 1057-1069, 1980.
9. Camps, M., A. Castello, P. Munoz, M. Monfar, X. Testar, M. Palacin, and A. Zorzano, Effect of diabetes and fasting on GLUT-4 (muscle/fat) glucose-transporter expression in insulin-sensitive tissues. Heterogeneous response in heart, red and white muscle, *Biochem. J.*, 282, 765-772, 1992.

10. Chappell, J. B. and B. H. Robinson, Penetration of the mitochondrial membrane by tricarboxylic acid anions, *Biochem. Soc. Symp.*, 27, 123-133, 1968.

11. Chatham, J. C. and J. R. Forder, A 13C-NMR study of glucose oxidation in the intact functioning rat heart following diabetes-induced cardiomyopathy, *J. Mol. Cell Cardiol.*, 25, 1203-1213, 1993.

12. Chen, V., C. D. Ianuzzo, B. C. Fong, and J. J. Spitzer, The effects of acute and chronic diabetes on myocardial metabolism in rats, *Diabetes*, 33, 1078-1084, 1984.

13. Dang, A. Q., F. H. Faas, and W. J. Carter, Effects of streptozotocin-induced diabetes on microsomal long-chain fatty acyl-CoA synthetase and hydrolase, *Lipids*, 19, 578-582, 1984.

14. Das, I., Effects of heart work and insulin on glycogen metabolism in the perfused rat heart, *Am. J. Physiol.*, 224, 7-12, 1973.

15. Denton, R. M. and P. J. Randle, Concentrations of glycerides and phospholipids in rat heart and gastrocnemius muscles. Effects of alloxan-diabetes and perfusion, *Biochem. J.*, 104, 416-422, 1967.

16. Depre, C., K. Veitch, and L. Hue, Role of fructose 2,6-bisphosphate in the control of glycolysis. Stimulation of glycogen synthesis by lactate in the isolated working rat heart, *Acta Cardiol.*, 48, 147-164, 1993.

17. Dhalla, N. S., G. N. Pierce, I. R. Innes, and R. E. Beamish, Pathogenesis of cardiac dysfunction in diabetes mellitus, *Can. J. Cardiol.*, 1, 263-281, 1985.

18. Ferber, S., J. Meyerovitch, K. M. Kriauciunas, and C. R. Kahn, Vanadate normalizes hyoperglycemia and phosphoenolpyruvate carboxykinase mRNA levels in ob/ob mice, *Metabolism*, 43, 1346-1354, 1994.

19. Finegan, B. A., A. S. Clanachan, C. S. Coulson, and G. D. Lopaschuk, Adenosine modification of energy substrate use in isolated hearts perfused with fatty acids, *Am. J. Physiol.*, 262, H1501-7, 1992.

20. Gabel, H., H. Bitter Suermann, C. Henriksson, J. Save Soderbergh, K. Lundholm, and H. Brynger, Streptozotocin diabetes in juvenile pigs. Evaluation of an experimental model, *Horm. Metab. Res.*, 17, 275-280, 1985.

21. Gamble, J. and G. D. Lopaschuk, Glycolysis and glucose oxidation during reperfusion of ischemic hearts from diabetic rats, *Biochim. Biophys. Acta*, 1225, 191-199, 1994.

22. Gamble, J. and G. D. Lopaschuk, Insulin inhibition of 5' AMP-activated protein kinase in the heart results in activation of acetyl CoA carboxylase and inhibition of fatty acid oxidation, *Metabolism*, 46, 1270-1274, 1997.

23. Gamble, J., L. A. Witters, and G. D. Lopaschuk, manuscript submitted.

24. Garcia, C. K., J. L. Goldstein, R. K. Pathak, R. G. Anderson, and M. S. Brown, Molecular characterization of a membrane transporter for lactate, pyruvate, and other monocarboxylates: implications for the Cori cycle, *Cell*, 76, 865-873, 1994.

25. Garvey, W. T., D. Hardin, M. Juhaszova, and J. H. Dominguez, Effects of diabetes on myocardial glucose transport system in rats: implications for diabetic cardiomyopathy, *Am. J. Physiol.*, 264, H837-H844, 1993.

26. Gertz, E. W., J. A. Wisneski, R. Neese, J. D. Bristow, G. L. Searle, and J. T. Hanlon, Myocardial lactate metabolism: evidence of lactate release during net chemical extraction in man, *Circulation*, 63, 1273-1279, 1981.

27. Gertz, E. W., J. A. Wisneski, W. C. Stanley, and R. A. Neese, Myocardial substrate utilization during exercise in humans. Dual carbon-labeled carbohydrate isotope experiments, *J. Clin. Invest.*, 82, 2017-2025, 1988.

28. Ghadiminejad, I. and E. D. Saggerson, A study of properties and abundance of the componenets of liver carnitine palmitoyltransferases in mitochondrial inner and outer membranes, *Biochem. J.*, 277, 611-617, 1991.

29. Glatz, J. F., E. van Breda, H. A. Keizer, Y. F. de Jong, J. R. Lakey, R. V. Rajotte, A. Thompson, G. J. van der Vusse, and G. D. Lopaschuk, Rat heart fatty acid-binding protein content is increased in experimental diabetes, *Biochem. Biophys. Res. Commun.*, 199, 639-646, 1994.

30. Goodwin, G. W., J. R. Arteaga, and H. Taegtmeyer, Glycogen turnover in the isolated working rat heart, *J. Biol. Chem.*, 270, 9234-9240, 1995.

31. Grinblat, L., L. F. Pacheco Bolanos, and A. O. Stoppani, Decreased rate of ketone-body oxidation and decreased activity of D-3-hydroxybutyrate dehydrogenase and succinyl-CoA:3-oxo-acid CoA-transferase in heart mitochondria of diabetic rats, *Biochem. J.*, 240, 49-56, 1986.

32. Grussner, R., R. Nakhleh, A. Grussner, G. Tomadze, P. Diem, and D. Sutherland, Streptozotocin-induced diabetes mellitus in pigs, *Horm. Metab. Res.*, 25, 199-203, 1993.

33. Hall, J. L., J. Henderson, L. A. Hernandez, L. A. Kellerman, and W. C. Stanley, Hyperglycemia results in an increase in myocardial interstitial glucose and glucose uptake during ischemia, *Metabolism*, 45, 542-549, 1996.

34. Hall, J. L., L. A. Hernandez, J. Henderson, L. A. Kellerman, and W. C. Stanley, Decreased interstitial glucose and transmural gradient in lactate during ischemia, *Basic. Res. Cardiol.*, 89, 468-486, 1994.

35. Hall, J. L., G. D. Lopaschuk, A. Barr, J. Bringas, R. D. Pizzurro, and W. C. Stanley, Increased cardiac fatty acid uptake with dobutamine infusion in swine is accompanied by a decrease in malonyl CoA levels, *Cardiovasc. Res.*, 32, 879-885, 1996.

36. Hall, J. L., W. L. Sexton, and W. C. Stanley, Exercise training attenuates the reduction in myocardial GLUT-4 in diabetic rats, *J. Appl. Physiol.*, 78, 76-81, 1995.

37. Hall, J. L., W. C. Stanley, G. D. Lopaschuk, J. A. Wisneski, R. D. Pizzurro, C. D. Hamilton, and J. G. McCormack, Impaired pyruvate oxidation but normal glucose uptake in diabetic pig heart during dobutamine-induced work, *Am. J. Physiol.*, 271, H2320-H2329, 1996.

38. Hansen, J. B. and C. M. Veneziale, Intracellular concentration of skeletal and cardiac muscle phosphofructokinase in diabetic and normal animals, *J. Lab. Clin. Med.*, 95, 133-143, 1980.

39. Hansford, R. G. and L. Cohen, Relative importance of pyruvate dehydrogenase interconversion and feed-back inhibition in the effect of fatty acids on pyruvate oxidation by rat heart mitochondria, *Arch. Biochem. Biophys.*, 191, 65-81, 1978.

40. Henning, S. L., R. B. Wambolt, B. O. Schonekess, G. D. Lopaschuk, and M. F. Allard, Contribution of glycogen to aerobic myocardial glucose utilization, *Circulation*, 93, 1549-1555, 1996.

41. Itoi, T. and G. D. Lopaschuk, The contribution of glycolysis, glucose oxidation, lactate oxidation, and fatty acid oxidation to ATP production in isolated biventricular working hearts from 2-week-old rabbits, *Pediatr. Res.*, 34, 735-741, 1993.

42. Jeffrey, F. M., V. Diczku, A. D. Sherry, and C. R. Malloy, Substrate selection in the isolated working rat heart: effects of reperfusion, afterload, and concentration, *Basic. Res. Cardiol.*, 90, 388-396, 1995.

43. Kerbey, A. L., P. M. Radcliffe, and P. J. Randle, Diabetes and the control of pyruvate dehydrogenase in rat heart mitochondria by concentration ratios of adenosine triphosphate/adenosine diphosphate, of reduced/oxidized nicotinamide-adenine dinucleotide and of acetyl-coenzyme A/coenzyme A, *Biochem. J.*, 164, 509-519, 1977.

44. Kerbey, A. L., P. J. Randle, R. H. Cooper, S. Whitehouse, H. T. Pask, and R. M. Denton, Regulation of pyruvate dehydrogenase in rat heart. Mechanism of regulation of proportions of dephosphorylated and phosphorylated enzyme by oxidation of fatty acids and ketone bodies and of effects of diabetes: role of coenzyme A, acetyl-coenzyme A and reduced and oxidized nicotinamide-adenine dinucleotide, *Biochem. J.*, 154, 327-348, 1976.

45. Keriakes, D. J., J. L. Naughton, B. Brundage, and N. B. Schiller, The heart in diabetes, *West. J. Med.*, 140, 583-593, 1984.

46. Knowlton, F. P. and E. H. Starling, Experiments on the consumption of sugar in the normal and the diabetic heart, *J. Physiol.*, XLIV, 146-163, 1912.

47. Kraegen, E. W., J. A. Sowden, M. B. Halstead, P. W. Clark, K. J. Rodnick, D. J. Chisholm, and D. E. James, Glucose transporters and *in vivo* glucose uptake in skeletal and cardiac muscle: fasting, insulin stimulation and immunoisolation studies of GLUT1 and GLUT4, *Biochem. J.*, 295, 287-293, 1993.

48. Kreisberg, R., Effect of diabetes and starvation on myocardial triglyceride and free fatty acid utilization, *Am. J. Physiol.*, 210, 379-384, 1966.

49. Kunau, W., V. Dommes, and H. Schulz, β-Oxidation of fatty acids in mitochondria, peroxisaomes and bacteria: a century of continued progress, *Prog. Lipid Res.*, 34, 267-342, 1995.

50. Kuo, T. H., F. Giacomelli, and J. Wiener, Oxidative metabolism of polytron vs. nagarse mitochondria in hearts of genetically diabetic mice, *Biochim. Biophysi. Acta*, 806, 9-15, 1985.

51. Kuo, T. H., K. H. Moore, F. Giacomelli, and J. Wiener, Defective oxidative metabolism of heart mitochondria from genetically diabetic mice, *Diabetes*, 32, 781-787, 1983.

52. Laughlin, M. R., J. Taylor, A. S. Chesnick, and R. S. Balaban, Nonglucose substrates increase glycogen synthesis *in vivo* in dog heart, *Am. J. Physiol.*, 267, H219-H223, 1994.

53. Liedtke, A. J., Alterations of carbohydrate and lipid metabolism in the acutely ischemic heart, *Prog. Cardiovasc. Dis.*, 23, 321-336, 1981.

54. Lopaschuk, G. D., Abnormal mechanical function in diabetes: relationship to altered myocardial carbohydrate/lipid metabolism, *Coronary Artery Dis.*, 7, 116-123, 1996.

55. Lopaschuk, G. D., J. R. Lakey, R. Barr, R. Wambolt, A. B. Thomson, M. T. Clandinin, and R. V. Rajotte, Islet transplantation improves glucose oxidation and mechanical function in diabetic rat hearts, *Can. J. Physiol. Pharmacol.*, 71, 896-903, 1993.

56. Lopaschuk, G. D., L. A. Witters, T. Itoi, R. Barr, and A. Barr, Acetyl-CoA carboxylase involvement in the rapid maturation of fatty acid oxidation in the newborn rabbit heart, *J. Biol. Chem.*, 269, 25871-25878, 1994.

57. Makinde, A., J. Gamble, and G. D. Lopaschuk, Upregualtion of 5'-AMP-activated protein kinase is responsible for the increase in myocardial fatty acid oxidation rates following birth in the newborn rabbit, *Circ. Res.*, 80, 482-489, 1997.

58. Manchester, J., X. Kong, J. Nerbonne, O. H. Lowry, and J. C. Lawrence, Jr., Glucose transport and phosphorylation in single cardiac myocytes: rate-limiting steps in glucose metabolism, *Am. J. Physiol.*, 266, E326-E333, 1994.

59. Marshall, M., Induction of chronic diabetes by streptozotocin in the miniature pig, *Res. Exp. Med. Berl.*, 175, 187-196, 1979.

60. McCormack, J. G., N. J. Edgell, and R. M. Denton, Studies on the interactions of Ca^{2+} and pyruvate in the regulation of rat heart pyruvate dehydrogenase activity. Effects of starvation and diabetes, *Biochem. J.*, 202, 419-427, 1982.

61. McCormack, J. G., A. P. Halestrap, and R. M. Denton, Role of calcium ions in regulation of mammalian intramitochondrial metabolism, *Physiol. Rev.*, 70, 391-425, 1990.

62. Mokuda, O., Y. Sakamoto, T. Ikeda, and H. Mashiba, Effects of anoxia and low free fatty acid on myocardial energy metabolism in streptozotocin-diabetic rats, *Ann. Nutr. Metab.*, 34, 259-265, 1990.

63. Morgan, H. E., E. Cadenas, D. M. Regan et al., Regulation of glucose uptake in muscle. II. Rate-limiting steps and effects of insulin and anoxia in heart muscle from diabetic rats, *J. Biol. Chem.*, 236, 262-268, 1961.

64. Murthy, V. K. and J. C. Shipp, Accumulation of myocardial triglycerides ketotic diabetes; evidence for increased biosynthesis, *Diabetes*, 26, 222-229, 1977.

65. Myears, D. W., B. E. Sobel, and S. R. Bergmann, Substrate use in ischemic and reperfused canine myocardium: quantitative considerations, *Am. J. Physiol.*, 253, H107-H114, 1987.

66. Neely, J. R. and H. E. Morgan, Relationship between carbohydrate and lipid metabolism and the energy balance of heart muscle, *Annu. Rev. Physiol.*, 36, 413-459, 1974.

67. Newsholme, E. A. and P. J. Randle, Regulation of glucose uptake by muscle. effects of fatty acids, ketone bodies and pyruvate and of alloxan diabetes, starvation, hypophysectomy and adrenalectomy, on the concentrations of hexose phosphates, nucleotides and inorganic phosphate in perfused rat heart, *Biochem. J.*, 93, 641-651, 1964.

68. Newsholme, E. A., P. J. Randle, and K. L. Manchester, Inhibition of the phosphofructokinase reaction in perfused rat heart by respiration of ketone bodies, fatty acids and pyruvate, *Nature*, 193, 270-271, 1962.

69. Nicholl, T. A., G. D. Lopaschuk, and J. H. McNeill, Effect of free fatty acids and dichloroacetate on isolated rat heart, *Am. J. Physiol.*, 261, 1053-1059, 1991.

70. Opie, L. H., Reperfusion injury and its pharmacologic modification, *Circulation*, 80, 1049-1062, 1989.

71. Opie, L. H., *The Heart: Physiology and Metabolism*, Raven Press, New York, 1991,

72. Opie, L. H. and P. Owen, Effect of glucose-insulin-potassium infusions on arteriovenous differences of glucose of free fatty acids and on tissue metabolic changes in dogs with developing myocardial infarction, *Am. J. Cardiol.*, 38, 310-321, 1976.

73. Osborn, B. A., J. T. Daar, R. A. Laddaga, F. D. Romano, and D. J. Paulson, Exercise training increases sarcolemmal GLUT-4 protein and mRNA content in diabetic heart, *J. Appl. Physiol.*, 82, 828-834, 1997.

74. Paulson, D. J. and M. F. Crass, III, Endogenous triacylglycerol metabolism in diabetic heart, *Am. J. Physiol.*, 242, H1084-H1094, 1982.

75. Paulson, D. J., R. Mathews, J. Bowman, and J. Zhao, Metabolic effects of treadmill exercise training on the diabetic heart, *J. Appl. Physiol.*, 73, 265-271, 1992.

76. Pierce, G. N., in *Heart Dysfunction in Diabetes*, G. N. Pierce, R. E. Beamish, and N. S. Dhalla, Eds., Boca Raton, FL, CRC Press, 1988,

77. Randle, P. J., Fuel selection in animals, *Biochem. Soc. Trans.*, 14, 799-806, 1986.

78. Randle, P. J., C. N. Hales, P. B. Garland, and E. A. Newsholme, The glucose-fatty acid cycle. its role in insulin sensitivity and the metabolic disturbances of diabetes mellitus, *Lancet*, 2, 785-789, 1963.

79. Randle, P. J., E. A. Newsholme, and P. B. Garland, Regulation of glucose uptake by muscle. effects of fatty acids, ketone bodies and pyruvate and of alloxan diabetes and starvation, on the uptake and metabolic fate of glucose in rat heart and diaphragm muscles, *Biochem. J.*, 93, 652-665, 1964.

80. Randle, P. J. and D. A. Priesman, in *Alpha-Keto Acid Dehydrogenase Complexes*, M. S. Patel, T. E. Roche, and R. A. Harris, Eds., Basel, Birkhausen Verlag, 1996, 151-161.

81. Reinauer, H., M. Adrian, P. Rosen, and F.-J. Schmitz, Influence of carnitine acyltransferase inhibitors on the performance and metabolism of rat cardiac muscle, *J. Clin. Chem. Clin. Biochem.*, 28, 335-339, 1990.

82. Rizza, R. A., M. F. Crass, III, and J. C. Shipp, Effect of insulin treatment *in vivo* on heart glycerides and glycogen of alloxan-diabetic rats, *Metabolism*, 20, 539-543, 1971.

83. Rodrigues, B., J. E. Braun, M. Spooner, and D. L. Severson, Regulation of lipoprotein lipase activity in cardiac myocytes from control and diabetic rat hearts by plasma lipids, *Can. J. Physiol. Pharmacol.*, 70, 1271-1279, 1992.

84. Rodrigues, B., M. C. Cam, and J. H. McNeill, Myocardial substrate metabolism: implications for diabetic cardiomyopathy, *J. Mol. Cell. Cardiol.*, 27, 169-179, 1995.

85. Rodrigues, B. and D. L. Severson, Acute diabetes does not reduce heparin-releasable lipoprotein lipase activity in perfused hearts from Wistar-Kyoto rats, *Can. J. Physiol. Pharmacol.*, 71, 657-661, 1993.

86. Rosen, P. and H. Reinauer, Inhibition of carnitine palmitoyltransferase I by phenylalkyloxiran-ecarboxylic acid and its influence on lipolysis and glucose metabolism in isolated, perfused hearts of streptozotocin-diabetic rats, *Metabolism*, 33, 177-185, 1984.

87. Russell, R. R., III, J. M. Mrus, J. I. Mommessin, and H. Taegtmeyer, Compartmentation of hexokinase in rat heart. A critical factor for tracer kinetic analysis of myocardial glucose metabolism, *J. Clin. Invest.*, 90, 1972-1977, 1992.

88. Russell, R. R., III and H. Taegtmeyer, Changes in citric acid cycle flux and anaplerosis antedate the functional decline in isolated rat hearts utilizing acetoacetate, *J. Clin. Invest.*, 87, 384-390, 1991.

89. Saddik, M., J. Gamble, L. A. Witters, and G. D. Lopaschuk, Acetyl-CoA carboxylase regulation of fatty acid oxidation in the heart, *J. Biol. Chem.*, 268, 25836-25845, 1993.

90. Saddik, M. and G. D. Lopaschuk, Triacylglycerol turnover in isolated working hearts of acutely diabetic rats, *Can. J. Physiol. Pharmacol.*, 72, 1110-1119, 1994.

91. Savabi, F., Mitochondrial creatine phosphokinase deficiency in diabetic rat heart, *Biochem. Biophys. Res. Commun.*, 154, 469-475, 1988.

92. Sochor, M., A.-M. Gonzales, and P. McLean, Regulation of alternative pathways of glucose metabolism in rat heart in alloxan diabetes: changes in the pentose phosphate pathway, *Biochem. Biophys. Res. Commun.*, 118, 110-116, 1984.

93. Sochor, M., S. Kunjara, M. Ali, and P. McLean, Vanadate treatment increases the activity of glycolytic enzymes and raises fructose 2,6-biphosphate concentration in hearts from diabetic rats, *Biochem. Int.*, 28, 525-531, 1992.

94. Stanley, W. C., Myocardial lactate metabolism during exercise, *Med. Sci. Sports Exerc.*, 23, 920-924, 1991.

95. Stanley, W. C., J. L. Hall, T. A. Hacker, L. A. Hernandez, and L. F. Whitesell, Decreased myocardial glucose uptake during ischemia in diabetic swine, *Metabolism*, 46, 168-172, 1997.

96. Stanley, W. C., J. L. Hall, K. R. Smith, G. D. Cartee, T. A. Hacker, and J. A. Wisneski, Myocardial glucose transporters and glycolytic metabolism during ischemia in hyperglycemic diabetic swine, *Metabolism*, 43, 61-69, 1994.

97. Stanley, W. C., L. A. Hernandez, D. Spires, J. Bringas, S. Wallace, and J. G. McCormack, Pyruvate dehydrogenase activity and malonyl CoA levels in normal and ischemic swine myocardium: effects of dichloroacetate, *J. Mol. Cell Cardiol.*, 28, 905-914, 1996.

98. Stanley, W. C., G. D. Lopaschuk, J. L. Hall, and J. G. McCormack, Regulation of myocardial carbohydrate metabolism under normal and ischaemic conditions. Potential for pharmacological interventions, *Cardiovas. Res.*, 33, 243-257, 1997.

99. Steigen, T. K., S. Pettersen, P. H. Guddal, and T. S. Larsen, Effects of hypothermia and rewarming on phospholipase C-evoked glycerol output in rat myocardial cells, *J. Mol. Cell Cardiol.*, 24, 457-464, 1992.

100. Sun, D., N. Nguyen, T. R. DeGrado, M. Schwaiger, and F. C3. Brosius, Ischemia induces translocation of the insulin-responsive glucose transporter GLUT4 to the plasma membrane of cardiac myocytes, *Circulation*, 89, 793-798, 1994.

101. Taegtmeyer, H., Energy metabolism of the heart: from basic concepts to clinical applications, *Curr. Probl. Cardiol.*, 19, 59-113, 1994.

102. Tahiliani, A. G. and J. H. McNeill, Diabetes-induced abnormalities in the myocardium, *Life. Sci.*, 38, 959-974, 1986.

103. Vrobel, T. R., C. R. Jorgensen, and R. J. Bache, Myocardial lactate and adenosine metabolite production as indicators of exercise-induced myocardial ischemia in the dog, *Circulation*, 66, 554-561, 1982.

104. Wall, S. R. and G. D. Lopaschuk, Glucose oxidation rates in fatty acid-perfused isolated working hearts from diabetic rats, *Biochim. Biophys. Acta*, 1006, 97-103, 1989.

105. Wang, X., A. J. Levi, and A. P. Halestrap, Kinetics of the sarcolemmal lactate carrier in single heart cells using BCECF to measure pHi, *Am. J. Physiol.*, 267, H1759-H1769, 1994.

106. Wheeler, T. J., Translocation of glucose transporters in response to anoxia in heart, *J. Biol. Chem.*, 263, 19447-19454, 1988.

107. Whitfield, C. F. and M. A. Osevala, Hexose transport modification of rat hearts during development of chronic diabetes, *J. Mol. Cell. Cardiol.*, 16, 1091-1099, 1984.

108. Wieland, O., E. Siess, F. H. Schulze-Wethmar, H. G. v. Funcke, and B. Winton, Active and inactive forms of pyruvate dehydrogenase in rat heart and kidney: effect of diabetes, fasting and refeeding on pyruvate dehydrogenase interconversion, *Arch. Biochem. Biophys.*, 143, 593-601, 1971.

109. Wilson, J. D., D. P. Dhall, C. J. Simeonovic, and K. J. Lafferty, Induction and management of diabetes mellitus in the pig, *Aust. J. Exp. Biol. Med. Sci.*, 64, 489-500, 1986.

110. Wisneski, J. A., E. W. Gertz, R. A. Neese, L. D. Gruenke, and J. C. Craig, Dual carbon-labeled isotope experiments using D-[6-14C] glucose and L-[1,2,3-13C3] lactate: a new approach for investigating human myocardial metabolism during ischemia, *J. Am. Coll. Cardiol.*, 5, 1138-1146, 1985.

111. Wisneski, J. A., W. C. Stanley, R. A. Neese, and E. W. Gertz, Effects of acute hyperglycemia on myocardial glycolytic activity in humans, *J. Clin. Invest.*, 85, 1648-1656, 1990.

112. Yeaman, S. J., The 2-oxo acid dehydrogenase complexes: recent advances, *Biochem. J.*, 257, 625-632, 1989.

113. Young, L. H., Y. Renfu, R. Russell, X. Hu, M. Caplan, J. Ren, G. I. Shulman, and A. J. Sinusas, Low-flow ischemia leads to translocation of canine heart GLUT-4 and GLUT-1 glucose transporters to the sarcolemma *in vivo*, *Circulation*, 95, 415-422, 1997.

114. Zaninetti, D., R. Greco Perotto, and B. Jeanrenaud, Heart glucose transport and transporters in rat heart: regulation by insulin, workload and glucose, *Diabetologia*, 31, 108-113, 1988.

3

Structural and Functional Consequences of Streptozotocin-Induced Diabetes on the Kidney

Kumar Sharma, Dong Cheol Han, András Mogyorósi, and Fuad N. Ziyadeh

CONTENTS

3.1 Introduction

The streptozotocin (STZ)-induced model of Type I diabetes mellitus in the rat has been the most widely studied model to demonstrate the hemodynamic and structural

TABLE 3.1

Renal Functional and Structural Changes in the STZ
Diabetic Rat

Renal Hemodynamic Alterations

Early glomerular hemodynamic alterations
  Single-nephron hyperfiltration
  Increased glomerular blood flow
  Increased intraglomerular pressure
Late glomerular hemodynamic alterations
  Increased glomerular basement membrane permeability
  Decreased glomerular filtration

Glomerular Structural Changes

Early glomerular lesions
  Glomerular hypertrophy
Late glomerular lesions
  Glomerular basement membrane thickening
  Mesangial matrix expansion

Tubular Structural Changes

  Tubular hypertrophy
  The Armanni–Ebstein lesion
  Tubular basement membrane thickening
  Tubulointerstitial fibrosis

---

alterations of the diabetic state on the kidney (Table 3.1). The mouse model of STZ-induced diabetes is far less well studied, mostly because of technical issues related to the relative resistance of this species to the induction of insulin deficiency by STZ[1] and to the difficulties in monitoring systemic and renal hemodynamic and functional parameters. This chapter will therefore mostly discuss the reported functional and structural changes in the kidney in the rat model during the early and late phases of the disease and will attempt to highlight the significant progress that this model has provided in the understanding of the pathogenesis and the clinical management of diabetic nephropathy in humans.

3.2   Renal Hemodynamic Alterations

3.2.1   Systemic Hemodynamic Alterations

Initial reports noted that STZ diabetes in the rat is associated with the development of systemic arterial hypertension as measured by the tail cuff method (employing an inflatable small cuff that interferes with the tail arterial blood flow and is connected to a sensor to identify the systolic pressure). A short duration of diabetes was found to be associated with a 10 to 20% increase in systolic pressure; however, subsequent studies using direct intra-arterial blood pressure monitoring did not demonstrate significant hypertension in this model.[2] This discrepancy has been attributed to lower muscle mass, fibrosis, or calcified vessels in the diabetic rat,[3] which result in artificially elevated blood pressure readings by the tail cuff plethysmography method. In fact, it is now recognized that the model of STZ-induced diabetes in the rat is characterized by chronic arterial vasodilation. The cause remains unknown, but reduced responsiveness to vasoconstrictors such as catecholamines (phenylephrine) has been demonstrated in aortic strips from diabetic rats.[4]

There also does appear to exist a systemic disturbance in vascular permeability in this model. Several studies have demonstrated that administration of radiolabeled albumin to the STZ rat within the first several weeks of diabetes leads to extravasation of radioactive material.[5,6] One study found that treatment with inhibitors of nitric oxide synthase (NOS) by L-arginine derivatives and aminoguanidine reversed the effect on permeability, suggesting that increased NO production in the diabetic state underlies enhanced permeability across the endothelium.[6] However, several studies have also demonstrated a protective effect of NO to maintain the endothelial barrier by inhibiting intercellular adhesion molecule (ICAM) expression and preventing neutrophil adhesion to the endothelium and the release of molecules that interfere with endothelial function.[7-9] Any alterations of systemic NO production and their functional consequences remain to be established in experimental diabetes.

3.2.2 Glomerular Hemodynamic Alterations

The studies led by Brenner and colleagues in the STZ diabetic rat have profoundly affected how physiologists and nephrologists understand the glomerular hemodynamics of diabetes. In the initial study by Hostetter and co-workers,[10] adult Munich-Wistar rats were given STZ 60 mg/kg in citrate buffer intravenously. The group that did not receive insulin was severely hyperglycemic (blood glucose >500 mg/dl), whereas the group that received 2 U of NPH insulin subcutaneously each evening for 3 weeks was moderately hyperglycemic (<400 mg/dl). Diabetic rats were studied by glomerular micropuncture 2 to 15 weeks after being made diabetic. The Munich-Wistar rat was used for these studies because the superficial glomeruli are accessible for direct glomerular micropuncture. These studies demonstrated that the moderately hyperglycemic STZ diabetic rat had increased single nephron GFR (SNGFR). It is important to note that inducing diabetes in the rat without administering insulin resulted in severe hyperglycemia, weight loss, marked osmotic diuresis, and a fall in SNGFR. Only when insulin was administered to attain moderate hyperglycemia and prevent weight loss were the hemodynamic characteristics of hyperfiltration discerned. The elevated SNGFR was found to be mediated by increased glomerular blood flow (Q_A) and an elevation of the glomerular capillary pressure (P_{GC}). The latter is mediated by relaxation of the afferent arteriole and relative constriction of the efferent arteriole. It is also important to note that both afferent and efferent arteriolar resistances decreased in the diabetic rat as compared with control; however, the degree of decrease was greater in the afferent arteriole than in the efferent arteriole. The net result is that the enhanced glomerular blood flow was permitted to enter the glomerulus via the relaxed afferent arteriole, and, since there was relatively less relaxation in the efferent arteriole, the hydrostatic pressure in the glomerular capillary increased. Plasma volume may play a role in the altered glomerular hemodynamics of diabetic rats; however, measurements of absolute blood volume were not different in the three groups of rats, although when factored per body weight there was an increase in blood volume in both diabetic groups as compared with control.[10]

The discrepant results regarding the GFR level in the severely hyperglycemic group as compared with the moderately hyperglycemic group[10] can be considered analogous to the clinical situation whereby patients with severe, uncontrolled diabetes (ketoacidosis or hyperglycemic nonketotic coma) may have an acute reduction in GFR. On the other hand, the GFR is typically elevated in the early phase of the disease in patients with Type I diabetes with moderate hyperglycemia on insulin treatment.

The micropuncture studies, which have been subsequently replicated by Brenner's group[2] and others,[11] form the basis for our current understanding of the development of glomerular hemodynamic stress in diabetic nephropathy; they also provide a rational basis to target treatment with angiotensin-converting enzyme inhibitors or low dietary protein. Based on observations in the STZ diabetic rat and in rats with ⅚ nephrectomy, the hemodynamic theory was proposed to explain the progressive nature of renal failure in diabetic nephropathy best.[12-14] Thus, the early increase in glomerular blood flow and glomerular capillary pressure would enhance the shear–stress effect on the glomerular capillary wall and the mesangium. This stress may lead to endothelial dysfunction, which somehow translates into alterations in glomerular basement membrane (GBM) structure and mesangial cell dysfunction that can lead to enhanced mesangial extracellular matrix (ECM) production. Eventually, progressive expansion of the mesangium will lead to loss of functioning filtration surface area and, hence, a fall in GFR. An exciting link can be invoked between the known intraglomerular hypertension of diabetic nephropathy and the stretch-induced production of the prosclerotic cytokine transforming growth factor-β.[15] In fact, the production of this growth factor can be stimulated in cultured mesangial cells exposed to either high glucose concentration[16,17] or cyclic stretch.[18]

3.2.3 Mechanisms of Glomerular Hyperfiltration

The possible causes for the enhanced glomerular blood flow and the decrease in afferent arteriolar resistance have been intensively studied by many investigators, but there are no definite answers regarding what mediates these changes. Plasma volume expansion is noted in several diabetic models and in patients with diabetes mellitus but plasma volume expansion (per unit of body weight) is also noted in the severely hyperglycemic rat, which has decreased glomerular blood flow and GFR.[10] Systemic levels of atrial natriuretic peptide (ANP) are elevated in the STZ diabetic rat,[19] and renal cortical mRNA levels for ANP are elevated in both untreated and insulin-treated STZ diabetic rats.[20] Inhibition of ANP by blocking antibodies or a receptor antagonist leads to a reduction in the elevated GFR.[21] Vasodilatory prostaglandins have also been implicated in diabetic hyperfiltration. Inhibiting prostaglandin production with indomethacin attenuates afferent arteriolar dilatation in STZ diabetic rats,[11] and isolated kidneys perfused with elevated glucose concentrations display a fall in renal vascular resistance, which is attenuated by indomethacin.[22] Glomeruli from STZ diabetic rats produce twice as much PGE2 as compared with control glomeruli.[23,24] NO appears to be an attractive mediator of glomerular hyperfiltration as it has a predominant action to decrease preglomerular vascular tone.[25] In fact, increased NO metabolites in the urine of STZ diabetic rats have been described.[26,27] Inhibition of intrarenal NOS with L-arginine analogs (N-monomethyl-L-arginine) leads to increased afferent arteriolar resistance and a decrease in hydraulic glomerular capillary ultrafiltration coefficient (K_f).[25] Administration of intrarenal N^G-nitro-L-arginine methyl ester to STZ diabetic rats reduces hyperfiltration and renal blood flow.[27] However, enhanced NO production by isolated glomeruli from STZ diabetic rats has not been demonstrated to date. Moreover, one study described impaired NO-dependent cyclic guanosine monophosphate generation in glomeruli from STZ diabetic rats.[28]

The most intensively studied factor that may underlie the altered renal hemodynamics in STZ diabetic rats is angiotensin II (AII), as this peptide has potent constrictor effects preferentially on the efferent arteriole. Relative efferent arteriolar constriction may be postulated to be due to increased intraglomerular AII production. One study demonstrated that ACE staining was increased in the glomerular endothelial cells of diabetic rats,[29] suggesting increased local production of AII. It may also be postulated that the afferent arteriole from STZ diabetic rats has reduced AII responsiveness, accounting for afferent vasodilatation. An elegant study employing *in vivo* video microscopy demonstrated appreciable dilatation predominantly in the afferent arteriole and to a much lesser degree in the efferent arteriole, as well as reduced AII responsiveness that was only partially restored by prostaglandin inhibition in STZ rats.[30]

It should be noted that the data examining the state of the renin–AII system (RAS) in the diabetic kidney have yielded conflicting results.[31] It has been demonstrated that in the early course of STZ diabetes in rats there is reduction in the density of glomerular AII receptors[32,33]; another group of investigators found an increased density of glomerular AII receptors but impaired contractile responsiveness of diabetic glomeruli to AII.[34] Another study, however, did not demonstrate a difference in AII-induced glomerular contraction in isolated glomeruli obtained from STZ diabetic rats.[35] Thus, it appears that in early diabetes (within 2 to 4 weeks) there is a reduction of glomerular AII receptors, whereas in established diabetes (>8 weeks) there is a normalization or increase in glomerular AII receptors[33,34] and these changes play some role in the responsiveness to AII. Insulin deficiency may also play a role in the decreased responsiveness to AII because mesangial cells (which possess smooth muscle–like properties) respond to AII in tissue culture by contraction only if insulin is added, but there is no contraction in the absence of insulin.[36] It has also been demonstrated that mesangial cells grown in high glucose exhibit an attenuated intracellular calcium rise in response to either AII or vasopressin.[37] It is not known whether insulin is similarly required for the responsiveness of vascular smooth muscle cells in the afferent arterioles to AII. Isolation and culture of smooth muscle cells from renal preglomerular resistance arterioles from normal animals have recently been performed; these cells have AII receptors and a brisk rise in intracellular calcium in response to AII.[38] It remains to be determined whether alterations in intracellular signaling pathways in vascular smooth muscle cells from STZ diabetic rats may underlie the reduced responsiveness of the afferent arteriole to vasoconstrictors such as AII.

3.2.4 The Renin–Angiotensin Axis

There have been divergent findings on the level of expression of the renin and angiotensinogen genes in the kidney in experimental diabetes mellitus.[31] For instance, Correa-Rotter et al.[39] found the level of expression of renal renin protein and mRNA not to be different between diabetic and normal rats; however, renal and liver angiotensinogen mRNA levels were lower in the diabetic group.[39] Kalinyak and co-workers,[40] although confirming that no significant differences in renal renin mRNA levels were detectable in rats 2 weeks after induction of diabetes as compared with controls, found also no differences in renal angiotensinogen transcript levels. Jaffa et al.[41] reported a 50% decrease in renal renin mRNA level 3 weeks after the induction of diabetes in rats compared with controls. In contrast, Anderson et al.[29] found a small increase in renal renin content and angiotensinogen expression 6 to 8 weeks after induction of diabetes in rats. This group also reported enhanced renal sensitivity to intrarenal administration of AII.[42] Several investigators have evaluated the renal RAS in other animal models of diabetes mellitus as an attempt to avoid the use of STZ, which can be potentially nephrotoxic.[43] A biphasic response was reported in the adult BB spontaneously diabetic rat, with an early increase in renal renin protein and mRNA content (at 2 months of diabetes) and a subsequent decrease (after 12 months of diabetes).[44] In the obese Zucker rat, a model of noninsulin-dependent (Type II) diabetes, plasma renin activity as well as renal renin protein content were significantly reduced at age 10 and 24 weeks compared with lean littermates.[45] The inconsistencies between the different studies are most likely explained by the various time points examined in the course of the disease rather than the type of diabetes itself. In addition, internephron heterogeneity of expression of the RAS components needs to be considered, as has recently been detected by *in situ* nucleic acid hybridization.[46] Several different intrarenal RASs can be envisioned within the different compartments of the kidney (e.g., vascular, glomerular, tubular, and interstitial). It is reasonable to conclude that at least one or more intrarenal RASs are generally activated early during the course of diabetes mellitus, at least to some modest degree.[46] Moreover, the nephroprotective effects of ACE inhibitors and AT_1-receptor blockers strongly argue for an increase in AII formation within the kidney in diabetes mellitus.

3.2.5 Interventions to Reduce Hemodynamic Stress

The concept of hemodynamic injury predicts that therapy aimed at reducing glomerular capillary pressure would be beneficial in protecting glomerular function and structure. The importance of glomerular hemodynamics in diabetic nephropathy is also underscored by the observation that uninephrectomy[47] and genetic susceptibility to hypertension[48-50] enhanced the development and severity of diabetic nephropathy in STZ diabetic rats. It has been shown by several investigators that inhibition of ACE activity leads to a decrease in glomerular capillary pressure.[2,51] This is due to preferential dilatation of the efferent arteriole, which results in matching the lowered resistance of the afferent arteriole and therefore in lowering of P_{GC}. Lowering the blood pressure with a regimen that does not include ACE inhibitors (reserpine, hydrochlorothiazide, hydralazine) also lowers P_{GC} in the early phase (6 to 10 weeks of diabetes), but does not protect against development of albuminuria in the late phase of diabetes (70 weeks).[2] Unfortunately, measurements of P_{GC} in the late phase have not been provided in this study. A separate study revealed that the calcium channel blocker nifedipine did not lower P_{GC} in STZ diabetic rats and also did not protect against albuminuria or glomerular injury.[52] Recent studies have found that lowering efferent arteriolar resistance with oral L-dopa and the dopamine receptor agonist, fenoldapam, also reduces hyperfiltration in STZ diabetic rats.[53,54] The reported beneficial effects of endothelin receptor blockade in reducing albuminuria and collagen gene expression in STZ diabetic rats[55] may also be due to altering glomerular hemodynamics; however, intrarenal micropuncture measurements have not been reported in this context.

Goldfarb et al.[56] demonstrated a significant reduction in glomerular hyperfiltration in STZ diabetic rats treated with either sorbinil (an aldose reductase inhibitor) or dietary myoinositol supplementation. In a study by Ghahary et al.,[57] aldose reductase activity from kidneys of STZ diabetic rats was significantly elevated after 3 months of diabetes. Northern hybridization showed upregulated mRNA encoding aldose reductase, suggesting that increased renal aldose reductase activity in these animals was likely due to pretranslational activation of the aldose reductase gene.[57]

High ambient glucose stimulates protein kinase C activation in many cell types,[58] including cultured mesangial cells,[59-62] through stimulation of *de novo* synthesis of diacylglycerol.[63,64] The oral administration of a novel agent that specifically inhibits protein kinase C-β isoform showed benefit in reducing hyperfiltration, albuminuria, and altered retinal blood flow in the early stages of STZ diabetes in rats.[65] Whether this form of therapy will also be beneficial for later stages of the disease is currently being investigated.

It is relevant to note here that results derived from examining the glomerular hemodynamics in the STZ diabetic rat model have been the principal impetus to perform important interventional studies in patients with diabetic nephropathy. For instance, the results of a major clinical trial have clearly revealed the preferential beneficial effect of ACE inhibition, compared with a regimen including diuretics and β blockers, in protection from the progressive decline in renal function in patients with Type I diabetes mellitus.[66] In addition, recent data suggest that short-acting dihydropyridine calcium channel blockers[67] do not protect against albuminuria in such patients, similar to what had been noted in STZ rats.[52] Loss of the beneficial effect of antihypertensive agents on reducing proteinuria by excess dietary salt intake was first demonstrated in STZ diabetic rats[68] and recently confirmed in human studies.[69] Such studies would probably not have been undertaken without the basic understanding of renal hemodynamics that has been originally described in the STZ diabetic rat.

3.3   Glomerular Structural Changes

3.3.1   Overview of Glomerular Lesions

Diabetic nephropathy in humans encompasses a host of structural alterations that are characterized by early hypertrophy of both glomerular and tubuloepithelial elements, thickening of the GBM and tubular basement membrane, progressive accumulation of ECM components in the glomerular mesangium, and less well recognized lesions such as progressive tubulointerstitial fibrosis and renal arteriosclerosis.[70-76] In the late phases of the disease, glomerular damage ultimately leads to frank proteinuria and systemic hypertension as well as to a marked reduction in GFR. Progressive tubulointerstitial fibrosis and renal arteriosclerosis also contribute to the renal failure.

3.3.2   Glomerular Hypertrophy

Significant enlargement of glomeruli is readily demonstrable in the early phases of STZ-induced diabetes in the rat. Rasch demonstrated a progressive increase in both kidney weight and glomerular volume in moderately hyperglycemic STZ diabetic rats during a period of 6 months of diabetes. These changes were reversible with strict glucose control by insulin treatment.[77] In severely hyperglycemic rats without insulin treatment, the glomerular volume relentlessly increased during the first 8 months of diabetes,[78,79] whereas later, no further increase was seen;[78] this resulted in identical glomerular volume in diabetic and control rats after 18 months. Moreover, in the 70-week study by Anderson et al.,[2] there was also no significant difference in the glomerular volume between the insulin-treated moderately hyperglycemic diabetic rats and the control rats at the end of the study.

3.3.3   Mesangial Matrix Expansion

Progressive expansion of the glomerular mesangial matrix is considered the most important lesion for the development of chronic renal failure in the diabetic population.[70,80] Diffuse intercapillary sclerosis correlates closely with the progressive decline in the glomerular capillary surface area available for filtration and, hence, is the structural counterpart of reduced GFR.[70,80]

Thickening of the GBM and modest expansion of the ECM in the mesangial area have both been demonstrated in long-term STZ diabetic rats. However, the lesions characteristic of many patients with advanced diabetic nephropathy, nodular and diffuse intercapillary glomerulosclerosis, have not been reported in this model.[79,81] Focal and segmental glomerulosclerosis, an uncommon finding in patients with diabetic nephropathy, has been reported in insulin-treated moderately hyperglycemic STZ diabetic rats,[2] as well as in untreated severely hyperglycemic STZ diabetic rats.[81] It should be noted that mild intercapillary glomerulosclerosis may develop with aging in the normal rat, but this lesion is seen infrequently, and only after 2 years of age.[82]

Glomerular histopathology in STZ diabetic rats is progressive with the duration of the disease. These light microscopic changes are periodic acid Schiff (PAS)-positive thickening of the glomerular mesangium (apparent after 4 to 6 months of diabetes) and focal and segmental distribution of mesangial matrix expansion.[81] Immunohistochemical studies have demonstrated progressive accumulation of IgG, IgM, and C3, within the mesangium.[81,83] Unlike the focal nature of the light microscopic changes, these immunohistochemical findings are diffuse and global. When IgG is exogenously administered, the diabetic mesangium shows impaired clearance of these macromolecular proteins. This phenomenon may underlie the increased accumulation of immunoglobulins.[84]

Electron microscopic examination by Weil et al.[83] revealed mesangial matrix expansion with electron-dense material in the mesangium, as well as some irregular barlike protrusions of the mesangial matrix (mesangial bar). The ratio of the mesangial volume in proportion to the glomerular volume (fractional mesangial volume) is increased from 12% in nondiabetic controls to 21% in diabetic rats after 9 months of diabetes.[79] In glomeruli from diabetic rats, although there is no major difference in the total glomerular capillary luminal surface, the percent of the surface of the glomerular capillary wall occupied by the mesangium exceeds that found in control animals.[79] This may result in a diminished capillary filtration surface.

Mesangial expansion is predominantly due to an overabundance of normal structural components of the mesangial ECM, including collagen Type IV, laminin, and fibronectin. Fukui et al.[85] reported that whole glomeruli from STZ diabetic rats demonstrate a significant increase in the steady-state mRNA levels encoding the α1 chain of Type IV collagen, fibronectin, and laminin B1 and B2. Yamamoto et al.[86] showed that glomerular staining for fibronectin and tenascin is also increased in long-term STZ diabetic rats.

The phenotypic expression of mesangial ECM such as the appearance of interstitial collagen Type III may also be altered in STZ diabetic rats.[87] Appreciable induction of gene expression for interstitial collagen types I and III was also demonstrated.[85] These fibrillar collagens are distinctly absent in glomeruli of nondiabetic animals *in vivo*. In the glomerular mesangium of STZ diabetic rats, immunohistochemical staining of vascular smooth muscle proteins show increased abundance of actomyosin,[88] α-smooth muscle actin,[89] caldesmon, and a myosin heavy-chain isoform.[90] This phenotypic dedifferentiation toward the embryonic phenotype may help explain mesangial cell activation and mesangial matrix expansion in the diabetic milieu.

3.3.4 Glomerular Basement Membrane Thickening

The exact biochemical and ultrastructural basis for the thickening of GBM and the increased permeability for macromolecules across the filtration barrier of the glomerular capillary wall remain only partly understood. A heterogeneous population of collagenous and noncollagenous proteins has been identified in the GBM. The most important constituent in quantitative terms is Type IV collagen. Other macromolecules include proteoglycans, namely, heparan sulfate proteoglycan (HSPG or perlecan) and structural glycoproteins (laminin, nidogen/entactin, and perhaps fibronectin).[73] It has been suggested that increased synthesis and/or decreased degradation of collagens and laminins are responsible for increased GBM thickness.[75] Hirose et al.[78] demonstrated progressive thickening of GBM in untreated STZ diabetic rats during 18 months of diabetes. Similar results were found in moderately hyperglycemic diabetic rats after 6 months of diabetes.[77] The thickness of GBM was reversible by strict blood glucose control with insulin.[77] Diffuse thickening of the GBM was highly variable from one capillary loop to another.[91] In a recent paper, Brees et al.[92] found no change in the content of Type IV collagen and nidogen/entactin but a significant increase in laminin and fibronectin in GBM extracts from rats after 3 months of STZ-induced diabetes.

Site-specific alterations in the composition of the GBM have been described in STZ diabetic rats. The protein A–gold immunocytochemical technique has revealed a relative increase in the labeling intensities of the $\alpha1(IV)$, $\alpha2(IV)$, and $\alpha3(IV)$ chains, but not of the $\alpha4(IV)$ chain of collagen Type IV. These changes were observed in the entire thickness of the GBM from diabetic animals,[93] whereas the labeling for $\alpha1(IV)$ and $\alpha2(IV)$ collagen occurs on the endothelial side of GBM in the nondiabetic control rats. In the kidneys of patients with diabetes, a relative decrease in the subendothelial density of $\alpha1(IV)$ and $\alpha2(IV)$, without similar changes in $\alpha3(IV)$ and $\alpha4(IV)$, has been found by immunofluorescence staining.[94]

By protein A–gold immunocytochemistry, endogenous IgG and albumin were localized to the subendothelial side of the GBM in normal control rats.[93,95] In contrast, IgG and albumin were present throughout the entire thickness of the GBM in 12-month-old STZ diabetic rats. These results suggest that the lamina densa may present the main barrier for the restriction of the passage of IgGs under normal conditions, but hyperglycemia may cause modification of this area and result in the loss of selective permeability of the GBM.[93]

3.3.5 Increased Glomerular Basement Membrane Permeability

The permeability defect causing frank proteinuria has been described as a loss of the size-selectivity as well as a loss of the charge-selectivity barriers in the GBM.[96] HSPG in the glomerulus is localized predominantly to the laminae rara of the GBM and is believed to govern the charge-permselective properties of the filtration barrier.[97] Several investigations have demonstrated a marked reduction in the number of anionic moieties in the diabetic GBM due to decreased incorporation of heparan sulfate into the core protein.[92,98-100] At the ultrastructural level, it is believed that the marked reduction in the content of the polyanionic HSPG may give rise to the charge-selectivity defect.[98,99,101] Expression of the mRNA and the core protein may also be altered. Whereas in the spontaneously diabetic KKay mouse the HSPG mRNA level is unaltered in whole renal cortex,[102] in isolated glomeruli of STZ diabetic rats the mRNA level is decreased after 4 weeks of diabetes and then increases with age exceeding the level in control rats at 24 weeks.[85] Future studies using other methods, such as *in situ* hybridization, are needed for more accurate analysis of HSPG mRNA expression in diabetic glomeruli.

In normal rats, basement membrane–specific chondroitin sulfate proteoglycan (CSPG) is localized to the basement membrane of Bowman's capsule and the mesangial matrix but not to the pericapillary GBM. However, in STZ diabetic rats, glomerular CSPG immunofluorescence staining can be found within the pericapillary GBM, where it forms a thin continuous rim that outlines the perimeter of affected capillaries.[101] Immunoelectron microscopy of diabetic glomeruli has revealed that CSPG tends to deposit within areas where the GBM is ostensibly thickened.[101] CSPG accumulation displaces endothelial cells from the GBM and results in loss of endothelial cell fenestration in some areas. Effacement of the epithelial podocyte foot processes is also observed.[101] Recent ultrastructural morphological studies with serial detergents revealed that the subendothelial layer is continuous with the mesangial matrix.[103] Hyperglycemia may cause altered metabolism of HSPG by glomerular cells and result in abnormal synthesis and/or removal of CSPG in the GBM by mesangial cells.

Recently, Pagtalunan et al.[104] demonstrated loss and fusion of podocytes (glomerular visceral epithelial cells) in Pima Indians with Type II diabetes with nephropathy. Broadening of podocyte foot processes was associated with a reduction in the number of podocytes per glomerulus and an increase in the surface area covered by the remaining podocytes. In STZ diabetic rats, increased widening of foot processes, which is reversible by islet transplantation, tends to occur with increasing proteinuria.[105] Osterby et al.[91] also demonstrated peculiar glomerular epithelial injury in alloxan diabetic rats. An increase in the number of lysosomal-like structures was found, particularly in glomerular epithelial cells of long-term STZ diabetes in rats.[95] Some of these structures appeared as myelinlike bodies surrounded by an impressive accumulation of Golgi complexes and endoplasmic reticulum.[91] It remains to be elucidated whether these alterations in the glomerular epithelial cell may contribute to progression of diabetic glomerulosclerosis in the STZ diabetic rat.

3.3.6 Mechanisms of Renal Matrix Accumulation

Both increased synthesis and/or decreased degradation rates have been proposed to explain ECM accumulation in the diabetic kidney. Several studies have reported increased mRNA levels of ECM constituents in the kidney cortex or isolated glomeruli of STZ diabetic rats.[75,76] However, one study of severely hyperglycemic, noninsulin-treated rats did not show an increase in $\alpha1(IV)$ collagen mRNA after 28 weeks of the disease.[106] In fact, a progressive decline in $\alpha1(IV)$ collagen mRNA level was seen with age in both the diabetic and nondiabetic animals. Nevertheless, this study described a two-fold increase in laminin B1 mRNA in the diabetic kidney cortex.[106] On the other hand, the mRNA levels encoding $\alpha1(IV)$ collagen, fibronectin, laminin B1, and laminin B2 were found to be significantly increased in isolated glomeruli of STZ diabetic rats during approximately the same period of diabetes.[85] A variably increased level of fibronectin mRNA in the renal cortex of STZ diabetic rats has also been demonstrated.[107] Thus, in general, most (but not all) studies indicate that the diabetic state stimulates the synthesis of collagen Type IV and other ECM molecules (such as fibronectin and laminin) in the kidney cortex and in isolated glomeruli at a relatively early time during the course of experimental diabetes, an effect partly related to increased mRNA levels encoding these molecules.

Matrix glycoprotein degradation rates may be decreased in diabetic renal disease[108] and this may contribute to the increased matrix accumulation in advanced stages of the disease. *In vivo* studies of GBM from STZ diabetic rats have shown that the turnover rate is significantly diminished compared with control animals.[109-111] The activities of several cortical enzymes involved in collagen degradation are also diminished in diabetes.[112-114] Other studies have reported that glomeruli isolated from diabetic rats have decreased proteinase activity,[115] encompassing two general classes of proteolytic enzymes, the metalloproteinases and the cathepsins.[116] Insulin treatment normalizes cathepsin activity but further decreases metalloproteinase activity.[116]

3.4 Tubular Structural Changes

The tubulointerstitial compartment in patients with Type I diabetes mellitus is characterized by early hypertrophy of tubuloepithelial elements as well as thickening of tubular basement membranes.[72,117,118] Progressive tubulointerstitial fibrosis develops much later in the course of the disease in those patients who are destined to suffer clinically significant diabetic nephropathy.[74,117]

The tubular histopathology may vary in STZ-induced diabetes mellitus in animals of different genetic background. For example, Honjo et al. showed that although DBA/2N mice and CD-1 mice both manifest cortical distal tubular lesions after 4 and 12 weeks of diabetes,[119] the characteristics of these changes are different. While distal tubular cells of DBA/2N mice show characteristic PAS-positive inclusions, CD-1 mice develop epithelial cell deformation and luminal dilatation of their distal tubules, and the Armanni–Ebstein lesions (see below) are only rarely found.

3.4.1 Renal Hypertrophy

In STZ-induced experimental diabetes in the rat, renal hypertrophy may be detected as early as 1 day after the onset of diabetes and it can be seen regularly after 60 h of diabetes.[120] The first sign of kidney hypertrophy is an increase in total RNA content of kidney extracts after 1 day of diabetes.[120] Renal hypertrophy is paralleled by an increase in the protein content of the kidney. The kidney weight increases by 15 to 20% 3 days after STZ administration and by 70 to 90% after 6 weeks. Later, the renal weight gain gradually tapers off.[121] It is the tubuloepithelial enlargement that largely accounts for kidney hypertrophy or nephromegaly in STZ diabetic rats. Proximal tubules, the major constituent of the kidney, show maximal increase in epithelial cell height after 4 days of diabetes, but later they mostly grow by increasing their diameter and length.[121,122] In a somewhat contradictory manner, Mayhew et al.[123] found that STZ-induced diabetic rats not treated with insulin have normal tubular volume after 16 weeks of diabetes. In this experiment, the tubules of untreated diabetic animals were of larger diameter but of shorter length than those in control rats. It should be noted, however, that in this study, the tubule volume/body weight ratio was significantly higher than in nondiabetic or insulin-treated diabetic controls.[123] In addition to cell hypertrophy, Romen and Takashi[124] also showed cell proliferation in convoluted segments of proximal tubules from STZ diabetic male Sprague-Dawley rats 6 days after the onset of diabetes. In the study of Rasch,[122] histological examination by light and electron microscopy showed that the proximal tubular epithelial cells of STZ diabetic female Wistar rats are normal by appearance and that pathologically changed cells are present only in the distal tubules, especially in the cortex and the outer stripe of the outer medulla. These cells either appear empty or show PAS-positive glycogen granules in their cytoplasm with decreased number of lysosomes, endocytic vacuoles, and basal cell membrane infoldings.[122] In other studies, Tucker et al.[125] demonstrated a decrease in proximal tubular brush border height in STZ-induced diabetic Munich-Wistar rats 50 to 70 days after the initiation of diabetes, and Kaneda et al.[126] found proximal tubular mitochondrial enlargement in STZ diabetic male Sprague-Dawley rats after 2 weeks of diabetes.

Diabetic renal hypertrophy is a result of increased accumulation of structural proteins and possibly other substances. Kidney protein mass is significantly increased in diabetic renal hypertrophy. In addition to upregulated protein synthesis,[120] decreased breakdown of proteins may contribute to this phenomenon. Olbricht and Geissinger[127] demonstrated increased cathepsin B and L activities in proximal tubules of STZ diabetic Sprague-Dawley rats 4 to 10 days following induction of diabetes.[127] This increased cathepsin activity parallels the early hypertrophy of the kidney, and both changes can be prevented by insulin treatment.[127] After 6 months, when renal hypertrophy is complete, proximal tubular cathepsin activities become similar to control values.[127] Zador et al.,[128] on the other hand, demonstrated significant increases in kidney weight and abundance of glucosylceramide and ganglioside GM3 after 16 days from the initiation of diabetes in STZ diabetic male rats, suggesting a role for glycosphingolipid accumulation in kidney hypertrophy in these animals. In STZ diabetic mice, the authors' group[1] have reported that both glomerular and total-kidney hypertrophy were significantly reduced in diabetic mice treated with neutralizing antitransforming growth factor-β antibodies. This growth factor, therefore, is an important contributor to diabetic renal hypertrophy because it has been shown to lead to hypertrophy of glomerular mesangial and proximal tubular cells in culture and is itself also stimulated by high ambient glucose in these cell types.[16,129]

3.4.2 The Armanni–Ebstein Lesion

The characteristic PAS-positive glycogen accumulation in the cytoplasm of tubular cells develops after a few weeks of diabetes in STZ-induced diabetic animals.[121] The Armanni–Ebstein lesion was first described by Armanni[130] in 1877. He assumed that glycogen accumulation is primarily a feature of epithelial cells of the collecting duct. Ebstein[131] localized the lesion to the descending limb of Henle's loop.[131] In STZ diabetic female Wistar rats, Holck and Rasch[132] found that the predominant location of the Armanni–Ebstein lesion is in the thick ascending limb of Henle's loop, especially in the cortical area and the macula densa segment excluding the macula densa cells themselves. Glycogen accumulation is also observed in the distal convoluted tubule, cortical collecting duct, and the initial part of the descending thin limb of Henle's loop. In STZ diabetic male Wistar rats, Bleasel and Yong[133] found that the early tubular degeneration (swelling and vacuolation of epithelial cell cytoplasm) occurs predominantly in the distal tubule. These changes are due to accumulation of fluid and glycogen granules in the cytoplasm. The investigators of this study point out that these changes represent a distinct difference compared with human diabetes where the proximal tubules are affected primarily and the accumulating material is lipid.[133] Interestingly, Reyes et al.[134] found that high cholesterol feeding in STZ diabetic female Sprague-Dawley rats prevents the development of the Armanni–Ebstein lesions, despite the presence of uncontrolled diabetes.

3.4.3 Tubular Basement Membrane Thickening

The structural abnormalities of the tubular basement membrane in diabetes may be conveniently divided into two stages. In the early phase of the disease, there appears to be an acute increase in membrane mass, which accompanies the development of renal hypertrophy without discernible abnormalities in morphology; this is followed by conspicuous thickening, which does not become apparent until several weeks have elapsed. Tubular (as well as glomerular) basement membrane thickening is a discrete structural feature of STZ-induced diabetic kidney disease.[83] These changes may be brought about by altered synthesis of key components of basement membranes. In the experiments of Poulsom et al.,[106] homogenized kidney tissue from STZ-induced diabetic male CDF rats showed a twofold increase in the mRNA levels encoding the B1 chain of laminin between 11 and 28 weeks of diabetes. This increase was not preventable by treatment with an aldose reductase inhibitor. In STZ-induced diabetic C57BL/6J mice, Rohrbach et al.[135] found that while total kidney laminin content was only slightly elevated, the level of the basement membrane–specific HSPG was only 20% of control. This significant decrease may underlie the increased porosity of basement membranes in diabetic kidney disease. Type IV collagen is another normal component of tubular and glomerular basement membranes. In the study by Ihm et al.,[136] 7 days after STZ injection in male Sprague-Dawley rats, renal proximal tubules of the deep cortex and the outer stripe of the medulla showed significantly upregulated collagen α1(IV) mRNA levels. This change occurred earlier than in the glomeruli, and it was ameliorated by insulin administration. Furthermore, Desjardins et al.[93] demonstrated increased α1(IV), α2(IV), and α3(IV) levels in the tubular basement membranes (as well as in GBM and Bowman's capsule) of STZ-induced diabetic male Sprague-Dawley rats. In STZ diabetic mice, the authors[1] have recently reported increased kidney mRNA levels for fibronectin and α1(IV) collagen after 6 to 9 days of induction of diabetes.

In addition to increased synthesis of collagen, there is evidence for decreased degradation of collagen in STZ diabetic animals.[108,137] Collagenolytic activity of kidney extracts from STZ diabetic rats is significantly lower than in control animals, and there is a negative correlation with blood glucose levels.[113] The activities of several renal cortical enzymes involved in collagen degradation are diminished in diabetes.[110,112,114] It is not clear if excess nonenzymatic glycation of collagenase is the key phenomenon behind this finding.

3.4.4 Tubulointerstitial Fibrosis

Fibrosis is a late structural change in STZ-induced diabetic nephropathy.[74,138] Although Weil et al.[83] did not describe tubulointerstitial fibrosis in STZ diabetic male Lewis rats after 12 months of diabetes, Zatz et al.[51] observed focal tubular atrophy with nonspecific round cell infiltration and fibrosis of the interstitium of untreated STZ diabetic male Munich-Wistar rats after 14 months of diabetes. Animals treated with enalapril in this study had only minor changes in the tubulointerstitial compartment.[51] Trachtman et al.[139] conducted a long-term (1-year) study in STZ diabetic male Sprague-Dawley rats examining the effect of antioxidant therapy on diabetic nephropathy. Besides its beneficial effects on proteinuria, glomerular hypertrophy, and glomerulosclerosis, taurine supplementation was reported to significantly decrease the development of tubulointerstitial fibrosis.[139]

The authors[74] have investigated the long-term changes in the renal interstitium in diabetes and have discovered tubulointerstitial changes that occur after 6 to 9 months of sustained hyperglycemia in STZ diabetic rats. By assaying for the presence of interstitial fibrosis, tubular cell atrophy, interstitial inflammatory infiltrates, or tubular dilation, it was found that 11 of 14 long-term diabetic rats demonstrated mild interstitial lesions whereas only 3 of 16 age-matched control animals on a normal diet manifested similar changes. Thus, it appears that tubular interstitial changes seen in patients with diabetes have their experimental counterpart in rats rendered diabetic with STZ.

3.5   Structural–Functional Correlates

Glomerular hypertrophy and the increased surface area available for filtration correlate with the early characteristic feature of glomerular hyperfiltration.[71,140] It remains intriguing that the increased thickness of the GBM[100,141] is actually associated with increased permeability of this membrane to macromolecules.[98] The latter phenomenon has been partly explained by decreased density of HSPG in the GBM.[97,98,135,142]

Progressive expansion of the glomerular mesangial matrix resulting in diffuse intercapillary sclerosis is the most important structural lesion of diabetic glomerulopathy in humans.[80] This lesion is also considered the most important for the development of chronic renal failure in the diabetic population. In fact, the degree of expansion of mesangial matrix in patients with Type I diabetes mellitus correlates closely with the progressive decline in the glomerular capillary surface area available for filtration and, hence, with the magnitude of the reduction in GFR.[70,71]

It is widely held that the characteristic glomerular lesion of diabetic nephropathy, in particular the expansion of the mesangial matrix, is a primary abnormality arising in the glomerulus and is largely responsible for the expression of the functional derangements that characterize the stage of overt dysfunction, namely, frank proteinuria, hypertension, and renal failure. However, progressive tubulointerstitial fibrosis and renal arteriosclerosis, less widely recognized lesions, are also important components of diabetic nephropathy, because they give rise to important alterations in tubular as well as glomerular function and because they often contribute significantly to the development of ischemic or obliterative, global glomerulosclerosis and thus to the marked reduction in GFR.[74,117,143] In fact, the degree of tubulointerstitial fibrosis in diabetic nephropathy in humans closely correlates with the magnitude of mesangial matrix expansion[70,74,117] and with the decline in GFR.[144] Thus, as with many different renal glomerular diseases, the severity of the accompanying tubular atrophy and interstitial fibrosis is an excellent predictor of impaired kidney function, measured principally as a reduction in GFR.[144]

Although structural changes in the tubules (including the Armanni–Ebstein lesions) have been localized mostly to the distal tubules of STZ-induced diabetic animals, structural–functional correlates of diabetic kidney disease are predominantly examined with regard to the proximal tubules. Tucker et al.[125] demonstrated a decrease in proximal tubular brush border height in STZ-induced diabetes in Munich-Wistar rats after 50 to 70 days from the initiation of diabetes. This morphological change appears concomitant with decreased proximal tubular albumin reabsorptive capacity and correlates with the appearance of microalbuminuria.[125] In STZ diabetic male Sprague-Dawley rats, Kaneda et al.[126] found a positive correlation between proximal tubular mitochondrial enlargement and microalbuminuria after 2 weeks of diabetes. They hypothesized that mitochondrial enlargement may lead to disturbed ATP metabolism and reduced active transport in proximal tubules and that this may have a role in the development of proteinuria.[126] Increased tubular Na^+,K^+-ATPase activity may also have an important role in kidney hypertrophy. Ku and Meezan[145] found that 5 to 7 weeks after STZ injection, tubules from Sprague-Dawley rats showed significantly increased Na^+,K^+-ATPase activity.[145] A similar increase in pump activity was not observed in the glomeruli of these animals.[145] The upregulation of Na^+,K^+-ATPase activity occurred after 4 days of diabetes in the outer medullary portion and after 7 days in the cortical regions of the kidney.[145] This phenomenon roughly coincides with the development of renal hypertrophy as measured by increases in kidney weight and kidney protein to DNA ratios.[146] Furthermore, with insulin treatment, both kidney hypertrophy and elevated Na^+,K^+-ATPase activity returned to control values.[147] In addition, Wald et al.[148] showed that Na^+,K^+-ATPase activity is increased along most of the nephron by 8 days of diabetes in STZ diabetic rats. The upregulation of the Na^+,K^+-ATPase was observed in the cortical and medullary thick ascending limbs of Henle's loop and in the distal convoluted tubule as early as 24 h after initiation of diabetes.[148]

An interesting yet unresolved puzzle is why STZ diabetic rats are resistant to gentamicin-induced renal injury.[149] After the administration of toxic doses of gentamicin, there is significantly decreased accumulation of the drug in the kidney cortex of STZ-induced diabetes in rats as compared with nondiabetic controls.[149] This phenomenon may be due to decreased expression of gp330 in the brush border membrane,[150] which likely acts as a receptor for gentamicin.

3.6   The Role of Hyperglycemia and Its Mediators

3.6.1   Effects of Hyperglycemia

Chronic hyperglycemia is likely responsible for almost all the glomerular and tubulointerstitial structural changes in diabetic nephropathy. This has been demonstrated by instituting tight glycemic control in STZ-induced diabetic animals either by insulin administration or pancreatic islet cell transplantation. For example, Cortes et al.[151] have shown that insulin prevents the augmented incorporation of orotate into RNA in the kidney cortex of diabetic rats. However, Seyer-Hansen[120] found that when insulin treatment is started after many weeks of diabetes there is no significant improvement in renal weight or RNA or DNA content in the kidneys of STZ diabetic rats. This was speculated to be likely due to the fact that strict glucose control is difficult to achieve by conventional insulin therapy in these animals.[120] When sufficient insulin therapy is started in STZ diabetic rats early enough (at day 2 following induction of diabetes), renal hypertrophy at day 10 can be completely prevented.[127] In other studies, insulin treatment prevents the increase in collagen $\alpha 1(IV)$ mRNA levels,[136] Na^+,K^+-ATPase activity,[147] and cathepsin B and L activities.[127] Insulin therapy can reverse the decrease in basement membrane HSPG synthesis[135] and the reduced AII receptor expression.[152] Such studies highlight the importance of hyperglycemia in the pathogenesis of the functional and structural alterations of the diabetic state in the kidney, but they do not rule out an independent, direct effect of insulin therapy in reversing these changes.

Rasch and Gotzsche[153] examined the effect of pancreatic islet transplantation on kidney hypertrophy and the Armanni–Ebstein lesion in STZ diabetic Lewis female rats. Animals were left diabetic for 4 weeks then transplanted with pancreatic islets. After 4 weeks, from islet cell transplantation, there were no glycogen-containing cells in the distal tubules of these animals, while in nontransplanted diabetic controls almost half of the distal tubular cells displayed the Armanni–Ebstein lesion. Although islet cell transplantation did not change the distal tubular length, it achieved partial normalization of kidney weight.[153] In a similar experiment by Gotzsche et al.,[154] pancreatic islet transplantation significantly decreased kidney weight and normalized renal RNA/DNA ratio in STZ diabetic animals.

3.6.2   Mediators of Hyperglycemia

High glucose may exert its deleterious effects by numerous pathways (Figure 3.1).[155] These include oxidative stress,[139,156] nonenzymatic glycation of proteins through early (Amadori)[157] and advanced reactions,[158,159] activation of the aldose reductase–dependent polyol pathway,[56,57,160] stimulation of protein kinase C activity,[65,76] as well as the increased activity of local growth factors such as AII and transforming growth factor-β.[1,152,161]

The salutary effects of taurine treatment are likely related to the demonstrated reduction in oxidative stress in the kidneys of these animals.[139] In contrast, it is very uncertain why in this study there was an unexpected deleterious effect of vitamin E supplementation (given as a mixture in the diet) on diabetic nephropathy.[139]

Mitsuhashi et al.[158] demonstrated by ELISA a 16-fold increase in advanced glycation end products (AGE) in the renal cortex of STZ diabetic male Wistar rats after 5 weeks of diabetes; after 20 weeks, AGE content of the kidney cortex was 45 times higher than that

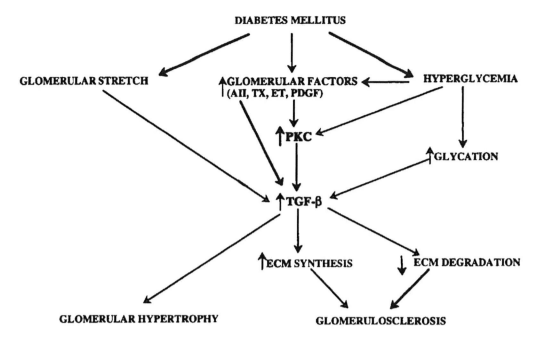

FIGURE 3.1

A working hypothesis emphasizing the central role of PKC activation and TGF-β overproduction in mediating glomerular hypertrophy and glomerulosclerosis in diabetic nephropathy. Note the convergence of several features of diabetes mellitus (hyperglycemia, enhanced production of glomerular vasoactive agents and growth factors, increased glycation of proteins, increased glomerular stretch) toward activation of the renal TGF-β system (TGF-β: transforming growth factor-β; PKC: protein kinase C; AII: angiotensin II; TX: thromboxane; ET: endothelin; PDGF: platelet-derived growth factor; ECM: extracellular matrix). (From Sharma, K., and Ziyadeh, F. N., *Semin. Nephrol.* 17, 80-92, 1997. Reprinted with permission from the publishers, W.B. Saunders Company, Philadelphia.)

of control rats. The increase in AGE content was less then 1.5-fold with fluorescence measurements.[158] Albuminuria, mesangial expansion, and tissue fluorescence in STZ diabetic rats are significantly retarded by administration of aminoguanidine (to reduce formation of AGE).[162] Treatment with aminoguanidine also ameliorates the GBM thickening observed in the diabetic rat.[163]

Sharma et al.[1] used high-dose STZ (200 mg/kg body weight intraperitoneally; two daily consecutive doses) to induce diabetes in mice. The mRNA expression of transforming growth factor-β1 as well as the Type II transforming growth factor-β receptor in the renal cortex of STZ-induced diabetic mice were increased as early as 3 days after the onset of diabetes, and these changes were associated with increased urinary levels of total (active plus latent) transforming growth factor-β1.[1] These changes also coincided with the appearance of kidney hypertrophy. Furthermore, α1(IV) collagen and fibronectin mRNA levels were also significantly increased after 9 days of diabetes. Of importance, this study demonstrated that treatment with a neutralizing monoclonal antibody against transforming growth factor-β prevented glomerular hypertrophy and reduced the increment in renal weight by approximately 50% without having any effect on the blood glucose concentration.[1] The increases in the mRNAs encoding transforming growth factor-β1, α1(IV) collagen and fibronectin were also significantly attenuated by treatment with the neutralizing transforming growth factor-β antibody. These results strongly suggest that upregulation of transforming growth factor-β and its Type II receptor may play an important role in kidney hypertrophy in STZ-induced diabetic animals.[1]

3.7   Concluding Remarks

The STZ diabetic rat has proved to be a very useful model to evaluate many of the hemodynamic and structural alterations induced by insulin-dependent diabetes mellitus on the kidney. This model has provided data that have clearly led to distinct improvements in the approach to treatment of patients principally based on the hemodynamic theory of diabetic kidney disease. However, since this model does not exactly reproduce the structural hallmark of diabetic nephropathy, namely, diffuse and/or nodular glomerulosclerosis, it remains to be established whether nonhemodynamic treatment strategies, which have been tried in this model to alter the pathological manifestations of diabetic kidney disease, will be as readily applicable to human diabetic nephropathy.

Acknowledgments

Supported in part by the National Kidney Foundation — Young Investigator Grant (K.S.), a KO8 grant DK02308 from the National Institutes of Health (K.S.), a fellowship grant from the Juvenile Diabetes Foundation International (A.M.), National Institutes of Health grants (DK-44513 and DK-45191 to F.N.Z., and training grant DK-07006), and the DCI-RED Fund. Dr. D. C. Han is visiting scholar at the University of Pennsylvania; he is supported by the Hyonam Kidney Laboratory, Soon Chun Hyang University, Seoul, Korea.

References

1. Sharma, K., Jin, Y., Guo, J., Ziyadeh, F. N., Neutralization of TGF-beta by anti-TGF-beta antibody attenuates kidney hypertrophy and enhanced extracellular matrix gene expression in streptozotocin-diabetic mice. *Diabetes*, 45, 522-530, 1996.
2. Anderson, S., Rennke, H. G., Garcia, D. L., Brenner, B. M., Short and long term effects of antihypertensive theraphy in the diabetic rat. *Kidney Int*, 36, 526-536, 1989.
3. Kusaka, M., Kishi, K., Sokabe, H., Does so-called streptozotocin hypertension exist in rats? *Hypertension*, 10, 517-521, 1987.
4. Pfaffman, M., Ball, C., Darby, A., Hilman, R., Insulin reversal of diabetes-induced inhibition of vascular contractility in the rat. *Am J Physiol*, 242, H490-H495, 1982.
5. Corbett, J. A., Tilton, R. G., Chang, K., Hasan, K. S., Ido, Y., Wang, J. L., Sweetland, M. A., Lancaster, J. R., Jr., Williamson, J. R., McDaniel, M. L., Aminoguanidine, a novel inhibitor of nitric oxide formation, prevents diabetic vascular dysfunction. *Diabetes*, 41, 552-556, 1992.
6. Tilton, R., Chang, K., Hasan, K., Smith, S., Petrash, J., Misko, T., Moore, W., Currie, M., Corbett, J., McDaniel, M. E. A., Prevention of diabetic vascular dysfunction by guanidines. Inhibition of nitric oxide synthase vs. advanced glycation end-product formation. *Diabetes*, 42, 221-232, 1993.
7. Gauthier, T., Scalia, R., Murohara, T., Guo, J., Lefer, A., Nitric oxide protects against leukocyte-endothelium interactions in the early stages of hypercholesterolemia. *Arterioscler Thromb Vasc Biol*, 15, 1652-1659, 1995.
8. Biffl, W., Moore, E., Moore, F., Barnett, C., Nitric oxide reduces endothelial expression of intercellular adhesion molecule (ICAM)-1. *J Surg Res*, 63, 328-332, 1996.

9. Khan, B., Harrison, D., Olbrych, M., Alexander, R., Medford, R., Nitric oxide regulates vascular cell adhesion molecule 1 gene expression and redox-sensitive transcriptional events in human vascular endothelial cells. *Proc Natl Acad Sci U.S.A.*, 93, 9114-9119, 1996.

10. Hostetter, T., Troy, J., Brenner, B., Glomerular hemodynamics in experimental diabetes mellitus. *Kidney Int*, 19, 410-415, 1981.

11. Jensen, P., Steven, K., Blaehr, H., Chriastiansen, J., Parving, H.-H., Effects of indomethacin on glomerular hemodynamics in experimental diabetes. *Kidney Int*, 29, 490-495, 1986.

12. Hostetter, T., Rennke, H., Brenner, B., The case for intrarenal hypertension in the initiation and progression of diabetic and other gomerulopathies. *Am J Med*, 72, 375-380, 1982.

13. Zatz, R., Meyer, T. W., Rennke, H. G., Brenner, B. M., Predominance of hemodynamic rather than metabolic factors in the pathogenesis of diabetic glomerulopathy. *Proc Natl Acad Sci U.S.A.*, 82, 5963-5967, 1985.

14. Zatz, R., Brenner, B., Pathogenesis of diabetic microangiopathy: The hemodynamic view. *Am J Med*, 80, 443-453, 1986.

15. Sharma, K., Ziyadeh, F. N., Hyperglycemia and diabetic kidney disease. The case for transforming growth factor-β as a key mediator. *Diabetes*, 44, 1139-1146, 1995.

16. Wolf, G., Sharma, K., Chen, Y., Ericksen, M., Ziyadeh, F. N., High glucose-induced proliferation in mesangial cells is reversed by autocrine TGF-β. *Kidney Int*, 42, 647-656, 1992.

17. Ziyadeh, F. N., Sharma, K., Ericksen, M., Wolf, G., Stimulation of collagen gene expression and protein synthesis in murine mesangial cells by high glucose is mediated by activation of transforming growth factor-β. *J Clin Invest*, 93, 536-542, 1994.

18. Riser, B. L., Cortes, P., Heilig, C., Grondin, J., Ladsonwofford, S., Patterson, D., Narins, R. G., Cyclic stretching force selectively upregulates transforming growth factor-β isoforms in cultured rat mesangial cells. *Am J Pathol*, 148, 1915-1923, 1996.

19. Ortola, F., Ballermann, B., Anderson, S., Mendez, R., Brenner, B., Elevated plasma atrial natriuretic peptide levels in diabetic rats, potential mediator of hyperfiltration. *J Clin Invest*, 80, 670-674, 1987.

20. Shin, S.-J., Lee, Y.-J., Tan, M.-S., Hsieh, T.-J., Tsai, J.-H., Increased atrial natriuretic peptide mRNA expression in the kidney of diabetic rats. *Kidney Int*, 51, 1100-1105, 1997.

21. Zhang, P., Mackenzie, H., Troy, J., Brenner, B., Effects of an atrial natriuretic peptide recceptor antagonist on glomerular hyperfiltration in diabetic rats. *J Am Soc Nephrol*, 4, 1564-1570, 1994.

22. Kasiske, B., O'Donnell, M., Keane, W., Glucose-induced increases in renal hemodynamic function: possible modulation by renal prostaglandins. *Diabetes*, 34, 360-364, 1985.

23. Kreisberg, J., Patel, P., The effects of insulin, glucose and diabetes on prostaglandin production by rat kidney glomeruli and cultured glomerular mesangial cells. *Prostaglandins Leukotrienes Med*, 11, 431-442, 1983.

24. Schambelan, M., Blake, S., Sraer, J., Increased prostaglandin production by glomeruli isolated from rats with streptozotocin-induced diabetes mellitus. *J Clin Invest*, 75, 404-412, 1985.

25. Deng, A., Baylis, C., Locally produced EDRF controls preglomerular resistance and ultrafiltration. *Am J Physiol*, 264, F212-215, 1993.

26. Bank, N., Aynedjian, H. S., Role of EDRF (nitric oxide) in diabetic renal hyperfiltration. *Kidney Int*, 43, 1306-1312, 1993.

27. Tolins, J., Shultz, P., Raij, L., Brown, D., Mauer, S., Abnormal renal hemodynamic response to reduced renal perfusion pressure in diabetic rats: role of NO. *Am J Physiol*, 265, F886-895, 1993.

28. Craven, P. A., Studer, R. K., DeRubertis, F. R., Impaired nitric oxide-dependent cyclic guanosine monophosphate generation in glomeruli from diabetic rats. *J. Clin Invest*, 93, 311-320, 1994.

29. Anderson, S., Jung, F., Ingelfinger, J., Renal renin–angiotensin system in diabetes: functional, immunohistochemical, and molecular biological correlations. *Am J Physiol*, 265, F477-486, 1993.

30. Inman, S., Porter, J., Fleming, J., Reduced renal microvascular reactivity to angiotensin II in diabetic rats. *Microcirculation*, 1, 137-145, 1994.

31. Wolf, G., Ziyadeh, F. N., The role of angiotensin II in diabetic nephropathy: Emphasis on nonhemodynamic mechanisms. *Am J Kidney Dis*, 29, 153-163, 1997.

32. Ballermann, B. J., Skorecki, K. L., Brenner, B. M., Reduced glomerular angiotensin II receptor density in early untreated diabetes mellitus in the rat. *Am J Physiol*, 247, F110-F116, 1984.

33. Wilkes, B., Reduced glomerular angiotensin II receptor density in diabetes mellitus in the rat: time course and mechanisms. *Endocrinology,* 120, 1291-1298, 1987.

34. Kikkawa, R., Kitamura, E., Fujiwara, Y., Arimura, T., Haneda, M., Y., S., Impaired contractile responsiveness of diabetic glomeruli to angiotensin II: a possible indication of mesangial dysfunction in diabetes mellitus. *Biochem Biophys Res Commun,* 136, 1185-1190, 1986.

35. Barnett, R., Scharschmidt, L., Ko, Y., Schlondorff, D., Comparison of glomerular and mesangial prostaglandin synthesis and glomerular contraction in two rat models of diabetes mellitus. *Diabetes,* 36, 1468-1475, 1987.

36. Kreisberg, J., Insulin requirement for contraction of cultured rat glomerular mesangial cells in response to angiotensin II: possible role for insulin in modulating glomerular hemodynamics. *Proc Natl Acad Sci U.S.A.,* 79, 4190-4192, 1982.

37. Mene, P., Pugliese, G., Pricci, F., DiMario, U., Cinotti, G. A., Pugliese, F., High glucose inhibits cytosolic calcium signaling in cultured rat mesangial cells. *Kidney Int,* 43, 585-591, 1993.

38. Zhu, Z., Arendshorst, W., Angiotensin II-receptor stimulation of cytosolic calcium concentration in cultured renal resistance arterioles. *Am J Physiol,* 271, F1239-F1247, 1996.

39. Correa-Rotter, R., Hostetter, T., Rosenberg, M., Renin and angiotensin gene expression in experimental diabetes mellitus. *Kidney Int,* 41, 796-804, 1992.

40. Kalinyak, J., Sechi, L., Griffin, C., Don, B., Tavangar, K., Kraemer, F., Hoffman, A., Schambelan, M., The renin–angiotensin system in streptozotocin-induced diabetes mellitus in the rat. *J Am Soc Nephrol,* 4, 1337-1345, 1993.

41. Jaffa, A., Chai, K., Cao, J., Chao, L., Mayfield, R., Effects of diabetes and insulin on expression of kallikrein and renin genes in the kidney. *Kidney Int,* 41, 789-795, 1992.

42. Kennefick, T., Oyama, T., Thompson, M., Vora, J., Anderson, S., Enhanced renal sensitivity to angiotensin actions in diabetes mellitus in the rat. *Am J Physiol,* 271, F595-F602, 1996.

43. Velasquez, M. T., Kimmel, P. L., Michaelis, O. E., Animal models of spontaneous diabetic kidney disease. *FASEB J,* 4, 2850-2859, 1990.

44. Everett, A., Scott, J., Wilfong, N., Marion, B., Rosenkranz, R., Inagami, T., Gomez, R., Renin and angiotensinogen expression during the evolution of diabetes. *Hypertension,* 19, 70-78, 1992.

45. Harker, C., O'Donnell, M., Kasiske, B., Keane, W., Katz, S., The renin–angiotensin system in the Type II diabetic obese zucker rat. *J Am Soc Nephrol,* 4, 1354-1361, 1993.

46. Rosenberg, M., Smith, L., Correa-Rotter, R., Hostetter, T., The paradox of the renin–angiotensin system in chronic renal disease. *Kidney Int,* 45, 403-410, 1994.

47. Steffes, M., Brown, D., Mauer, S., Diabetic glomerulopathy following unilateral nephrectomy in the rat. *Diabetes,* 27, 35-41, 1978.

48. Cooper, M., Macmillan, A., Bach, L., Jerums, G., Doyle, A., Genetic hypertension accelerates nephropathy in the streptozotocin diabetic rat. *Am J Hypertension,* 1, 5-10, 1988.

49. Cooper, M., Allen, T., O'Brien, R., Papazoglou, D., Clarke, B., Jerums, G., Doyle, A., Nephropathy in model combining genetic hypertension with experimental diabetes. *Diabetes,* 39, 1575-1579, 1990.

50. Cooper, M., Rumble, J., Allen, T., O'Brien, R., Jerums, G., Doyle, A., Antihypertensive therapy in a model combining spontaneous hypertension with diabetes. *Kidney Int,* 41, 898-903, 1992.

51. Zatz, R., Dunn, B. R., Meyer, T. W., Anderson, S., Rennke, H. G., Brenner, B. M., Prevention of diabetic glomerulopathy by pharmacological amelioration of glomerular capillary hypertension. *J Clin Invest,* 77, 1925-1930, 1986.

52. Anderson, S., Rennke, H., Brenner, B., Zayas, M., Lafferty, H., Troy, J., Sandstorm, D., Nifedipine vs. fosinopril in uninephrectomized diabetic rats. *Kidney Int,* 41, 891-897, 1992.

53. Barthelmebs, M., Vailly, B., Velly, J., Grima, M., Imbs, J.-L., L-Dopa and streptozotocin-induced diabetic nephropathy in rats. *Am J Hypertension,* 3, 72S-74S, 1990.

54. Barthelmebs, M., Vailly, B., Grima, M., Velly, J., Stephan, D., Froehly, S., Imbs, J.-L., Effects of dopamine prodrugs and fenoldopam on glomerular hyperfiltration in streptozotocin-induced diabetes in rats. *J Cardiovasc Pharmacol,* 18, 243-253, 1991.

55. Nakamura, T., Ebihara, I., Fukui, M., Tomino, Y., Koide, H., Effect of a specific endothelin receptor A antagonist on mRNA levels for extracellular matrix components and growth factors in diabetic glomeruli. *Diabetes,* 44, 895-899, 1995.

56. Goldfarb, S., Ziyadeh, F. N., Kern, E. F. O., Simmons, D. A., Effects of polyol-pathway inhibition and dietary *myo*-inositol on glomerular hemodynamic function in experimental diabetes mellitus in rats. *Diabetes*, 40, 465–471, 1991.
57. Ghahary, A., Luo, J., Gong, Y., Chakrabarti, S., Sima, A. F. A., Murphy, L. J., Increased renal aldose reductase activity, immunoreactivity, and mRNA in streptozotocin-induced diabetic rats. *Diabetes*, 38, 1067-1071, 1989.
58. Xia, P., Inoguchi, T., Kern, T. S., Engerman, R. L., Oates, P. J., King, G. L., Characterization of the mechanism for the chronic activation of diacylglycerol-protein kinase C pathway in diabetes and hyperglycemia. *Diabetes*, 43, 1122-1129, 1994.
59. Kikkawa, R., Haneda, M., Uzu, T., Togawa, M., Koya, D., Kajiwara, N., Shigeta, Y., Translocation of protein kinase Cα and ζ in rat glomerular mesangial cells cultured under high glucose conditions. *Diabetologia*, 37, 838-841, 1994.
60. Williams, B., Schrier, R. W., Glucose-induced protein kinase C activity regulated arachidonic acid release and eicosanoid production by cultured glomerular mesangial cells. *J Clin Invest*, 92, 2889-2896, 1993.
61. Ayo, S. H., Radnik, R. A., Glass, W. F., II, Garoni, J. A., Rampt, E. R., Appling, D. R., Kreisberg, J. I., Increased extracellular matrix synthesis and mRNA in mesangial cells grown in high-glucose medium. *Am J Physiol*, 260, F185-F191, 1991.
62. Fumo, P., Kuncio, G. S., Ziyadeh, F. N., PKC and high glucose stimulate collagen alpha1(IV) transcriptional activity in a reporter mesangial cell line. *Am J Physiol*, 267, F632-F638, 1994.
63. Craven, P. A., Davidson, C. M., DeRubertis, F. R., Increase in diacylglycerol mass in isolated glomeruli by glucose from *de novo* synthesis of glycerolipids. *Diabetes*, 39, 667-674, 1990.
64. Ayo, S. H., Radnik, R., Garoni, J. A., Kreisberg, J., High glucose increases diacylglycerol mass and activates protein kinases C in mesangial cell culture. *Am J Physiol*, 261, F571-F577, 1991.
65. Ishii, H., Jirouesk, M. R., Koya, D., Takagi, C., Xia, P., Clermont, A., Bursell, S.-E., Kern, T. S., Ballas, L. M., Heath, W. F., Stramm, L. E., Feener, E. P., King, G. L., Amelioration of vascular dysfunctions in diabetic rats by an oral PKC β inhibitor. *Science*, 272, 728-731, 1996.
66. Lewis, E. J., Hunsicker, L. G., Bain, R. P., Rohde, R. D., The effect of angiotensin-converting-enzyme inhibition on diabetic nephropathy. *N Engl. J. Med*, 329, 1456-1462, 1993.
67. O'Donnel, M. P., Kaseske, B. L., Keane, W. F., Glomerular hemodynamic and structural alterations in experimental diabetes mellitus. *FASEB J*, 2, 2339-2347, 1988.
68. Fabris, B., Jackson, B., Johnston, C., Salt blocks the renal benefits of ramipril in diabetic hypertensive rats. *Hypertension*, 17, 497-503, 1991.
69. Bakris, G., Smith, A., Effects of sodium intake on albumin excretion in patients with diabetic nephropathy treated with long-acting calcium antagonists. *Ann Intern Med.* 125(3): 201-204, 1996.
70. Mauer, S. M., Steffes, M. W., Ellis, E. N., Sutherland, D. E. R., Brown, D. M., Goetz, F. C., Structural-functional relationships in diabetic nephropathy. *J Clin Invest*, 74, 1143-1155, 1984.
71. Osterby, R., Parving, H., Nyberg, G., Jorgensen, H., Lokkegaard, H., Svalander, C., A strong correlation between glomerular filtration rate and filtration surface in diabetic nephropathy. *Diabetologia*, 31, 265-270, 1988.
72. Steffes, M. W., Bilous, R. W., Sutherland, D. E. R., Mauer, S. M., Cell and matrix components of the glomerular mesangium in Type I diabetes mellitus. *Diabetes*, 41, 679-684, 1992.
73. Ziyadeh, F. N., Goldfarb, S., Kern, E. F. O. Diabetic nephropathy: Metabolic and biochemical mechanisms, in *The Kidney in Diabetes*, B. M. Brenner and J. H. Stein, Eds., Churchill Livingstone, New York, 1989, 87-113.
74. Ziyadeh, F. N., Goldfarb, S., The renal tubulointerstitium in diabetes mellitus. *Kidney Int*, 39, 464-475, 1991.
75. Ziyadeh, F. N., The extracellular matrix in diabetic nephropathy. *Am J Kidney Dis*, 22, 736-744, 1993.
76. Ziyadeh, F. N., Mediators of hyperglycemia and the pathogenesis of matrix accumulation in diabetic renal disease. *Miner Electrolyte Metab*, 21, 292-302, 1995.
77. Rasch, R., Prevention of diabetic glomerulopathy in streptozotocin diabetic rats by insulin treatment. Kidney size and glomerular volume. *Diabetologia*, 16, 125-128, 1979.

78. Hirose, K., Osterby, R., Nozawa, M., Gundersen, H. J. G., Development of glomerular lesions in experimental long-term diabetes in the rat. *Kidney Int*, 21, 689-695, 1982.

79. Steffes, M. W., Brown, D. M., Basgen, J. M., Mauer, S. M., Amelioration of mesangial volume and surface alterations following islet transplantation in diabetic rats. *Diabetes*, 29, 509-515, 1980.

80. Steffes, M. W., Osterby, R., Chavers, B., Mauer, S. M., Mesangial expansion as a central mechanism for loss of kidney function in diabetic patients. *Diabetes*, 38, 1077-1081, 1989.

81. Mauer, S. M., Michael, A. F., Fish, A. J., Brown, D. M., Spontaneous imunoglobulin and complement deposition in glomeruli of diabetic rats. *Lab Invest*, 27, 488-494, 1972.

82. Lamson, B. G., Billings, M. S., Ewell, L. H., Bennett, L. R., Late effects of total-body roentgen irradiation. IV. Hypertension and nephrosclerosis in female Wistar rats surviving 1000r hypoxic total-body irradiation. *Arch Pathol*, 66, 322, 1958.

83. Weil, R., Nozawa, M., Koss, M., Reemtsma, K., McIntosh, R., The kidney in streptozotocin diabetic rats. Morphologic, ultrastructural, and function studies. *Arch Pathol Lab Med*, 100, 37-49, 1976.

84. Mauer, S. M., Steffes, M. W., Chern, M., Brown, D. M., Mesangial uptake and processing of macromolecules in rats with diabetes mellitus. *Lab Invest*, 41, 401, 1979.

85. Fukui, M., Nakamura, T., Ebihara, I., Shirato, I., Tomino, Y., Koide, H., ECM gene expression and its modulation by insulin in diabetic rats. *Diabetes*, 41, 1520-1527, 1992.

86. Yamamoto, T., Nakamura, T., Noble, N. A., Ruoslahti, E., Border, W. A., Expression of transforming growth factor beta is elevated in human and experimental diabetic nephropathy. *Proc Natl Acad Sci U.S.A.*, 90, 1814-1818, 1993.

87. Abrass, C. K., Peterson, C. V., Raugi, G. S., Phenotypic expression of collagen types in mesangial matrix of diabetic and nondiabetic rats. *Diabetes*, 37, 1695-1702, 1988.

88. Scheinman, J., Steffes, M. W., Brown, D. M., Mauer, S. M., The immunohistopathology of glomerular antigen. III. Increased mesangial actomyosin in experimental diabetes in the rat. *Diabetes*, 27, 632-637, 1978.

89. Young, B. A., Johnson, R. J., Alpers, C. E., Eng, E., Gordon, K., Floege, J., Couser, W. G., Cellular events in the evolution of experimental diabetic nephropathy. *Kidney Int*, 47, 935-944, 1995.

90. Makino, H., Kashihara, N., Sugiyama, H., Kanao, K., Sekikawa, T., Okamoto, K., Maeshima, Y., Ota, Z., Nagai, R., Phenotypic modulation of the mesangium reflected by contractile proteins in diabetes. *Diabetes*, 45, 488-495, 1996.

91. Osterby, R., Lundbaek, K., Olsen, T. S., Orskov, H., Kidney lesions in rats with severe long term alloxan diabetes. *Lab Invest*, 17, 675-692, 1967.

92. Brees, D. K., Hutchison, F. N., Cole, G. J., Williams, J. C., Differential effects of diabetes and glomerulonephritis on glomerular basement membrane composition. *Proc Soc Exp Biol Med*, 212, 69-77, 1996.

93. Desjardins, M., Gros, F., Wieslander, J., Gubler, M. C., Bendayan, M., Immunogold studies of monomeric elements from the globular domain (NC1) of Type IV collagen in renal basement membranes during experimental diabetes in the rat. *Diabetologia*, 33, 661-670, 1990.

94. Kim, Y., Kleppel, M. M., Butkowski, R., Mauer, S. M., Wieslander, J., Michael, A. F., Differential expression of basement membrane collagen chains in diabetic nephropathy. *Am J Pathol*, 138, 413-420, 1991.

95. Bendayan, M., Gingra, D., Charest, P., Distribution of endogenous albumin in the glomerular wall of streptozotocin-induced diabetic rats as revealed by high-resolution immunocytochemistry. *Diabetologia*, 29, 868-875, 1986.

96. Scandling, J., Myers, B., Glomerular size-selectivity and microalbuminuria in early diabetic glomerular disease. *Kidnet Int*, 41, 840-846, 1992.

97. Stow, J., Sawada, H., Farquhar, M., Basement membrane heparan sulfate proteoglycans are concentrated in the laminae rarae and podocytes of rat renal glomerulus. *Proc Natl Acad Sci U.S.A.*, 82, 3296-300, 1985.

98. Kanwar, Y. S., Linker, A., Farquhar, M. G., Increased permeability of glomerular basement membrane to ferritin after removal of glycosaminoglycans (heparan sulfate) by enzyme digestion. *J Cell Biol*, 86, 688-693, 1980.

99. Kanwar, Y. S., Rosenzweig, L. J., Linker, A., Decreased *de novo* synthesis of glomerular pro-teoglycan in diabetes: biochemical and autoradiographic evidence. *Proc Natl Acad Sci U.S.A.*, 80, 2272-2275, 1983.

100. Cohen, M. P., Klepser, H., Wu, V. Y., Heparan sulfate of glomerular basement membrane is undersulfated in experimental diabetes and is not corrected with aldose reductase inhibition. *Diabetes*, 37, 1324-1327, 1988.

101. McCarthy, K. J., Abrahamson, D. R., Bynum, K. R., St. John, P. L., Couchman, J. R., Basement membrane–specific chondroitin sulfate proteoglycan is abnormally associated with the glom-erular capillary basement membrane of diabetic rats. *J Histochem Cytochem*, 42, 473-484, 1994.

102. Ledbetter, S., Copeland, E., Noonan, D., Vogeli, G., Hassell, J., Altered steady-state mRNA levels of basement membrane proteins in diabetic mouse kidneys and thromboxane synthase inhibition. *Diabetes*, 39, 196-203, 1990.

103. Makino, H., Yamasaki, Y., Hironaka, K., Ota, Z., Glomerular extracellular matrices in rat diabetic glomerulopathy by scanning electron microscopy. *Virchows Arch B Cell Pathol Incl Mol Pathol*, 62, 19-24, 1992.

104. Pagtalunan, M. E., Miller, P. L., Jumping-Eagle, S., Nelson, R. G., Myers, B. D., Rennke, H. G., Coplon, N. S., Sun, L., Meyer, T. W., Podocyte loss and progressive glomerular injury in Type II diabetes. *J Clin Invest*, 99, 342-348, 1997.

105. Steffes, M. W., Leffert, J. D., Basgen, J. M., Brown, D. M., Mauer, S. M., Epithelial cell foot process width in intact and uninephrectomized diabetic and nondiabetic rats. *Lab Invest*, 43, 225-230, 1980.

106. Poulsom, R., Kurkinen, M., Prockop, D. J., Boot-Hanford, R. P., Increased steady-state levels of laminin B1 mRNA in kidneys of long-term streptozotocin-diabetic rats. No effect of aldose reductase inhibitor. *J Biol Chem*, 263, 10072-10076, 1988.

107. Roy, S., Sala, R., Cagliero, E., Lorenzi, M., Overexpression of fibronectin induced by diabetes or high glucose: phenomenon with a memory. *Proc Natl Acad Sci U.S.A.*, 87, 404-408, 1990.

108. Mohanam, S., Bose, S. M., Influence of streptozotocin- and alloxan-induced diabetes in the rat on collagenase and certain lysosomal enzymes in relation to the degradation of connective tissue proteins. *Diabetologia*, 25, 66-70, 1983.

109. Cohen, M. P., Surma, M. L., Wu, V. Y., In vivo biosynthesis and turnover of glomerular basement membrane in diabetic rats. *Am J Physiol*, 242, F385-F389, 1982.

110. Lubec, G., Leban, J., Peyroux, J., Sternberg, M., Pollack, A. O., Latzka, M., Coradello, H., In vivo biosynthesis and turnover of glomerular basement membrane in diabetic rats. *Nephron*, 30, 357-360, 1982.

111. Romen, W., Lange, H. W., Hempel, R., Heck, T., Studies on collagen metabolism in rats. II. Turnover and amino acid composition of the collagen of glomerular basement membrane in diabetes mellitus. *Virchow Arch*, 36, 313-320, 1981.

112. Lubec, G., Pollak, A., Reduced susceptibility of nonenzymatically glucosylated glomerular basement membrane to proteases. *Renal Physiol*, 3, 4-8, 1980.

113. Lubec, G., Leban, J., Peyroux, J., Sternberg, M., Pollack, A., Latzka, M., Coradello, H., Reduced collagenolytic activity of rat kidneys with streptozotocin diabetes. *Nephron*, 30, 357-363, 1982.

114. Cohen-Forterre, L., Mozere, G., Andre, J., Sternberg, M., Studies on kidney sialidase in normal and diabetic rats. *Biochim Biophys Acta*, 801, 138-145, 1984.

115. Teshner, M., Schaefer, R. M., Svarnas, A., Heidland, U., Heidland, A., Decreased proteinase activity in isolated glomeruli of streptozotocin diabetic rats. *Am J Nephrol*, 9, 464-469, 1989.

116. Reckelhoff, J. F., Tyart, V. L., Mitias, M. M., Walcott, J. L., STZ-induced diabetes results in decreased activity of glomerular cathepsin and metalloproteinase in rats. *Diabetes*, 42, 1425-1432, 1993.

117. Lane, P. H., Steffes, M. W., Fioretto, P., Mauer, S. M., Renal interstitial expansion in insulin-dependent diabetes mellitus. *Kidney Int*, 43, 661-667, 1993.

118. Ziyadeh, F. N., Renal tubular basement membrane and collagen Type IV in diabetes mellitus. *Kidney Int*, 43, 114-120, 1993.

119. Honjo, K., Doi, K., Doi, C., Mitsuoka, T., Histopathology of streptozotocin-induced diabetic DBA/2N and CD-1 mice. *Lab Anim*, 20, 298-301, 1986.

120. Seyer-Hansen, K., Renal hypertrophy in streptozotocin diabetic rats. *Clin Sci Mol Med*, 51, 551-555, 1976.
121. Seyer-Hansen, K., Renal hypertrophy in experimental diabetes mellitus. *Kidney Int*, 23, 643-646, 1983.
122. Rasch, R., Tubular lesions in streptozotocin diabetic rats. *Diabetologia*, 27, 32-37, 1984.
123. Mayhew, T. M., Sharma, A. K., McMallum, K. N. C., Effects of continuous subcutaneous insulin infusion on renal morphology in experimental diabetes. I. Blood glucose levels, body size, kidney weight and glomerulotubular morphometry. *J Pathol*, 151, 147-155, 1987.
124. Romen, W., Takashi, A., Autoradiographic studies on the proliferation of glomerular and tubular cells of the rat kidney in early diabetes. *Virchows Arch Cell Pathol*, 40, 339-345, 1982.
125. Tucker, B. J., Rasch, R., Blantz, R. C., Glomerular filtration and tubular reabsorption of albumin in preproteinuric and proteinuric diabetic rats. *J Clin Invest*, 92, 686-694, 1993.
126. Kaneda, K., Iwao, J., Sakata, N., Takebayashi, S., Correlation between mitochondrial enlargement in renal proximal tubules and microalbuminuria in rats with early streptozotocin-induced diabetes. *Acta Pathol Jpn*, 42, 855-860, 1992.
127. Olbricht, C. J., Geissinger, B., Renal hypertrophy in streptozotocin diabetic rats: role of proteolytic lysosomal enzymes. *Kidney Int*, 41, 966-972, 1992.
128. Zador, I. Z., Deshmukh, G. D., Kunkel, R., Johnson, K., Radin, N. S., Shayman, J. A., A role for glycosphingolipid accumulation in the renal hypertrophy of streptozotocin-induced diabetes mellitus. *J Clin Invest*, 91, 797-803, 1993.
129. Rocco, M., Chen, Y., Goldfarb, S., Ziyadeh, F. N., Elevated glucose stimulates TGF-β gene expression and bioactivity in proximal tubule. *Kidney Int.*, 41, 107-114, 1992.
130. Armanni, L., Fuenf Autopsien mit histologischen Untersuchungen und klinischer Epicrise, in *Der Diabetes Mellitus*. Cantani A, Ed. Denickes Verlag, Berlin, 1877, 315-329.
131. Ebstein, W., Uber Druesenepithelnekrosen beim Diabetes mellitus mit besonderer Beruecksichtigung des diabetischen Koma. *Dtsch Arch Klin Med*, 30, 143-185, 1881.
132. Holck, P., Rasch, R., Structure and segmental localization of glycogen in the diabetic rat kidney. *Diabetes*, 42, 891-900, 1993.
133. Bleasel, A. F., Yong, L. C. J., Streptozotocin induced diabetic nephropathy and renal tumors in the rat. *Experientia*, 38, 129-130, 1982.
134. Reyes, A. A., Kissane, J., Klahr, S., A high cholesterol diet ameliorates renal tubular lesions in diabetic rats. *Proc Soc Exp Biol Med* 194, 177-185, 1990.
135. Rohrbach, D., Wagner, C., Star, V., Martin, G., Brown, K., Yoon, J.-W., Reduced synthesis of basement membrane heparan sulfate proteoglycan in streptozotocin-induced diabetic mice. *J Biol Chem*, 258, 11672-11677, 1982.
136. Ihm, C. G., Lee, G. S. L., Nast, C. C., Artishevsky, A., Guillermo, R., Levin, R. J., Glassock, R. J., Adler, S. G., Early increased procollagen α1(IV) mRNA levels in streptozotocin induced diabetes. *Kidney Int*, 41, 768-777, 1992.
137. Wong, A. P., Cortez, S. L., Baricos, W. H., Role of plasmin and gelatinase in extracellular matrix degradation by cultured rat mesangial cells. *Am J Physiol*, 32, F1112-F1118, 1992.
138. Ziyadeh, F. N., Goldfarb, S. The diabetic renal tubulointerstitium, in *Tubulointerstial and Cystic Diseases of the Kidney, Current Topics in Pathology* (Series), S. Dodd., Eds., Vol. 88, Springer-Verlag, Berlin, 1995, 175-201.
139. Trachtman, H., Futterweit, S., Maesaka, J., Ma, C., Valderrama, E., Fuchs, A., Tarectecan, A. A., Rao, P. S., Sturman, J. A., Boles, T. H., Fu, M.-X., Baynes, J., Taurine ameliorates chronic streptozotocin-induced diabetic nephropathy in rats. *Am J Physiol*, 269, F429-F438, 1995.
140. Osterby, R., Gundersen, H. J. G., Fast accumulation of basement membrane material and the rate of morphological changes in acute experimental diabetic glomerular hypertrophy. *Diabetologia*, 18, 493-500, 1980.
141. Osterby, R., Gundersen, H. J., Glomerular basement membrane thickening in streptozotocin diabetic rats despite treatment with an aldose reductase inhibitor. *J Diabetic Complications*, 3, 149-153, 1989.
142. Vernier, R. L., Steffes, M. W., Sisson-Ross, S., Mauer, S. M., Heparan sulfate proteoglycan in the glomerular basement membrane in type 1 diabetes mellitus. *Int Soc Nephrol*, 41, 1070-1080, 1992.

143. Deckert, T., Parving, H. H., Thomsen, O. F., Jorgensen, H. E., Brun, C., Thomsen, A. C., Renal structure and function in Type I (insulin-dependent) diabetic patients. *Diabetic Nephropathy,* 4, 163-168, 1986.

144. Bader, R., Bader, H., Grund, K., Markensen-Haen, S., Christ, H., Bohle, A., Structure and function of the kidney in diabetic glomerulosclerosis: correlations between morphologic and functional parameters. *Pathol Res Pract,* 167, 204-216, 1980.

145. Ku, D. D., Meezan, E., Increased renal tubular sodium pump and Na⁺-K⁺-adenosine triphosphate in streptozotocin-diabetic rats. *J Pharmacol Exp Ther,* 229, 664-670, 1984.

146. Ku, D. D., Sellers, B. M., Meezan, E., Development of renal hypertrophy and increased renal Na,K-ATPase in streptozotocin-diabetic rats. *Endocrinology,* 119, 672-679, 1986.

147. Ku, D. D., Roberts, R. B., Sellers, B. M., Meezan, E., Regression of renal hypertrophy and elevated renal Na⁺, K⁺-ATPase activity after insulin treatment in streptozotocin-diabetic rats. *Endocrinology,* 120, 2166-2173, 1987.

148. Wald, H., Scherzer, P., Popovtzer, M. M., Enhanced renal tubular ouabain-sensitive ATPase in streptozotocin diabetes mellitus. *Am J Physiol,* 251, F164-F170, 1986.

149. Vaamonde, C. A., Bier, R., Gouvea, W., Alpert, H., Kelley, J., Pardo, V., Effect of duration of diabetes on the protection observed in the diabetic rat against gentamicin-induced acute renal failure. *Miner Electrolyte Metab,* 10, 209-216, 1984.

150. Farquhar, M. G., The unfolding story of megalin (gp330): now recognized as a drug receptor. Editorial. *J Clin Invest,* 96, 1184, 1995.

151. Cortes, P., Dumler, F., Venkatachalam, K. K., Goldman, J., Sastry, K. S. S., Venkatachalam, H., Bernstein, J., Levin, N. W., Alterations in glomerular RNA in diabetic rats: roles of glucagon and insulin. *Kidney Int,* 20, 491-499, 1981.

152. Cheng, H. F., Burns, K. D., Harris, R. C., Reduced proximal tubule angiotensin II receptor expression in streptozotocin-induced diabetes mellitus. *Kidney Int,* 46, 1603-1610, 1994.

153. Rasch, R., Gotzsche, O., Regression of glycogen nephrosis in experimental diabetes after pancreatic islet transplantation. *APMIS,* 96, 749-754, 1988.

154. Gotzsche, O., Gundersen, H. J. G. G., Osterby, R., Irreversibility of glomerular basement membrane accumulation despite reversibility of renal hypertrophy with islet transplantation in early experimental diabetes. *Diabetes,* 30, 481-485, 1981.

155. Sharma, K., Ziyadeh, F. N., Biochemical events and cytokine interactions linking glucose metabolism to the development of diabetic nephropathy. *Semin Nephrol,* 17, 80-92, 1997.

156. Tilton, R. G., Baier, L. D., Harlow, J. E., Smith, S. R., Ostrow, E., Williamson, J. R., Diabetes-induced glomerular dysfunction: links to a more reduced cytosolic ratio of NADH/NAD+. *Kidney Int,* 41, 778-788, 1992.

157. Cohen, M. P., Ziyadeh, F. N., Role of Amadori-modified nonenzymatically glycated serum proteins in the pathogenesis of diabetic nephropathy. *J Am Soc Nephrol,* 7, 1-8, 1996.

158. Mitsuhashi, T., Nakayama, H., Itoh, T., Kuwajima, S., Aoki, S., Atsumi, T., Koike, T., Immunochemical detection of advanced glycation end products in renal cortex from STZ-induced diabetic rat. *Diabetes,* 42, 826-832, 1993.

159. Bucala, R., Cerami, A., Vlassara, H., Advanced glycosylation end products in diabetic complications. Biochemical basis and prospects for therapeutic intervention. *Diabetes Reviews,* 3, 258-268, 1995.

160. Bleyer, A., Fumo, P., Snipes, E. R., Goldfarb, S., Simmons, D. A., Ziyadeh, F. N., Polyol pathway mediates high glucose-induced collagen synthesis in proximal tubule. *Kidney Int,* 45, 659-666, 1994.

161. Ziyadeh, F. N., Fumo, P., Rodenberger, C. H., Kuncio, G. S., Neilson, E. G., Role of PKC and cAMP/PKA in high glucose-stimulated transcriptional activation of collagen α1(IV) in glomerular mesangial cells. *J Diabetes Complications,* 9, 255-261, 1995.

162. Soulis-Liparota, T., Cooper, M., Papazoglou, D., Clarke, B., Jerums, G., Retardation by aminoguanidine of development of albuminuria, mesangial expansion, and tissue fluorescence in streptozocin-induced diabetic rat. *Diabetes,* 40, 1328-1334, 1991.

163. Ellis, E. N., Good, B. H., Prevention of glomerular basement membrane thickening by aminoguanidine in experimental diabetes mellitus. *Metabolism,* 40, 1016-1019, 1991.

4

Physiological and Pathological Consequences of Streptozotocin Diabetes on the Heart

Brian Rodrigues and John H. McNeill

CONTENTS

4.1 Introduction

With the discovery of insulin, mortality from acute complications such as diabetic ketoacidosis has been practically eliminated and the quality of life of many patients with diabetes has improved. However, the prolongation of survival of patients with diabetes is accompanied by the development of chronic degenerative complications, which include retinopathy, renal failure, neuropathy, and cardiovascular disease.

Clinical studies have confirmed that the incidence of heart disease is much greater among diabetics, and is the leading cause of death in these patients.[1,2] The cardiac disease includes a lower stroke volume, cardiac index, and ejection fraction, and a higher left ventricular end diastolic pressure.[3-5] Factors that have been implicated in the development of cardiovascular dysfunction during diabetes include atherosclerosis of the coronary arteries,[6] macroangiopathy, and autonomic neuropathy.[7] However, it has also become apparent that these factors, although important, are not exclusive determinants of the cardiac problems associated with diabetes. Indeed, a significant number of patients with diabetes who do not develop atherosclerosis continue to suffer from cardiomegaly, left ventricular dysfunction, and clinically overt congestive heart failure.[3-5,8] This suggests that a specific cardiac muscle disease, i.e., diabetic cardiomyopathy, may also occur during diabetes[9,10] and could be a causal factor in producing the increase in mortality and morbidity of diabetes.

In animal models, diabetes is produced by injection of chemical agents like alloxan or streptozotocin (STZ). These toxins selectively induce β-cell necrosis in the pancreas and provide relatively permanent diabetes. With time, these diabetic animals also develop myocardial abnormalities. Stroke volume, stroke work, cardiac output, peak left ventricular pressure, and rate of rise and fall of ventricular pressure (±dP/dt) are all depressed, whereas left ventricular compliance is increased in cardiac muscle preparations from these diabetic animals.[11-16] Another model of diabetes that is closely related to human insulin-dependent diabetes mellitus (IDDM) is the spontaneously diabetic Bio Breeding (BB). In this animal, diabetes develops spontaneously with the appearance of symptoms including weight loss, hypoinsulinemia, hyperglycemia, and ketoacidosis and leads to death if not treated with exogenous insulin.[17] If BB diabetic rats are maintained with a low dose of insulin (such that the rats are severely hyperglycemic, hypoinsulinemic, and hyperlipidemic) and heart function is measured 6 weeks after the onset of diabetes, they exhibit depressed left ventricular developed pressure, cardiac contractility, and ventricular relaxation rates when compared with BB nondiabetic littermates.[18] Thus, irrespective of chemical or spontaneous diabetes, animal models show the development of cardiac failure similar to that seen in human patients with diabetes. Given the parallel observations in both humans and diabetic animals that cardiac dysfunction is not accompanied by a significant reduction in myocardial oxygenation and coronary flow or the presence of major vessel disease, it can be proposed that chronic diabetes mellitus can negatively alter myocardial function independent of vascular defects.

4.2   Etiology of Diabetic Cardiomyopathy

Several etiological factors have been put forward to explain the development of diabetic cardiomyopathy, which include metabolic, biochemical, and ultrastructural changes.

4.2.1   Metabolic Changes

4.2.1.1   Supply of Fatty Acids

In the early stages of diabetes, alterations in both fuel supply and utilization by the heart tissue may be the initiating factor for the development of diabetic cardiomyopathy. Mitochondrial generation of ATP in the heart is through the oxidation of various substrates that include glucose, free fatty acids (FFA), lactate, and ketone bodies.[19] The breakdown of glucose or glycogen to pyruvate (glycolysis) provides some energy. However, it is the subsequent entry of pyruvate into the mitochondria and its conversion into acetyl coenzyme A (CoA) that provides the majority of energy obtained from glucose. Acetyl CoA can also be derived from amino acids and FFA. In fact, the heart muscle of rat is known to account for the largest consumption of FFA with respect to body weight.[20] The heart has a limited potential to synthesize FFA. Hence, FFA are supplied to cardiac cells from several sources: (1) lipolysis of endogenous triglyceride (TG) within the cardioadipocyte or cardiomyocyte; (2) lipolysis of adipose tissue triglyceride with subsequent entry of FFA into the blood where they are carried to the heart, usually bound to albumin; and (3) lipolysis of circulating triglyceride in chylomicrons and very low density lipoproteins (VLDL) by coronary endothelial-bound lipoprotein lipase (LPL). Vascular endothelial-bound LPL is the rate-limiting enzyme that determines the clearance of plasma TG and partially regulates FFA supply to the tissues; hence, it is also called heparin-releasable "functional" LPL.[21] As endothelial cells cannot synthesize LPL, the enzyme is synthesized by the parenchymal cells of a variety of extrahepatic tissues, including adipose, heart, skeletal muscle, brain, and ovary. In the adult heart, LPL is synthesized and processed in myocytes and is translocated onto heparan sulfate proteoglycan (HSPGs) binding sites on the luminal surface of endothelial cells,[22] where it actively metabolizes lipoproteins. Chylomicrons and VLDL bind transiently to endothelium-binding lipolysis sites where heparin-releasable endothelial LPL hydrolyzes the TG core to FFA and 2-monoacylglycerol,[23] which are then transported into the heart for numerous metabolic and structural tasks.

In diabetes, because of inadequate glucose transport and oxidation, energy production in the heart is almost entirely via β-oxidation of FFA, a process that may have deleterious effects on myocardial function. Despite this excessive use of FFA, the approximate contribution of FFA from exogenous or endogenous sources toward β-oxidation in the diabetic heart is not known. In an insulin-deficient state, adipose tissue lipolysis is enhanced, resulting in elevated circulating FFA.[24] In addition, an increased activity of myocardial enzymes that catalyze the synthesis of TG, together with a rise in CoA levels, promotes the production of TG during diabetes.[25] Subsequent hydrolysis of this augmented TG store could also lead to high tissue FFA levels.[26,27] These processes serve to guarantee FFA supply to the diabetic heart to compensate for the diminished contribution of glucose as an energy source. Considering these mechanisms that enhance cardiac FFA levels, the relative contribution of cardiac LPL activity to the delivery of FFA to the diabetic heart is unknown. An additional caveat is that available information on the influence of diabetes on heart LPL is inconclusive. Thus, LPL immunoreactive protein or activity has been reported to be unchanged,[28-30] increased,[31-34] or decreased[35-39] in the diabetic rat heart. In part, this variability between different studies could be due to the diversity in the rat strains used, the dosage of STZ used to induce diabetes, and the duration of the diabetic state. In addition, many of the above investigations utilized procedures that did not distinguish between the heparin-releasable component (localized on capillary endothelial cells that is implicated in the hydrolysis of circulating TG) and cellular (i.e., non-heparin-releasable pool that represents a storage form of the enzyme) pools of cardiac LPL as cellular LPL activity or protein levels have largely been obtained using whole heart homogenates.

The authors have demonstrated that in rats with moderate diabetes induced by 55 mg/kg STZ, there was an elevated peak heparin-releasable LPL activity at 2 and 12 weeks after diabetes induction.[40] It was hypothesized that the enhanced heparin-releasable LPL activity in D55 rat hearts may be due to an increased synthesis of the enzyme in the cardiomyocytes.[41] Interestingly, the higher heparin-releasable LPL activity in D55 rats was not secondary to an expanded cellular pool, which was dramatically reduced. At present, the mechanism for the enhanced heparin-releasable LPL pool at the endothelial surface is not fully understood, but could involve the increased vectorial transfer of LPL from the myocyte to the endothelial cell via several HSPG sites,[42] an enhanced intermediate interstitial pool of LPL, an increased number of HSPG sites on the endothelial surface, or an altered turnover of LPL at the endothelial cells. Alternatively, any changes in the activation state of the heparin-releasable LPL during diabetes cannot be ruled out. It should be noted that a 90-min insulin treatment of 2-week diabetic rats had no effect on the cellular LPL store. Interestingly, peak heparin-releasable LPL activity was reduced to control levels, suggesting a direct effect of insulin in displacing LPL from its binding sites. In support, insulin was demonstrated to release LPL from 3T3-L1 adipocytes, possibly via the phospholipase C–catalyzed hydrolysis of a glycosylphosphatidylinositol membrane anchor.[43,44] More recently, however, the authors did not observe any release of LPL in response to insulin perfusion of the isolated whole heart.[45] Hence, a mechanism for the acute effect of insulin *in vivo* in reducing the heparin-releasable LPL activity in moderate diabetes has yet to be determined. It is believed that this increased enzyme activity could lead to an accelerated hydrolysis of lipoprotein-TG, providing an additional source of FFA that could have deleterious effects in the diabetic heart. However, as compositional changes in circulating lipoproteins have also been reported during diabetes, making them poorer substrates for the enzyme,[46] the role of an enhanced cardiac LPL in FFA supply to the diabetic heart is still unclear.

4.2.1.2   Consequences of Excessive Utilization of Fatty Acids

An increase in the supply and oxidation of FFA of endogenous or exogenous origin is one of the characteristic disorders of diabetes. It is postulated that FFA can exert adverse electrophysiological, biochemical, and mechanical effects in the heart. These include

1. An increased susceptibility to arrhythmias,[47-50]

2. Esterification to complex lipids and hence higher tissue levels of triglyceride,

3. An increased requirement of oxygen for catabolism,

4. Reduction in both the basal and insulin-stimulated glucose transport and metabolism,[51]

5. Modification of the structure of sarcolemmal and other subcellular membranes thereby altering membrane fluidity and molecular dynamics,[52]

6. Inhibition of critical enzyme systems such as Ca^{2+}-ATPase of sarcoplasmic reticulum, and Na^+, K^+-ATPase, Na^+/Ca^{2+} exchange and Ca^{2+} pump in myocardial sarcolemma,[53-55]

7. Inhibition of the adenine nucleotide translocator in isolated mitochondria leading to a reduction in the myocardial levels of ATP,[56]

8. Mediation of an increase in α_1-response[57,58] leading to a mobilization of Ca^{2+} from intracellular stores, and

9. Interacting with voltage-dependent Ca^{2+} channels.[59,60]

A consequence of these effects is an aberrant intracellular handling of Ca^{2+} with subsequent alterations in membrane permeability; activation of Ca^{2+}-stimulated proteases, phospholipases, and lysosomal enzyme activities; mitochondrial calcification with depletion of cellular ATP stores; cell death; and eventual cardiac dysfunction.[61-63] The role of calcium is further supported by the observation that treatment of STZ diabetic rats with verapamil, a calcium channel blocker that is known to depress the entry of Ca^{2+} into the cell, was capable of decreasing the severity of the cardiomypopathy.[64,65] Overall, there appears to be a lipid paradox in that low concentrations of FFA are essential for the proper functioning of the heart, whereas excessive amounts are potentially deleterious.

4.2.1.3   Altered Carbohydrate Metabolism

Intracellular glucose disposal occurs through several major pathways. Nonoxidative glucose disposal primarily reflects the conversion to glycogen, whereas the oxidative pathway involves the complete oxidation of glucose-derived carbon atoms to carbon dioxide or the conversion to fatty acids in lipogenic tissues.[66] The major metabolic action of insulin is its stimulation of glucose oxidation. Insulin achieves this effect by controlling the transport of glucose and does so by inducing a rapid, reversible translocation of glucose transporter proteins from a latent intracellular pool to the plasma membrane.[67] Activation of glucose transport by insulin leads to enhanced glycolytic rates and glycogen deposition, and these effects contribute in large part to the hypoglycemic action of insulin *in vivo*. In the absence of insulin, the major restriction to glucose utilization by the heart is the slow rate of glucose transport across the sarcolemmal membrane into the myocardium, probably as a result of a cellular depletion of glucose transporters.[68] Eckel and Reinauer[69] have reported that in insulin-deficient rats, it was the insulin-responsive glucose transporter (GLUT-4) that was specifically reduced in cardiomyocytes. The diabetes-associated reduction in glucose transporter protein/activity is poorly understood. It has been demonstrated that the activity of the glucose transporter *in vitro* is influenced by the composition (specifically membrane lipid) and structure of cell membranes.[70] Since the diabetic state is associated with hypertriglyceridemia and a considerable alteration in fatty acid profile of membranes, it could explain the decrease in glucose transporters and a reduction in insulin-stimulated cardiac glucose utilization.[71] In support of this concept, cardiomyocytes cultured in the presence of palmitate exhibit a largely reduced insulin responsiveness that is partially restored by the inhibition of fatty acid oxidation.[72]

Glucose oxidation in the diabetic heart is markedly impaired, not only as a result of impaired glucose transport into the myocyte but also by a reduced rate of phosphorylation of glucose within the cell. The reduced phosphorylation, in turn, probably results from an increased metabolism of FFA.[73] For instance, during diabetes, when plasma FFA levels are high, the heart preferentially oxidizes this substrate. This excessive oxidation of FFA is then at least partly responsible for the insulin resistance and depression of glucose uptake and oxidation, a notion introduced by the classic studies of Randle and colleagues.[51] They suggested that an increased availability of FFA could increase the TCA cycle activity and thus citrate concentration. The citrate formed may inhibit phosphofructokinase, thereby decreasing the rate of glycolysis, and this, in turn, results in an impairment of glucose uptake and oxidation. The reduction in substrate flow through the glycolytic pathway results in an eventual increase in the tissue levels of glucose-6-phosphate, which then activates glycogen synthase and inhibits phosphorylase; these changes in enzyme activity appear to account for glycogen accumulation, as the small amount of glucose that is taken up is diverted to glycogen.[74] Another explanation for the reduced oxidation of glucose by the diabetic heart is that the activity of pyruvate dehydrogenase complex is also depressed, again possibly as a result of an increased fatty acid oxidation, which results in an increased acetyl CoA/CoA ratio. The end result is an impaired pyruvate oxidation. Subsequent studies by Wall and Lopaschuk[75] confirmed the findings of Randle and his colleagues. These authors demonstrated that in the presence of relevant concentrations of fatty acids, myocardial glucose oxidation is essentially abolished in chronically STZ diabetic rats. Furthermore, they showed that fatty acids inhibit glucose oxidation to a much greater extent than glycolysis, such that, in the presence of high concentrations of fatty acids, rates of glycolysis are more than 13 times the rate of glucose oxidation, thus supporting the concept that fatty acid inhibition of glucose utilization occurs to a greater extent at the level of pyruvate dehydrogenase than at the level of phosphofructokinase. The authors have also observed a reduction in basal glucose oxidation in cardiac myocytes isolated from acutely diabetic rats. In addition, the inhibitory effect of fatty acids is demonstrated when incubation with exogenous oleate further reduced basal and insulin-stimulated glucose oxidation in both control and diabetic myocytes. Interestingly, in control myocytes, the inhibitory effect of oleate on basal glucose oxidation was reversed by washing, whereas the inhibition of insulin-stimulated glucose oxidation remained.[76] Additional evidence that changes in FFA metabolism can affect carbohydrate metabolism have come from the demonstration that pharmacological agents that strongly inhibit the activity of CPT 1 and therefore the hepatic oxidation of long-chain fatty acids — e.g., 2-tetradecylglycidic acid; 2[5(4-chlorophenyl) pentyl oxirane-2-carboxylic acid; etomoxir; B 827-33 — can correct derangements such as fatty acid–induced inhibition of glucose oxidation and are effective hypoglycemic agents in fasted or diabetic animals.[77,78] The hypoglycemic potency of agents that act in this manner appears to be independent of the actions of insulin and is suggested to be either due to their ability to increase glucose oxidation and utilization by insulin-sensitive tissues[79] by reactivating the pyruvate dehydrogenase complex or to a suppression of hepatic gluconeogenesis (when hepatic oxidation of fatty acid is blocked, the liver must oxidize carbohydrates and a diversion of carbohydrate from the gluconeogenic to the oxidative pathway could account for the observed fall in plasma glucose.[80] In addition, fatty acid oxidation supplies ATP and acetyl CoA, which are necessary for hepatic glucose production, and inhibition of fatty acid oxidation, therefore, seems to reduce the fasting blood glucose level. A switch from predominantly fatty acid to carbohydrate oxidation could then explain the salutary effects of these drugs on cardiac performance.[81,82] Other agents that directly alter lipid metabolism have also been shown to have similar effects. For example, acute administration of nicotinic acid (a potent inhibitor of fatty acid lipolysis) has been shown to lower elevated plasma FFA, fatty acid oxidation, and plasma glucose levels in diabetic rats.[83]

4.2.2 Biochemical Changes

Various biochemical changes in the myocardium have also been characterized in animal models of diabetes. The more prominent systems affected, which are known to regulate calcium homeostasis and hence cardiac function, are the sarcolemma and sarcoplasmic reticulum.

4.2.2.1 *Sarcolemma*

The cardiac contraction and relaxation cycle is generally viewed as a consequence of raising and lowering the intracellular concentration of free calcium. The importance of the sarcolemma in this beat-by-beat phenomenon is well documented.[84] Heart sarcolemma is composed of a basement and plasma membrane. The basement membrane is located on the extracytoplasmic side of the bilayered plasma membrane.[85] Several enzyme and nonenzymatic systems are associated with the plasma membrane and are involved in the regulation of myocardial ion transport and contractility.[86,87] When the cardiac cell is depolarized, there is an influx of calcium through the sarcolemma, resulting in contraction; relaxation, on the other hand, is partly achieved by calcium efflux through the sarcolemma. Some sarcolemmal bound proteins that have been identified as playing important roles either directly or indirectly in myocardial calcium transport are Na^+-K^+-ATPase, Ca^{2+}-Mg^{2+}ATPase (Ca^{2+} pump), and adenylate cyclase.[88] Other calcium transporters such as the Na^+–Ca^{2+}-exchanger also appear to have regulatory roles in cardiac contraction.[89] Thus, from a functional point of view, the sarcolemma contains a variety of systems that play important roles in the regulation of myocardial contraction. Hence, any alteration in the composition and/or structure of this subcellular organelle can change its ability to transport calcium effectively, and, as a result, the cardiac contraction and relaxation process can be significantly altered.

Heart failure associated with diabetes mellitus appears to be accompanied by alterations in sarcolemmal phospholipids.[90] In addition to their role as major structural constituents of cell membranes, phospholipids bind calcium[91] and also influence the activity of several enzyme systems via transmembrane methylation. During this process, membrane-bound enzymes convert phosphatidylethanolamine to phosphatidylcholine by transferring three methyl groups to the amino polar head of the phospholipid.[92] The activities of adenylate cyclase[93] and sarcolemmal-calcium pump[94] have been reported to be enhanced during this phenomenon. Phospholipid methylation has been reported to be depressed in the diabetic rat heart and, therefore, may be involved in the cardiac dysfunction of diabetics.[95]

Sarcolemmal Na^+-K^+-ATPase is considered to control the movement of sodium and potassium across the cell membrane. Myocardial contraction is initiated when an action potential depolarizes the sarcolemma. The action potential is triggered by an increase in sodium permeability that results in membrane depolarization. The outward movement of potassium down its concentration gradient achieves repolarization. It is evident, therefore, that a pump system is required to propel sodium out of the cell and potassium back into the cell to maintain the electrochemical gradient necessary to produce a resting membrane potential in order to establish the appropriate environment for subsequent action potentials. Depression of this sodium pump will alter the resting membrane potential and subsequently cardiac contraction. Indeed, Na^+-K^+-ATPase activity has been reported to be depressed in diabetic failing hearts.[96] It must be pointed out that inhibition of the Na^+-K^+-ATPase system by agents such as cardiac glycosides is believed to be associated with an increase in intracellular calcium concentration and an increase in cardiac contractility. Thus, the role of the depressed Na^+-K^+-ATPase activity in explaining the diminished force of contraction under the pathophysiological situation of diabetes is unclear at present.

The adenylate cyclase system mediates catecholamine and other hormonal effects on cells. It consists of at least three distinct components: the receptor, which binds the hormone or neuro-transmitter; the catalytic moiety, which converts ATP to cyclic AMP (cAMP); and the guanine nucleotide (GTP) regulatory protein, which binds and hydrolyzes GTP and which functionally couples the receptor to the catalytic moiety (adenylate cyclase). Upon agonist binding to the receptor, and of GTP to GTP regulatory protein, the catalytic unit is activated and catalyzes the conversion of ATP to cAMP. cAMP not only regulates myocardial metabolism, but also modulates myocardial contractility by energizing several membrane systems and the contractile apparatus due to phosphorylation induced by protein kinases. Thus, any alteration in this enzyme complex will affect the normal functioning of the myocardium. In diabetic hearts, a decrease in response to β-stimulation[97] together with a reduced cAMP accumulation has been reported. Interestingly, adenylate cyclase activity has been reported to be either unaffected[98] or attenuated[99] in these hearts, suggesting that the reduced sensitivity to catecholamines may involve an additional defect upstream of the adenylate cyclase/G protein system. An alteration in adrenergic receptor density is also believed to be involved in this abnormality.[100]

Cardiac contraction is triggered by membrane depolarization and the resulting calcium entry into the sarcoplasm from the extracellular space, as well as calcium release from the sarcoplasmic reticular terminal cistenae.[101] The sarcolemma also plays an important role in calcium removal from the sarcoplasm during the relaxation phase of the cardiac contractile process. Sarcolemmal calcium mobilization appears to be achieved by different transporting systems, one being the Na^+–Ca^{2+}-exchanger. It is believed to transport calcium in[102] and out[103] of the cell in exchange for sodium, and appears to be involved in myocardial contraction and relaxation. The Ca^{2+}-pump is another sarcolemmal transporter that transports calcium from the sarcoplasm to the extracellular environment and, therefore, is believed to be involved in cardiac relaxation. Both the Na^+-Ca^{2+}-exchanger and Ca^{2+}-pump of sarcolemma have been reported to be defective in the diabetic myocardium[104] and, therefore, appear to be involved in the altered calcium transport in the heart during this pathological condition.

4.2.2.2 Mitochondria

Mitochondria are the chief source of myocardial ATP. This energy, produced by oxidative phosphorylation, is distributed to a number of energy-utilizing systems of the cell; for example, Na^+-K^+-ATPase and the Ca^{2+}-pump of sarcolemma and sarcoplasmic reticulum. Although the main function of mitochondria is to generate energy, these organelles have also been reported to accumulate calcium actively under *in vitro* conditions. Despite their calcium-accumulating ability, it is generally believed that mitochondria do not play a major role in the regulation of cytoplasmic calcium during the contraction–relaxation cycle.[105] The main criticisms against their involvement in effecting relaxation by lowering cytoplasmic calcium concentration are based on their low affinity for that ion, as well as the very slow rate in which they transport physiological levels of intracellular calcium. Despite these observations, the calcium-accumulating activity of mitochondria may act as a reservoir or "sink" to modulate intracellular calcium stores when concentrations of calcium are pathologically elevated. One drawback to mitochondrial calcium transport is that it competes with its energy-producing activity. This therefore suggests that during pathological conditions, when the myocardium is confronted with abnormal levels of calcium, mitochondria may not only have to provide ATP for extramitochondrial functions but also transport more calcium via a pathway that competes with ADP phosphorylation. Calcium transport by mitochondria appears to be altered in the heart during diabetes, an effect reversed by 2 weeks of insulin therapy.[106]

There are also reports of an alteration in the respiratory activity (which is coupled to ATP production) in mitochondria from diabetic hearts and includes an altered phosphorylation of creatinine in the presence of succinate or malate,[107] a depression of succinate dehydrogenase activity,[108] and an attenuation of ATP production.[109] Low tissue ATP levels may eventually impair normal cellular function and may therefore be involved in the genesis of cardiomyopathy during diabetes

4.2.2.3 Sarcoplasmic Reticulum

Calcium transport by the sarcoplasmic reticulum (SR) is a major mechanism by which intramyocardial levels of Ca^{2+}- and, thereby, tension development — are modulated. Participation of the SR in such regulatory processes depends on the ability to sequester calcium by an energy-consuming process and, as a consequence, promote relaxation of myofibrils.[110] SR membranes contain a K^+-sensitive Ca^{2+}-dependent ATPase enzyme[111] that transports Ca^{2+} from the sarcoplasm into the vesicles of sarcoplasmic reticulum with a high velocity and affinity.[112] Hence, the SR participates in the relaxation of the heart by actively accumulating calcium from the cytoplasmic space, and any alteration in the capacity of this membrane to sequester Ca^{2+} efficiently would, therefore, be expected to have an important impact on the contractile performance of the heart. In this regard, cardiac SR function is depressed in diabetic animals[113-115] and could explain the slowing of the rate at which affected ventricular muscle can relax.

4.2.2.4 Contractile Proteins

Another prominent system closely associated with contractility, which is altered by diabetes, is the contractile proteins. A number of studies have shown that the isoenzyme distribution shifts from the normally predominant isoenzyme V_1 form to the less active

V_3 form in diabetic rats with a corresponding decrease in Ca^{2+}-ATPase activities of myosin and actomyosin.[116-117] This could then account for the decreased shortening velocity of cardiac muscle.

It should be noted that most of the above changes were observed in isolated whole hearts obtained from animals that had been made moderately diabetic with 55 to 60 mg/kg STZ. More recently, Ren and Davidoff[118] demonstrated that, in rats made severely diabetic with 100 mg/kg STZ, abnormalities in isolated myocyte shortening and relengthening were already present after 4 to 6 days of diabetes as a result of impaired Ca^{2+} sequestration or extrusion. Interestingly, the same authors reported that when isolated normal ventricular myocytes were cultured in a low-insulin/high-glucose medium, an abnormal ventricular relaxation (similar to the effects of *in vivo* diabetes) was inducible in 1 day and likely depended on impaired Ca^{2+} sequestration and/or extrusion.[119]

4.2.3 Ultrastructural Changes

Hearts from chronically diabetic rats were observed to have mitochondrial clumping and disruption with intramitochondrial dense-staining particles; loss of contractile protein and disrupted banding; sarcolemmal and SR changes; edematous focal areas adjacent to the SR; capillary changes like thickening of lamina densa, loss of lamina lucida, an increased number of micropinocytic vesicles in the capillary walls; and increased lipid levels.[120] The above changes were paralleled by a depression in cardiac function. With a progressive deterioration in myocardial ultrastructure, there was no further worsening of cardiac performance. Some, but not all, of these ultrastructural changes could be reversed by insulin treatment.[121]

4.3   Conclusion

The incidence of mortality from cardiovascular diseases is higher in patients with diabetes. The cause of this accelerated cardiovascular disease is multifactorial, and, although atherosclerotic cardiovascular disease in association with well-defined risk factors has an influence on morbidity and mortality in diabetics, myocardial cell dysfunction independent of vascular defects has also been defined. In studying the latter, factors that lie at one end of the spectrum include generalized metabolic changes like hyperglycemia, hypoinsulinemia, and hyperlipidemia. At the other end are changes at the molecular level within the heart, such as depressed myosin ATPase activity, decreased ability of the SR to take up calcium, as well as depression of other membrane enzymes, for example, Na^+-K^+-ATPase and Ca^{2+}-ATPase. Recently, clinical and animal studies have suggested that cardiac dysfunction could be more closely linked to major abnormalities in carbohydrate and lipid metabolism. Specifically, these changes include an increased fatty acid utilization or lack of glucose oxidation in the diabetic heart, which can account for the accumulation of various acyl carnitine and CoA derivatives, abnormalities in calcium homeostasis, and heart dysfunction. Given the supportive data so far, the study of the relationship between glucose transport and utilization with TG breakdown and utilization should be examined in greater detail. However, there is little dispute that an attempt should be made to lower raised serum TG and FFA levels in diabetes. This could decrease the reliance of the heart on fatty acids and, hence, overcome the accumulation of toxic fatty acid intermediates and remove the fatty acid inhibition of myocardial glucose utilization. Glucose oxidation in the diabetic heart is important for the following reasons:

1. Glycolytically produced ATP may be preferentially used by membrane ion pumps, such as sarcolemmal ATPases, and any depletion of ATP produced by glycolysis could damage the integrity of cellular membranes.
2. Increasing flux through the pyruvate dehydrogenase complex will prevent the accumulation of glycolytic products such as lactate.
3. Fatty acids are known to have an "oxygen-wasting" effect when compared with carbohydrates, which results in an increased myocardial oxygen consumption for any given level of cardiac work, i.e., an increase in O^2 consumed per ATP produced. Since metabolic changes have severe effects on cardiac function, the maintenance of normal levels of circulatory fatty acids and TGs should be added to the criteria of management of diabetes.

Acknowledgments

Some of the studies described in this chapter were supported by grants from the Heart and Stroke Foundation of B.C. and Yukon, MRC (Canada), and the Canadian Diabetes Association.

References

1. Kannel, W. B. and McGee, D. L., Diabetes and cardiovascular disease: the Framingham study, *JAMA*, 241, 2035, 1979.
2. Palumbo, P. J., Elveback, C. R., and Conolly, D. C., Coronary artery disease and congestive heart failure in the diabetic: epidemiological aspects, the Rochester Diabetes Project, in *Clinical Cardiology and Diabetes*, Scott, R. C., Ed., Futura, New York, 1981, 13.
3. Hamby, R. I., Zoneraich, S., and Sherman, L., Diabetic cardiomyopathy, *JAMA*, 229, 1749, 1974.
4. Regan, T. J., Lyons, M. M., and Ahmed, S. S., Evidence for cardiomyopathy in familial diabetes mellitus, *J. Clin. Invest.*, 60, 885, 1977.
5. D'Elia, J. A., Weinrauch, L. A., Healy, R. W., Libertino, R. W., Bradley, R. F., and Leland, O. S., Myocardial dysfunction without coronary artery disease in diabetic renal failure, *Am. J. Cardiol.*, 43, 193, 1979.
6. Young, L. H., Ramahi, T. M., and McNulty, P. H., Heart disease in diabetes mellitus: a clinical and metabolic perspective, *Diabetes Nutr. Metab.*, 7, 233, 1994.
7. Ledet, B., Neubauer, B., Christensen, N. J., and Lundback, K., Diabetic cardiopathy, *Diabetologia*, 16, 207, 1979.
8. Ahmed, S. S., Jaferi, G. A., Narang, R. M., and Regan, T. J., Preclinical abnormality of left ventricular function in diabetes mellitus, *Am. Heart J.*, 89, 153, 1975.
9. Fein, F. S. and Sonnenblick, E. H., Diabetic cardiomyopathy, *Prog. Cardiovasc. Res.*, 27, 255, 1985.
10. Galderisi, M., Anderson, K. M., Wilson, P. W. F., and Levy, D., Echocardiographic evidence for the existence of a distinct diabetic cardiomyopathy (the Framingham Heart Study), *Am. J. Cardiol.*, 68, 85, 1991.
11. Regan, T. J., Ettinger, P. O., Khan, M. I., Jesran, M. U., Lyons, M. M., Oldewurtel, H. A., and Weber, M., Altered myocardial function and metabolism in chronic diabetes mellitus without ischemia in dogs, *Circ. Res.*, 35, 222, 1974.
12. Miller, T. B., Jr., Cardiac performance of isolated perfused hearts from alloxan diabetic rats, *Am. J. Physiol.*, 236, 808, 1979.

13. Vadlamudi, R. V. S. V., Rodgers, R. L., and McNeill, J. H., The effect of chronic alloxan and streptozotocin diabetes on isolated rat heart performance, *Can. J. Physiol. Pharmacol.*, 60, 902, 1982.

14. Fein, F. S., Miller-Green, B., and Sonnenblick, E. H., Altered myocardial mechanics in diabetic rabbits, *Am. J. Physiol.*, 248, 729, 1985.

15. Rodrigues, B. and McNeill, J. H., Cardiac function in spontaneously hypertensive diabetic rats, *Am. J. Physiol.*, 251, 571, 1986.

16. Okayama, H., Hamada, M., and Hiwada, K., Contractile dysfunction in the diabetic-rat heart is an intrinsic abnormality of the cardiac myocyte, *Clin. Sci.*, 86, 257, 1994.

17. Marliss, E. B., Nakhooda, A. F., Poussier, P., and Sima, A. A. F., The diabetic syndrome of the "BB" wistar rat: possible relevance to Type I (insulin-dependent) diabetes in man, *Diabetologia*, 22, 225, 1982.

18. Rodrigues, B. and McNeill, J. H., Cardiac dysfunction in isolated perfused hearts from spontaneously diabetic BB rats, *Can. J. Physiol. Pharmacol.*, 68, 514, 1990.

19. van der Vusse, G. J., Glatz, J. F. C., Stam, H. C. G., and Reneman, R. S., Fatty acid homeostasis in the normoxic and ischemic heart, *Physiol. Rev.*, 72, 881, 1992.

20. Neely, J. R. and Morgan, H. E., Relationship between carbohydrate and lipid metabolism and the energy balance of heart muscle, *Annu. Rev. Physiol.*, 36, 413, 1974.

21. Eckel, R. H., Lipoprotein lipase. A multifunctional enzyme relevant to common metabolic diseases, *N. Engl. J. Med.*, 320, 1060, 1989.

22. O'Brien, K. D., Ferguson, M., Gordon, D., Deeb, S. S., and Chait, A., Lipoprotein lipase is produced by cardiac myocytes rather than interstitial cells in human myocardium, *Arterioscler. Thromb.*, 14, 1445, 1994.

23. Hamosh, M. and Hamosh, P., Lipoprotein lipase: its physiological and clinical significance, *Mol. Aspects Med.*, 6, 199, 1983.

24. Rodrigues, B., Braun, J. E. A., Spooner, M., and Severson, D. L., Regulation of lipoprotein lipase activity in cardiac myocytes from control and diabetic rats by plasma lipids, *Can. J. Physiol. Pharmacol.*, 70, 1271, 1992.

25. Murthy, V. K., Bauman, M. D., and Shipp, J. C., Regulation of triacylglycerol lipolysis in the perfused hearts of normal and diabetic rats, *Diabetes*, 32, 718, 1983.

26. Kenno, K. A. and Severson, D. L., Lipolysis in isolated myocardial cells from diabetic rat hearts, *Am. J. Physiol.*, 249, 1024, 1985.

27. Chattopadhayay, J., Thompson, E. W., and Schmid, H. H. O., Elevated levels of nonesterified fatty acids in the myocardium of alloxan diabetic rats, *Lipids*, 25, 307, 1990.

28. Elkeles, R. S. and Hambley, J., The effects of fasting and streptozotocin on hepatic triglyceride lipase activity in the rat, *Diabetes*, 26, 58, 1977.

29. Veeraraghavan, K., Murthy, K., Bauman, M. D., and Shipp, J., Regulation of triacylglycerol lipolysis in the perfused hearts of normal and diabetic rats, *Diabetes*, 32, 718, 1983.

30. Inadera, H., Tashiro, J., Okubo, Y., Ishikawa, K., Shirai, K., Saito, Y., and Yoshida, S., Response of lipoprotein lipase to calorie intake in streptozotocin-induced diabetic rats, *Scand. J. Clin. Invest.*, 52, 797, 1992.

31. Raurama, R., Kuusela, P., and Hietanen, E., Adipose, muscle, and lung tissue lipoprotein lipase activities in young streptozotocin treated rats, *Horm. Metab. Res.*, 12, 591, 1980.

32. Stam, H., Schoonderwoerd, K., Breeman, W., and Hulsman, W., Effects of hormones, fasting and diabetes on triglyceride lipase activity in rat heart and liver, *Horm. Metab. Res.*, 16, 293, 1984.

33. Nomura, T., Hagino, H., Gotoh, M., Iguchi, A., and Sakamoto, N., The effects of streptozotocin diabetes on tissue specific lipase activities in the rat, *Lipids*, 19, 594, 1984.

34. Tavangar, K., Murata, Y., Pedersen, M. E., Goers, J. F., Hoffman, A. R., and Kraemer, F. B., Regulation of lipoprotein lipase in the diabetic rat, *J. Clin. Invest.*, 90, 1672, 1992.

35. O'Looney, P., Maten, M. V., and Vahouny, G. V., Insulin-mediated modifications of myocardial lipoprotein lipase and lipoprotein metabolism, *J. Biol. Chem.*, 258, 12994, 1983.

36. Deshaies, Y., Geloen, A., Paulin, A., and Bukowiecki, L. J., Restoration of lipoprotein lipase activity in insulin-deficient rats by insulin infusion is tissue-specific, *Can. J. Physiol. Pharmacol.*, 69, 746, 1990.

37. Braun, J. E. A. and Severson, D. L., Lipoprotein lipase release from cardiac myocytes is increased by decavanadate but not insulin, *Am. J. Physiol.*, 262, 663, 1992.

38. Rodrigues, B. and Severson, D. L., Acute diabetes does not reduce heparin-releasable lipoprotein lipase activity in perfused hearts from Wistar-Kyoto rats, *Can. J. Physiol. Pharmacol.*, 71, 657, 1993.

39. Liu, L. and Severson, D. L., Myocardial lipoprotein lipase activity: regulation by diabetes and fructose-induced hypertriglyceridemia, *Can. J. Physiol. Pharmacol.*, 73, 369, 1995.

40. Rodrigues, B., Cam, M. C., Jian, K., Lim, F., Sambandam, N., and Shepherd, G., Differential effects of streptozotocin-induced diabetes on cardiac lipoprotein lipase activity, *Diabetes*, 46, 1346, 1997.

41. Camps, L., Reina, M., Lobera, M., Vilard, S., and Olivecrona, T., Lipoprotein lipase: cellular origin and functional distribution, *Am. J. Physiol.*, 258, 673, 1990.

42. Blanchette-Mackie, E. J., Masuno, H., Dwyer, N. K., Olivecrona, T., and Scow, R. O., Lipoptoetin lipase in myocytes and capillary endothelium of heart: immunocytochemical study, *Am. J. Physiol.*, 256, 818, 1989.

43. Spooner, P. M., Chernick, S. S., Garrison, M. M., and Scow, R. O., Insulin regulation of lipoprotein lipase acitivity and release in 3T3-L1 adipocytes, *J. Biol. Chem.*, 254, 10021, 1979.

44. Chan, B. L., Lisanti, M. P., Rodriguez-Boulan, E., and Saltiel, A. R., Insulin stimulated release of lipoprotein lipase by metabolism of its phosphatidylinositol anchor, *Science*, 241, 1670, 1988.

45. Sambandam, N., Chen, X., Cam, M. C., and Rodrigues, B., Cardiac lipoprotein lipase in the spontaneously hypertensive rat, *Cardiovasc. Res.*, 33, 460, 1997.

46. Mamo, J. C. L., Hirano, T., Sainsbury, A., Fitzgerald, A. K., and Redgrave, T. G., Hypertriglyceridemia is exacerbated by slow lipolysis of triacylglycerol-rich lipoproteins in fed but not fasted streptozotocin diabetic rats, *Biochim. Biophys. Acta*, 1128, 132, 1992.

47. Opie, L. H., Effect of fatty acid on contractility and rhythm of the heart, *Nature* (London), 227, 1055, 1970.

48. Willebrands, A. F., Terivelle, H. F., and Tarserson, S. J. A., The effect of a high molar FFA/albumin ratio in the perfusion medium on rhythm and contractility of the isolated heart, *J. Mol. Cell. Cardiol.*, 5, 259, 1973.

49. Fields, L. E., Daugherty, A., and Bergmann, S. R., Effect of fatty acid on performance and lipid content of hearts from diabetic rabbits, *Am. J. Physiol.*, 250, 1079, 1986.

50. Kurien, V. A. and Yates, P. A., The role of free fatty acids in the production of ventricular arrhythmias after acute coronary artery occlusion, *Eur. J. Clin. Invest.*, 1, 225, 1971.

51. Randle, P. J., Hales, C. N., Garland, P. B., and Newsholme, E. A., The glucose fatty acid cycle: its role in insulin sensitivity and the metabolic disturbances of diabetes mellitus, *Lancet*, 1, 785, 1963.

52. Katz, A. M. and Messineo, F. C., Lipid membrane interactions and the pathogenesis of ischemic damage in the myocardium, *Circ. Res.*, 48, 1, 1981.

53. Adams, R. J., Cohen, D. W., Gupte, S., Johnson, J. D., Wallick, E. T., Wang, T., and Schwartz, A., *In vitro* effects of palmityl carnitine on cardiac plasma membrane Na^+, K^+-ATPase and sarcoplasmic reticulum Ca^{2+}-ATPase and Ca^{2+} transport, *J. Biol. Chem.*, 254, 12404, 1979.

54. Kramer, J. H. and Weglicki, W. B., Inhibition of sarcolemmal Na^+, K^+-ATPase by palmitoyl carnitine: potentiation by propranolol, *Am. J. Physiol.*, 248, 75, 1985.

55. Dhalla, N. S., Kolar, F., Shah, K. R., and Ferrari, R., Effects of some L-carnitine derivatives on heart membrane ATPases, *Cardiovasc. Drugs Ther.*, 5, 25, 1991.

56. Vaartjes, W. J., Kemp, A., Jr., Souverijon, J. H. M., and Van Den Gergh, S. G., Inhibition by fatty acyl esters of adenine nucleotide translocator in rat-liver mitochondria, *FEBS Lett.*, 23, 303, 1972.

57. Heathers, G. P., Yamada, K. A., Kanter, E. M., and Corr, P. B., Long-chain acylcarnitines mediate the hypoxia-induced increase in α_1-adrenergic receptors on adult canine myocytes, *Circ. Res.*, 61, 735, 1987.

58. Hodgkin, D. D., Boucek, R. J., Purdy, R. E., Pearce, W. J., Fraser, I. M., and Gilbert, R. D., Dietary lipids modify receptor- and non-receptor-dependent components of α_1-adrenoceptor-mediated contraction, *Am. J. Physiol.*, 261, 1465, 1991.

59. Inoue, D. and Pappano, A. J., L-Palmitylcarnitine and calcium ions act similarly on excitatory ionic currents in avian ventricular muscle, *Circ. Res.*, 52, 625, 1983.
60. Spedding, M. and Mir, A. K., Direct activation of Ca^{2+} channels by palmitoyl carnitine, a putative endogenous ligand, *Br. J. Pharmacol.*, 92, 457, 1987.
61. Orrenius, S., McConkey, D. J., Bellomo, G., and Cicotera, P., Role of Ca^{2+} in toxic cell killing, *TIPS*, 10, 281, 1989.
62. Levy, J., Gavin, J. R., and Sowers, J. R., Diabetes mellitus: a disease of abnormal cellular calcium metabolism, *Am. J. Med.*, 96, 260, 1994.
63. Patel, M. B., Zhang, P. L., Patel, A. C., and Patel, K. P., Altered pressure-volume relation of right atrium and venoatrial junction in diabetic rats, *Am. J. Physiol.*, 263, 1017, 1992.
64. Afzal, N., Ganguly, P. K., Dhalla, K. S., Pierce, G. N., Singal, P. K., and Dhalla, N. S., Beneficial effects of verapamil in diabetic cardiomyopathy, *Diabetes*, 37, 936, 1988.
65. Afzal, N., Pierce, G. N., Elimban, V., Beamish, R. E., and Dhalla, N. S., Influence of verapamil on some subcellular defects in diabetic cardiomyopathy, *Am. J. Physiol.*, 256, 453, 1989.
66. DeFronzo, R. A., Jacot, E., Jequier, E., Maeder, E., Wahren, J., and Felber, J. P., The effect of insulin on the disposal of intravenous glucose: results from indirect calorimetry and hepatic and femoral venous catheterization, *Diabetes*, 30, 1000, 1981.
67. Suzuki, K. and Kono, T., Evidence that insulin causes translocation of glucose transport activity to the plasma membrane from intracellular storage site, *Proc. Natl. Acad. Sci. U.S.A.*, 77, 2542, 1980.
68. Kobayashi, M. and Olefsky, J. M., Effects of streptozotocin-induced diabetes on insulin binding, glucose transport and intracellular glucose metabolism in isolated rat adipocytes, *Diabetes*, 28, 87, 1979.
69. Eckel, J. and Reinauer, H., Insulin action on glucose transport in isolated cardiac myocytes: signaling pathways and diabetes induced alterations, *Biochem. Soc. Trans.*, 18, 1135, 1990.
70. Zuniga-Guarjardo, S., Steiner, G., and Zinman, B., Insulin resistance and action in hypertriglyceridemia, *Diabetes Res. Clin. Pract.*, 14, 55, 1991.
71. Bieger, W. P., Michel, G., Barwich, D., Biehl, K., and Wirth, A., Diminished insulin receptors on monocytes and erythrocytes in hypertriglyceridemia, *Metabolism*, 33, 982, 1984.
72. Eckel, J., Asskamp, B., and Reinauer, H., Induction of insulin resistance in primary cultured adult cardiac myocytes, *Endocrinology*, 129, 345, 1991.
73. Das, I., Effects of heart work and insulin on glycogen metabolism in the perfused rat heart, *Am. J. Physiol.*, 224, 7, 1993.
74. Chen, V. and Ianuzzo, C. D., Dosage effect of streptozotocin on rat tissue enzyme activities and glycogen concentration, *Can. J. Physiol. Pharmacol.*, 60, 1251, 1982.
75. Wall, S. R. and Lopaschuk, G. D., Glucose oxidation rates in fatty acid-perfused isolated working hearts from diabetic rats, *Biochim. Biophys. Acta*, 1006, 97, 1989.
76. Rodrigues, B., Cam, M. C., and McNeill, J. H., Myocardial substrate metabolism: implications for diabetic cardiomyopathy, *J. Mol. Cell. Cardiol.*, 27, 169, 1995.
77. Tutwiler, G. F., Kirsh, T., Mohrbacher, R. J., and Ho, W., Pharmacologic profile of methyl 2-tetradecylglycidate (McN-3716) — an orally effective hypoglycemic agent, *Metab. Clin. Exp.*, 27, 1539, 1978.
78. Rosen, P. and Reinauer, P., Inhibition of carnitine palmitoyltransferase 1 by phenylalkyloxiranecarboxylic acid and its influence on lipolysis and glucose metabolism in isolated, perfused hearts of streptozotocin-diabetic rats, *Metabolism*, 33, 177, 1984.
79. Martin, C., Odeon, R., Cohen, R., and Beylor, M., Mechanisms of the glucose lowering effect of a carnitine palmitoyl transferase inhibitor in normal and diabetic rats, *Metabolism*, 40, 420, 1991.
80. Wolf, H. P. O. and Engel, D. W., Decrease of fatty acid oxidation, ketogenesis and gluconeogenesis in isolated perfused rat liver by phenylalkyl oxirane carboxylate (B807-27) due to inhibition of CPT 1 (EC2.3.1.21), *Eur. J. Biochem.*, 146, 359, 1985.
81. Dillmann, W. H., Methyl palmoxirate increases Ca^{2+}-myosin ATPase activity and changes myosin isozyme distribution in the diabetic heart, *Am. J. Physiol.*, 248, 602, 1985.
82. Lopaschuk, G. D., Wall, S. R., Olley, P. M., and Davies, N. J., Etomoxir, a carnitine palmitoyltransferase 1 inhibitor, protects hearts from fatty acid-induced ischemic injury independent of changes in long chain acylcarnitine, *Circ. Res.*, 63, 1036, 1988.

83. Reaven, G. A., Chang, H., and Hoffman, B. B., Additive hypoglycemic effects of drugs that modify free-fatty acid metabolism by different mechanisms in rats with streptozotocin-induced diabetes, *Diabetes*, 37, 28, 1988.

84. Langer, G. A., Events at the cardiac sarcolemma: localization and movement of contractile-dependent calcium, *Fed. Proc.*, 35, 1274, 1976.

85. Langer, G. A., The structure and function of the myocardial cell surface, *Am. J. Physiol.*, 235, H461, 1978.

86. Dhalla, N. S., Das, P. K., and Sharma, G. P., Subcellular basis of cardiac contractile failure, *J. Mol. Cell. Cardiol.*, 10, 363, 1978.

87. Schwartz, A., Active transport in mammalian myocardium, in *The Mammalian Myocardium*, Langer, J. A. and Brady, A. J., Eds, John Wiley & Sons, New York, 1974, 81.

88. Caroni, P. and Carafoli, E., The Ca^{2+}-pumping ATPase of heart sarcolemma, *J. Biol. Chem.*, 256, 3263, 1981.

89. Philipson, K. D., Bersohn, M. M., and Nishimoto, A. Y., Effects of pH on Na^+-Ca^+ exchange in canine cardiac sarcolemmal vesicles, *Circ. Res.*, 50, 287, 1982.

90. Pierce, G. N., Kutryk, M. J. B. V., and Dhalla, N. S., Alterations in calcium binding and composition of the cardiac sarcolemmal membrane in chronic diabetes, *Proc. Natl. Acad. Sci. U.S.A.*, 80, 5412, 1983.

91. Philipson, K. D., Bers, D. M., and Nishimoto, A. Y., The role of phospholipids in the Ca^{2+}-binding of isolated cardiac sarcolemma, *J. Mol. Cell. Cardiol.*, 12, 1159, 1980.

92. Strittmatter, W. J., Hirata, F., and Axelrod, J., Regulation of β-adrenergic receptor by methylation of membrane phospholipids, in *Advances in Cyclic Nucleotide Research*, Vol. 14, Dumont, J. E., Greengard, P., and Robison, G. A., Eds., Raven Press, New York, 1981, 83.

93. Hirata, F. and Axelrod, J., Phospholipid methylation and biological signal transmission, *Science*, 209, 1082, 1980.

94. Strittmatter, W. J., Hirata, F., and Axelrod, J., Increased Ca^{2+}-ATPase activity associated with methylation of phospholipids in human erythrocytes, *Biochem. Biophys. Res. Commun.*, 88, 147, 1979.

95. Ganguly, P. K., Rice, K. M., Panagia, V., and Dhalla, N. S., Sarcolemmal phosphatidylethanolamine N-methylation diabetic cardiomyopathy, *Circ. Res.*, 55, 504, 1984.

96. Pierce, G. N. and Dhalla, N. S., Sarcolemmal Na^+-K^+-ATPase activity in diabetic rat heart, *Am. J. Physiol.*, 245, 241, 1981.

97. Tsuchida, K., Watajima, H., and Otomo, S., Calcium current in rat diabetic ventricular myocytes, *Am. J. Physiol.*, 267, 2280, 1994.

98. Wichelaus, A., Russ, M., Petersen, S., and Eckel, J., G protein expression and adenylate cyclase regulation in ventricular cardiomyocytes from STZ diabetic rats, *Am. J. Physiol.*, 267, 548, 1994.

99. Smith, C. I., Pierce, G. N., and Dhalla, N. S., Alterations in adenylate cyclase activity due to streptozotocin-induced diabetic cardiomyopathy, *Life Sci.*, 34, 1223, 1984.

100. Heyliger, C. E., Pierce, G. N., Singal, P. K., Beamish, R. E., and Dhalla, N. S., Cardiac alpha- and beta-adrenergic receptor alterations in diabetic cardiomyopathy, *Basic Res. Cardiol.*, 77, 610, 1982.

101. Philipson, K. D., Bers, D. M., Nishimoto, A. Y., and Langer, G. N., Binding of Ca^{2+} and Na^{2+} to sarcolemmal membranes: relation to control of myocardial contractility, *Am. J. Physiol.*, 238, H373, 1980.

102. Drummond, G. I., The role of the sarcolemma in cardiac function, *Tex. Rep. Biol. Med.*, 39, 37, 1979.

103. Reuter, H. and Seitz, N., The dependence of calcium efflux from cardiac muscle on temperature and external ion composition, *J. Physiol.*, 195, 451, 1968.

104. Makino, N., Dhalla, K. S., Eliban, V., and Dhalla, N. S., Heart sarcolemmal Na^+–Ca^{2+} exchange and Ca^{2+}-pump activities in chronic diabetes, *Fed. Proc.*, 44, 2451, 1985.

105. Katz, A. M., Excitation-contraction coupling, in *Physiology of the Heart*, Raven Press, New York, 1977, 137.

106. Pierce, G. N. and Dhalla, N. S., Heart mitochondrial function in chronic experimental diabetes in rats, *Can. J. Cardiol.*, 1, 48, 1985.

107. Goranson, E. S. and Erulkar, S. D., The effect of insulin on the aerobic phosphorylation of creatinine in tissues from alloxan-diabetic rats, *Arch. Biochem.*, 24, 40, 1949.
108. Chen, V. and Ianuzzo, C. D., Dosage effect of streptozotocin on rat tissue enzyme activities and glycogen concentration, *Can. J. Physiol. Pharmacol.*, 60, 1251, 1982.
109. Haugaard, E. S. and Haugaard, N., Diabetic metabolism. I. Carbohydrate utilization and high energy phosphate formation in heart homogenate from normal and alloxan-diabetic rats, *J. Biol. Chem.*, 239, 705, 1964.
110. Reuter, H., Exchange of calcium ions in the mammalian myocardium, *Circ. Res.*, 34, 599, 1974.
111. MacLennan, D. H., Purification and properties of an adenosine triphosphatase from sarcoplasmic reticulum, *J. Biol. Chem.*, 245, 4508, 1970.
112. Chamberlain, B. K., Levitsky, D. L., and Fleischer, S., Isolation and characterization of canine cardiac sarcoplasmic reticulum with improved Ca^{2+} transport properties, *J. Biol. Chem.*, 258, 6602, 1983.
113. Penpargkul, S., Fein, F., Sonnenblick, E. H., and Scheuer, J., Depressed cardiac sarcoplasmic reticulum function from diabetic rats, *J. Mol. Cell. Cardiol.*, 13, 303, 1981.
114. Ganguly, P. K., Pierce, G. N., Dhalla, K. S., and Dhalla, N. S., Defective sarcoplasmic reticular calcium transport inn diabeteic cardiomyopathy, *Am. J. Physiol.*, 244, E528, 1983.
115. Bouchard, R. A. and Bose, D., Influence of experimental diabetes on sarcoplasmic reticulum function in rat ventricular muscle, *Am. J. Physiol.*, 260, 341, 1991.
116. Dillmann, W. H., Diabetes mellitus induces changes in cardiac myosin of the rat, *Diabetes*, 29, 579, 1980.
117. Malhotra, A., Penpargkul, S., Fein, F. S., Sonnenblick, E. H., and Scheuer, J., The effect of streptozotocin-induced diabetes in rats on cardiac contractile proteins, *Circ. Res.*, 49, 1243, 1981.
118. Ren, J. and Davidoff, A. J., Diabetes rapidly induces contractile dysfunctions in isolated ventricular myocytes, *Am. J. Physiol.*, 272, 148, 1997.
119. Davidoff, A. J. and Ren, J., Low insulin and high glucose induce abnormal relaxation in cultured adult rat ventricular myocytes, *Am. J. Physiol.*, 272, 159, 1997.
120. Jackson, C. V., McGarth, G. M., Tahiliani, A. G., Vadlamudi, R. V. S. V., and McNeill, J. H., A functional and ultrastructural analysis of experimental diabetic rat myocardium: manifestation of cardiomyopathy, *Diabetes*, 34, 876, 1985.
121. McGarth, G. M. and McNeill, J. H., Cardiac ultrastructural changes in streptozotocin-induced diabetic rats: effects of insulin treatment, *Can. J. Cardiol.*, 2, 164, 1986.

5

The Effects of Experimental Diabetes on the Cytochrome P450 System and Other Metabolic Pathways

Costas Ioannides, Peter R. Flatt, and Christopher R. Barnett

CONTENTS

0-8493-1667-7/99/$0.00+$.50
© 1999 by CRC Press LLC

The human body is continuously exposed to a myriad of, structurally very diverse, chemicals, both naturally occurring and anthropogenic. Some of these are taken voluntarily, e.g., drugs and food additives, but the vast majority are taken involuntarily, e.g., atmospheric pollutants and dietary chemicals which may be inherent to the diet, contaminants, or generated during the cooking process. Exposure to such chemicals is unavoidable. The body cannot exploit these chemicals either by using them as a source of energy or by converting them to forms that can function as structural building units. Many of these chemicals possess biological activity that, in some cases, can prove beneficial, as, for example, in the treatment of disease, but in many cases they are detrimental and can lead to diseases such as cancer. Hundreds of chemicals have been linked to human disease, either following strong epidemiological evidence or extrapolation of experimental evidence obtained in animals. No living organism could sustain such a relentless exposure to chemicals unless it was endowed by effective protecting mechanisms.

The initial response of the body to the presence of a foreign chemical is to eliminate it, an objective the body achieves through excretion, primarily through the kidney and bile. However, as most chemicals that find their way into the body are lipophilic, this process is inefficient. To enhance the hydrophilicity of these compounds, and thus ensure a more rapid elimination through excretion, the body has developed a number of enzyme systems adept at metabolizing these foreign compounds, frequently referred to as xenobiotics, to more polar and, consequently, more readily excretable metabolites. Such metabolism, moreover, terminates the biological activity of chemicals since the metabolites, in contrast to the parent compounds, are unable to react with receptors and macromolecules to elicit a biological response. A paradox of xenobiotic metabolism is that deactivation is not always the outcome, but may result in the production of deleterious reactive intermediates. This chapter will be divided into two parts; the first part will deal briefly with xenobiotic metabolism and the major enzyme systems involved, whereas the second part will discuss in detail how these enzyme systems are perturbed by diabetes mellitus.

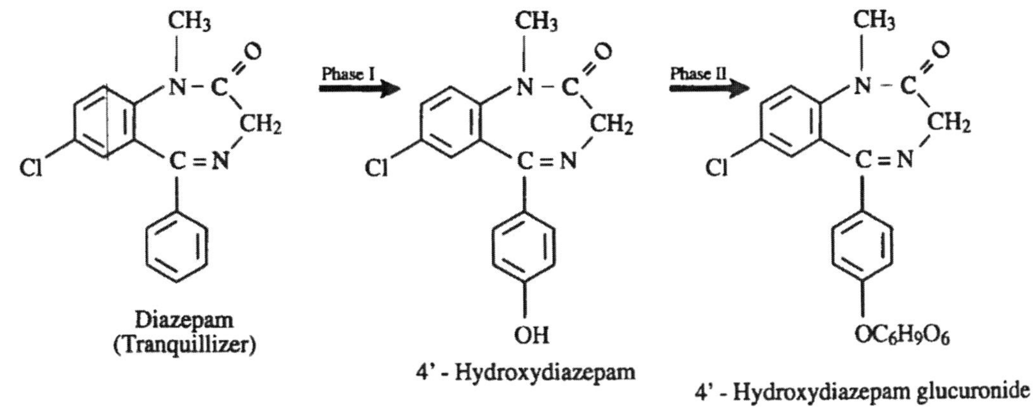

FIGURE 5.1
Phase I and Phase II metabolism of diazepam.

5.1 Xenobiotic Metabolism

5.1.1 Nature of Xenobiotic Metabolism

The metabolism of xenobiotics, including drugs, proceeds through two phases; Phase I encompasses pathways that involve largely the incorporation of an oxygen into the substrate, giving it a more polar character, as a first step in its elimination. The hydrophilicity of the substrate is further enhanced by the Phase II reactions, where the product of the Phase I metabolism is conjugated with hydrophilic endogenous substrates such as glucuronic acid, sulfate, aminoacids, and the tripeptide glutathione. Indeed, a function of Phase I metabolism is to prepare the chemical for Phase II metabolism by introducing or unmasking functional groups such as –OH, –COOH, etc., to which the endogenous substrates may be attached. These, highly polar and biologically inactive, conjugated metabolites are more readily excreted from the human body than the parent compounds. Chemicals that already possess a group that can participate in a conjugation reaction may bypass Phase I metabolism (Figure 5.1).

5.1.2 Bioactivation of Chemicals

The vast majority of chemicals that express toxicity are per se innocuous and chemically unreactive, thus precluding any interactions with cellular components. To express their toxicity, they must be metabolically converted to highly reactive intermediates, potent electrophiles with electron-deficient centers, which can interact covalently with vital cellular macromolecules such DNA, RNA, lipids, and proteins. That is to say, these chemicals acquire through metabolism the necessary reactivity that allows them to interact with cellular components. Such chemicals, referred to as *indirect acting*, will manifest toxicity only if the body possesses the necessary enzyme systems to convert them to their reactive form(s); such reactive forms are epoxides, carbonium ions, and nitrenium ions (Figure 5.2). Numerous adducts have been isolated resulting from the interaction of reactive intermediates with DNA, RNA, and protein. The process by which an innocuous chemical is converted to a reactive intermediate is known as *metabolic activation* or *bioactivation*. Clearly, with some chemicals, metabolism confers adverse biological activity (Figure 5.3). A relatively small number of chemicals are inherently reactive, and can interact with cellular macromolecules to elicit toxicity without prior requirement for metabolism; such chemicals are termed *direct acting*. Indirect-acting chemicals are endowed with higher toxic potential than direct-acting chemicals, since the reactive forms of the former are generated within the cell, in close proximity to macromolecules, e.g., DNA, with which they can readily interact, and are not required to gain entry into the cell. For such chemicals, toxicity and carcinogenicity are inextricably associated with their metabolism. In contrast, direct-acting chemicals may be effectively neutralized during their transport from the site of entry into the body to the target site. Moreover, in this case, metabolism almost invariably leads to deactivation and attenuation of toxicity.

The generated reactive intermediates may interact with DNA to form adducts which, if they escape the repair mechanisms of the cell, may be fixed and passed to the progeny, thus giving rise to a mutation (see Figure 5.3). This constitutes the first stage in the complex process of carcinogenesis, termed *initiation*, and entails irreversible DNA damage (genotoxicity). Initiation is followed by the poorly understood, long-term stages of promotion and progression leading to the appearance of a tumor. Cells may detach from a tumor in one tissue and be transported to other tissues to induce secondary tumors, the process known as *metastasis*. Reactive intermediates of chemicals may also induce DNA damage through an alternative mechanism that involves interaction with molecular oxygen to produce superoxide anions which, in the presence of traces of iron salts, can be transformed to the highly reactive hydroxyl radical (OH), a powerful oxidant. The hydroxyl radical, as well as other reactive oxygen species, can cause cellular damage similar to that resulting from the covalent interaction of the reactive species of chemicals with cellular components; they oxidize DNA to induce mutations, oxidize lipids to form lipid peroxides which appear to play an important role in the promotion and progression stages of chemical carcinogenesis, and also oxidize proteins. It is of interest that reactive oxygen species are currently being implicated it the etiology and progression of a number of major chronic diseases, including atherosclerosis, cancer, diabetes, and rheumatoid arthritis.[1-3]

The reactive intermediates of chemicals may also interact covalently with proteins, disturbing physiological homeostasis, leading to cell death. In the last decade, it has also become apparent that reactive intermediates can also function as haptens, conferring on proteins antigenic potential and eliciting immunotoxicity.[4] Drugs such as tienilic acid, dihydralazine, and halothane are metabolically converted by the cytochrome P450–dependent mixed-function oxidases (see below) to metabolites that bind covalently to proteins to generate neoantigens resulting in the production of autoantibodies. Subsequent exposure to these drugs provokes an autoimmune response leading to hepatitis.

5.1.3   Deactivation of Chemicals

As already discussed, in most cases metabolism of a chemical results in loss of biological activity and, consequently, is viewed as deactivation. As such, these processes constitute a major defense mechanism against chemicals; such deactivation pathways predominate in the metabolism of chemicals. A second line of defense is also available to deal with chemicals that have, paradoxically, been converted to toxic, reactive intermediates. This defensive mechanism involves nucleophilic constituents of the cell, the most prominent of which is the simple tripeptide glutathione which, through the nucleophilic –SH group of the cysteine moiety, interacts and neutralizes electrophiles, thus impeding their

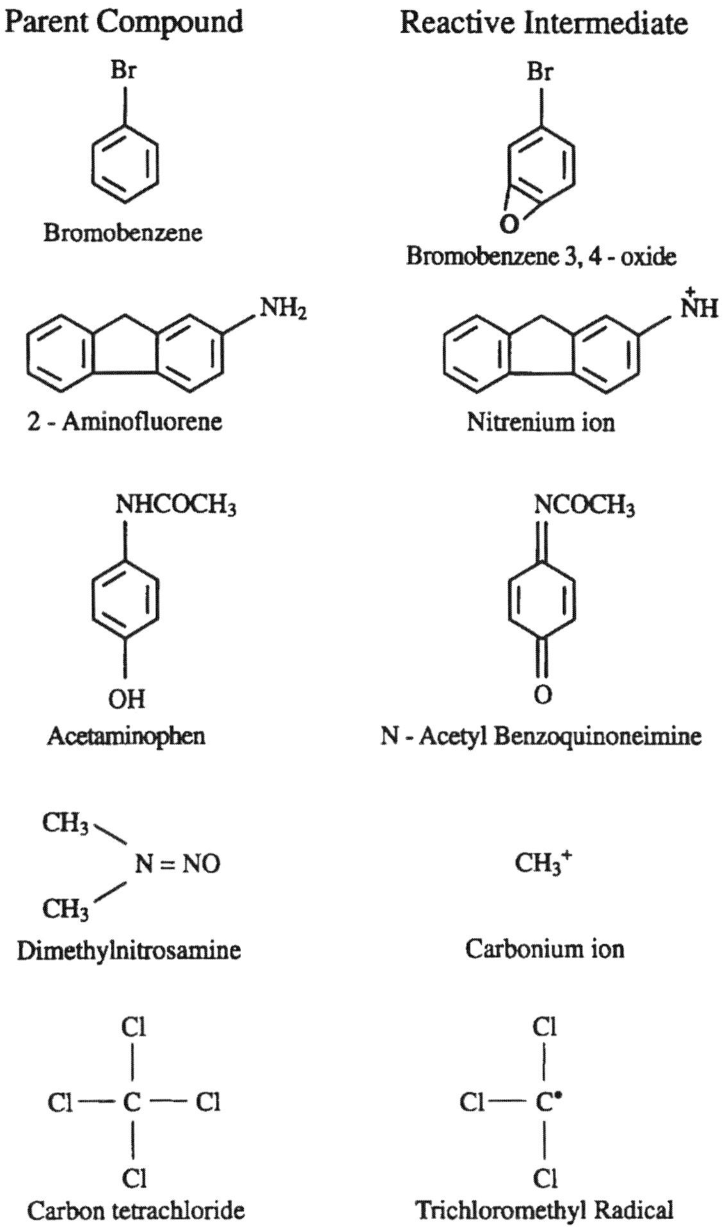

Parent Compound

Reactive Intermediate

Br

Bromobenzene

Br

Bromobenzene 3, 4 - oxide

NH$_2$

2 - Aminofluorene

$\overset{+}{N}H$

Nitrenium ion

NHCOCH$_3$

OH

Acetaminophen

NCOCH$_3$

O

N - Acetyl Benzoquinoneimine

CH$_3$
      N = NO
CH$_3$

Dimethylnitrosamine

CH$_3^+$

Carbonium ion

Cl
|
Cl — C — Cl
|
Cl

Carbon tetrachloride

Cl
|
Cl — C$^\bullet$
|
Cl

Trichloromethyl Radical

FIGURE 5.2
Toxic chemicals and their reactive intermediates.

interaction with cellular components. The conjugation of reactive nucleophiles with glutathione is catalyzed by the ubiquitous glutathione *S*-transferases. Depletion of glutathione, e.g., following exposure to megadoses of drugs or long-term ingestion of inadequate diets, exacerbates the toxicity of chemicals that are dependent on this pathway for their deactivation. The toxin bromobenzene is activated by oxidation to form an epoxide, which is normally detoxicated through interaction with glutathione to yield a glutathionyl conjugate. As a result, bromobenzene toxicity is markedly potentiated in animals where glutathione has been depleted by starvation (Figure 5.4). A number of other

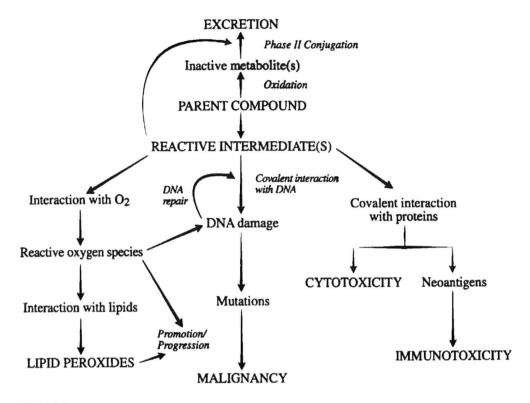

FIGURE 5.3
Bioactivation of chemicals.

enzyme systems protect the cell against reactive oxygen species; such systems are superoxide dismutase, which converts the superoxy anion to H_2O_2, and glutathione peroxidase and catalase that break down H_2O_2 and other peroxides to water (Figure 5.5). Moreover, the cells contain a number of antioxidants, such as vitamins A, E, and C, which also play an important role in the detoxication of reactive oxygen species.

5.1.4 Importance of Activation/Deactivation Balance

Clearly, a chemical is metabolized through a number of pathways, most of which lead to deactivation and, by making the chemical more hydrophilic, facilitate its elimination through excretion. However, some routes of metabolism, frequently just a single one, may produce a reactive intermediate, which, if it bypasses or overwhelms the protective mechanisms, is capable of inducing toxicity. The amount of reactive intermediate formed, and hence the manifestation of toxicity, is dependent on the rates of the competing pathways of activation and deactivation. If an animal species favors the activation of a chemical, then it will be susceptible to its toxicity, whereas if deactivation predominates, it will be resistant. For example, the rat is relatively resistant to the toxicity of acetaminophen (paracetamol) because its ability to form the reactive intermediate by oxidation is limited, whereas the hamster, an animal species that readily converts it to the reactive intermediate, is very susceptible.[5] Furthermore, the guinea pig is refractive to the carcinogenicity of 2-acetylaminofluorene because it is unable to catalyse the first step in its activation.[6] Clearly, toxicity is not simply a consequence of the intrinsic molecular

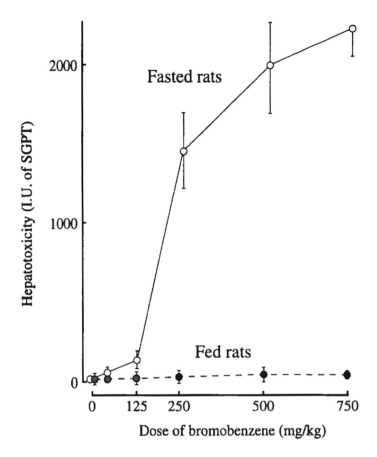

FIGURE 5.4
Bromobenzene toxicity in fed and fasted rats. (Adapted from Reference 138).

$$2GSH + H_2O_2 \xrightarrow{\text{\textit{Glutathione peroxidase}}} GSSG + 2H_2O$$

$$2H_2O_2 \xrightarrow{\text{\textit{Catalase}}} 2H_2O + O_2$$

$$O_2^{\cdot} + O_2^{\cdot} + 2H^+ \xrightarrow{\text{\textit{Superoxide dismutase}}} H_2O_2 + O_2$$

FIGURE 5.5
Enzyme systems protecting against reactive oxygen species.

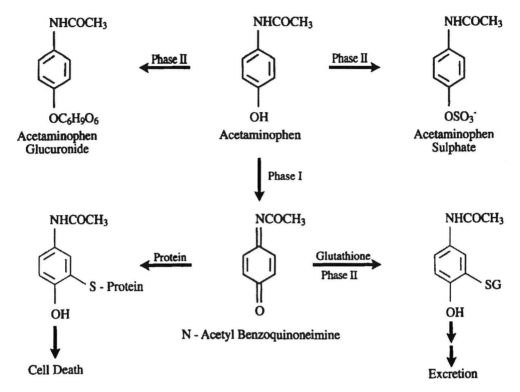

FIGURE 5.6
Metabolism of acetaminophen.

structure and physicochemical properties of the chemical, but is also largely dependent on the nature and levels of the enzymes present in the animal at the time of exposure.

Activation pathways, in most cases, represent a minor route of metabolism so that the generation of reactive metabolites is minimal, the low levels formed are effectively detoxicated by the defensive mechanisms, and consequently no toxicity is apparent. Under certain conditions, however, the activation pathways assume greater importance, leading to enhanced production of reactive intermediates, overwhelming the deactivation pathways, thus increasing the likelihood of an interaction with vital cellular macromolecules and of the ensuing toxicity. Such a situation may arise during drug overdosage, where the major deactivation pathway is saturated, so that metabolism is pushed through the normally minor activation pathway. For example, the mild analgesic drug acetaminophen, at therapeutic doses, is effectively deactivated through conjugate formation with glucuronide and sulfate (Figure 5.6); to a very small extent it undergoes oxidation to a reactive intermediate (*N*-acetyl benzoquinoneimine), which is detoxicated by conjugation with glutathione. During overdosage, as in suicide attempts, the acetaminophen conjugation pathways are saturated as a result of unavailability of sulfate and UDP-glucuronic acid, essential cofactors for these conjugations; the rate of consumption of these endogenous substrates exceeds their rate of supply. The consequence is that more of the drug is metabolized by oxidation, and the increased amounts of the reactive intermediate deplete cellular glutathione, so that the defensive mechanism falters, allowing the reactive intermediate to interact covalently with hepatic proteins leading to hepatotoxicity. Indeed, treatment of this condition involves supplying the body with precursors of cysteine, e.g., *N*-acetylcysteine and methionine, the limiting aminoacid in the biosynthesis of glutathione.

Activation pathways can also be stimulated in cases where the enzyme systems involved are induced as a result of previous exposure to other chemicals. Induction of the xenobiotic-metabolizing enzymes is a common phenomenon encountered not only in animals but also in humans. Such inducing agents are abundant in the environment, being present in the air people breathe, especially in polluted urban areas, and in the diet, being inherent to the food, e.g., caffeine, or contaminants generated during cooking, e.g., polycyclic aromatic hydrocarbons. For example, the cytochrome P450 proteins responsible for the conversion of acetaminophen to its reactive intermediate are induced as a result of previous chronic exposure to alcohol. As a result, chronic alcoholics are more susceptible to the hepatotoxicity of this drug.

5.1.5 Fate of Reactive Intermediates

As the liver contains the highest concentration of most xenobiotic-metabolizing enzyme systems, it is the most prominent tissue in the bioactivation of chemicals, whereas other tissues, having a more-restricted number of enzymes generally present at much lower levels, play a more limited role in the production of chemical reactive intermediates. Under such circumstances, it would be logical to expect that the liver would be the principal target of toxic manifestations. In reality, however, toxicity is encountered in many tissues, many of which have minimal or no ability to activate chemicals. It appears that reactive intermediates can be sufficiently stable to be exported from the liver to other tissues. The site of benzene toxicity, expressed through metabolite(s), is the bone marrow, but attempts to detect metabolizing activity have failed, suggesting that the liver, a tissue that readily activates benzene, supplies the reactive metabolites to the bone marrow. The mechanisms through which reactive intermediates leave the hepatocyte and are transported to other tissues have not been elucidated.

5.1.6 Enzymes Involved in the Metabolism of Chemicals

A number of enzyme systems contribute to the Phase I metabolism of chemicals, both activation and deactivation, including the cytochrome P450–dependent mixed-function oxidases, flavin monooxygenases, and the prostaglandin synthases. Almost every enzyme system concerned with the metabolism of chemicals has also the potential to catalyze the formation of reactive intermediates.

5.1.6.1 Cytochromes P450

The cytochrome P450–dependent mixed-function oxidases are by far the most important enzyme system in the metabolism of xenobiotics. Almost every lipophilic chemical that finds its way into the body is, at least partly, subject to metabolism catalysed by this enzyme system. This versatile oxygenase inserts oxygen into specific sites in organic molecules to make them polar and prepare them for Phase II metabolism. It displays unprecedented substrate specificity, being efficient in metabolising structurally very diverse chemicals, of markedly different molecular shape and size. The metabolic function of the cytochrome P450 system is not confined to xenobiotics, but extends to vital endogenous substrates. It plays an important role in the metabolism of steroid hormones, both in their biosynthesis and catabolism, eicosanoids such as prostaglandins, fatty acids such as arachidonic acid, and vitamins such as vitamins A and D. The cytochrome P450–dependent mixed-function oxidase system comprises an electron transport chain consisting of the flavoprotein cytochrome P450 reductase and the haemoprotein

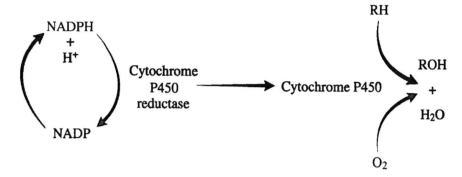

FIGURE 5.7
The cytochrome P450 electron transport chain.

cytochrome P450, which functions as a terminal oxidase (Figure 5.7). It catalyses the incorporation of one atom of molecular oxygen to the substrate (RH) while the second atom forms water.

$$RH + NADPH + H^+ + O_2 \rightarrow ROH + NADP^+ + H_2O$$

No single enzyme protein could accommodate such a diversity of substrates, so it is not surprising that the cytochrome P450 system exists as a superfamily of enzyme proteins, being subdivided into families that comprise one or more subfamilies, each containing one or more proteins (isoforms). Families are denoted with the prefix CYP, followed by an arabic number representing the family, a capital letter for the subfamily, and another arabic number showing the individual cytochrome P450 protein; for example, CYP2E1 denotes cytochrome P450 family two, subfamily E, protein one. Each cytochrome P450 protein is characterized by its own substrate specificity, even stereospecificity, and this allows the use of chemical probes, selectively metabolized by a single isoform, to monitor the activity of individual enzymes. Small structural changes in the amino acid sequence can result in significant alteration of substrate specificity and catalytic activity of individual cytochrome P450 proteins. As polyclonal antibodies against most xenobiotic-metabolizing cytochrome P450 isoforms are now readily available, they are readily used to determine the tissue apoprotein levels of cytochromes P450. Of the various families of cytochrome P450, CYP1, CYP2, and CYP3 are by far the most important in xenobiotic metabolism. Table 5.1 outlines some of the more important characteristics, including their role in drug metabolism and in the bioactivation of chemicals.

Cytochromes P450 are tightly regulated by hormones such as growth hormone and the sex hormones, but levels can also be modulated by exposure to chemicals; such chemicals can induce or inhibit cytochrome P450 activity, leading to interactions that can be of major toxicological relevance. As already discussed, alcoholics, by virtue of their ability to readily catalyze the oxidation of acetaminophen to its reactive intermediate, are vulnerable to the toxicity of this drug. Alcohol is a selective inducer of CYP2E1, one of the major cytochrome P450 isoforms catalyzing this activation pathway, and this is the underlying mechanism for this interaction. Chemicals, including drugs such as cimetidine and ketoconazole, can inhibit cytochrome P450 activity and, consequently, lead to adverse drug interactions when coadministered with other drugs that are dependent on this enzyme system for their metabolism and elimination. Inhibition of metabolism leads, on repeated administration, to accumulation and the appearance of side effects commensurate with overdosage.

TABLE 5.1

Characteristics of the Xenobiotic-Metabolizing Cytochrome P450 Proteins

Family	Subfamily	Role in Drug Metabolism	Example of Drug Substrates	Role in Metabolic Activation	Example of Activated Chemicals
CYP1	A	Limited	Theophylline Imipramine	Very extensive	Benzo(a)pyrene 4-Aminobiphenyl
CYP2	A	Limited	Coumarin Propranolol	Limited	6-Aminochrysene DMN
	B	Limited	Benzphetamine Hexobarbitone	Limited	Cyclophosphamide Cocaine
	C	Extensive	Mephenytoin Tolbutamide	Very limited	Tienilic acid
	D	Extensive	Debrisoquine Bufuralol	Very limited	NNK
	E	Extensive	Chlorzoxazone Enflurane	Extensive	Acetaminophen Benzene
CYP3	A	Extensive	Dapsone Erythromycin	Limited	Aflatoxin B_1 Senecionine
CYP4	A	None	—	None	—
	B	None	—	Very limited	Aminofluorene 4-Ipomeanol

DMN, dimethylnitrosamine; NNK, 4-(methylnitrosamino)-1-(3-pyridyl)-1-butanone.

5.1.6.1.1 CYP1 Family

CYP1 is one of the smallest cytochrome P450 families comprising two subfamilies, namely, CYP1A and CYP1B. The latter has only recently been described and little is known at present about its regulation and substrate specificity. In contrast, CYP1A has received enormous attention, being one of the first to be identified and purified from the liver of animals and humans; moreover, this subfamily, which consists of two isoforms, A1 and A2, plays a major role in the bioactivation of chemicals, including some of the major classes of human carcinogens. The principal feature of CYP1A substrates is a planar molecular configuration. The CYP1A family is ubiquitous and appears to be the most conserved within the phylogenetic tree, the human proteins having similar substrate specificity to their rodent counterparts, alluding to a major role for this subfamily in a vital biological function.[7] Furthermore, it is extensively induced by exposure to a variety of chemicals, e.g., the human CYP1A is induced by smoking, exposure to drugs such as omeprazole, environmental pollutants such as polychlorinated biphenyls, and by the consumption of foods rich in indoles, such as cruciferous vegetables, or meat broiled in charcoal and thus contaminated by polycyclic aromatic compounds, products of the incomplete combustion of organic material.[8]

The activity of no other cytochrome P450 protein has been so closely linked to human cancer incidence. High levels of CYP1A activity in lymphocytes has been directly correlated with susceptibility to lung cancer.[9] Extensive studies conducted by the IARC in Lyon established good positive relationships between lung cancer and CYP1A1 activity in the lung of smokers.[10] Moreover, CYP1A activity has been related inversely to survival in human breast cancer.[11]

5.1.6.1.2 CYP2 Family

This is a one of largest families of cytochrome P450 comprising at least five subfamilies:

CYP2A — The major function of this subfamily is in steroid metabolism, and its role in the metabolism of xenobiotics is very limited, coumarin being the principal substrate so far identified. The human proteins are CYP2A6 and the closely related CYP2A7, and at least in the liver constitute minor isoforms, comprising some 1% of the total cytochrome P450 content. CYP2A6 contributes to the 4-hydroxylation of the anticancer drug cyclophosphamide, which in this case leads to the formation of the biologically active acrolein and phosphoramide mustard. At least in animals, CYP2A is inducible.

CYP2B — One of the first subfamilies to be purified from the liver of animals, CYP2B has been extensively studied and shown to display broad substrate specificity.[13] Although it metabolizes a large number of known chemical carcinogens, it tends to convert these to inactive metabolites and it is generally unable to convert them to their reactive intermediates.[8] An activating role has, however, been ascribed to it in certain instances as in the case of certain long-chain aliphatic nitrosamines and drugs like cocaine and cyclophosphamide, where it acts as the major catalyst for the bioactivation of this anticancer drug to the pharmacologically active form in humans. Like CYP2A, in humans it is a minor form representing less than 2% of the total liver cytochrome P450, the isoforms being CYP2B6 and CYP2B7.

CYP2C — This is a large subfamily that plays an important role in the metabolism of many drugs such as tolbutamide, warfarin, hydantoins, and diclofenac.[14] It also catalyzes the activation of the diuretic drug tienilic acid to form a protein-interacting intermediate which is responsible for its immunotoxicity (see above). An important aspect of this family is its genetic polymorphism, resulting in slow and fast metabolizers of drugs such as tolbutamide and mephenytoin.

CYP2D — This is the first cytochrome P450 family shown to contain isoforms that are subject to genetic polymorphism.[15] A polymorphism in the expression of human CYP2D6, a protein catalyzing the hydroxylation of the antihypertensive drug debrisoquine, has been established. About 5 to 10% of Caucasians lack an active form of this protein and are thus unable to metabolize debrisoquine and other drugs that rely on this isoform for their metabolism, such as bufurarol, sparteine, and dextromethorphan; patients lacking this protein show an exaggerated response when taking such drugs.

CYP2E — This subfamily is very active in the metabolism of low-molecular-weight compounds including short-chain alcohols and organic solvents, such as ether and chloroform.[16] It is active in the bioactivation of many chemical carcinogens such as benzene, nitrosamines such as dimethylnitrosamine, carcinogenic halogenated hydrocarbons such as carbon tetrachloride and vinyl chloride, and drugs such as acetaminophen. It mediates the metabolic activation of the anesthetic halothane to form a trifluoroacetyl intermediate, an active metabolite that interacts covalently with hepatic proteins forming neoantigens that are responsible for the hepatitis associated with this drug (see above). A major and important characteristic of CYP2E is its high propensity to generate reactive oxygen species, which have been linked to many chronic human diseases, such as cancer, cardiovascular disease, and diabetes mellitus. Reactive oxygen species are not only genotoxic, but can also enhance cellular proliferation and dysplastic growth, thus stimulating the promotional stage of carcinogenesis. CYP2E may therefore facilitate carcinogenesis by two distinct mechanisms, namely, the oxidative activation of chemicals and by the generation of reactive oxygen species. It has been purified from human liver, and it appears to have similar substrate preferences to the corresponding rat and rabbit protein. In common with the CYP1A, CYP2E appears also to be one of the most-conserved subfamilies among animal species. It is an inducible protein, and human CYP2E1 is elevated in chronic alcoholics.

5.1.6.1.3 CYP3 Family

CYP3 is the most abundant family in human liver and as a consequence plays a pivotal role in the metabolism of xenobiotics.[17] It is the most important family in the metabolism and deactivation of drugs in humans. Substrates include major drugs, such as erythromycin, cyclosporin, dapsone, tamoxifen, warfarin, nifedipine, and lovastatin. The major human form is CYP3A4, but other isoforms have also been detected, one of which, CYP3A7, is expressed only in the fetus and disappears shortly before birth. It is an inducible subfamily, and the human proteins are induced by barbiturates, dexamethasone, rifampicin, and troleandomycin.

5.1.6.1.4 CYP4 Family

Six subfamilies have been identified so far of which three, namely, CYP4A, CYP4B, and CYP4F, are found in humans.[18] No major role in the metabolism of xenobiotics has been ascribed to this family, its principal function being in the metabolism of endogenous substrates such as fatty acids and eicosanoids. However, a protein belonging to this family, namely, CYP4B1, expressed in the lungs of rodents, activates a number of aromatic amines. What prompted considerable interest in this family is the observation that peroxisomal proliferators, a major group of nongenotoxic rodent carcinogens that increase the number and size of peroxisomes and cause cellular proliferation, also induce this enzyme. It has now been established that peroxisomal proliferation, as exemplified by an increase in palmitoyl coenzyme A (CoA) oxidation, and CYP4A induction are coordinately regulated by the same receptor.[19] Many drugs, such as fibrate hypolipidemic drugs, and anti-inflammatories, such as ibuprofen and benoxaprofen, all stimulate CYP4 activity in addition to giving rise to peroxisomal proliferation.[20-22]

5.1.6.2 Peroxidases

Physiologically, the most important peroxidase is the glycoprotein prostaglandin synthetase, an enzyme found in the seminal vesicles, kidney, bladder, and lung but which is, however, absent from the liver.[23,24] Its physiological function is to convert arachidonic acid to prostaglandin H_2, which then proceeds to form thromboxanes, prostaglandins, and prostacyclins (Figure 5.8). The prostaglandin synthetase system comprises two activities, a fatty acid cyclooxygenase that converts arachidonic acid to the peroxide prostaglandin G_2, and a hydroperoxidase, which reduces the peroxide to the alcohol, prostaglandin H_2. During this second step chemicals may be metabolized to reactive forms by either the peroxidase activity or the peroxyl radicals generated. Xenobiotics metabolized by this enzyme system include drugs, such as acetaminophen, and carcinogenic aminocompounds, such as the occupational human carcinogen benzidine and the dietary carcinogen IQ (2-amino-3-methylimidazo[4,5-*f*]quinoline).

5.1.6.3 FAD Monooxygenases

Similar to the cytochromes P450, these multigene enzymes are also located in the endoplasmic reticulum and require oxygen and NADPH for their function.[25,26] They are capable of catalyzing the N- and S-oxidation of xenobiotics but, in contrast to cytochromes P450, they are unable to catalyze C-oxidations. A number of forms have been described, capable of oxidizing compounds to both reactive and less active metabolites.

5.1.6.4 Other Phase I Enzyme Systems

Although most chemicals are metabolized by oxidation, with some chemicals reduction can be an important route of metabolism and bioactivation. Nitroreductases and azoreductases catalyze the reduction of nitrocompounds to hydroxylamines and reduction of diazo bonds to the corresponding amines, respectively. In addition to mammalian

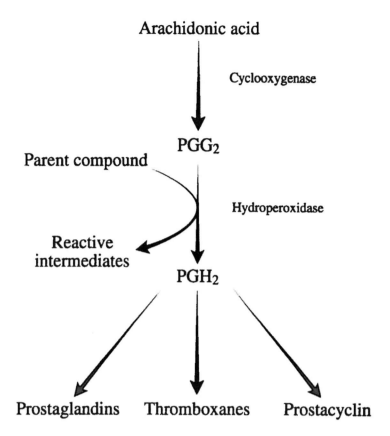

FIGURE 5.8
Bioactivation of chemicals by the prostaglandin synthetase system.

tissues, reductases are found in microorganisms that normally inhabit the gastrointestinal tract, so that a chemical may be subjected to metabolism before being absorbed.

5.1.6.5   Phase II Enzyme Systems

5.1.6.5.1   Epoxide Hydrolase

Epoxides are reactive intermediates of many xenobiotics and are usually formed following the oxidation of olefinic bonds by cytochromes P450. The epoxide hydrolases add water to these epoxides to convert them to the corresponding, less-reactive vicinal dihydrodiols, which are then excreted after conjugation with such substrates as sulfate and glucuronic acid (Figure 5.9). There are multiple forms of this enzyme and are encountered in the microsomes and cytosol.[27] Similar to the cytochrome P450 enzymes, epoxide hydrolases are inducible by xenobiotics.

5.1.6.5.2   Glutathione Conjugation

Conjugation with the simple tripeptide glutathione, catalyzed by the glutathione transferases, constitutes the most effective defensive mechanism through which the body protects itself from chemical insult.[28] For this reason, it is encountered in many organs at high concentrations; in the liver, the principal site of generation of reactive intermediates, it is present in concentrations as high as 10 mM. The sulfhydryl group of the cysteine acts as a nucleophile, attacking and neutralizing electrophiles, and in this way glutathione

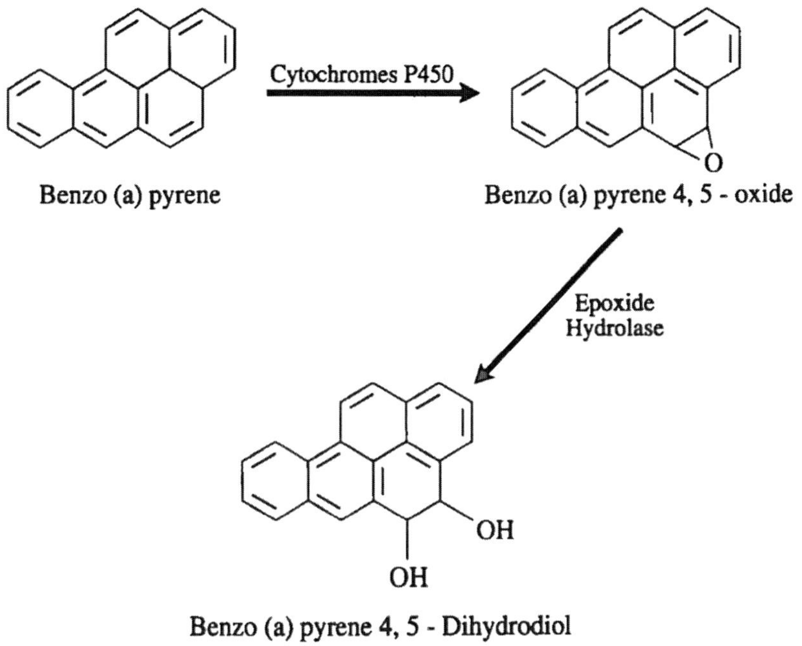

FIGURE 5.9
Epoxide hydrolase in the metabolism of benzo(a)pyrene.

protects critical cellular components from chemical injury. Indeed, the current search for chemicals with anticarcinogenic potential is frequently based on their ability to stimulate the detoxication of chemical carcinogens by glutathione conjugation. Glutathione S-transferases, catalyzing the conjugation with glutathione, are widespread enzymes present in most tissues and are localized in the cytosol and microsomes. Multiple forms are present and the soluble enzymes are divided into five gene families. Although the consequence of glutathione conjugation is largely one of detoxication, in a few cases, e.g., haloalkenes such as ethylene dibromide, the glutathione conjugate may be further processed enzymically to generate toxic intermediates.[29] The conjugate translocates into the kidney, where the glutamyl and glycine moieties are removed by the enzyme γ-glutamyl transpeptidase. The resulting cysteine conjugate, in addition to being detoxicated by acetylation to a mercapturic acid, is also activated by the pyridoxal phosphate-containing β-lyase to generate a reactive thiol, considered to be the ultimate toxic entity.

5.1.6.5.3 Acetylation

Acetylation is a major route of metabolism for aminocompounds and hydrazines, including drugs such as hydralazine and isoniazid; it involves the transfer of the acetyl group from acetyl CoA to amino, sulfhydryl, and hydroxyl groups, catalyzed by N-acetylases residing in the cytosol.[30] At least two forms of the enzyme exist *in humans*, namely, NAT1 and NAT2. They are capable of catalyzing N-acetylation, O-acetylation, and N,O-acyltransfer, these pathways being particularly important in the bioactivation of aminocompounds. These enzymes are subject to genetic polymorphism, with the population being divided into slow and rapid acetylators.

5.1.6.5.4 Sulfate Conjugation

Sulfotransferases are ubiquitous enzymes that catalyze the transfer of the activated form of sulfate (3′-phosphoadenosine-5′-phosphosulfate) to amino or hydroxyl groups, a very common pathway in xenobiotic metabolism.[31] Although in most cases sulfate conjugation is a detoxication reaction, insertion of sulfate to hydroxylamines generates unstable N-sulfonoxy metabolites, which break down spontaneously, forming highly electrophilic nitrenium ions that interact with DNA to produce mutations. In humans, two forms have been recognized, a thermostable and a thermolabile form. Unlike most other xenobiotic-metabolizing systems, sulfotransferases appear not to be readily inducible by exposure to chemicals.

5.1.6.5.5 *Glucuronide conjugation*

Similar to sulfate conjugation, conjugation of products of Phase I metabolism with glucuronic acid, in its activated form of uridinediphosphoglucuronic acid (UDPGA), is a frequent pathway of xenobiotic metabolism. In most cases it acts as a deactivation pathway conferring hydrophilicity to the accepting substrate, thus facilitating its excretion. Multiple forms of glucuronosyl transferases have been recognized in many animal species and in humans. They are found in many tissues, with the liver having the highest content located in the endoplasmic reticulum.[32]

5.2   Modulation of Xenobiotic Metabolism by Diabetes Mellitus

The levels and nature of the xenobiotic-metabolizing enzyme systems may be modulated by a number of physiological factors, e.g., pregnancy, and environmental factors, such as dietary habits and previous exposure to other chemicals. A population exposed regularly to high levels of chemicals are patients suffering from chronic diseases, who are usually treated by an array of drugs to combat individual symptoms. Not only the disease itself, but the chronic intake of drugs to treat the disease is likely to perturb the various xenobiotic-metabolizing enzymes. For example, women suffering from tuberculosis did not receive adequate protection from the contraceptive pill; the intake of the antituberculosis drug rifampicin stimulated the CYP3A subfamily of cytochromes P450, leading to enhanced steroid deactivation and loss of contraceptive protection.[33] Moreover, chronic diseases may be accompanied by marked changes in dietary habits, such as substantial loss of appetite, further complicating the picture. Thus, chronic disease associated with drug treatment and changes in food intake may exert a marked effect on the enzyme systems that metabolize drugs and other chemicals. Bearing this in mind, it is incomprehensible that the effects of disease on drug metabolism have not received the attention they clearly merit. The few studies that have been carried out were limited to animal models of the disease, and studies in human patients are scarce despite the fact that there are currently available relatively simple techniques to monitor the activity of important enzyme systems, such as individual forms of cytochromes P450.

Failure to appreciate quantitative as well as qualitative changes, i.e., altered isoform profiles, may lead to two adverse situations, especially when the drugs concerned are characterized by a narrow therapeutic index. On the one hand, increased metabolic capacity will mean lower plasma levels that rapidly decrease; the consequence is a less-intense and shorter pharmacological effect than envisaged. In extreme cases, the effect may be totally abolished. On the other hand, suppression of drug-metabolizing activity will lead to higher plasma drug levels and, on repeated administration, the drug will accumulate with the possible appearance of adverse affects normally associated with overdosage. Clearly, an understanding of the effects of disease on drug metabolism is essential, in that it will allow appropriate precautions to be taken to alter the dose regimen to ensure that the desirable effect is maintained and the likelihood of toxicity is minimized. Alternatively, it may be possible to select other drugs where metabolism is catalyzed by enzyme systems whose activity is not influenced by the disease.

It is well established that major drug-metabolizing systems, such as the cytochrome P450–dependent mixed-function oxidases, are tightly regulated by hormones and other chemical mediators. Chronic diseases are frequently accompanied by pronounced and sustained changes in the circulating levels of such hormones, and it is logical to expect that such diseases may provoke meaningful changes in drug-metabolizing activities. Diabetes mellitus is a disease characterized by marked physiological and biochemical changes, and a number of studies have established unequivocally that this disease causes pronounced pharmacological and toxicologically relevant changes in metabolic capacity.

5.2.1 Insulin-Dependent Diabetes Mellitus (IDDM)

Syndromes resembling human diabetes develop spontaneously in many animal species, but may also be provoked by diabetogenic chemicals; the most extensively used are streptozotocin and, to a lesser extent, alloxan. None of these models of insulin-dependent diabetes mellitus (IDDM) mimics all the characteristics encountered in the human form of the disease but, nevertheless, allow studies to be carried out to elucidate the mechanisms responsible for the many physiological and biochemical changes accompanying this form of diabetes. Animals in which diabetes has been chemically induced may survive for several months in the absence of an exogenous supply of insulin, and in this respect they differ markedly from the human disease, where daily administration of insulin is indispensable.

5.2.1.1 *The Metabolism of Drugs and Other Xenobiotics in IDDM*

The first reports linking the induction of IDDM with changes in xenobiotic metabolism appeared in the early 1960s. Dixon et al.[34] investigated the metabolism of three drugs, hexobarbital, codeine, and chlorpromazine, in the liver of rats treated with alloxan; the metabolism of all three substrates was markedly suppressed by this treatment. As a consequence, the sleeping time induced by a single dose of hexobarbital was prolonged in the animals treated with alloxan. Interestingly, all these changes were reversed by treatment with insulin, indicating that the effects elicited by alloxan were due to the induction of the diabetic state rather than to the diabetogen itself. Another observation supporting this conclusion was the fact that the effects of alloxan on drug metabolism were not transient, but persisted for at least 3 months after treatment with the diabetogen.[35] Not all substrates responded to induction of diabetes in the same way; when aniline was utilized as the model substrate, its *in vitro* hepatic metabolism, in contrast to the other substrates studied, was increased. Clearly, the effect of diabetes on xenobiotic metabolism in the liver was dependent on the nature of the substrate. These studies were confirmed and extended to include other substrates,[36] and, in addition, it was noted that the effect of alloxan treatment on xenobiotic metabolism was sex-specific. For example, alloxan treatment suppressed the metabolism of hexobarbital only in the male rat. Sex-specific effects were also reported by other workers[37] who observed that aryl hydrocarbon hydroxylase activity was depressed in the female but was unaffected in the male diabetic rat. Mice were refractive to treatment with alloxan, in that hexobarbital and aniline hydroxylation, expressed per nanomole of cytochrome P450, were not altered by treatment with alloxan.[38,39]

In the late 1970s, similar studies were conducted using the less-toxic nitrosamide strep-tozotocin as the diabetogenic agent.[40,41] As previously observed with alloxan, hepatic metabolism of hexobarbital was suppressed with the sleeping time extended in rats by pretreatment with streptozotocin. Metabolism of aniline was enhanced, and all biochemical changes were antagonized by treatment with insulin.[41] Moreover, two nondiabetogenic analogs of streptozotocin failed to influence the metabolism of the same substrates,[41] thus establishing beyond doubt that it is the diabetic state and not the diabetogen that is responsible for the changes in hepatic xenobiotic metabolism. Finally, a comparison of the streptozotocin-induced diabetic rat with the spontaneous diabetic BB rat (see Chapter 12) from which insulin therapy was withdrawn for 4 days revealed no differences in xenobiotic metabolism between the two animal models of the disease.[37]

The influence of diabetes on xenobiotic metabolism is not confined to the liver; changes were evident in the intestinal and pulmonary metabolism of model substrates, but the effects did not always parallel those seen in the liver. For example, the oxidation of the carcinogen benzo(a)pyrene, commonly known as the aryl hydrocarbon hydroxylase (AHH), rose in the liver and intestine of rats exposed to streptozotocin, but decreased in the lungs and was unaffected in the kidney.[42] Other workers reported a decrease in the metabolism of benzo(a)pyrene in the liver of diabetic rats,[37] and, when the metabolism of benzo(a)pyrene was determined by an HPLC procedure, the level of all metabolites generated by the liver was suppressed by the induction of diabetes with streptozotocin.[43] Generally, a decrease in activity is observed in studies where animals were killed 4 days or earlier following the administration of the diabetogen; under such conditions, interpretation of the data is complicated by the hepatotoxicity of the diabetogen per se which may mask the effects of diabetes. Similarly, tissue-specific differences have been reported when 7-ethoxycoumarin was employed as the model substrate, its deethylation being increased in the liver and intestine but, conversely, diminished in the lungs.[44]

The largely *in vitro* studies were subsequently followed by *in vivo* studies where the pharmacokinetic characteristics of drugs were compared in control and diabetic animals. In alloxan-induced diabetic rabbits, the plasma levels of the antidiabetic drug chlorpropamide were higher compared with normal animals.[45] As this drug is largely excreted unchanged, the higher plasma levels were attributed to impaired renal function and increased protein binding. When the sulfonamide sulfadimethoxine was used as the model drug, plasma levels in the β phase were higher in the diabetic rabbits; similarly, the levels of the N-acetylated metabolite rose in the diabetic rabbits; these effects also appear to be the consequence of increased protein binding and impaired renal excretion. The choice of these drugs did not allow any effects of diabetes on drug metabolism to be evaluated. However, when phenacetin was studied, higher levels of the drug were present in the plasma of alloxan-induced diabetic rabbits compared with controls; in contrast, the plasma levels of the deethylated metabolite were lower. In the urine, more of the drug was excreted in the parent form in the diabetic animal, whereas less was present as the deethylated metabolite or its conjugated forms.[46] All the above differences between normal and diabetic rabbits were effectively antagonized by treatment with insulin. Since in these studies kidney function tests and histological examination revealed that the kidneys were unaffected by the treatment with alloxan, it may be confidently concluded that the metabolism of phenacetin was impaired in the diabetic animals. Indeed, when the metabolism of this drug was investigated using hepatic microsomal preparations, metabolism was lower in diabetic animals but near normal in diabetic animals treated with insulin.

The pharmacokinetic characteristics of the immunosuppressant cyclosporin, a drug with a narrow therapeutic range, were also influenced by the induction of IDDM using streptozotocin.[47] The diabetic animals, 8 days following the diabetogen administration, displayed lower clearance and prolonged plasma half-life of cyclosporine, both effects being counteracted by insulin treatment. Similarly, the clearance of aminopyrine was reduced and is half-life extended in rats treated with either alloxan or streptozotocin.[48] Plasma levels of the drug were higher in the diabetic animal suggesting suppressed metabolism; indeed the authors established that the N-demethylation of aminopyrine by hepatic microsomes was lower in the diabetic animals. In contrast, the clearance of diflunisal, a nonsteroidal anti-inflammatory drug, was enhanced and its half-life shortened in streptozotocin-treated rats, the effects being reversed by administration of insulin.[49] When the extensively metabolized diazepam was investigated in streptozotocin-treated rats, no differences in the metabolism of this drug, either oxidation or conjugation, were observed.[50] However, in these experiments the metabolism of diazepam was studied only 24 h following streptozotocin administration, and consequently the effects of diabetes on the drug-metabolizing systems may not have been fully manifested. Moreover, metabolic capacity may have been modulated by the hepatotoxicity of streptozotocin that persists for 1 week following administration.[51,52] It is evident from the above studies that the effect of IDDM on drug metabolism and pharmacokinetics cannot be predicted since it depends on the nature of the drug in question.

5.2.1.2 Expression of Cytochrome P450 Proteins in IDDM

The late 1970s witnessed rapid development and increased understanding of the complexities of the cytochrome P450 system. Isoforms were isolated and purified from the livers of animals and humans, their tissue distribution and inducibility determined immunologically following the production of antibodies to the purified proteins, and the substrate specificity of individual proteins was assessed in reconstituted systems. It had become clear that the term *cytochrome P450* encompassed a multitude of enzyme proteins. The initial observations on the differential effects of diabetes on xenobiotic metabolism could now be rationalized in terms of differential modulation of individual cytochrome P450 isoforms.

Past and Cook[53] analyzed electrophoretically hepatic microsomes from alloxan-treated rats and observed changes, both increases and decreases, in the cytochrome P450 region between control and diabetic animals. Thus, it was established that the effects of diabetes on cytochromes P450 are isoform specific and demonstrated for the first time the potential of a pathological state to modulate the expression of cytochromes P450; their studies were confirmed by other groups.[37] The same workers isolated a "diabetes"-inducible form of cytochrome P450 from the liver of diabetic rats, with high turnover toward aniline, a substrate whose p-hydroxylation is consistently increased in diabetic animals.[54,55] This protein was apparently absent from normal rats or diabetic rats treated with insulin. It was initially believed to be a unique form of cytochrome P450 induced by IDDM, but it was subsequently realized that this protein was identical with the ethanol-inducible CYP2E1.

A systematic study of the effects of diabetes on the expression of hepatic xenobiotic-metabolizing cytochromes P450 was carried out by Barnett et al.,[59] by adopting a somewhat different approach to the induction of diabetes to eliminate the effects of the diabetogen itself, in this case streptozotocin. In their studies, four groups of animals were always employed. One served as control; the second received a single dose of the diabetogen streptozotocin; the third received daily subcutaneous doses of insulin in addition to the single dose of streptozotocin, to assess whether or not any effects elicited are due to the diabetic state; and finally the fourth group received simultaneous administration of nicotinamide with the streptozotocin. Nicotinamide, when concurrently administered with streptozotocin, blocks the diabetogenic effects of the nitrosamide, presumably by preventing the depletion of NAD^+ within the pancreatic B-cells,[56] thus making it possible to discern the effects of diabetes from those of the diabetogen per se. All animals were killed 21 days after treatment with the diabetogen so that the transient toxicity associated with streptozotocin was avoided.[52] In these studies, diabetic animals developed the expected symptoms of polyphagia and polydipsia. All animals showed body weight gain with the streptozotocin group displaying the least gain; animals that received nicotinamide simultaneously with the streptozotocin exhibited the same body weight growth as the control group. Finally, the body weight gain in the group injected with streptozotocin and treated with insulin was intermediate between that seen in the control and streptozotocin-treated groups.[57] Animals receiving the streptozotocin only developed severe hyperglycemia, whereas mild hyperglycemia was evident in the groups that received nicotinamide or insulin in addition to the diabetogen.

Two approaches were used to monitor changes in cytochrome P450 proteins: the first employed established chemical probes metabolized selectively by specific cytochrome P450 isoforms, and the second involved immunological analysis of solubilized microsomes by Western blot. This second approach demonstrates whether any changes in cytochrome P450 activities induced by IDDM were the result of changes in the enzyme protein levels or involved other mechanisms, e.g., interference with the electron transport mechanism. It is pertinent to emphasize at this stage that IDDM is associated with a doubling in the specific content of cytochrome P450 indicating the presence of higher levels of enzyme protein.[57]

5.2.1.2.1 CYP1 Family

Induction of diabetes by streptozotocin led to a near trebling in the hepatic deethylations of ethoxycoumarin and ethoxyresorufin, two substrates selective for the CYP1A family.[57] Daily treatment of diabetic animals with subcutaneous injections of insulin reversed both activities to near control values. Western blot analysis revealed that of the two isoforms belonging to the CYP1A subfamily, diabetes selectively enhanced the levels of CYP1A2.[58] The increase in CYP1A2 activity was not a transient event but persisted for at least 12 weeks following the injection of the diabetogen.[59] Similar increases in CYP1A2 were noted when alloxan was employed as the diabetogen.[60] A similar picture emerged in studies conducted in the spontaneous diabetic BB rat when insulin was withdrawn for 5 days: a modest increase in the O-deethylation of ethoxyresorufin was evident in rats up to 12 weeks old, but no significant difference was seen in 24-week-old animals.[61] Elevated levels of CYP1A in the liver were also observed in streptozotocin-treated hamsters.[62] As CYP1A2 is not expressed in the lung and kidneys, induction of diabetes by treatment with streptozotocin did not modulate the low levels of O-dealkylation of the CYP1A substrates ethoxy- and methoxy-resorufin.[63]

Consequent to the hepatic increase in the levels of CYP1A2, postmitochondrial (S9) preparations from diabetic rats were more effective than those from normal animals in converting the two heterocyclic amines Trp-P-1 (3-amino-1,4-dimethyl-5H-pyrido[4,3-*b*]indole) and Trp-P-2 (3-amino-1-methyl-5H-pyrido[4,3-*b*]indole) to metabolites that induce a mutagenic response in the Ames mutagenicity test;[57] both of these compounds relying on CYP1A2 for their activation. Similar findings were reported when the diabetogen was alloxan, in that hepatic microsomal preparations from diabetic animals were more efficient in the bioactivation of the heterocyclic amines Glu-P-1 (2-amino-6-methyldipyrido[1,2-*a*:3′,2′-d]imidazole), IQ (2-amino-3-methylimidazo[4,5-*f*]quinoline), and MeIQx (2-amino-3,8-dimethylimidazo[4,5-*f*]quinoxaline),[64] all of which are selectively bioactivated by the CYP1A2 isoform. Moreover, the same authors established a very good correlation (r = 0.879) between CYP1A2 levels in the microsomes and mutagenic potency. All the above increases were successfully antagonized by insulin therapy. Clearly, it is likely diabetic animals may be more susceptible to the carcinogenicity of such chemicals, unless detoxication mechanisms are concurrently induced. Since CYP1A2 plays a major role in the bioactivation of many planar carcinogens, particularly those containing an exocyclic amino group, in both animals and humans, it may be inferred that the patient with uncontrolled diabetes may display enhanced sensitivity to such chemicals.[65] CYP1A1 levels are not modulated by IDDM, and consequently the bioactivation of polycyclic aromatic hydrocarbons such as benzo(a)pyrene and 3-methylcholanthrene, whose major catalyst is CYP1A1, was not perturbed by the disease.[66]

5.2.1.2.2   CYP2A Subfamily

Induction of diabetes in rats by the administration of streptozotocin is accompanied by a rise in hepatic, CYP1A2-mediated, 7α-hydroxylation of testosterone, the effect being antagonized by insulin administration.[67] Western blot analysis of microsomes from diabetic rats revealed that the proteins CYP2A1 and CYP2A2 are differentially modulated by the disease, the latter being downregulated and the former upregulated, the effects being reversible by treatment with insulin.[67,68]

Moreover, the 7α-hydroxylation of testosterone was increased in streptozotocin-treated diabetic rats but the CYP2A2-mediated 15α-hydroxylation was unaltered.[60,69]

5.2.1.2.3   CYP2B Subfamily

The O-dealkylation of pentoxyresorufin, an activity with high specificity for the CYP2B subfamily, was markedly increased in diabetic rats, 21 days after the administration of streptozotocin,[57] and this effect was accompanied by corresponding increases in the apoprotein levels.[58] An increase over control values was still evident some 12 weeks following administration of the diabetogen, but was less marked compared with the effect seen during the first 3 to 4 weeks.[59] Similarly, testosterone 16β-hydroxylase activity, a diagnostic probe for the CYP2B subfamily, was also elevated in the diabetic rat. The hepatic levels of only one of the isoforms belonging to this subfamily, namely, CYP2B1, rose in the diabetic rat, whereas CYP2B2 was not modulated by the disease.[60,70] In the spontaneous diabetic BB rat, withdrawal of the daily insulin therapy resulted in only a modest increase in the O-dealkylation of the CYP2B substrate pentoxyresorufin.[61] Surprisingly, in the hamster, treatment with streptozotocin-suppressed hepatic CYP2B levels.[62] Whether this reflects a true species difference or the higher susceptibility of the hamster to the toxicity of the diabetogen remains to be elucidated. Dealkylation of pentoxyresorufin in the lung and kidney was not influenced by the induction of IDDM in rats with streptozotocin,[63] whereas in the hamster kidney pentoxyresorufin O-dealkylase and CYP2B levels were suppressed.[62]

5.2.1.2.4   CYP2C Subfamily

CYP2C6 and CYP2C7 levels rose in the liver of animals rendered diabetic by the administration of streptozotocin.[67] In contrast, the expression of another member of this subfamily, CYP2C11, was drastically suppressed in IDDM animals, by as much as 95%, as determined by employing the probes 2α- and 16α-hydroxylation of testosterone.[67-71] Moreover, mRNA levels paralleled the changes in apoprotein levels indicating that the suppression of this isoform by IDDM occurs at a pretranslational stage.[70] CYP2C12 is a female-specific isoform, not normally present in the male rat; low apoprotein levels were, however, detected in streptozotocin-induced diabetic male rats.[68] Finally, the apoprotein levels of CYP2C13 in the liver were decreased markedly, by about 85%, in diabetic rats.[68,71] In studies conducted in the spontaneously diabetic BB rat, no changes could be detected in the apoprotein levels of CYP2C7, and only a modest decrease was apparent in CYP2C11.[71,72] Clearly, the CYP2C subfamily is sensitive to chemically induced IDDM, but the nature of the effect is isoform specific.

5.2.1.2.5 *CYP2D Subfamily*

Western blot analysis of rat hepatic microsomes employing antibodies to the human CYP2D6 recognized a single protein, which was not modulated by the onset of streptozotocin-induced diabetes; similarly, bufurarol hydroxylase, an activity associated with this subfamily was also unaffected.[73]

5.2.1.2.6 *CYP2E Subfamily*

The perturbation of the levels of the CYP2E1 by diabetes has been the subject of many studies since this protein is associated with high aniline *p*-hydroxylase activity, the first activity recognized as being upregulated following administration of various diabetogens. It is most frequently monitored using as probes the *N*-demethylation of the carcinogen dimethylnitrosamine, at low substrate concentrations, or the oxidation of *p*-nitrophenol to nitrocatechol. The hepatic levels of this isoform increased following the induction of IDDM, both in male and female rats, but the effect was prevented by the simultaneous administration of nicotinamide with streptozotocin, and reversed by insulin therapy.[57,67,68,70,74-76] The extent of induction of this isoform by IDDM decreased with time, but was clearly detectable 12 weeks after administration of streptozotocin.[59] An increase in CYP2E1 activity was also observed in the spontaneously diabetic BB rat from which insulin treatment was withdrawn for 4 to 5 days.[61,69,71,75] The activity of the CYP2E1 enzyme *p*-nitrophenol hydroxylase was doubled in such animals by the 4th week of age, and this increase was maintained for at least 24 weeks.[61] A rise in hepatic CYP2E1 activity and apoprotein levels has also been reported in streptozotocin-treated hamsters.[62]

Immunological studies established that the levels of CYP2E1 apoprotein were also elevated in the lung and kidney of streptozotocin-induced diabetic rats, 7 days after diabetogen administration.[77] However, in a subsequent study,[63] an increase in apoprotein levels was observed only in the kidney, but a decrease was evident in the lung; in this study animals were sacrificed 21 days after treatment with streptozotocin. An increase in kidney apoprotein levels has also been reported by others, in both rat[67] and hamsters[62] exposed to streptozotocin.

CYP2E1 mRNA levels were also increased in chemically induced diabetic animals, not only in the liver but also in the lung and kidney, and the increase, at least in the liver, was abolished by treatment with insulin.[75,76] The diabetes-mediated increase in hepatic CYP2E1 mRNA levels appears to be the result of stabilization rather than of enhanced transcription.[76] In recent studies,[77] the streptozotocin-induced increase in CYP2E1 activity and apoprotein levels in the liver of rats was completely abolished by administration of ascorbic acid in the drinking water of the animals, after the onset of diabetes. This effect was specific to this cytochrome P450 protein, and the other isoforms were not influenced by the ascorbic acid treatment. The treatment of the diabetic animals with ascorbic acid ameliorated biochemical symptoms of the disease such as hyperketonemia and hypertriglyceridemia. It has been suggested,[7] that the lower triglyceride levels in animals treated with ascorbic acid may lead to reduced oxidation and lower circulating ketone levels, leading to the lower CYP2E1 levels[77] (see below).

As already discussed, CYP2E1 is involved in the metabolism of small molecular weight compounds, having a collision diameter of less than 6.5 Å.[79] As a result, animals suffering from IDDM are susceptible to the toxicity of small-molecular-weight toxins, which depend on CYP2E1 for their activation. The hepatotoxicity of dimethylnitrosamine was markedly elevated in rats rendered diabetic by treatment with streptozotocin.[80] Commensurate with these observations is the fact that the diabetic rats metabolized dimethylnitrosamine more effectively than the normal animals.[43] In addition, hepatic postmitochondrial preparations from streptozotocin-induced diabetic rats displayed higher capacity than corresponding controls in metabolically converting two nitrosamines, nitrosopiperidine and nitrosopyrrolidine, to mutagenic intermediates in the Ames test, the effect being successfully antagonized by daily insulin administration.[66] As a result of the elevated CYP2E1 activity in the diabetic animals, the hepatotoxicity of haloalkanes, such as carbon tetrachloride and 1,1,2-trichloroethane, was also more marked in diabetic rats, as indicated by serum enzymes and histological evaluation, even 90 days after the administration of streptozotocin.[81-83] The hepatic injury provoked by a dose of 25 ml/kg of carbon tetrachloride in rats with IDDM, was in fact greater than that induced by a dose of 400 ml/kg in normal animals.[81] However, in certain cases, diabetes can offer protection against the toxicity of chemicals. Diabetic rats are resistant to the hepatotoxicity of acetaminophen apparently because of the higher activity of deactivation pathways such as glucuronide and, to a lesser extent, sulfate conjugation, and an increased capacity to detoxicate, via glutathione conjugation, the reactive intermediate generated from the oxidation of the drug.[84] All the effects are reversed by insulin treatment.

5.2.1.2.7 CYP3 Family

After 3 weeks of treatment of rats with streptozotocin, an increase was evident in the hepatic N-demethylations of erythromycin and ethylmorphine, two activities associated with the CYP3A subfamily; these effects were antagonized by insulin and were not manifested when nicotinamide was administered concurrently with the diabetogen.[85] The activities of these enzymes correlated with the apoprotein levels in Western blot analysis. The increase in CYP3A1 activity was transient and was not detectable by 4 weeks after injection of the diabetogen.[59] A similar increase has been reported in hepatic CYP3A2 apoprotein levels and in the associated activities of testosterone 2β- and 6β-hydroxylase 2 weeks after the administration of the diabetogen.[67] Other workers reported,[68] in contrast, lower apoprotein levels in diabetic rats. Withdrawal of insulin from BB rats for 5 days prior to sacrifice resulted in an increase in the N-demethylation of ethylmorphine in 4-week-old animals; the increase became less pronounced as the disease progressed and was only just detectable in 24-week-old animals.[61]

5.2.1.2.8 CYP4 Family

IDDM induced by streptozotocin in rats was accompanied by a marked increase in the hepatic ω-hydroxylation of lauric acid, the effect being reversed by treatment with insulin.[67,85] The increase in the ω-hydroxylation of lauric acid was paralleled by a rise in CYP4A1 apoprotein levels.[85] Both activity and apoprotein levels declined with the progress of the disease but the increase was still detectable 12 weeks after the administration of streptozotocin.[59] Lauric acid hydroxylase activity was also elevated in the BB rat, which also declined with the progress of the disease, but was still detectable in 24-week-old animals.[61] Similarly, CYP4A2 and CYP4A3 apoprotein levels were increased in the hepatic microsomes from diabetic rats.[67]

The expression of the CYP4A subfamily in the kidney was also influenced by the diabetic state. CYP4A2 and CYP4A3, but not CYP4A1 levels, were elevated and a doubling in the ω-hydroxylation of lauric acid was noted.[63,67] No lauric acid hydroxylase activity was detectable in the lungs of either control or streptozotocin-induced diabetic rats.[63]

TABLE 5.2

IDDM-Induced Changes in Cytochrome P450 Expression in Rats

Cytochrome P450 Isoform	Tissue	Modulation of Expression	Ref.
CYP1A2	Liver	↑	57,58,60,61,62
CYP2A1	Liver	↑	60,67,68,69
CYP2A2	Liver	↓	68
CYP2B	Liver	↑	59,60,61,62,70
	Kidney	←	62,63
		↓ in the hamster	
	Lung	↓	63
CYP2C6	Liver	↑	67
CYP2C7	Liver	↑ or →	67,72
CYP2C11	Liver	↓	67 — 71
CYP2C12	Liver	↑	68
CYP2C13	Liver	↓	68,71
CYP2D	Liver	←	73
CYP2E1	Liver	↑	57,61,62,67-71,74-76
	Kidney	↑	62,63,67,77
	Lung	↑ or ↓	63,77
CYP3A1	Liver	↑	59,61,85
CYP3A2	Liver	↑ or →	67,68
CYP4A1	Liver	↑	59,61,85
CYP4A2	Liver	↑	67
	Kidney	↑	63,67
CYP4A3	Liver	↑	67
	Kidney	↑	62,67

Note: ↑, increase; ↓, decrease; ←, no change.

5.2.1.2.9 Other Cytochrome P450 Isoforms

The expression of the cytochrome P450 proteins, whose primary function is the metabolism of endogenous substrates, in IDDM has received very little attention. Cholesterol 7α-hydroxylase (CYP7), the rate-limiting step in the catabolism of cholesterol to bile acids was higher in the liver of rats made diabetic by streptozotocin treatment; the effect was successfully antagonized by insulin.[86] Similarly, the 12α-hydroxylation of 5β-cholestane-3α,7α-diol, a pathway involved in bile acid biosynthesis, was elevated in IDDM rats.[87] Pathways of hepatic steroid metabolism are also differentially modulated by the induction of IDDM in rats using streptozotocin.[88]

The diabetes-induced changes in hepatic and extrahepatic cytochrome P450 expression are summarized in Table 5.2.

5.2.1.3 Underlying Mechanisms in IDDM-Induced Changes in Cytochrome P450 Expression

IDDM is a chronic and complex disease that is accompanied by many physiological changes, one or more of which may contribute, at least partly, to the changes in the expression of cytochromes P450.

5.2.1.3.1 Hypoinsulinemia

A feasible mechanism responsible for the IDDM effects on cytochrome P450 expression is a direct effect of insulin, so that depletion of the hormone may be a major contributory mechanism. However, addition of insulin *in vitro* to incubation mixtures did not reverse the changes in drug metabolism induced by diabetes.[89] Moreover, treatment of control animals with insulin did not influence the metabolism of chemicals that are modulated by the onset of IDDM.[41] In more recent studies,[90] treatment of rats with insulin gave rise to a dose-dependent, but modest, increase in the O-deethylation of ethoxyresorufin, i.e., the same effect seen in the hypoglycemic IDDM rats. The same workers demonstrated that in insulinoma-bearing rats, characterized by marked and sustained hyperinsulinemia, only the oxidation of p-nitrophenol and lauric acid hydroxylation were depressed, but the O-dealkylation of ethoxyresorufin was increased and that of pentoxyresorufin was unaffected. Clearly, although a direct effect of insulin cannot be excluded in the case of some cytochrome P450 isoforms, it is very unlikely that hypoinsulinemia alone can explain the IDDM changes in cytochrome P450 expression. It is pertinent to point out, however, that incorporation of insulin *in vitro* into the incubation mixtures attenuated cholesterol 7α-hydroxylase activity in both normal and diabetic rats, alluding to a direct effect of insulin on enzyme activity.[86] Furthermore, in studies conducted using hepatoma cells, exposure of the cells to insulin resulted in a decrease in CYP2B and CYP2E proteins, which was preceded by similar changes in the corresponding mRNA levels.[91] In addition, insulin suppressed the induction of CYP2B apoprotein and mRNA levels in cultured rat hepatocytes.[92] At this stage, the possible direct effect of insulin on cytochrome P450 expression in diabetic animals needs to be further addressed and clarified in view of conflicting evidence.

5.2.1.3.2 Hyperphagia

A classical symptom of IDDM is hyperphagia, and it is conceivable that the greater calorific intake may be a contributing factor in the changes in cytochrome P450 expression. This appears unlikely since in studies where diabetic animals were pair-fed the normal food intake and treated with carbon tetrachloride, they still displayed a similar degree of hepatotoxicity as diabetic animals receiving the same diet *ad libitum*.[82]

5.2.1.3.3 Hyperglycemia

A major biochemical characteristic of IDDM is marked and sustained hyperglycemia, and the persistent high glucose levels in the serum may be involved in the regulation of cytochromes P450. All available experimental evidence, however, does not support this hypothesis. Hyperglycemia induced by the intraperitoneal administration of glucose modulated only modestly the metabolism of cytochrome P450 substrates, but the effects were not always comparable with those provoked by IDDM.[93] For example, a consistent effect of IDDM, in both male and female rats, is an increase in the p-hydroxylation of aniline, whereas following glucose administration a decrease was observed. Moreover, hyperglycemia induced by a 24-h infusion of a 40% glucose solution did not influence the oxidation of hexobarbital, which is suppressed in diabetic animals.[40] When hyperglycemia was induced in animals by treatment with the diabetogen N-methylacetamide, where hypoinsulinemia is not encountered as insulin is produced and released by the pancreas but an insulin-resistant state occurs where insulin is unable to reduce blood glucose levels, no changes in hepatic hexobarbital oxidase activity were observed. In contrast, treatment with other diabetogens such as streptozotocin and 6-aminonicotinamide led to a decrease in this activity.[40] Finally, blood glucose levels in alloxan-induced diabetic animals did not relate to the increase in p-hydroxylation of aniline; the increase in this activity was similar in animals that differed by nearly threefold in blood glucose levels.[35] On the basis of the available experimental evidence, it may be concluded that hyperglycemia is not a factor contributing to the IDDM-induced changes in cytochromes P450.

5.2.1.3.4 Hyperglucagonemia

Continuous infusion of glucagon to mice for 5 days modulated the levels of hepatic metabolism of cytochrome P450 model substrates.[94] However, the effects of glucagon were not always the same as those induced by treatment with streptozotocin, implying that the role of glucagon, if any, in the diabetes-induced changes in hepatic cytochrome P450 expression may be isoform specific. No correlation between the degree of hyperglucagonemia in diabetic animals and changes in the cytochrome P450 profile has so far been reported, but this possible mechanism merits further investigation, and its true contribution to the effects elicited by diabetes cannot at present be critically evaluated.

5.2.1.3.5 Hyperketonemia and Hyperlipidemia

The observation by many researchers that conditions characterized by high levels of circulating ketones, such as starvation and high alcohol intake, bring about changes in the levels in cytochrome P450 proteins similar to those established in IDDM prompted considerable work into evaluating the role of ketone bodies in the IDDM-induced changes in cytochrome P450 expression. To discern the effects of hyperketonemia from the other biochemical changes that are present in diabetes, animals were made hyperketonemic by the administration of medium-chain triacylglycerides. These animals remained normoglycemic, and the cytochrome P450 profile was established in the liver and compared with that encountered in IDDM animals. Similar to IDDM, oral administration of medium-chain triacylglycerides caused an increase in the activities and apoprotein levels of CYP1A2, CYP2B, CYP2E1, and CYP4A1; in contrast, no changes were seen in CYP3A.[58,85,95] These data indicate that hyperketonemia may have a role to play in the IDDM-induced changes in hepatic cytochromes P450, but the effect is isoform specific, from which it may be inferred that additional mechanisms are also operative. Moreover, the changes induced by hyperketonemia were less pronounced than those elicited by IDDM, despite the same degree of hyperketonemia.

In the above studies no distinction was made between the effects of ketones from any direct effects of the triglycerides. To achieve this distinction, hepatic expression of cytochromes P450 was determined in rats that were treated with acetone[96]; a rise in CYP1A2, CYP2B, and CYP2E1 activities and apoprotein levels was noted. Surprisingly, 1,3-butanediol at the same dose of 15 mmol/kg failed to stimulate the expression of these isoforms. However, an increase in CYP2E1 activity was observed when a higher dose was employed.[97] Induction of CYP2B and CYP2E1 by treatment with acetone has also been reported by other groups.[98-100] Furthermore, partial normalization of ketone and lipid levels in diabetic animals restored CYP2E1 and partially CYP2B levels.[70] Moreover, in long-term IDDM, hepatic CYP2E1 activity correlated well with the plasma ketone levels.[59] A role for hyperketonemia in the IDDM-induced changes in hepatic CYP2E1 is further supported by observations that, in the BB rat, CYP2E1 activity correlated with plasma 3-hydroxybutyrate levels.[72] CYP4A1 was unaffected by acetone treatment,[96] alluding to a direct triglyceride effect in the induction of this activity in the triglyceride-induced hyperketonemia. Indeed, it is established that fatty acids stimulate CYP4A expression,[101,102] and this observation has been recently confirmed in studies where exposure of primary cultured rat hepatocytes to fatty acids, but not ketones, enhanced CYP4A mRNA levels.[103] Moreover, administration of vanadate to IDDM rats, a process that reverses hyperketonemia and hyperlipidemia, diminished the levels of CYP4A1 and its mRNA.[104] Following treatment of rats with acetone, CYP3A was unchanged, confirming the lack of involvement of hyperketonemia in the diabetes-induced increase in this activity.[96]

Compatible with the role of ketone bodies in CYP2E1 induction, the hepatotoxicity of dimethylnitrosamine was potentiated, not only in IDDM rats but also in animals that were subjected to fasting or treated with acetone or isopropanol, which is metabolized to acetone.[80] Similarly, the toxicity of haloalkanes, such as carbon tetrachloride, chloroform, 1,1-dichloroethylene, and 1,1,3-trichloroethylene, was potentiated in rats pretreated with acetone or 1,3-butanediol, which induces ketosis by being converted to acetoacetate, acetone, and 3-hydroxybutyrate.[105-108] In concordance with the above, the metabolism of chloroform was increased in animals treated with acetone, as a result of an increase in CYP2E1 activity.[99] Moreover, hepatic preparations from rats rendered hyperketonemic by the dietary administration of triacylglycerols, like similar preparations from IDDM animals, were more efficient in catalyzing the CYP1A2-mediated bioactivation of Glu-P-1 and Trp-P-2 and the CYP2E1-mediated activation of nitrosopiperidine and nitrosopyrrolidine to mutagens in the Ames test.[109] The experimental evidence implicating hyperketonemia as an important factor responsible partly for the diabetes-induced changes in hepatic cytochromes P450 is clearly overwhelming. It has been suggested that ketones are converted to fatty acids that may be responsible for the effect of ketones on the cytochrome P450 system, at least in the case of CYP2B.[103]

All the above studies provide strong experimental evidence that the high circulating levels of ketones in IDDM, directly or indirectly, are largely responsible for the increase in CYP2E1 levels, and also contribute to the increases in other cytochrome P450 proteins, such as CYP1A2 and CYP2B.

5.2.1.3.6 Impairment of Hormonal Homeostasis

Marked changes in the secretion patterns and circulating levels of hormones, including growth hormone, thyroid hormone, and sex hormones, many of which play prominent roles in regulating cytochrome P450 expression, are seen in IDDM. Consequently, it is not unexpected that the changes in cytochromes P450 induced by diabetes have their etiology partly in the altered hormone levels.

Plasma levels of growth hormone in IDDM are very low as a result of impaired secretion,[110] and the decline in the plasma levels of this hormone may be responsible for the upregulation of CYP3A expression in the liver.[85] In hypophysectomized rats, CYP3A mRNA levels in the liver accumulated but were reversed by injection of human growth hormone.[111] The contribution of the low levels of growth hormone in the induction of CYP2E1 is less clear. Elevated CYP2E1 apoprotein levels in the livers of hypophysectomized rats, partially reversed by growth hormone administration has been reported,[112] but administration of the hormone to male diabetic rats failed to reverse the increased CYP2E1 levels.[68] In addition, an increase in hepatic CYP2E1 in IDDM is seen in both male and female rats despite their markedly different patterns of secretion. Other cytochrome P450 proteins are also increased in the liver of hypophysectomized rats, including isoforms belonging to the CYP2A and CYP2B subfamilies, whereas the level of CYP2C11 is suppressed, these changes being similar to those occurring in diabetic animals.[60,113] However, human growth hormone administration to diabetic animals failed to antagonize the diabetes-induced changes in CYP2C11.[68]

Onset of IDDM in rats is accompanied by a decline in the circulating plasma levels of testosterone,[68,114] raising the possibility that the levels of this hormone may have a role in provoking the changes in the activity of cytochromes P450 in diabetic animals. Initial studies where the effect of diabetes was assessed using the N-demethylation of aminopyrine, a substrate in whose metabolism a number of cytochrome P450 isoforms participate, showed that testosterone could not reverse the decrease in activity elicited by various

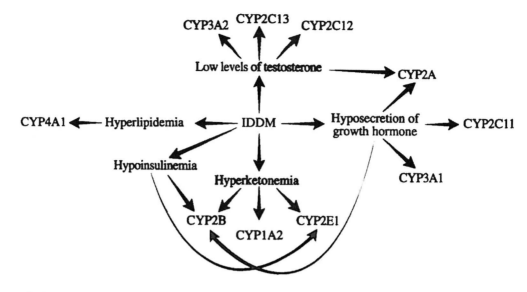

FIGURE 5.10
Mechanisms of the IDDM-induced changes in cytochrome P450.

diabetogens.[114] However, in subsequent, more-detailed studies looking at individual cytochrome P450 isoforms, administration of testosterone to diabetic rats reversed the changes in hepatic CYP2A2, CYP2C12, CYP2C13, and, to a lesser extent, CYP2C11 without modulating the growth hormone secretion profile of these animals.[68]

In male rats that have undergone thyroidectomy, hepatic CYP2A1 levels were doubled, and this effect was reversed by the administration of T_3 (triiodothyronine).[115] However, in diabetic animals circulating levels of T_3 appear unchanged, whereas T_4 levels are markedly lower than control levels.[68]

5.2.1.4   Other Phase I Enzyme Systems

Hepatic flavin monooxygenase activity, determined using the S-oxidation of thiobenzamide as probe, doubled in rats and mice treated with streptozotocin.[116] No studies have been carried out to establish whether this increase in activity is due to the diabetic state rather than a property of the diabetogen. However, since increased activity was seen in animals killed 2 weeks after the diabetogen, it is likely that the diabetic state is responsible for the effect, but it remains to be demonstrated unequivocally. To the authors' knowledge, the effect of diabetes on the prostaglandin synthase system has not been investigated.

Figure 5.10 illustrates schematically the various mechanisms involved in the regulation of cytochrome P450 proteins in IDDM.

5.2.1.5   Phase II Conjugation Reactions

The response of Phase II enzyme systems to the onset of IDDM has not been studied in depth; most published work is restricted to investigations using a limited range of substrates with no attempt to delineate specific changes to individual isoforms.

5.2.1.5.1 Glucuronidation

The influence of IDDM on the glucuronidation of endogenous and exogenous chemicals is substrate specific, implying selective modulation of isoforms. In rats treated with streptozotocin, the hepatic microsomal glucuronide conjugation of 1-naphthol and testosterone declined, whereas that of diethylstilbestrol increased and in the case of estrone no change was evident.[81] In support of these observations, hepatocytes from diabetic rats were markedly less effective than control hepatocytes in catalyzing the glucuronidation of 1-naphthol and phenolphthalein, both effects being counteracted by insulin.[117] In this study, intracellular levels of UDP-glucuronic acid, an essential and rate-limiting factor in glucuronidation, were lower in the diabetic animals, and this could be a contributory factor in the suppressed glucuronidation capacity. When mice were injected with streptozotocin, the glucuronidation of bilirubin was increased whereas that of *p*-nitrophenol was unaffected.[118] In these studies no attempt was made to distinguish the effects of diabetes from those of the diabetogen per se.

5.2.1.5.2 Sulfation

The sulfation of 1-naphthol by intact rat hepatocytes derived from IDDM animals did not differ from controls.[117]

5.2.1.5.3 Acetylation

Contradictory results were obtained in the two models of IDDM when the *N*-acetylation of sulfamethazine was investigated; no difference was observed in animals treated with streptozotocin,[118] whereas higher activity was found in the diabetic BB rat compared with controls.[119] In another study,[48] *N*-acetyltransferase activity in rats made diabetic with alloxan or streptozotocin was significantly lower than controls. Whether or not diabetes modulates differentially the forms of this enzyme remains to established. It is noteworthy that in streptozotocin-induced IDDM the hepatocellular levels of CoA are increased.[120]

5.2.1.5.4 Glutathione Conjugation

Cytosolic glutathione *S*-transferase activity determined in the liver of mice using the broad-specificity 1-chloro-2,4,-dinitrobenzene as the accepting substrate was doubled following treatment with streptozotocin.[121,122] This effect persisted even when nicotinamide was administered to the animals prior to the streptozotocin, a procedure that prevents the onset of IDDM. Moreover, this activity was not stimulated when alloxan was employed as the diabetogen. Consequently, the increase in activity brought about with the streptozotocin treatment was ascribed to the diabetogen itself rather than to the diabetic condition.[122] In rats, cytosolic activity determined using three substrates, namely, 1-chloro-2,4,-dinitrobenzene, sulfobromophthalein, and ethacrynic acid, was suppressed 3 months following the induction of diabetes with streptozotocin, but no difference or a slight decrease was evident 1 month or earlier after the administration of the diabetogen.[81,123] A decrease in glutathione conjugation may reflect suppressed transferase activity or unavailability of glutathione for conjugation; in the *in vitro* studies an excess of glutathione is added to the incubation system. It is pertinent to point out, however, that lower levels of glutathione were reported in rat hepatocytes compared with control animals,[117] but this decrease was not reported by other workers.[124] When cytosolic glutathione *S*-transferase activity was determined in extrahepatic tissues using 1-chloro-2,4,-dinitrobenzene, induction of IDDM by streptozotocin increased the activity modestly in the kidney with no effect in the lung; glutathione levels and glutathione reductase activity, the enzyme responsible for maintaining glutathione in the reduced form, were not altered in both tissues.[63]

5.2.1.5.5 Hydration of Epoxides

The hydration of epoxides is catalyzed by epoxide hydrolases, which are localized in the microsomes and cytosolic fractions of the cell. When the microsomal activity was monitored using as substrate benzo(α)pyrene 4,5-oxide, activity was markedly enhanced in mice treated with streptozotocin.[121] When the microsomal activity was monitored utilizing styrene oxide as the substrate a transient decline in activity was described in streptozotocin-treated rats.[81,123] In contrast, when the cytosolic epoxide hydrolase activity was measured using *trans*-stilbene oxide, activity was increased following treatment of rats with either alloxan or streptozotocin and the effect was antagonized by insulin.[122]

5.2.2   Noninsulin-Dependent Diabetes Mellitus

The model employed in studies aimed at establishing whether or not drug metabolism is influenced by noninsulin-dependent diabetes mellitus (NIDDM) is the spontaneously obese hyperglycemic (ob/ob) mouse, an animal that displays many features of the human form of the disease. No significant differences in the metabolism of various cytochrome P450 substrates were observed between ob/ob mice and their normal lean littermates.[125,126] However, the ob/ob mice exhibited substantially reduced hepatic glutathione S-transferase activity, determined using 1,chloro-2,4-dinitrobenzene, which was accompanied by lower glutathione content, implying a diminished capacity to detoxicate electrophiles.[126]

5.2.3   Xenobiotic Metabolism in Human Diabetes

The small number of studies in which drug pharmacokinetics were studied in patients with diabetes demonstrated impaired ability to eliminate these drugs, even when the diabetic condition was treated with insulin. The drug antipyrine has been used extensively as a probe to detect changes in hepatic metabolism, since this is the principal site of its metabolism. Although this drug relies on cytochromes P450 for its metabolism, several isoforms are involved so that no information on specific cytochrome P450 proteins can be obtained. In one study,[127] antipyrine plasma half-life was generally shorter in individuals with diabetes on various treatments such as insulin and chlorpropamide; it appears no distinction was made in this study between patients with IDDM and patients with NIDDM. In contrast, in a later study[128] it was reported that the salivary half-life of antipyrine was higher in a group of ten patients with uncontrolled diabetes, both IDDM and NIDDM, compared with controls. Following insulin therapy for 15 days the difference in antipyrine half-life between subjects with diabetes and controls was abolished. In a study confined to patients with IDDM, no difference was seen in the metabolism of this drug compared with controls.[129] When phenacetin was used as the model drug, the metabolism of this drug was impaired in five individuals with diabetes as evidenced by the larger amounts of the parent drug and the lower paracetamol, the deethylated metabolite of paracetamol, and its conjugated metabolites excreted in the urine compared with healthy volunteers.[130] Moreover, stabilization of the diabetic condition with insulin administration tended to restore the urinary metabolic pattern of phenacetin to that observed in controls. When the elimination of tolbutamide was investigated,[131] no difference in the plasma half-life was seen between ten patients with diabetes and seven healthy subjects. In *in vitro* studies, aryl hydrocarbon hydroxylase activity in liver biopsy samples was higher in NIDDM.[132] These studies illustrate that in the diabetic state, drug biotransformation may be significantly altered, but no generalizations can be made as the effect depends on the nature of the drug, probably reflecting specific changes in certain cytochrome P450 proteins.

The expression of individual cytochrome P450 isoforms in patients with diabetes has not yet been systematically addressed. In a pioneering study,[133] CYP2E1 expression was determined in peripheral lymphocytes of 14 patients with IDDM, whose control of the disease was poor as exemplified by the high levels of glycosylated hemoglobin (HbA1). In seven healthy teenage subjects, CYP2E1 levels were very low or undetectable but were clearly higher in the 14 teenagers with IDDM diabetes. Moreover, a direct correlation was noted between levels of glycosylated hemoglobin and lymphocyte CYP2E1 levels. Interestingly, in one patient where diabetic control was improved, a parallel drop in CYP2E1 to normal levels was seen. This study provides unequivocal evidence that cytochromes P450 are perturbed in human IDDM and that degree of change is related to the quality of management and severity of the condition.

The metabolism of theophylline (1,3-dimethylxanthine) was investigated in groups of eight patients with IDDM and appropriate controls.[134] Interest in this drug lies in the fact that its N-demethylations, important routes of its metabolism, are specifically catalyzed by CYP1A2, thus allowing the expression of this isoform in patients with IDDM to be determined. In contrast, a number of cytochrome P450 isoforms, including CYP2E1, contribute to its hydroxylation to 1,3-dimethyluric acid. The pharmacokinetic characteristics of theophylline and the formation clearance of its metabolites in the patients with diabetes did not differ from controls. However, the free fraction of plasma theophylline in the plasma was higher in the subjects with diabetes compared with controls. In the group with diabetes, a direct correlation was established between glycosylated hemoglobin levels and theophylline clearance, and formation clearance of two of the metabolites, 3-methyluric acid and 1,3-dimethyluric acid.[134] These observations suggest that patients with poorly controlled diabetes may display increased theophylline metabolism, presumably as a result of increased CYP1A2 and CYP2E1 activity, as established in the experimental studies.[57,58]

5.3 Conclusions

Strong experimental evidence has accumulated indicating that, in animal models, IDDM modulates the enzyme systems responsible for the metabolism of drugs and other xenobiotic compounds. The cytochrome P450–dependent mixed-functions oxidases are the most susceptible enzymes to the onset of IDDM. Marked changes have been documented in animals with uncontrolled IDDM, sufficiently pronounced to be of major toxicological relevance. Only limited studies have been conducted in humans with diabetes, but even these few investigations have established that the individuals with diabetes are likely to be subject to changes in the cytochrome P450 profile, similar to those encountered in the animal models. Moreover, these changes were directly related to the degree of control of the disease as indicated by the blood levels of glycosylated hemoglobin. Current therapeutic approaches to diabetes are not ideal, and patients may experience periods of marked hyperglycemia, ketosis, and hyperlipidemia that may lead to alterations in cytochrome P450 expression. Thus, it is conceivable that the patient with diabetes may be especially susceptible to the toxicity of certain chemicals as a result of higher capacity to convert these to their reactive intermediates that manifest their toxicity.

CYP2E1 activity is enhanced in subjects with poorly controlled diabetes and, in view of the propensity of this isoform to generate deleterious reactive oxygen species, it may have some bearing on some of the complications of diabetes, such as nephropathy and retinopathy. These conditions may be brought about by excess production of reactive oxygen species leading to oxidative stress. Both of these long-term complications of diabetes have been linked to damage initiated by reactive oxygen species and the generation of lipid peroxides.[2,135-137] The increase in CYP2E1 and CYP4A activities, the latter not yet demonstrated in human diabetes, may be viewed as an adaptive response of the body to combat the more immediate adverse effects of hyperketonemia and hyperlipidemia, by stimulating the catabolism of acetone and fatty acids, respectively.

References

1. Oberley, L. W. and Oberley, T. D., Reactive oxygen species in the aetiology of cancer, in *Drugs, Diet and Disease*. Vol. 1, *Mechanistic Approaches to Cancer*, Ioannides, C. and Lewis, D. F. V., Eds., Ellis Horwood, London, 1995, 47.
2. Baynes, J. W., Reactive oxygen in the aetiology and complications of diabetes, in *Drugs, Diet and Disease*. Vol. 2, *Mechanistic Approaches to Diabetes*, Ioannides, C. and Flatt, P. R., Eds., Ellis Horwood, London, 1995, 201.
3. Parke, A. L., Ioannides, C., Lewis, D. F. V., and Parke, D. V., Molecular pathology of drug–disease interactions in chronic autoimmune inflammatory diseases, *Inflammopharmacology*, 1,3, 1991.
4. Pirmohamed, M. and Park, B. K., Cytochromes P450 and immunotoxicity, in *Cytochromes P450: Metabolic and Toxicological Aspects*, Ioannides, C., Ed., CRC Press, Boca Raton, FL, 1996, 329.
5. Ioannides, C., Steele, C. M., and Parke, D. V., Species variation in the metabolic activation of paracetamol to toxic intermediates: role of cytochrome P-450 and P-448, *Toxicol. Lett.*, 16, 167, 1983.
6. Kawajiri, K., Yonekawa, H., Hara, E., and Tagashira, Y., Biochemical basis for the resistance of guinea pigs to the carcinogenesis by 2-acetylaminofluorene, *Biochem. Biophys. Res. Commun.*, 85, 275, 1978.
7. Kawajiri, K. and Hayashi, S.-I., The CYP1 family, in *Cytochromes P450: Metabolic and Toxicological Aspects*, Ioannides, C., Ed., CRC Press, Boca Raton, FL, 1996, 77.
8. Ioannides, C. and Parke, D. V., The cytochrome P450I gene family of microsomal haemoproteins and their role in the metabolic activation of chemicals, *Drug Metab. Rev.*, 22, 1, 1990.
9. Karki, N. T., Pokela, R., Nuutinen, L., and Pelkonen, O., Aryl hydrocarbon hydroxylase in lymphocytes and lung tissue from lung cancer patients and controls, *Int. J. Cancer*, 39, 565, 1987.
10. Bartsch, H., Castegnaro, M., Rojas, M., Camus, A.-M., Alexandrov, K., and Lang, M., Expression of pulmonary cytochrome P4501A1 and carcinogen adduct formation in high risk subjects for tobacco-related lung cancer, *Toxicol. Lett.*, 64/65, 477, 1992.
11. Pyykko, K., Tuimala, R., Aalto, L., and Perkio, T., Is aryl hydrocarbon hydroxylase activity a new prognostic indicator for breast cancer? *Br. J. Cancer*, 63, 596, 1991.
12. Chang, T. K. H. and Waxman, D. J., The CYP2A subfamily, in *Cytochromes P450: Metabolic and Toxicological Aspects*, Ioannides, C., Ed., CRC Press, Boca Raton, FL, 99, 1996.
13. Nims, R. W. and Lubet, R. A., The CYP2B subfamily, in *Cytochromes P450: Metabolic and Toxicological Aspects*, Ioannides, C., Ed., CRC Press, Boca Raton, FL, 1996, 135.
14. Richardson, T. H. and Johnson, E. F., in *Cytochromes P450: Metabolic and Toxicological Aspects*, Ioannides, C., Ed., CRC Press, Boca Raton, FL, 1996, 161.
15. Gonzalez, F. J., The CYP2D subfamily, in *Cytochromes P450: Metabolic and Toxicological Aspects*, Ioannides, C., Ed., CRC Press, Boca Raton, FL, 1996, 183.
16. Ronis, M. J. J., Lindros, K. O., and Ingelman-Sundberg, M., The CYP2E subfamily, in *Cytochromes P450: Metabolic and Toxicological Aspects*, Ioannides, C., Ed., CRC Press, Boca Raton, FL, 1996, 211.
17. Maurel, P., The CYP3 family, in *Cytochromes P450: Metabolic and Toxicological Aspects*, Ioannides, C., Ed., CRC Press, Boca Raton, FL, 1996, 329.
18. Lake, B. G. and Lewis, D. F. V., The CYP4 family, in *Cytochromes P450: Metabolic and Toxicological Aspects*, Ioannides, C., Ed., CRC Press, Boca Raton, FL, 1996, 271.

19. Johnson, E. F., Palmer, C. N. A., Griffin, K. J., and Hse, M.-H., Role of the peroxisome proliferator-activated receptor in cytochrome P450 4A gene regulation, *FASEB J.*, 10, 1241, 1996.
20. Gibson, G. G., Comparative aspects of the mammalian cytochrome P450 IV gene family, *Xenobiotica*, 19, 1123, 1989.
21. Rekka, E., Ayalogu, E. O., Lewis, D. F. V., Gibson, G. G., and Ioannides, C., Induction of hepatic microsomal CYP4A activity and of peroxisomal β-oxidation by two non-steroidal anti-inflammatory drugs, *Arch. Toxicol.*, 68, 73, 1994.
22. Ayrton, A. D., Ioannides, C., and Parke, D. V., Induction of the cytochrome P450I and IV families and peroxisomal proliferation in the liver of rats treated with benoxaprofen. Possible implications in its hepatotoxicity, *Biochem. Pharmacol.*, 42, 109, 1991.
23. Eling, T. E. and Curtis, J. F., Xenobiotic metabolism by prostaglandin H synthase, *Pharmacol. Ther.*, 53, 261, 1992.
24. Smith, B. J., Curtis, J. F., and Eling, T. E., Bioacivation of xenobiotics by prostaglandin H synthase, *Chem. Biol. Interact.*, 79, 245, 1991.
25. Ziegler, D. M., Flavin-containing monooxygenases: enzymes adapted for multisubstrate specificity, *TIPS Rev.*, 11, 1990, 321.
26. Hines, R. N., Cashman, J. R., Philpot, R. M., Williams, D. E., and Ziegler, D. M., The mammalian flavin-containing monooxygenases; molecular characterization and regulation of expression, *Toxicol. Appl. Pharmacol.*, 125, 1, 1994.
27. Oesch, F., Significance of various enzymes in the control of reactive metabolites, *Arch. Toxicol.*, 60, 174, 1987.
28. Awasthi, Y. C., Sharma, R., and Singhal, S. S., Human glutathione S-transferases, *Int. J. Biochem.*, 26, 295, 1994.
29. Monks, T. J., Anders, M. W., Dekant, W., Stevens, J. L., Lau, S. S., and van Bladeren, P. J., Glutathione conjugate mediated toxicities, *Toxicol. Appl. Pharmacol.*, 106, 1, 1990.
30. Evans, D. P., N-Acetyltransferase, *Pharmacol. Ther.*, 42, 157, 1989.
31. Falany, C. N., Sulfation and sulfotransferases. 3. Enzymology of human cytosolic sulfotransferases, *FASEB J.*, 11, 206, 1997.
32. Mulder, G. J., Glucuronidation and its role in regulation of biological activity or rats, *Annu. Rev. Pharmacol. Toxicol.*, 32, 25, 1992.
33. Bolt, H. M., Interactions between clinically used drugs and oral contraceptives, *Environm. Health Perspect*, 102, 35, 1994.
34. Dixon, R. L., Hart, L. G., and Fouts, J. R., The metabolism of drugs by liver microsomes from alloxan-diabetic rats, *J. Pharmacol. Exp. Ther.*, 133, 7, 1961.
35. Dixon, R. L., Hart, L. G., Rogers, L. A., and Fouts, J. R., The metabolism of drugs by liver microsomes from alloxan-diabetic rats: long-term diabetes, *J. Pharmacol. Exp. Ther.*, 142, 312, 1963.
36. Kato, R. and Gillette, J. R., Sex differences in the effects of abnormal physiological states on the metabolism of drugs by rat liver microsomes, *J. Pharmacol. Exp. Ther.*, 150, 285, 1965.
37. Warren, B. L., Pak, R., Finlayson, M., Tontovnik, L., Sunahara, G., and Bellward, G., Differential effects of diabetes on microsomal metabolism of various substrates. Comparison of streptozotocin and spontaneously diabetic Wistar rats, *Biochem. Pharmacol.*, 32, 327, 1983.
38. Kato, R., Onoda, K.-I., and Takanaka, A., Species difference in drug metabolism by liver microsomes in alloxan diabetic or fasted animals. (I) The activity of drug-metabolizing enzymes and electron transport system, *Jpn. J. Pharmacol.*, 20, 546, 1970.
39. Kato, R., Onoda, K.-I., and Takanaka, A., Species difference in drug metabolism by liver microsomes in alloxan diabetic or fasted animals. (II) The substrate interaction with cytochrome P450 in drug oxidation, *Jpn. J. Pharmacol.*, 20, 554, 1970.
40. Ackerman, D. M. and Leibman, K. C., Effect of experimental diabetes on drug metabolism in the rat, *Drug Metab. Dispos.*, 5, 405, 1977.
41. Reinke, L. A., Stohs, S. J., and Rosenberg, A. H., Altered activity of hepatic mixed-function monooxygenase enzymes on streptozotocin-induced diabetic rats, *Xenobiotica*, 8, 611, 1978.
42. Stohs, S. J., Reinke, L. A., Hassing, J. M., and Rosenberg, A. H., Benzo(a)pyrene metabolism by hepatic and extrahepatic tissues in stereptozotocin diabetic rats, *Drug Metab. Dispos.*, 7, 49, 1979.

43. Peng, R., Tennant, P., Lorr, N. A., and Yang, C. S., Alterations of microsomal monooxygenase systems and carcinogen metabolism of streptozotocin-induced diabetes in rats, *Carcinogenesis*, 4, 703, 1983.

44. Al-Turk, W. A., Stohs, S. J., and Roche, E. B., Altered metabolism of ethoxycoumarin by hepatic, pulmonary and intestinal microsomes from streptozotocin-diabetic rats, *Drug Metab. Dispos.*, 8, 44,1980.

45. Nishimata, T., Yata, N., and Kamada, A., Pharmacokinetic behaviour of chlorpropamide and sulfadimethoxine in alloxan diabetic rabbits, *Chem. Pharm. Bull.*, 26, 3363, 1978.

46. Dajani, R. M. and Kayyali, S. Y., The biotransformation of acetophenetidine in the alloxan-diabetic rabbit, *Comp. Gen. Pharmacol.*, 4, 23, 1973.

47. D'Souza, M. J., Solomon, H. M., Fowler, L. C., and Pollock, S. H., Pharmacokinetics of cyclosporine in streptozotocin-induced diabetic rats, *Drug Metab. Dispos.*, 16, 78, 1988.

48. Toda, A., Shimeno, H., Nagamatsu, A., and Shigematsu, H., Effects of experimental diabetes on aminopyrine metabolism in rats, *Xenobiotica*, 17, 1075, 1987.

49. Lin, J. H., Deluna, F. A., Tocco, D. J., and Ulm, E. H., Effect of experimental diabetes on elimination kinetics of diflunisal in rats, *Drug Metab. Dispos.*, 17, 147, 1989.

50. Andrews, S. M. And Griffiths, L. A., The metabolism and disposition of [2-14C]diazepam in the streptozotocin-diabetic rat, *Xenobiotica*, 14, 751, 1984.

51. Kazumi, T., Yoshimo, G., Fujii, S., and Baba, S., Tumorigenic action of streptozotocin on the pancreas and kidney in male Wistar rats, *Cancer Res.*, 38, 2144, 1978.

52. Laguens, R. P., Candela, S., Hernandez, R. E., and Gagliardino, J. J., Streptozotocin-induced liver damage in mice, *Horm. Metab. Res.*, 12, 197, 1980.

53. Past, M. R. and Cook, D. E., Alterations in hepatic microsomal cytochrome P450 heme-proteins in diabetic rats, *Res. Commun. Chem. Pathol. Pharmacol.*, 27, 329, 1980.

54. Past, M. R. and Cook, D. E., Effect of diabetes on rat liver cytochrome P450. Evidence for a unique diabetes-dependent liver cytochrome P450, *Biochem. Pharmacol.*, 31, 3329, 1982.

55. Past, M. R. and Cook, D. E., Drug metabolism in a reconstituted system by diabetes-dependent hepatic cytochrome P450, *Res. Commun. Chem. Pathol. Pharmacol.*, 37, 81, 1982.

56. Schein, P. S., Cooney, D. A., and Vernon, M. L., The use of nicotinamide to modify the toxicity of streptozotocin in diabetes without loss of anti-tumour activity, *Cancer Res.*, 27, 2324, 1967.

57. Ioannides, C., Bass, S. L., Ayrton, A. D., Trinick, J., Walker, R., and Flatt, P. R., Streptozotocin-induced diabetes modulates the metabolic activation of chemical carcinogens, *Chem. Biol. Interact.*, 68, 189, 1988.

58. Barnett, C. R., Flatt, P. R., and Ioannides, C., Induction of hepatic microsomal P450I and IIB proteins by hyperketonemia, *Biochem. Pharmacol.*, 40, 393, 1990.

59. Barnett, C. R., Flatt, P. R., and Ioannides, C., Modulation of the rat hepatic cytochrome P450 composition by long-term streptozotocin-induced insulin-dependent diabetes, *J. Biochem. Toxicol.*, 9, 63, 1994.

60. Yamazoe, Y., Murayama, N., Shimada, M., Yamauchi, K., and Kato, R., Cytochrome P450 in livers of diabetic rats: regulation by growth hormone and insulin, *Arch. Biochem. Biophys.*, 268, 567, 1989.

61. Barnett, C. R., Flatt, P. R., Bone, A. J., and Ioannides, C., Hepatic cytochrome P450 profile in BB rats with spontaneous insulin-dependent diabetes mellitus, in *Biochemistry, Biophysics and Molecular Biology of Cytochrome P450*, Lechner, M. C., Ed., John Libbey Eurotext, Paris, 547, 1994.

62. Chen, T.-L., Chen, S.-H., Tai, T.-Y., Chao, C.-C., Park, S. S., Guengerich, F. P., and Ueng, T.-H., Induction and suppression of renal and hepatic cytochrome P450-dependent monooxygenases by acute and chronic streptozotocin diabetes in hamsters, *Arch. Toxicol*, 70, 202, 1996.

63. Irizar, A. and Ioannides, C., Extrahepatic expression of P450 proteins in insulin-dependent diabetes mellitus, *Xenobiotica*, 25, 941, 1995.

64. Yamazoe, Y., Abu-Zeid, M., Yamouchi, K., Murayama, N., Shimada, M., and Kato, R., Enhancement by alloxan-induced diabetes of the rate of metabolic activation of three pyrolysate carcinogens via increase in P-448-H content in rat liver, *Biochem. Pharmacol*, 37, 2503, 1988.

65. Ioannides, C. and Parke, D. V., The cytochrome P450I gene family of microsomal hemoproteins and their role in the metabolic activation of chemicals, *Drug Metab. Rev.*, 22, 1, 1990.

66. Flatt, P. R., Bass, S.L., Ayrton, A. D., Trinick, J., and Ioannides, C., Metabolic activation of chemical carcinogens by hepatic preparations from streptozotocin-treated rats, *Diabetologia*, 32, 135, 1989.
67. Shimojo, N., Ishizaki, T., Imaoka, S., Funae, Y., Fujii, S., and Okuda, K., Changes in amounts of cytochrome P450 isozymes and levels of catalytic activities in hepatic and renal microsomes of rats with streptozotocin-induced diabetes, *Biochem. Pharmacol.*, 46, 621, 1993.
68. Thummel, K. E. and Schenkman, J., Effects of testosterone and growth hormone treatment on hepatic microsomal P450 expression in the diabetic rat, *Mol. Pharmacol.*, 37, 119, 1990.
69. Favreau, L. V. and Schenkman, J. B., Decrease in the levels of a constitutive cytochrome P-450 (RLM5) in hepatic microsomes of diabetic rats, *Biochem. Biophys. Res. Commun.*, 142, 623, 1987.
70. Donahue, B. S. and Morgan, E. T., Effects of vanadate on hepatic cytochrome P-450 expression in streptozotocin-induced diabetes, *Drug Metab. Dispos.*, 18, 1992, 519.
71. Favreau, L. V. and Schenkman, J. B., Composition changes in hepatic microsomal cytochrome P-450 during onset of streptozotocin-induced diabetes and during insulin treatment, *Diabetes*, 37, 577, 1988.
72. Bellward, G. D., Chang, T., Rodrigues, B., McNeill, J. H., Maines, S., Ryan, D. E., Levin, N., and Thomas, P. E., Hepatic cytochrome P-450j induction in the spontaneously diabetic BB rat, Mol. Pharmacol., 33, 140, 1988.
73. Irizar, A. and Ioannides, C., unpublished data
74. Thomas, P. E., Bandiera, S., Maines, S. L., Ryan, D. E., and Levin, W., Regulation of cytochrome P450j — a high affinity N-nitrosodimethylamine demethylase in rat hepatic microsomes, *Biochemistry*, 26, 2280, 1987.
75. Dong, Z., Hong, J., Ma, Q., Li, D., Bullock, J., Gonzalez, F. J., Park, S. S., Gelboin, H. V., and Yang, C. S., Mechanisms of induction of cytochrome P-450$_{ac}$ (P-450j) in chemically induced and spontaneous diabetic rats, *Arch. Biochem. Biophys.*, 263, 29, 1988.
76. Favreau, L. V., Machoff, D. M., Mole, J. E., and Schenkman, J., Responses to insulin by two forms of rat hepatic microsomal cytochrome P-450 that undergo major (RLM6) and minor (RLM5b) elevations in diabetes, *J. Biol. Chem.*, 262, 14319, 1987.
77. Song, B. J., Matsunaga, T., Hardwick, J. P., Park, S. S., Veech, R. L.,Yang, C. S., Gelboin, H. V., and Gonzalez, F. J., Stabilization of cytochrome P450j messenger ribonucleic acid in the diabetic rat, *Mol. Endocrinol.*, 1, 542, 1987.
78. Clarke, J., Snelling, J., Ioannides, C., Flatt, P. R., and Barnett, C. R., Effect of vitamin C supplementation on hepatic cytochrome P450 mixed-function oxidase activity in streptozotocin-diabetic rats, *Toxicol. Lett.*, 89, 249, 1996.
79. Lewis, D. F. V., Ioannides, C., and Parke, D. V., Validation of a novel molecular orbital approach (COMPACT) for the prospective safety evaluation of chemicals by comparison with rodent carcinogenicity and *Salmonella* mutagenicity data evaluated by the US/NTP, *Mutat. Res.*, 21, 61, 1993.
80. Lorr, N. A., Miller, K. W., Chung, H. R., and Yang, C. S., Potentiation of the hepatotoxicity of N-nitrosodimethylamine by fasting, diabetes, acetone and isopropanol, *Toxicol. Appl. Pharmacol.*, 73, 423, 1984.
81. Watkins, J. B., III, Sanders, R. A., and Beck, L. V., The effect of long-term streptozotocin-induced diabetes on the hepatotoxicity of bromobenzene and carbon tetrachloride and hepatic biotransformation in rats, *Toxicol. Appl. Pharmacol.*, 93, 329, 1988.
82. Hanasono, G. K., Cote, M. G., and Plaa, G. L., Potentiation of carbon tetrachloride-induced hepatotoxicity in alloxan- or streptozotocin-diabetic rats, *J. Pharmacol. Exp. Ther.*, 192, 592, 1975.
83. Hanasono, G. K., Witschi, H., and Plaa, G. L., Potentiation of the hepatotoxic responses to chemicals in alloxan-diabetic rats, *Proc. Soc. Exp. Biol. Med.*, 149, 903, 1975.
84. Price, V. F. and Jollow, D. J., Increased resistance of diabetic rats to acetaminophen-induced hepatotoxicity, *J. Pharmacol. Exp. Ther.*, 220, 504, 1982.
85. Barnett, C. R., Gibson, G. G., Wolf, C. R., Flatt, P. R., and Ioannides, C., Induction of cytochrome P450III and P450IV family proteins in streptozotocin-induced diabetes, *Biochem. J.*, 268,765, 1990.
86. Subbiah, M. T. R. and Yunker, R. L., Cholesterol 7α-hydroxylase of rat liver: an insulin sensitive enzyme, *Biochem. Biophys. Res. Commun.*, 124, 896, 1984.

87. Hansson, R., Effect of diabetes, starvation, ethanol and isoniazid on rat liver microsomal 12α-hydroxylase activity involved in bile acid biosynthesis, *Biochem. Pharmacol.*, 38, 3386, 1989.

88. Skett, P., Sex-dependent effect of streptozotocin-induced diabetes mellitus on hepatic steroid metabolism in the rat, *Acta Endocrinol.*, 111, 217, 1986.

89. Reinke, L. A., Stohs, S. J., and Rosenberg, H., Increased aryl hydrocarbon hydroxylase activity in hepatic microsomes from streptozotocin-diabetic rats, *Xenobiotica*, 12, 769, 1979.

90. Barnett, C. R., Wilson, J., Wolf, C. R., Flatt, P. R., and Ioannides, C., Hyperinsulinemia causes a preferential increase in hepatic P4501A2 activity, *Biochem. Pharmacol.*, 43, 1255, 1992.

91. De Waziers, I., Garlatti, M., Bouguet, J., Beaune, P. H., and Barouki, R., Insulin downregulates P4502B and 2E expression at the post-transcriptional level in the rat hepatoma cell line, *Mol. Pharmacol.*, 47, 474, 1995.

92. Yoshida, Y., Kimura, N., Oda, H., and Kakinuma, A., Insulin suppresses induction of CYP2B1 and CYP2B2 gene expression by phenobarbital in adult rat cultured hepatocytes, *Biochem. Biophys. Res. Commun.*, 229, 182, 1996.

93. Hartshorn, R. D., Demers, L. M., Sultatos, L. G., Vesell, E. S., Max Lang, C., and Hughes, H. C., Jr., Effects of chronic parenteral carbohydrate administration on hepatic drug metabolism in rat, *Pharmacology*, 18, 103, 1979.

94. Rouer, E., Beaune, P., Augereau, C., and Leroux, J.-P., The effect of different hyperglucago-naemic states on monooxygenase activities and isozymic patterns of cytochrome P450 in mouse, *Biosci. Rep.*, 5, 335, 1985.

95. Barnett, C. R., Flatt, P. R., and Ioannides, C., Role of ketone bodies in the diabetes-induced changes in hepatic mixed-function oxidase activities, *Biochim. Biophys. Acta*, 967, 250, 1988.

96. Barnett, C. R., Petrides, L., Wilson, J., Flatt, P. R., and Ioannides, C., Induction of rat hepatic mixed-function oxidases by acetone and other physiological ketones: their role in diabetes-induced changes in cytochrome P450 proteins, *Xenobiotica*, 22, 1441, 1992.

97. Li, D., Brady, J. F., Lee, M. J., and Yang, C. S., Effect of 1,3-butanediol on rat liver microsomal NDMA demethylation and other monooxygenase activities, *Toxicol. Lett.*, 45, 141, 1989.

98. Johansson, I., Ekstrom, G., Scholte, B., Puzycki, D., Jornvall, H., and Ingelman-Sunsberg, M., Ethanol-, fasting- and acetone-inducible cytochromes P450 in rat liver: regulation and characteristics of enzymes belonging to the IIB and IIE gene subfamilies, *Biochemistry*, 27, 1925, 1988.

99. Brady, J. F., Li, D., Ishizaki, H., Lee, M., Ning, S. M., Xiao, F., and Yang, C. S., Induction of cytochromes P450IIE1 and P450IIB1 by secondary ketones and the role of P450IIE1 in chloroform metabolism, *Toxicol. Appl. Pharmacol.*, 100, 342, 1989.

100. Wu, D. and Cederbaum, A. I., Combined effects of streptozotocin-induced diabetes plus 4-methylpyrazole treatment on rat liver cytochrome P4502E1, *Arch. Biochem. Biophys.*, 312, 175, 1993.

101. Kaikaus, R. M., Chan, W. K., Lysenko, N., Ray, R., Ortiz de Montellano, P. R., and Bass, N. M., Induction of peroxisomal fatty acid β-oxidation and liver fatty acid-binding protein by peroxisome proliferators. Mediation via the cytochrome P-450IVA1 ω-hydroxylase pathway, *J. Biol. Chem.*, 268, 9593, 1993.

102. Tollet, P., Strömstedt, M., Frøyland, L., Berge, R. K., and Gustaffson, J.-Å., Pretranslational regulation of cytochrome P4504A1 by free fatty acids in primary cultures of rat hepatocytes, *J. Lipid Res.*, 35, 248, 1994.

103. Zangar, R. C. and Novak, R. F., Effects of fatty acids and ketone bodies on cytochromes P450 2B, 4A and 2E1 expression in primary cultured hepatocytes, *Arch. Biochem. Biophys.*, 337, 217, 1997.

104. Ferguson, N. L., Donahue, B. S., Tenney, K. A., and Morgan, E. T., Pretranslational induction of CYP4A subfamily gene products in diabetic rats and reversal by oral vanadate treatment, *Drug Metab. Dispos.*, 21, 745, 1993.

105. Hewitt, W. R. and Plaa, G. L., Potentiation of carbon tetrachloride-induced hepatotoxicity by 1,3-butanediol, *Toxicol. Appl. Pharmacol.*, 47, 177, 1979.

106. Hewitt, W. R. and Plaa, G. L., Dose-dependent modification of 1,1-dichloroethylene toxicity by acetone, *Toxicol. Lett.*, 16, 145, 1983.

107. Hewitt, W. R., Miyajima, H., Cote, M. G., and Plaa, G. L., Modification of haloalkane-induced hepatotoxicity by exogenous ketones and metabolic ketosis, *Fed. Proc.*, 39, 3118, 1980.

108. MacDonald, J. R., Gandolfi, A. J., and Sipes, I. G., Acetone potentiation of 1,1,2-trichloroethane hepatotoxicity, *Toxicol. Lett.*, 13, 57, 1982.

109. Barnett, C. R., Flatt, P. R., and Ioannides, C., Hyperketonemia markedly modulates the metabolic activation of chemical carcinogens, *Chem. Biol. Interact.*, 74, 281, 1990.

110. Tannenbaum, G. S., Growth hormone secretory dynamics in the streptozotocin diabetes: evidence of a role for endogenous somatostatin, *Endocrinology*, 18, 76, 1981.

111. Lemoine, A., Marie, S., and Cresteil, T., Expression of cytochrome P450 isozymes in the liver of hypophysectomized rats, *Eur. J. Biochem.*, 177, 597, 1988.

112. Williams, M. T. and Simonet, L. C., Effects of growth hormone on cytochrome P450, *Biochem. Biophys. Res. Commun.*, 155, 392, 1988.

113. Waxman, D. J., Morissey, J. J., and Leblanc, G. A., Hypophysectomy differentially alters P-450 protein levels and enzyme activities in rat liver: pituitary control of hepatic NADPH cytochrome P-450 reductase, *Mol. Pharmacol.*, 35, 519, 1989.

114. Chawalit, K., Sretarugsa, P., and Thithapandha, A., Comparative effects of diabetogenic agents on hepatic drug metabolism, *Drug Metab. Dispos.*, 10, 81, 1982.

115. Yamazoe, Y., Ling, X., Murayama, N., Gong, D., Nagata, K., and Kato, R., Modulation of hepatic level of microsomal testosterone 7α-hydroxylase, P-450a (P450IIA), by thyroid hormone and growth hormone in rat liver, *J. Biochem.*, 108, 599, 1990.

116. Rouer, E., Rouet, P., Delpech, M., and Leroux, J.-P., Purification and comparison of liver microsomal flavin-containing monooxygenase from normal and streptozotocin-diabetic rats, *Biochem. Pharmacol.*, 18, 3455, 1988.

117. Grant, M. H. and Duthie, S. J., Conjugation reactions in hepatocytes isolated from streptozotocin-induced diabetic rats, *Biochem. Pharmacol.*, 36, 3647, 1987.

118. Lindsay, R. M. and Baty, J. D., The effects of streptozotocin-induced diabetes on the *in vivo* acetylation and the *in vitro* blood N-acetyltransferase activity of the adult Sprague-Dawley rat, *Biochem. Pharmacol.*, 39, 1193, 1990.

119. Lindsay, R. M. and Baird, J. D., The effect of diabetes on the *in vivo* acetylation capacity of the spontaneously diabetic, insulin-dependent BB/Edinburgh Wistar rat, *Biochem. Pharmacol.*, 41, 425, 1991.

120. Xiaotao, Q. and Hall, S. D., Enantioselective effects of experimental diabetes mellitus on the metabolism of ibuprofen, *J. Pharmacol. Exp. Ther.*, 274, 1192, 1995.

121. Rouer, E., Mahu, J. L., Dansette, P., and Leroux, J.-P., UDP-glucuronosyl transferase, epoxide hydrolase and glutathione S-transferase activities in the liver of diabetic mice, *Biochim. Biophys. Acta*, 676, 274, 1981.

122. Agius, C. and Gidari, A. S., Effects of streptozotocin on the glutathione S-transferases of mice liver cytosol, *Biochem. Pharmacol.*, 34, 811, 1985.

123. Thomas, H., Schladt, L., Knehr, M., and Oesch, F., Effect of diabetes and starvation on the activity of rat liver epoxide hydroxylases, glutathione S-transferases and peroxisomal β-oxidation, *Biochem. Pharmacol.*, 38, 4291, 1989.

124. McLennan, S. V., Heffernan, S., Wright, L., Rae, C., Fisher, E., Yue, D. K., and Turtle, J. R., Changes in hepatic glutathione metabolism in diabetes, *Diabetes*, 40, 344, 1991.

125. Rouer, E. and Leroux, J.-P., Liver microsomal cytochrome P450 and related monooxygenase activities in genetically hyperglycemic (ob/ob and db/db) and streptozotocin-treated mice, *Biochem. Pharmacol.*, 29, 1959, 1980.

126. Barnett, C. R., Abbott, R. A., Bailey, C. J., Flatt, P. R., and Ioannides, C., Cytochrome P450-dependent mixed-function oxidase and glutathione S-transferase activities in spontaneous obesity diabetes, *Biochem. Pharmacol.*, 43, 1868, 1992.

127. Daintith, H., Stevenson, I. H., and O'Malley, K., Influence of diabetes mellitus on drug metabolites in man, *Int. J. Clin. Pharmacol.*, 13, 55, 1976.

128. Murali, K. V., Adithan, C., Shashindran, C. H., Gambhir, S. S., and Chandrasekar, S., Antipyrine metabolism in patients with diabetes mellitus, *Clin. Exp. Pharmacol. Physiol.*, 10, 7, 1983.

129. Salmela, P. I., Sotaniemi, E. A., and Pelkonen, O. R., The evaluation of the drug-metabolising capacity in patients with diabetes mellitus, *Diabetes*, 29, 788, 1980.

130. Dajani, R. M., Kayyali, S. R., Saheb, S. E., and Birbari, A., A study on the physiological disposition of acetophenetidine by diabetic man, *Comp. Gen. Pharmacol.*, 5, 1, 1974.

131. Ueda, H., Sakurai, T., Ota, M., Nakajima, A., Kamii, K., and Maezawa, H., Disappearance rate of tolbutamide in normal subjects and in diabetes mellitus, liver cirrhosis, and renal disease, *Diabetes*, 12, 414, 1963.
132. Sotaniemi, E. A., Arranto, A. J., Salmela, P. I., Stengard, J. H., and Pelkonen, O. R., Hepatic microsomal enzyme activity in patients with noninsulin-dependent diabetes mellitus (NID-DM) and its clinical significance, *Acta Endocrinol.*, 262, 125, 1984.
133. Song, B. J., Veech, R. L., and Saenger, P., Cytochrome P450IIE1 is elevated in lymphocytes from poorly controlled insulin-dependent diabetics, *J. Clin. Endocrinol. Metab.*, 71, 1036, 1990.
134. Korrapati, M., Vestal, R. E., and Loi, C.-M., Theophylline metabolism in healthy nonsmokers and in patients with insulin-dependent diabetes mellitus, *Clin. Pharmacol. Ther.*, 57, 413, 1995.
135. Paller, M. S., Hoydal, J. R., and Ferris, T. F., Oxygen free radicals in ischemic acute renal failure in the rat, *J. Clin. Invest.*, 74, 1156, 1984.
136. Armstrong, D. and Al-Awadi, F., Lipid peroxidation and retinopathy in streptozotocin-induced diabetes, *Free Radical Biol. Med.*, 11, 433, 1991.
137. Wolff, S. P., Diabetes mellitus and free radicals, *Br. Med. Bull.*, 49, 642, 1993.
138. Pessayre, D., Dolder, A., Artigou, J. Y., Wandscheer, J.-C., Descatoire, V., Degott, C., and Benhamou, J. P., Effect of fasting on metabolite-mediated hepatotoxicity in the rat, *Gastroenterology*, 77, 264, 1979.

6

Nerve and Retinal Changes in Experimental Diabetes

Subrata Chakrabarti

CONTENTS

0-8493-1667-7/99/$0.00+$.50
© 1999 by CRC Press LLC

6.1   Introduction

Diabetes and its complications are problems of enormous proportion. It is estimated that 5% of the world population is affected by diabetes.[1] In 1995, in the U.S. there are an estimated 16 million people with diabetes.[2] The estimated total cost of direct and indirect care for the population in the U.S. with diabetes was $92 billion in 1992.[2]

Long-term complications are a major cause of morbidity among patients with diabetes and about 60 to 70% of patients with diabetes have mild to severe forms of nerve damage.[2] Severe forms of diabetic nerve disease are a major cause of lower extremity amputation,[2] and diabetic neuropathy can affect both somatic and automonic nerves, causing a variety of symptoms.

It has been estimated that 12,000 to 24,000 new cases of blindness are caused by diabetes in the U.S. each year.[2] Although all structural components of the eye are affected in diabetes, retinopathy is the most important occular complication. Diabetic retinopathy is the leading cause of blindness in people 25 to 74 years old.[3] Retinopathy accounts for a 25-fold increase in the incidence of blindness in patients with Type I diabetes and a three to threefold increase in those with Type II diabetes compared with age-matched control populations.[4]

Although extensive research has been carried out in these two areas over the last three decades, the pathogenesis of these diabetic complications is not clear. To gain insight into the natural history of chronic diabetic complications, reproduction of the lesions in animal models is necessary. Data from various controlled animal experiments may provide desirable perspectives for the development of preventive or interventional therapeutic approaches. In chronic diabetic complications, where the pathogenesis is poorly understood, animal experiments are of immense importance as they offer unique advantages by enabling sequential studies at the molecular, biochemical, functional, and structural levels to pinpoint complex mechanisms in the dynamic development of the disease. Much of the knowledge regarding the pathogenesis of diabetic retinopathy and neuropathy stems from experiments in various animal models in which the lesions of these diabetic complications have been reproduced.

This chapter will briefly discuss human diabetic neuropathy and retinopathy and address various abnormalities in animal models of these diabetic complications and how they may enter into the complex pathogenetic web of this disorder. Both diabetic and galactosemic animals have been used in the study of diabetic complications. In the investigation of diabetic neuropathy, spontaneous or chemically diabetic rats are the predominant models. However, several strains of diabetic mice have also been used. The majority of the experiments in diabetic retinopathy have been carried out in diabetic dogs and rats. Galactosemic dogs and rats are important, as diabetes-like lesions are produced in these models, whcih provide specific model systems for the study of polyol pathway as well as other biochemical pathways activated secondarily to hyperhexosemia.

6.2 Diabetic Neuropathy in Humans

Diabetic neuropathy can be broadly classfied as mononeuropathy or polyneuropathy. Mononeuropathies can involve isolated single nerves or may affect multiple nerves (mononeuritis multiplex). These neuropathies may affect peripheral or cranial nerves.[5,6]

Polyneuropathies can affect the sensory, motor, or autonomic nervous system. Acute sensory neuropathy clinically manifests as a painful condition with complete recovery. Proximal motor neuropathies, also known as amyotrophy, are manifested as acute onset of pain and weakness of proximal muscle. Chronic sensorimotor polyneuropathy is the most common type of neuropathy. It is manifested as progressive glove-and-stocking anesthesia, paresthesia, or hyperasthesia, with impaired balance, propioception, and vibration. Although motor weakness is not pronounced, wasting of small muscle and loss of reflex activity are also manifested. As a long-term effect, foot ulceration and neuropathic changes may develop. Electrophysiologically impaired nerve conduction velocity is a key feature. Autonomic neuropathy may produce bladder, bowel, or gastric motility problems and postural hypotension.[5,6]

6.2.1 Pathology

Mononeuropathy is vascular in etiology and is manifested as infarction of nerve fibers secondary to an ischemic event. In the case of polyneuropathy, progressive loss of nerve fibers is the pathological hallmark of diabetic neuropathy.[5,6] Loss of nerve fibers roughly corresponds to the neurological deficit and delayed conduction velocity. The morphological findings further include segmental demyelination and remyelination and axonal degeneration. All structural subsets of the peripheral nerve, including the axonal cell body, manifest a series of lesions. Simultaneously, microangiopathic alterations, such as thickening of capillary basement membrane, develop in the endoneurial microvessels. The combined effects of all these changes ultimately manifest as clinical peripheral neuropathy.[5-8]

6.2.2 Pathogenesis

Hyperglycemia is possibly the primary pathogenetic factor in the development of all chronic diabetic complications; diabetic neuropathy is no exception. Several biochemical changes may develop in the cellular constituents of the peripheral nerve as a result of hyperglycemia.[7-8] Although some of the biochemical changes are universal to all organs affected by diabetic complications, others are peculiar to particular organ system such as peripheral nerve. The alterations include polyol-myoinositol-related metabolic defect, nonenzymatic glycation, altered carnitine and prostaglandin metabolism, defective synthesis of vasoactive factors, and neurotrophic factors alteration.[7-9] These changes will be described in detail in section 6.3.4 describing biochemical alterations in animal models. The biochemical changes may affect neuronal, glial, and vascular components of the nerves, and altered blood rheology may have its superimposed effect.[10] Although no direct relationship of rheological alteration with that of diabetic neuropathy has been detected, several rheological abnormalities, such as increased blood viscosity, fibrinogen levels, and red cell aggregation and decreased red cell deformability, have been demonstrated in diabetes.[10,11] Rheological alteration can contribute significantly toward loss of blood flow in the peripheral nerve.[10-12] Microscopically thrombotic occlusion of capillaries has been demonstarted in human diabetic neuropathy.[13] A complex interplay among all these factors may lead to neuronal functional deficit and, subsequently, to a cascade of structural alterations and may manifest clinically as diabetic neuropathy.

6.3   Animal Models of Diabetic Neuropathy

In contrast to the diverse animal models used for the study of diabetic retinopathy (see below), experimental work in diabetic neuropathy is largely limited to rodent models. The experiments are mainly directed toward the understanding of distal sensorimotor polyneuropathy and autonomic neuropathy. The animal models consists of models for both Type I and Type II diabetes.

6.3.1   Structural and Functional Changes in the Peripheral Nerve in Models of Type I Diabetes

Both spontaneously diabetic BB/W rats and streptozotocin (STZ)-induced diabetic rats have been investigated. Structural studies have been performed both at the light microscopic and at the ultrastructural level. The STZ diabetic rat is a well-studied model of diabetic neuropathy. Atrophy of the myelinated fiber is a reproducible, predominant lesion of the peripheral nerve in this model.[14-17] Single-nerve-fiber preparations have shown that nodal abnormalities, such as paranodal demyelination, segmental demyelination, and axonal degeneration, are produced in this model.[18-20] It is of interest to note that the lesions in this model are pronounced if the diabetes is induced after puberty,[21] when fiber atrophy is produced as early as 1 month after the onset of diabetes. This finding also suggests that, similarly to diabetic retinopathy, sex hormones may play an additional role in the genesis of diabetes-induced nerve damage.[22] The reduced fiber size secondary to axonal atrophy is severe distally compared with the proximal portion of the nerve in short-term diabetes.[18,23-25] With progression, however, the proximal portion showed similar changes.[24,25] This particular pathological change probably represents a structural component of axonal transport defect seen in diabetes.[24,25] Axonal pathology in STZ diabetic rats is manifested ultrastructurally in the form of dystrophic changes of the cytoskeleton, from accumulation of smooth ER and membrane-bound organelles to a complete wallerian degeneration.[18,26,27] Slowing of axonal transport of neurofilaments has been demonstrated in this model.[28-31] Both axonal transport defect and axonal atrophy in the peripheral nerve can be prevented by correction of hyperglycemia by insulin treatment or by islet transplantation and adjuvant therapy, such as aldose reductase (AR) inhibitor, myoinositol supplementation, methylcobalamin, and prostaglandin E1 analog.[19,20,32-33,36]

The spontaneously diabetic BB rat has been studied in depth by Sima et al.[37-60] Diabetes in this model is characterized by autoimmune destruction of β-cells.[52] Progressive nerve fiber loss has been reproducibly demonstrated in this model (Figure 6.1).[38,39,43] This model has been successfully used in the study of symmetric polyneuropathy and proximal motor neuropathy, as well as autonomic neuropathy.[36-60] Progressive nodal and paranodal changes in this model are similar to the human diabetic neuropathy.[42,43,46,49,50,55] The changes are manifested as axonal swelling, increased intraxonal Na^+, development of axoglial dysjunction, depression of nodal Na^+ channels, paranodal demyelination, remyelination, and distal wallerian degeneration.[42,43,46,49,50] Axoglial dysjunction probably represents initial demyelination, causes lateral migration of Na^+ channels, and can be completely prevented by

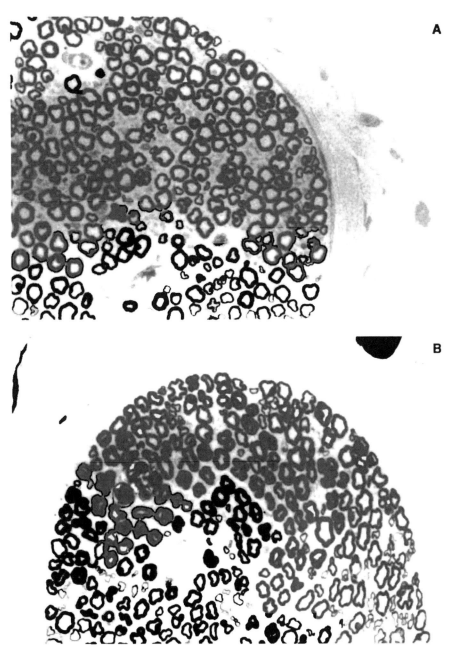

FIGURE 6.1
Photomicrographs of sural nerve from a nondiabetic BB/W rat (A) and an age-matched diabetic BB/W rat with 8-month duration of diabetes (B). Note marked axonal atrophy and wallerian degeneration in B. Magnification ×720 for both micrograrphs. (Courtesy of Dr. A. A. F. Sima, Department of Pathology, Wayne State University, Detroit, MI.)

treatment with an AR inhibitor or by pancreatic islet transplantation.[19,39-43,46,49] Metabolic defects secondary to hyperglycemia leading through a Na^+-K^+- ATPase-dependent mechanism have been suggested to be responsible for these nodal changes.[39-43,50,55] If hyperglycemia is corrected at the time of onset of diabetes by intensive insulin treatment, paranodal swelling, increased intraaxonal Na^+, and loss of nerve conduction velocity can all be completely corrected.[41-43,55] On the other hand, if the intervention is delayed in chronically diabetic animals, metabolic correction only partially restores nerve conduction velocity loss due to the development of structural changes, such as axonal atrophy and fiber loss.[37,39,40,46,55] In the neuronal microvasculature, thickening of the capillary basement membrane and loss of charge selective barrier, which may lead to increased permeability, are present in these animals.[56] A significant fiber loss is present in this model after long-term diabetes.[36,37,55] An impaired regeneration of nerve fibers in diabetic BB rats is associated with reduced expression of insulin-like growth factor-I (IGF-I) and nerve growth factor (NGF) and impaired immune response to nerve injury.[44,45,49] AR inhibitor treatment, however, was able to correct this impaired regeneration.[44] Similarly to the sensory and motor nerves, the autonomic nervous system in the BB rat shows dystrophic changes in the proximal axon and distal axonal atrophy in both sympathetic and parasympathetic nerves.[51,53,54,57,59] These lesions in the somatosensory nerves of the BB rat are similar to those in STZ diabetic rats, and a similar pathogenetic mechanism may be responsible for the pathogenesis of these changes.[7] However, in addition to the metabolic defects, non-enzymatic glycation of proteins and cross-linking may be another factor in the genesis of axonopathy in the rats.[59,60] The BB rat further shows a central sensory neuropathy, which is less severe than the simultaneously occurring peripheral neuropathy accompanied by dystrophic changes in the proximal axons and in the ganglion cells of the retina.[61,62]

Functional changes of peripheral neuropathies have been extensively demonstrated in rodent diabetes. In the study of peripheral neuropathy, slowing of motor nerve conduction velocity is the major functional alteration. A wide range of pharmaceutical agents, such as insulin, AR inhibitors, myoinositol, Ca^{2+} channel blocker, hyperbaric oxygen, and ganglioside, were found to prevent slowing of nerve conduction velocity, autonomic disturbance, and axoplasmic transport in rats with chemical or spontaneous diabetes.[40-43,49,55,62-127] Several additional treatment modalities such as essential fatty acid, prostaglandin E1 analog, ACTH analog, α-glucosidase inhibitor, methylcobolamine, and acetylcarnitine, were found to prevent loss of nerve conduction velocity.[62-127] These data suggest that although hyperglycemia is a key initiating event, it may subsequently lead to several biochemical abnormalities, all of which may contribute in part to loss of nerve conduction velocity. Several of these factors possibly act through reduced neurofilament synthesis, transport, and subsequent axonal atrophy.[7] Impaired low- and high-molecular-weight neurofilament mRNA expression has been demonstrated in the dorsal root ganglion cells of STZ diabetic rats.[128,129]

Study of the autonomic nervous system in diabetic BB/W rats showed the presence of cardiac sinus arrythmia, which can be prevented by AR inhibitor treatment.[58,130] The BB rat and the STZ rats both develop urinary bladder dysfunction, which can be corrected by ganglioside therapy.[104,106,107,131,132] BB rats further show increased latencies of visual evoked potentials, which can be corrected by AR inhibitor treatment.[62]

As ischemia has been proposed to be a pathogenetic factor in the genesis of diabetic neuropathy, endoneurial blood flow has been measured in the peripheral nerves of diabetic rats. In STZ-induced diabetic rats, increased vascular resistance and reduced endoneurial blood flow and oxygen tension have been demonstrated in the peripheral nerve.[133,34] In diabetic rats, reduced endoneurial blood flow and nerve conduction velocity have been shown to be prevented by several vasoactive substances. The list of the drugs include prostaglandins, α-adrenergic blockers, essential fatty acids, angiotensin-converting enzyme inhibitor, Ca^{2+} channel blockers, endothelin (ET) receptor blockers.[113,135-140] In acute diabetes, however, discordant data have been obtained regarding whether the endoneurial blood flow and vascular permeability are increased or decreased in diabetes.[9,141-148] Various methods used for measurement of blood flow as well as the various time points at which measurements were made may in part be responsible for such discrepancies.[9,82,141-148] The data, however, are indicative of loss of microvascular autoregulation in the peripheral nerve in diabetes.[7-9] The results from the experimental studies with regard to blood flow suggest that hypoxia is an important effect of diabetic dysmetabolism, be it via direct vasoconstriction[7-9] or via other metabolic defects leading to a "hyperglycemic pseudohypoxia."[141] In keeping with this view, it has been demonstrated that several vasoactive substances, such as noradrenergic antagonist, Ca^{2+} channel antagonist, angiotensin-converting enzyme inhibitor, ET-1 antagonist, and prostanoid analogs, are effective in simultaneous prevention of the alteration of blood flow and reduced nerve conduction velocity.[133-150] It is of further interest to note that in STZ diabetic rats, but not in the age-matched normal rats, vasoactive peptide ET-1 was found to have a major role in the production of nerve perfusion deficit and treatment with a specific ET-1 antagonist can prevent such deficit and reduced nerve conduction velocity.[139]

6.3.2 Structural and Functional Changes in the Peripheral Nerve in Models of Type II Diabetes

The models of Type II diabetes used for the study of diabetic neuropathy include db/db mice and GK rats. In db/db mice, decreased nerve conduction velocity, axonal and nerve fiber atrophy, Schwann cell changes, and vascular changes such as thickening of the basement membrane have been demonstrated.[151-155] Some investigators, however, have failed to demonstrate axonal atrophy.[156] The changes in this model are relatively mild. An Na^+-K^+-ATPase-dependent mechanism may be responsible for the pathogenesis of neuropathy in this model.[157]

The GK rat is a nonobese, hyperglycemic, noninsulin-dependent model of diabetes. This model demonstrates loss of nerve conduction velocity and myelinated nerve fiber atrophy without axonal atrophy.[158] Using freeze-fracture studies, a reduction of intramembranous particles in the myelin sheath has been demonstrated.[158] Interestingly, vascular changes such as thickening of basement membrane, which are not prominent features in STZ or BB rats, have been demonstrated in these animals.[158] It is further to be noted that although axonal atrophy is present in the peripheral nerves in Type II models, it is not a prominent feature compared with the Type I models.[7]

6.3.3 Structural and Functional Changes in the Peripheral Nerve in Galactosemic Models

The importance of galactosemic animal models is due to the fact that the activated polyol pathway mechanism is significant in the development of diabetic neuropathy. Although biochemical changes in these animals are different from those of diabetic animals (see below), morphological and functional changes such as slowing of nerve conduction velocity and myelinated nerve fiber atrophy similar to the diabetic animals have been demonstrated in this model.[159,160] In contrast to the diabetic animals, where axonal atrophy is the predominant lesion, galactosemic animals show Schwann cell abnormalities and demyelination.[159,160]

6.3.4 Biochemical Changes in the Peripheral Nerve

Degree and duration of antecedent hyperglycemia is the key initiating event in the pathogenesis of diabetic neuropathy. DCCT trials have shown that intensive insulin treatment effectively delays the onset and slows the progression of diabetic neuropathy.[161,162]

Traditionally, pathogenetic hypotheses with regard to diabetic peripheral neuropathy have been grouped under "metabolic theories" and "vascular theories."[7-9] However, the metabolic abnormalities secondary to hyperglycemia affect both the vascular and nonvascular components of the peripheral nerve. The subsequent alterations are also interdependent. Several biochemical abnormalities may be triggered secondarily to hyperglycemia. Although similar abnormalities may occur in various target organs of diabetic complications, the effects of these alterations may be tissue specific. The abnormalities in the peripheral nerve in diabetes include augmented polyol-myoinositol-related metabolic defect, impaired fatty acid metabolism, nonenzymatic glycation, oxidative stress, protein kinase C (PKC) abnormalities, and alteration of growth factors.[7-9] As the neuronal tissue is not dependent on insulin for glucose uptake, the vascular, neuronal, and glial cells are all affected. A complex interaction of the biochemical and subsequently developed functional abnormalities interact and finally manifest as loss of nerve fibers and clinical diabetic retinopathy. In this section some of these mechanisms will be discussed as they apply to the pathogenesis of diabetic neuropathy.

6.3.4.1 Augmented Polyol Pathway, Myoinositol Depletion, and Their Consequences

Augmented polyol pathway activity is a well-studied mechanism of diabetic complications. The key enzyme AR2 has a high k_m for glucose. However, under hyperglycemic conditions, particularly in tissues where glucose uptake is not dependent on insulin, glucose can be metabolized to sorbitol by the enzyme AR2 and then to fructose by sorbitol dehydrogenase.[163-166] Experimental evidence in both the STZ rat and the BB/W rat shows that this may be one of the important pathogenetic mechanisms.[7-9,66-82,164,167-170] AR has been localized in the Schwann cell, particularly arround the nodal region and in the microvasculature of the peripheral nerve.[167] Augmented AR2 mRNA, protein, and enzyme reacitvity are present in the peripheral nerve from diabetic BB/W rats. All these changes are correctable by euglycemia achieved by insulin treatment, whereas AR inhibitor prevented only AR enzyme activity.[168] Accumulation of intracellular sorbitol causes an increase in intracellular osmotic pressure and a reciprocal depletion of myoinositol and taurine.[169-171] In animals with spontaneous or chemical diabetes, myoinositol causes deranged phosphoinositide metabolism and subsequent impaired activation of PKC activity, ultimately translating to impaired nerve Na^+-K^+-ATPase activity.[55,164,172-178] Nerve Na^+-K^+-ATPase activity and impaired conduction velocity in diabetic rats are corrected by myoinositol supplementation, ARI inhibitors, and prostacyclins.[43,110-112,177,178] On the other hand, myoinositol derangement may not be a primary mechanism, as AR inhibitor treatment can correct nerve functional deficit in spite of decreased tissue myoinositol levels.[179,180] It is of further interest to note that in long-term diabetes, to maintain tissue osmolality, the AR gene may be downregulated.[128,181]

Similarly to the hyperglycemic conditions, in experimental galactosemia, galactitol accumulates in the tissue due to polyol pathway activation as it cannot be metabolized further. Loss of nerve conduction velocity in these animals is further associated with myoinositol and taurine depletion.[7,170,182-183] However, in contrast to diabetic animals, galactosemic rats show a high Na^+-K^+-ATPase activity,[182,183] indicating that although the response to polyol pathway activation is different in this model it may lead to similar structural changes.

6.3.4.2 Altered Redox Potential

Augmented polyol pathway activity may have other far-reaching effects. Increased $NADH^+$/NAD ratio as a result of increased glycolysis and an activated polyol pathway may lead to tissue changes similar to hypoxia and has been termed *pseudohypoxia*.[141] The effects include reduced fatty acid oxidation and decreased neuronal Na$^+$-K$^+$-ATPase activity.[141] Depletion of NADPH may inhibit nitric oxide (NO) generation as NO synthase and AR2 share the same cofactor. Experimental NO inhibitors in normal rats produce slower nerve conduction velocity.[138] Free radical generation in diabetes is favored by an increased NADH$^+$/NAD ratio.[141] Increased free radical generation in the diabetic endothelium may destroy NO.[184] PKC alteration (see below) may further modulate NO activity.[141] Based on these findings, it appears that the beneficial effects of AR inhibitors on the reduced nerve conduction velocity in diabetes may be in part mediated through the effect on NO generation.[9] Experimental evidence supports the interrelationship between AR and NO. For example, AR inhibitor treatment in diabetic rats improves blood flow and nerve conduction velocity deficit, along with endothelium-dependent relaxation to normal levels.[184-186] Furthermore, AR inhibitor–mediated prevention of neuropathy can be reversed by treatment with l-NAME, an NO synthase inhibitor, in spite of high sorbitol and decreased myoinositol levels.[8,9,186]

Abnormal fatty acid metabolism has been implicated in the pathogenesis of neuropathy. The increased NADH$^+$/NAD ratio inhibits β-oxidation of long-chain fatty acids and the accumulation of these long-chain fatty acids as esters of coenzyme A and carnitine.[141,187-190] These acyl esters can modulate enzyme activity of Na$^+$-K$^+$-ATPase, PKC, etc. Furthermore, the increased NADH/NAD ratio may affect prostaglandin metabolism by increasing the synthesis of vasoconstricting thromboxane and reducing the synthesis of vasodilatory prostacyclins.[141,191] This view is supported by the evidence that treatment with acetylcarnitine is effective in blocking nerve conduction velocity deficit in the diabetic rat.[97,98] Reduced superoxide dismutase and glutathione synthase may further increase oxidative stress in diabetes.[65] It has been shown that antioxidant therapy prevents diabetes-induced reduced blood flow and nerve conduction velocity.[65,126,127,147]

6.3.4.3   Nonenzymatic Glycation

Nonenzymatic modification of tissue proteins by physiological hexoses *in vivo* is an important secondary mechanism in the pathogenesis of diabetic retinopathy.[192] Glucose and fructose generated as end products of polyol pathway activity take part in nonenzymatic glycation of proteins.[60,192-194] Advanced glycation end products (AGE) accumulate in the tissues as a function of time and sugar concentration. AGEs may change the functional and structural properties of proteins and contribute to pathophysiological alterations in diabetes.[60,192,193] AGEs may affect signal transduction pathways and the levels of soluble signals, such as cytokines, hormones, and free radicals, directly affecting protein functions in target tissues.[60,195] Basement membrane proteins, myelin, tubulin, and neurofilaments all undergo glycation in hyperglycemia.[196-200] In the peripheral nerve, this mechanism role plays an important through its effects on structural proteins, free radical generation, and NO depletion.[60,141,195-200] Aminoguanidine, an inhibitor of nonenzymatic glycation has been demonstrated to improve motor nerve conduction velocity and the blood flow deficit in diabetic rats.[118,120,201]

6.3.4.4   DAG-PKC Pathway

Impaired phosphoinositide metabolism in the peripheral nerve may lead to impaired activity of PKC and Na$^+$-K$^+$-ATPase. This is in sharp contrast to the retinal findings, where an activation of PKC has been established (see below). Peripheral nerves from diabetic animals show reduced diacylglycerol (DAG) levels.[202] Furthermore, PKC inhibitors prevent diabetes-induced reduced neuronal Na$^+$-K$^+$-ATPase.[203] In a recent study decreased DAG and PKC activity and nerve conduction velocity in association with increased blood flow and albumin permeation have been demonstrated. All these changes are preventable by treatment with acetylcarnitine.[204] These data demonstrate that biochemical alterations in hyperglycemia may vary in target organs of diabetic complications depending on the tissue microenvironment.

6.3.4.5 Growth Factor Abnormalities

Growth factor abnormalities may develop secondarily to diabetic dysmetabolism by a direct effect of hyperglycemia or by a PKC-mediated pathway or via defective phosphoinositide metabolism.[8,205] NGF is a physiological requirement for maintaining neuronal integrity. Reduced NGF levels, however, have been demonstrated in STZ diabetic rats and in diabetic mice.[206-208] Decreased NGF transport has been demonstrated in the somatic sensory nerve.[209] Simultaneously, mRNA expression for NGF receptor trk1 and NGF-dependent genes such as substance P and calcitonin gene–related peptide are decreased.[210-214] Several of these changes are normalized by metabolic correction with insulin.[210] Functionally, externally administered NGF and the compounds that stimulate NGF synthesis are effective in improving diabetes-induced reduction in nerve conduction velocity deficit.[215,216] Another neurotrophic factor, neurotrophin-3, mRNA has recently been reported to be reduced in the muscle of diabetic rats, supplementation of which selectively improves sensory loss in diabetes.[210] Among the other growth factors, reduced serum IGF-I levels and decreased IGF-1 mRNA in the non-neuronal tissues have been demonstrated in STZ diabetic rats.[217-220] The present data support the notion that deficient neurotrophism is an important pathogenetic factor in diabetic neuropathy. A detailed analysis of the role of growth factors is, however, necessary for the better understanding of their role in the pathogenesis of diabetic neuropathy and to develop potential targeted therapies.

The data obtained from these biochemical pathways are complex but interactive and may involve vascular, neuronal, as well as glial components of the peripheral nerves. The functional deficit of one component may modulate the function of another component. For example, alteration of blood flow may produce changes in tissue oxygen tension and neuronal functional deficit. On the other hand, alteration of autonomic function secondary to diabetic dysmetabolism may change nerve blood flow. Hence, it is conceivable that interaction of all these factors ultimately leads to structural changes in the nerve and produces symptoms of clinical diabetic neuropathy. A simplified outline of the putative pathogenetic mechanisms is presented in Figure 6.2.

6.4   Diabetic Retinopathy in Humans

Although diabetes mellitus was first described around 1000 B.C., diabetic retinopathy was recognized relatively recently by Jager in 1855 following the discovery of the ophthalmoscope.[221] Duration of diabetes appears to be a major risk factor for the development of retinopathy. The incidence of retinopathy varies from nil with a diabetes duration of less than 5 years to 71% with diabetes of more than 10-years duration.[222,223] Elevated glycated hemoglobin is an important predictive marker for the development of retinopathy.[161,223] Other risk factors for the development of diabetic retinopathy include poor blood glucose control, hypertension, renal disease, pregnancy, and tobacco and alcohol consumption.[224] However, hyperglycemia in poorly controlled diabetes is the primary pathogenetic factor leading to clinical retinopathy and other complications of diabetes.[162] Good blood glucose control by intensive insulin therapy delays the onset and progression of diabetic retinopathy.[161]

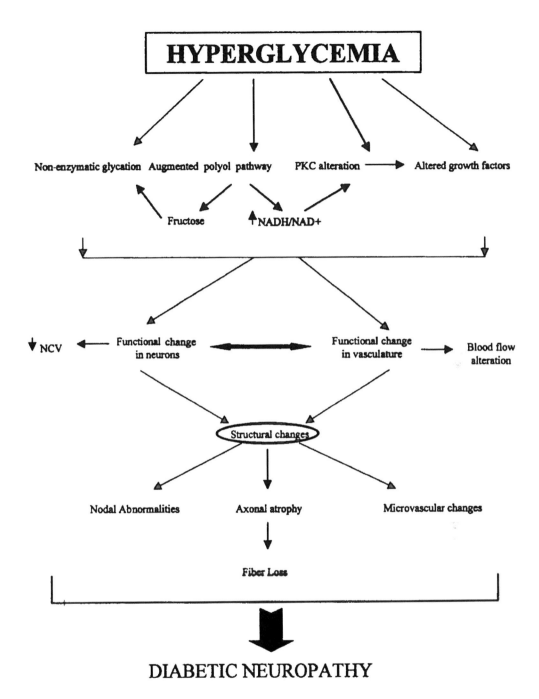

FIGURE 6.2
An outline of putative pathogenetic mechanisms leading to diabetic neuropathy.

6.4.1 Pathology

Human diabetic retinopathy is classified into progressive stages, namely, background (nonproliferative) retinopathy, severe or advanced background (preproliferative) retinopathy, and proliferative retinopathy. Background retinopathy consists of capillary microangiopathy, macular edema and soft exudate, and retinal hemorrhages and exudate. Capillary microangiopathy structurally shows basement membrane thickening, loss of pericytes, microvascular obstruction, permeability changes, and microaneurysms. Cotton wool spots (soft exudate), representing microinfracts of the nerve fiber layer, were once considered an important predictor of proliferative diabetic retinopathy. However, this has not been substantiated.[224] Profuse retinal hemorrhages and exudate, venous dilatation and beading, widespread capillary nonperfusion, and intraretinal microvascular abnormalities (IRMA), consisting of telangiectatic vessels shunting blood around areas of nonperfusion, are the characteristic features of preproliferative retinopathy. Patients with these lesions are prone to develop proliferative retinopathy. Proliferative retinopathy is characterized by neovascularization. New blood vessels form on the optic disk, within the retina, on the retinal surface, or inside the vitreous. Neovascularization eventually leads to bleeding, fibrosis, and tractional retinal detachment. An outline of lesions in the various stages of diabetic retinopathy is presented in Figure 6.3.

6.4.2 Pathogenesis

Hyperglycemia is the initiating factor leading to several biochemical alterations in the target organs of diabetic complications.[60,141,205,222] Sustained hyperglycemia initiates systemic coagulation abnormalities and several secondary biochemical pathways in the target organs of diabetic complications. The secondary mechanisms include augmented polyol pathway activity, redox imbalances and oxidative stress, alterations of DAG–PKC pathway and nonenzymatic glycation.[60,141,192,205] These biochemical pathways have been widely studied in experimental animals and will be discussed in Section 6.5.3.

The systemic coagulation abnormalities in the course of diabetes mellitus may further impact on the functional and structural integrities of the retina. The result is an imbalance between thrombus formation and dissolution, in favor of the former.[225] Oxidative stress due to free radical generation in diabetes is correlated with hemostatic alterations.[226] Nonenzymatic glycation of fibrin and platelet membrane further potentiates thrombotic activity.[225,227] Increased plasma levels of fibrinogen, factor VII, VIII, and von Willebrand factor have been demonstrated in diabetes.[228-230]

The concerted effects of these abnormalities resulting from long-term hyperglycemia lead to alterations of cellular synthetic activities and enzyme action, alterations in the gene expression of extracellular matrix proteins and other proteins, blood flow and permeability abnormalities, structural changes, cell death, and the development of clinical diabetic retinopathy.[205,231,232] Development of background retinopathy sets the stage for subsequent development of retinal ischemia, upregulation and/or release of several vasoproliferative factors, leading to proliferation of new vessels. Recently described vascular endothelial growth factor (VEGF) is a key candidate responsible for neovascularization.[233] Increased levels of VEGF have been demonstrated in intraocular fluids of patients with neovascularization.[233] VEGF is further of importance as a permeability factor in background retinopathy.[232-234] The list of vasoproliferative factors include transforming growth factor β (TGF-β), fibroblast growth factor (FGF), IGF, tumor necrosis factor-α (TNF-α), Platelet-derived growth factor (PDGF), epidermal growth factor (EGF), etc.[205,235,236] These factors stimulate endothelial cell proliferation and neovascularization of the ischemic retina. A detailed description of neovascularization factors will not be attempted here.

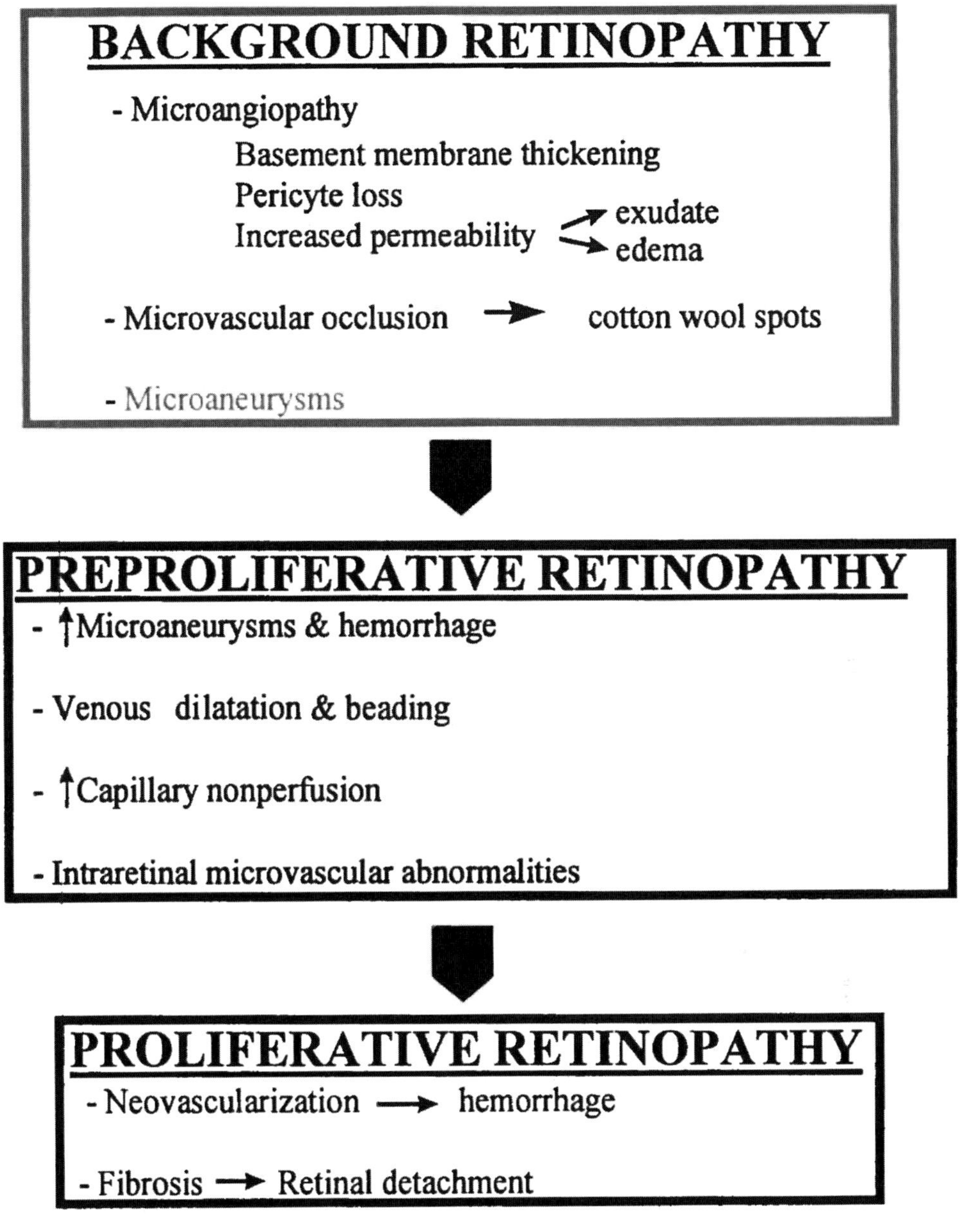

BACKGROUND RETINOPATHY

- Microangiopathy

      Basement membrane thickening

      Pericyte loss

      Increased permeability   exudate / edema

- Microvascular occlusion ⟶ cotton wool spots

- Microaneurysms

PREPROLIFERATIVE RETINOPATHY

- ↑Microaneurysms & hemorrhage

- Venous dilatation & beading

- ↑Capillary nonperfusion

- Intraretinal microvascular abnormalities

PROLIFERATIVE RETINOPATHY

- Neovascularization ⟶ hemorrhage

- Fibrosis ⟶ Retinal detachment

FIGURE 6.3
An outline of various lesions in different stages of diabetic retinopathy.

6.5 Diabetic Retinopathy in Animals

Animal experiments have been important in understanding the pathology and pathogenesis of human diabetic retinopathy. In this chapter, structural, biochemical, and functional changes in diabetic retinopathy will be addressed. Both diabetic and galactosemic animals have been used as models for diabetic retinopathy.

6.5.1 Retinal Structural Lesions in Animal Models

Retinal structural lesions have been produced in both diabetic and galactosemic animals. Prevention of these changes by inhibition of specific biochemical pathways has provided indirect evidence for their role in the genesis of diabetic retinopathy.

6.5.1.1   Diabetic Dogs

Diabetic dogs are the best models for diabetic retinopathy. Histopathologically characteristic features of background and proliferative diabetic retinopathy have repeatedly been produced in diabetic dogs.[237] Lesions of diabetic retinopathy develop and progress in this model irrespective of the methodologies used for the production of diabetes such as pancreatectomy, alloxan, growth hormones, or whether or not diabetes is of idiopathic origin.[237-240] Diabetic dogs demonstrated progressive, early retinal lesions of diabetic retinopathy, such as, basement membrane thickening, pericyte loss, capillary leakage, capillary occlusion, and loss of microvascular smooth muscle cells. Further, advanced retinopathic changes such as microaneurysms, intraretinal microvascular abnormalities, and retinal neovascularization have consistently been produced in diabetic dogs.[237-241] The dog model has unequivocally demonstrated a definitive role of hyperglycemia in the development of diabetic retinopathy.[239,240] Retinopathy was effectively prevented when strict blood glucose control was initiated shortly after onset of hyperglycemia. However, complete prevention was not achieved when strict blood glucose control was initiated after a longer period of preceding hyperglycemia.[239,240] Virtually similar results were obtained in human diabetic retinopathy.[161] Treatment with AR inhibitors has failed to prevent the progression of retinopathy in this model[242] suggesting activation of multiple biochemical mechanisms secondary to hyperglycemia and polyol pathway activation (see below), which in themselves are not responsive to AR inhibition. It is interesting to note that distribution of retinal lesions may vary in different retinal quadrants in the diabetic dog.[243] The exact reason for this variation is not known; however, it is possible that local microenvironmental factors in various sectors of the retina may have a modulatory influence on the development of retinopathy.

6.5.1.2   Diabetic Rats

Although small laboratory animals do not develop advanced retinal lesions such as neovascularization, early microangiopathic lesions have repeatedly been produced in rats. These early lesions are important in the study of the pathogenetic mechanisms and the development of preventive strategies.

The STZ-induced diabetic rat is the most extensively studied diabetic rat model. Early microangiopathic lesions, such as basement membrane thickening, loss of capillary pericytes, acellular capillaries, endothelial cell proliferation, and rare microaneurysms,[244-248] are demonstrated. Euglycemia achieved by pancreatic islet cell transplantation can prevent microangiopathic changes in STZ diabetic rats.[248,249] In STZ diabetic rats, increased permeability across the retinal pigment epithelium due to breakdown of the blood retinal barrier in association with structural alterations of the retinal pigment epithelium was observed. These changes are preventable by tight control of blood glucose by insulin therapy and syngeneic islet cell transplantation.[250-252] Progressive intracellular AGE accumulation is associated with pericyte loss in STZ diabetic rats.[253] Aminoguanidine, an

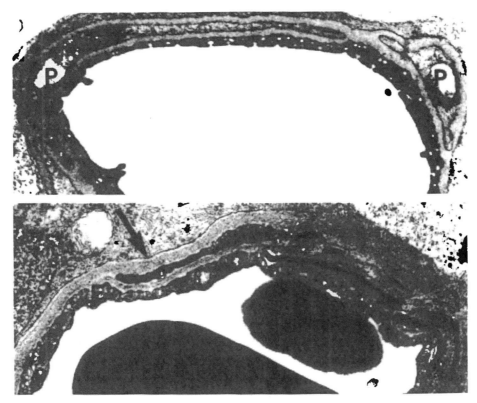

FIGURE 6.4
Retinal capillary electron micrographs from a nondiabetic BB/W rat (top) and an age-matched diabetic BB/W rat with 8-month duration of diabetes (bottom). Note thickening and laminated appearence of basement membrane in bottom panel compared with top panel. E = endothelial cell, P = pericyte, magnification × 22,000 for both micrographs.

inhibitor of nonenzymatic glycation, is only effective in preventing the late changes of diabetic retina, suggesting that AGE-associated changes are time dependent.

The spontaneously diabetic BB/W rat shows basement membrane thickening, pericyte degeneration and loss, platelet microthrombi, retinal pigment epitheliopathy, and thickening of the vitreoretinal border membrane[256-259] (Figure 6.4). Similar to the STZ rat, retinal lesions in this animal were prevented by good blood glucose control by insulin or acarbose, an α-glucosidase inhibitor, indicating the role of hyperglycemia in the pathogenesis of these lesions.[260,261] Capillary basement membrane and Bruch's membrane thickening in the diabetic BB/W rat are associated with an absolute loss of anionic sites, provided by the proteoglycans, resulting in a loss of the charge-selective barrier function of the basement membrane, which is important in the pathogenesis of diabetes-induced hyperpermeability.[56] AR inhibitor treatment and myoinositol supplementation prevented basement membrane thickening in the BB/W rat in the superficial capillary bed but not in the deep capillary bed.[260,262] This interesting observation indicates that local microenvironmental factors such as oxygen tension and/or hemodynamic pressure may modulate the effects of hyperglycemia on the microvasculature.

Several diabetic retinal lesions were demonstrated in other rat models of diabetes. The list includes alloxan diabetes rats and rats with diabetes induced by pancreatectomy and by growth hormone.[263-266] The lesions are of early microangiopathic nature and are similar to those in previously discussed models.

6.5.1.3   Other Diabetic Animal Models

Some of the diabetic retinopathic changes have been demonstrated in diabetic monkeys following long-term alloxan-induced diabetes ,[267,268] as well as in spontaneously diabetic monkeys.[269] However, very few studies have been carried out in diabetic monkeys, and the usefulness of primates as models of diabetic retinopathy has yet to be established. The list of other animal models used in the study of diabetic retinopathy is impressive and includes models such as diabetic carp.[270] However, in general, these models do not offer any advantages over the diabetic dog or rat models.

The body of information generated from small-animal models of diabetes further confirms the role of hyperglycemia as the primary culprit and the involvement of multiple secondary biochemical mechanisms responsible for the development of structural lesions in the retina in diabetes.

6.5.1.4   Galactosemic Animal Models

Galactosemic animals provide an opportunity to investigate effects of hyperhexosemia in isolation from hormonal alterations in diabetes and have a special role in the study of diabetic complications. Augmented polyol pathway activity and other biochemical mechanisms, triggered secondarily to hyperhexosemia, have been investigated in this model. Retinal structural lesions similar to those of diabetic retinopathy have been produced in the retina of galactosemic animals.[271,272,273] Both galactosemic rats and dogs have been used. Galactosemic dogs produce advanced retinal structural lesions similar to diabetic dogs.[271-273] Treatment with AR inhibitors to prevent galactose-induced retinal lesions has shown discordant results. Although complete prevention of retinal lesions in the dog were reported by some investigators,[273,274] others failed to demonstrate similar results.[242] The reason for these divergent results is not clear. Differences in the severity of galactosemia and the different AR inhibitors used for treatment may be possible variables. Early microangiopathic lesions such as basement membrane thickening were prevented by AR inhibitors in galactosemic rats.[275-278] It has been claimed that chronically galactosemic rats develop IRMA and microaneurysms.[277] Some investigators, however, failed to find unequivocal microaneurysms in galactosemic rats.[237]

6.5.2   Retinal Functional Alterations in Animal Models

Diabetic rats have been used to study functional abnormalities, such as retinal blood flow, permeability alteration, and retinal electrophysiological changes. Both the STZ diabetic rat and the BB/W rat have been investigated. In human diabetes, retinal blood flow is initially decreased, followed by an increase when background retinopathy is present.[205] Retinal blood flow studies in STZ and BB/W rats have resulted in conflicting data about whether blood flow is increased or decreased.[279,280] Variation in the methods used in the detection of blood flow abnormalities, as well as duration and/or severity of diabetes, may be responsible for such discrepancies. Furthermore, alteration in blood flow has been suggested to be heterogeneous in the retina of diabetic rats.[281] Treatment with various pharmaceutical agents, such as insulin, AR inhibitors, sorbitol dehydrogenase inhibitors, NO synthase inhibitor, antioxidants, acetyl-L-carnitine, aminoguanidine, has been found to prevent, at least in part, retinal blood flow abnormalities.[187,282-288] Recently, a specific inhibitor of the β isoform of PKC has shown to prevent retinal circulatory abnormalities in STZ diabetic rats in parallel with inhibition of the increased PKC activities, indicating important roles of PKC in the pathogenesis of vascular abnormalities.[289]

Increased vascular permeability is another characteristic alteration of human diabetic retinopathy. Macular edema and hard exudate seen in background retinopathy are formed as a result of increased permeability. Such changes have been demonstrated in association with increased retinal polyol accumulation both in the STZ rat and in the BB/W rat.[284,290] Treatment with an AR inhibitor was able to prevent these changes.[290] Breakdown of the blood retinal barrier secondary to retinal pigment epitheliopathy was demonstrated both in the STZ diabetic rats and in the BB/W rat.[251,256,258] In the BB/W rat such changes were associated with increased AR immunoreactivity in the retinal pigment epithelium.[258] VEGF has recently been shown to be important to the genesis of increased retinal vascular permeability. VEGF-induced increased permeability is mediated through a PKC-dependent mechanism and can be inhibited by treatment with a specific inhibitor β2 isoform of PKC.[234]

The retina in the STZ rat shows electrophysiological abnormalities of oscillatory potentials contributed by the Müller cells and the a- and b-waves of the electroretinogram, generated by the neuronal retina. These changes were prevented by AR inhibitor treatment. These data suggest an early neuronal alteration in the retina similar to human diabetes.[291,292] A progressive alteration of c-wave amplitude, contributed by the retinal pigment epithelium, was demonstrated in STZ diabetic rats and prevented by both AR inhibitor treatment and myoinositol supplementation.[293] In the BB/W rat prolonged latencies of the visual evoked potentials are associated with dystrophic changes in retinal ganglion cells and atrophy of the myelinated fibers of optic nerve and axoglial dysjunctions.[61,62] Treatment with an AR inhibitor was effective in preventing the visual evoked potential abnormalities and axoglial dysjunctions but not the axonal atrophy, suggesting that several biochemical mechanisms may be involved in the generation of advanced lesions of the optic nerves.[62]

6.5.3 Retinal Biochemical Alterations in Animal Models

Experiments in animal diabetes have demonstrated that hyperglycemia is the primary insult in the pathogenesis of diabetic retinopathy.[222] Several biochemical pathways, however, may be activated secondary to hyperglycemia. Although these pathways may appear isolated and diverse at the outset, there are significant interactions and they may act synergistically to produce the functional and structural effects of diabetes. The pathways include augmented polyol pathway activity, altered redox state, PKC activation, and nonenzymatic glycation.[141,205,237] The following sections will briefly comment on some of the salient features.

6.5.3.1 *Polyol Pathway*

Augmented polyol pathway activity is a widely studied mechanism in several target organs of diabetic complications.[7-9,165,167,168,222] As discussed previously, excessive cellular glucose is metabolized by this pathway to sorbitol and fructose.[165] The enzyme AR is present in the dog and rat retinal microvasculature, and isolated microvessels from the dog retina show hexitol-producing activity.[167,294-296] Increased retinal AR mRNA and AR immunoreactivity were demonstrated in the diabetic BB/W rat.[168] Furthermore, some of the diabetes-induced structural changes can be prevented by AR inhibitor treatment.[260,277] However, unlike the ocular lens, the amount of sorbitol in the retina, accumulated secondary to polyol pathway activation, is very low. Furthermore, diabetes-induced vascular dysfunctions in the retina can be prevented by inhibiting sorbitol dehydrogenase in spite of high sorbitol levels.[141,193,282] Hence, rather than direct accumulation of sorbitol, other consequences of the polyol pathway activation may be of importance in the pathogenesis. Both glucose and fructose, the latter produced as an end product of the polyol pathway, are potent nonenzymatic glycators.[60,192-194] Polyol pathway activation may further lead to increased NADH/NAD+ ratio, resulting in a redox imbalance in such target organs of diabetic complications as the retina.[141]

6.5.3.2   Redox Imbalance

In hyperglycemia, as mentioned earlier, increased glycolysis in the tissues and an augmented polyol pathway activity cause an increase of the NADH/NAD+ ratio.[141] This alteration has been termed pseudohypoxia, as it is similar to that seen in hypoxia. An increased NADH/NAD+ ratio may lead to alterations in lipid peroxidation, DAG synthesis, and defective DNA repair.[141,187] Increased DAG synthesis further activates PKC in the retina.[144,205] Redox imbalances have been demonstrated in the retina, which may favour increased free radical generation, increased prostaglandin synthesis, and decreased NO synthesis.[141,187]

6.5.3.3   DAG-PKC Pathway

Increased PKC activities are seen in several vascular target organs of diabetic complications including the retina.[205] Hyperglycemia-induced DAG-mediated PKC synthesis has been demonstrated in the retina.[297,298] High glucose levels alone or with an increased NADH/NAD+ ratio resulting from increased polyol pathway activity lead to an increase in DAG synthesis, which is a potent PKC activator.[205,297,298] Augmented PKC and decreased Na+-K+-ATPase activity in the retina of STZ diabetic rats can be prevented by a specific inhibitor of the β isoform of PKC.[289,298,299] Recently, it was demonstrated that hyperhexosemia induces increased DAG levels and PKC activation in the retina and aorta of both diabetic and galactosemic dogs, as well as decreased Na+-K+-ATPase and Ca++-Mg++-Mg-ATPase activity in these tissues.[300,301] PKC is involved in several important vascular functions such as blood flow and permeability.[302] Diabetes-induced retinal blood flow alterations can be prevented by treatment with a specific inhibitor of β-isoform of PKC.[286] Recently, the same inhibitor has been found to inhibit VEGF-induced increased retinal vascular permeability.[286] Furthermore, PKC is a regulator of several growth factors, such as PDGF, EGF, and IGF, which may be important in mediating the later effects of diabetic retinopathy, such as endothelial proliferation and neovascularization.[205]

6.5.3.4   Nonenzymatic Glycation

Nonenzymatic modification of tissue proteins by physiological hexoses *in vivo* is an important secondary mechanism in the pathogenesis of diabetic retinopathy.[60,192-195] Glucose and fructose generated as end products of polyol pathway activity take part in nonenzymatic glycation of proteins.[60,192-195] In chronic hyperglycemia, AGEs accumulate in the tissues as a function of time and sugar concentration. AGEs may change the functional and structural properties of proteins and contribute to pathophysiological alterations in diabetes.[192-195] AGEs may affect signal transduction pathways and the levels of soluble signals, such as cytokines, hormones, and free radicals, and can directly affect protein functions in target tissues.[60,192-195] In vascular endothelial cells, AGE formation may affect gene expression of thrombomodulin and ET-1[303,304] and may modify growth factors such as bFGF.[60] In the microvasculature, AGEs may interfere with extracellular matrix organization and matrix cell interaction.[305] AGEs may induce permanent abnormalities of extracellular matrix proteins and intracellular proteins, and may stimulate cytokines and reactive oxygen species through AGE receptors.[60,192-195] Diabetes-induced structural and functional changes in the retina are prevented by aminoguanidine, an inhibitor of nonenzymatic glycation.[254,255,283]

The symphony of these biochemical alterations may further cause inhibition of fatty acid oxidation, increased prostaglandin synthesis, inhibition of NO activity, and possible alteration of vasoactive peptides, such as ETs, and growth factors expression.[141,205] PKC is an important regulator of ETs and several growth factors.[205,306] In the STZ diabetic rat, increased retinal ET-1 mRNA expression has been demonstrated.[307] Increased immunocytochemically detectable ET-1 and ET-3 proteins have further been noted in the retina of the diabetic BB/W rat.[308] Alterations of several growth factors, such as bFGF, IGF-I mRNA has been demonstrated in the retina of the STZ diabetic rat.[309] Growth factor alterations, crucial in the development of advanced retinopathic changes such as neovascularization, have recently been reviewed.[310,311]

Interaction of these biochemical alterations leads to such functional changes as retinal blood flow and permeability defects. Subsequently, structural changes develop in the microvasculature, and clinical retinopathy is manifested. Based on these animal studies, a simplified outline of putative sequence of events leading to diabetic retinopathy is given in Figure 6.5.

6.6 Effects of Experimental Treatments on Nerve and Retinal Changes in Diabetes

Various treatment modalities that have been carried out in animals to prevent the retinal and neuronal lesions in diabetes fall broadly within two groups. One group of treatments is directed to correct or reduce hyperglycemia by insulin injection, islet cell transplantation or adjuvant treatment by agents such as α-glucosidase inhibitors. Another group of therapies uses inhibitors of specific biochemical pathways. The data emerging from various treatments reveal the importance of specific biochemical abnormalities in the development of diabetic retinopathy and neuropathy. In addition, these experiments provide the first step toward the development of adjuvant therapies for human diabetic neuropathy and retinopathy. The effects of specific treatments were discussed under each type of lesion. Overall, it is evident that by correcting hyperglycemia, structural, functional, or biochemical nerve and retinal lesions can be at least ameliorated in both human and in animal diabetes provided the treatment is initiated early in the disease process. The major specific treatments include AR inhibitors, aminoguanidine and PKC inhibitors, and vasoactive compounds. By using these blockers, important pathogenetic mechanisms have been elucidated and confirmed. Animal models are therefore invaluable for further exploration of efficacy and development of specific therapies to prevent and/or treat these chronic diabetic complications.

6.7 Results Derived from Animal Models

Data from various animal models have imparted an enormous body of knowledge regarding the pathogenesis of chronic diabetic complications. It is now clear that

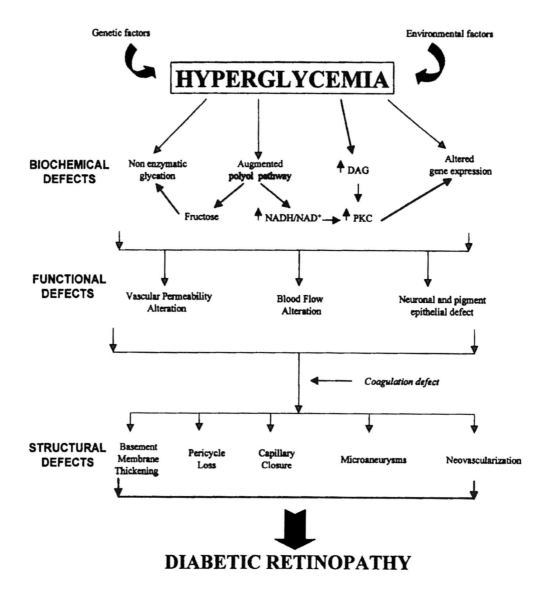

FIGURE 6.5
An outline of putative sequence of events leading to clinical diabetic retinopathy.

hyperglycemia is the key initiating event in the genesis of diabetic retinopathy.[141,161,237] However, development of retinal lesions is probably further influenced by individual genetic makeups and environmental factors (e.g., smoking).[224,235] Current data indicate activation of multiple interactive mechanisms, such as augmented polyol pathway activity, nonenzymatic glycations, and PKC alterations, in the development of retinal lesions in diabetes. This may, in part, explain the failure of some clinical trials with a single agent blocking a particular pathway and the success of glycemic control in the prevention of diabetic complications.[312,313]

Similar to studies of the retina, study of the peripheral nerve has demonstrated activation of multiple biochemical pathways secondary to dysmetabolism. As more is learned regarding diabetic neuropathy the pathogenetic theories, *vascular* and *metabolic* are becoming unified as various mechanistic aspects of a single pathogenetic hypothesis.[7-9] DCCT trial has demonstrated the importance of hyperglycemia in the pathogenesis of neuropathy,[161] although clinical trials with adjuvant therapies such as AR inhibitors have not been completely successful. However, the importance of the polyol pathway has been learned and, further, it has been learned that multiple interactive mechanisms are simultaneously at work leading to neuropathy.[311]

6.8 Conclusion and Future Directions

Animal models offer a unique advantage to study a disease process in a longitudinal fashion. Further studies using the models of chronic diabetic complications are needed to pinpoint biochemical abnormalities and their interrelationships in the development of early and late functional and structural abnormalities of chronic diabetic complications and to develop adjuvant treatment strategies. A largely underexplored area in diabetic retinopathy is altered gene expression. A high blood glucose level by itself, as well as through secondary mechanisms such as augmented polyol pathway, nonenzymatic glycation, PKC activation, perturbed Ca^{2+} metabolism, and altered ecosianoid production, may affect expression of several vasoactive genes such as ETs, NO synthase, and VEGF, and other growth factors and cytoskeletal protein genes.[128,129,141,205,235,236,310,311] In a recent study, it was shown that hyperhexosemia-induced cataract formation and thrombotic occlusion of retinochoroidal vessels develop rapidly in transgenic mice with human AR cDNA.[314] Diabetes-induced biochemical changes may further alter the expression of extracellular matrix protein genes.[315-319] By using mRNA differential display techniques, several genes with diverse functions have been identified in the retinal capillary pericytes, which are altered by exposure to high glucose levels.[320] Increased expression of collagen IV and fibronectin mRNA has been demonstrated in human diabetic retinopathy, in the retina of galactosemic rats, as well as in the cultured retinal capillary pericytes and endothelial cells in the hyperhexosemic condition.[319-323] Transgenic mice with upregulated human AR2 gene showed enhanced polyol pathway activity and neuronal functional and structural changes following galactose feeding.[7,8,324] In addition, if these mice are made diabetic by STZ injection, they show severe conduction-velocity deficit compared with littermates.[314,324] Altered gene expressions may play major roles in the genesis of structural lesions, such as basement membrane thickening and neovascularization, or functional defects, such as vascular dysfunctions and axonal transport deficit. Abnormal gene expressions secondary to hyperglycemia, insulin deficiency, or systemic hyperinsulinism may be conceptually important pathogenetic mechanisms in the development of diabetic neuropathy and retinopathy. Exploration and manipulation of genetic expressions is a potentially important area of future research. A detailed analysis of such mechanisms will further open up possibilities of gene therapy along with good blood glucose control and other adjuvant therapies in the treatment of diabetic neuropathy and retinopathy.

Acknowledgment

This work was supported by a grant from the Canadian Diabetes Association in honor of Florence Langille. The author is grateful to Cheryl Campbell and Diana Deng for their help in preparation of this manuscript.

References

1. Cantagallo, A., Epidemiologia della retinopatia diabetica, *Med. Prev. Comm.*, 128, 1, 1989.
2. NIH Publication No. 96-3926, 1995.
3. Benson, W. E., Tasman, W., Duane, T. D., Diabetes mellitus and the eye, in *Duane's Clinical Ophthalmology*, Tasman, W. and Jaeger, E. A., Eds., Lippincott, Philadelphia, 1990, chap. 30, 1-29.
4. Report on the Second National Diabetes Research Conference: Progress and promise in diabetes research, NIH Publication No. 84-661, 1984, 21-86.
5. Thomas, P. K., Diabetic neuropathy: models, mechanisms and mayhem, *Can. J. Neurol. Sci.*, 19, 1, 1992.
6. Boulton, A. J. M., Pathogenesis of diabetic neuropathy, in *The Diabetes Annual*, Marshall, S.M., Home, P.D., Alberti, K.G.M.M., Krall, L.P., Eds., Elsevier Science, Amsterdam, Chapter 11, p192, 1993.
7. Yagihashi, S., Pathology and pathogenetic mechanisms of diabetic neuropathy, *Diabetes Metab. Rev.*, 11, 193, 1995.
8. Stevens, M. J., Feldman, E. L., Greene, D. A., The etiology of diabetic neuropathy: The combined roles of metabolic and vascular defect, *Diabetic Med.*, 12, 566, 1995.
9. Cameron, N. E., Cotter, M. A., Metabolic and vascular factors in the pathogenesis of diabetic neuropathy, *Diabetes*, 46 (Suppl. 2), 531, 1997.
10. Bauersachs, R. M., Shaw, S., Ziedler, A., Meiselman, J. J., Red blood cell aggregation and blood viscosity in poorly controlled type 2 diabetes mellitus, *Clin. Hemorheol.*, 9, 935, 1989.
11. Low, P. A., Tuck, R. R., Takeuchi, M., Nerve microenvironment in diabetic neuropathy, in *Diabetic Neuropathy*, Dyck, P. J., Thomas, P. K., Asbury, A. K., Winegrad, A. I., Porte, D., Jr., Eds., Saunders, Philadelphia, 1987, 266
12. MacRury, S. M., Lockhart, J. C., Small, M., Weir, A. I., MacCuish, A. C., Lowe, G. D. O., Do rheological variables play a role in diabetic peripheral neuropathy? *Diabetic Med.*, 8, 232, 1991.
13. Faberberg, S. E., Diabetic neuropathy: a clinical and histological study of the significance of vascular affection, *Acta Med. Scand.*, 164 (Suppl. 345), 1, 1959.
14. Yagihashi, S., Sugimoto, K., Wada, R., Different neuropathic patterns between Type I and Type II animal models, in *Pathogenesis and Treatment of NIDDM and its Related Problems*, Sakamoto, N., Alberti, K. G. M. M., Hotta, N., Eds., Elsevier, Amsterdam, 1994, 401.
15. Sharma, A. K., Thomas, P. K., Animal models: pathology and pathophysiology, in *Diabetic Neuropathy*, Dyck, P. J., Thomas, P. K., Asbury, A. K., Winegrad, A. I., Porte, D., Jr., Eds., Saunders, Philadelphia, 1987, 237.
16. Jakobsen, J., Lundbaek, K., Neuropathy in experimental diabetes: an animal model, *Br. Med. J.*, 2, 278, 1976.
17. Jakobsen, J., Axonal dwindling in early experimental diabetes. I. A study of cross sectioned nerves, *Diabetologia*, 12, 539, 1976.
18. Yagihashi, S., Kamijo, M., Watanabe, K., Reduced myelinated fibre size correlates with loss of axonal neurofilaments in peripheral nerve of chronically streptozotocin diabetic rats, *Am. J. Pathol.*, 136, 1365, 1990.
19. Sima, A. A. F., Zhang, W.-X., Tai, J., Tze, W. J., Nathaniel, V., Diabetic neuropathy in STZ induced diabetic rat and effect of allogenic islet cell transplantation: a morphometric analysis, *Diabetes*, 37, 1129, 1988.
20. Yagihashi, S., Kamijo, M., Ido, Y., Mirrlees, D. J., Effects of long-term aldose reductase inhibition on development of experimental diabetic neuropathy: ultrastructural and morphometric studies of sural nerve in streptozotocin-induced diabetic rats, *Diabetes*, 39, 690, 1990.
21. Lowitt, S., Malone, J., Korthals, J., Salen, A., Miranda, C., Differential depression of nerve conduction velocity (NCV) determined by the age at which streptozotocin (ST2) was administered, *Diabetes*, 43 (Suppl. 1), 109A, 1994.

22. Williamson, J. R., Chang, K., Tilton, R. G., Prater, C., Jeffrey, J. R., Weigel, C., Sherman, W. R., Eades, D. M., Kilo, C., Increased vascular permeability in spontaneously diabetic BB/W rats and in rats with mild vs. severe streptozotocin induced diabetes: prevention by aldose reductase inhibition and castration, *Diabetes*, 36, 813, 1987.

23. Medori, R., Autilio-Gambetti, L., Monaco, S., Gambetti, P., Experimental diabetic neuropathy: impairment of slow transport with changes in axon cross-sections area, *Proc. Natl. Acad. Sci. U.S.A.*, 82, 7716, 1985.

24. Medori, R., Autilio-Gambetti, L., Jenich, H., Gambetti, P., Changes in axon size and slow axonal transport are related in experimental diabetic neuropathy, *Neurology* 38, 597, 1988.

25. Yagihashi, S., Axonal cytoskeleton and diabetic neuropathy, *Diabetic Med.*, 10 (Suppl. 2), 1075, 1993.

26. Schmidt, R. E., Plurad, S. B., Modert, C. W., Experimental diabetic autonomic neuropathy: characterization in streptozotocin-diabetic Sprague-Dawley rats, *Lab. Invest.*, 49, 538, 1983.

27. Schmidt, R. E., Scharp, D. W., Axonal dystrophy in experimental diabetic neuropathy, *Diabetes*, 31, 761, 1982.

28. Sidenius, P., Jakobsen, J., Axonal transport in early experimental diabetes, *Brain Res.*, 173, 315, 1979.

29. Jakobsen, J., Sidenius, P., Decreased axonal transport of structural proteins in streptozotocin diabetic rats, *J. Clin. Invest.*, 66, 292, 1980.

30. Sidenius, P., Jakobsen, J., Reversibility and preventability of the decrease in slow axonal transport velocity in experimental diabetes, *Diabetes*, 31, 689, 1982.

31. Takenaka, T., Inomata, K., Horie, H., Slow axoplasmic transport of labelled protein in sciatic nerves of streptozotocin-diabetes rats and methylcobalamin treated rats, in *Diabetic Neuropathy*, Goto, Y., Horiuchi, A., Kogure, K., Eds, Excerpta Medica, Amsterdam, 1982, 99.

32. Jakobsen, J., Early and preventable changes of peripheral nerve structure and function in insulin deficient diabetic rats, *J. Neurol. Neurosurg. Psychiatry*, 42, 509, 1979.

33. Sonobe, M., Yasuda, H., Hisanaga, T., Maeda, K., Yamasha, M., Kawabata, T., Kikkawa, R., Taniguchi, Y., Shigeta, Y., Amelioration of nerve Na(+)-K(+)-ATPase activity independently of myo-inositol level by PGE1 analogue OP-1206, alpha-CD in streptozocin-induced diabetic rats, *Diabetes*, 40, 726, 1991.

34. Larsen, J. R., Sidenius, P., Slow axonal transport of structural polypeptides in rat, early changes in streptozotocin diabetes and effect of insulin treatment, *J. Neurochem.*, 52, 390, 1989.

35. Tomlinson, D. R., Sidenius, P., Larsen, J. R., Slow component of axonal transport, nerve myo-inositol, and aldose reductase inhibition in streptozotocin-diabetic rats, *Diabetes*, 34, 398, 1986.

36. Green, D. A., DeJesus, P. V., Winegrad, A. I., Effects of insulin and dietary myo-inositol on impaired motor nerve conduction velocity in acute streptozotocin diabetes, *J. Clin. Invest.*, 55, 1326, 1975.

37. Sima, A. A. F., Hay, K., Functional aspects and pathogenetic considerations of the neuropathy in the spontaneously diabetic BB-Wistar rat, *Neuropathol. Appl. Neurobiol.*, 7, 341, 1981.

38. Sima, A. A. F., Bouchier, M., Christensen, H., Axonal atrophy in sensory nerves of the diabetic BB-Wistar rat, a possible early correlate of human diabetic neuropathy, *Ann. Neurol.*, 13, 264, 1983.

39. Sima, A. A. F., Lorusso, A. C., Thibert, P., Distal symmetric polyneuropathy in the spontaneously diabetic BB-Wistar rat: an ultrastructural and teased fibre study, *Acta Neuropathol.*, 58, 39, 1982.

40. Sima, A. A. F., Lattimer, S. A. Yagihashi, S., Greene, D. A., "Axo-glial dysjunction": a novel structural lesion that accounts for poorly reversible slowing of nerve conduction in the spontaneously diabetic BB-rat, *J. Clin. Invest.*, 77, 474, 1986.

41. Sima, A. A. F., Brismar, T., Reversible diabetic nerve dysfunction: structural correlates to electrophysiological abnormalities, *Ann. Neurol.*, 18, 21, 1985.

42. Brismar, T., Sima, A. A. F., Greene, D. A., Reversible and irreversible nodal dysfunction in diabetic neuropathy, *Ann. Neurol.*, 21, 504, 1987.

43. Greene, D. A., Chakrabarti, S., Lattimer, S. A., Sima, A. A. F., Role of sorbitol accumulation and myo-inositol depletion in paranodal swelling of large myelinated nerve fibers in the insulin-deficient spontaneously diabetic biobreeding rat reversal by insulin replacement, an aldose reductase inhibitor and myo-inositol, *J. Clin. Invest.*, 79, 1479, 1987.

44. Kamijo, M., Merry, A. C., Cherian, P. V., Akdas, G., Sima, A. A. F., Nerve fibre regeneration following axotomy in the diabetic BB/W rat: the effect of ARI-treatment, *J. Diab. Compl.* 10, 183, 1996.

45. Ristic, H., Merry, A. C. Kamijo, M., Sima, A. A. F., Impaired functional maturation of regenerated nerve fibers in the BB/W-rat is not corrected by ARI-treatment, *Diabetes*, 44 (Suppl. 1), 63A, 1995.

46. Sima, A. A. F., Brismar, T., Yagihashi, S., Neuropathies encountered in the spontaneously diabetic BB Wistar rat, in *Diabetic Neuropathy*, Dyck, P. J., Thomas, P. K., Asbury, A. K., Winegrad, A. I., Porte, D., Jr., Eds. Saunders, Philadelphia, 1987, 253.

47. Sima, A. A. F., Yagihashi, S., Distal central axonopathy in the spontaneously diabetic BB- Wistar rat: a sequential ultrastructural and morphometric study, *Diabetes Res. Clin. Pract.*, 1, 289, 1986.

48. Sima, A. A. F., Zhang, W-X., Cherian, P. V., Chakrabarti, S., Impaired visual evoked potential and primary axonopathy of the optic nerve in the diabetic BB/W rat, *Diabetologia*, 35, 602, 1992.

49. Sima, A. A. F., Prashar, A., Zhang, W-X, Chakrabarti, S., Green, D. A., Preventive effect of long term aldose reductase inhibition (Ponalrestat) on nerve conduction and sural nerve structure in the spontaneously diabetic BB-rat, *J. Clin. Invest.*, 85, 1410, 1990.

50. Greene, D. A., Yagihashi, S., Lattimer, S. A., Sima, A. A. F., Nerve Na^+-K^+-ATPase, conduction and myo-inositol in the insulin deficient BB rat, *Am. J. Physiol.*, 247, E534, 1984.

51. Yagihashi, S., Sima, A. A. F., Diabetic autonomic neuropathy in the BB-rat: ultrastructural and morphometric changes in sympathetic nerves, *Diabetes*, 34, 558, 1985.

52. Marliss, E. B., Nakhooda, E. F., Poussier, P., Sima, A. A. F., The diabetic syndrome of the "BB" Wistar rat: possible relevance to Type I (insulin dependent) diabetes in man, *Diabetologia*, 22, 225, 1982.

53. Yagihashi, S., Sima, A. A. F., Diabetic autonomic neuropathy in the BB-rat: ultrastructural and morphometric changes in parasympathetic nerves, *Diabetes*, 35, 733, 1986.

54. Yagihashi, S., Sima, A. A. F., Neuroaxonal and dendritic dystrophy in diabetic autonomic neuropathy: classification and topographic distribution in the BB rat, *J. Neuropathol. Exp. Neurol.*, 45, 545, 1986.

55. Sima, A. A. F., Can the BB-rat help to unravel diabetic neuropathy? Annotation. *Neuropathol. Appl. Neurobiol.*, 11, 253, 1985.

56. Chakrabarti, S., Ma, N., Sima, A. A. F., Anionic sites in diabetic basement membranes and their possible role in diffusion barrier abnormalities, *Diabetologia*, 34, 301, 1991.

57. Yagihashi, S., Sima, A. A. F., The distribution of structural changes in sympathetic nerves in the diabetic BB-rat, *Am. J. Pathol.*, 121, 138, 1985.

58. Zhang, W.-X., Chakrabarti, S., Greene, D. A., Sima, A. A. F., Diabetic autonomic neuropathy in BB-rats: the effect of ARI treatment on heart-rate variability and vagus nerve structure, *Diabetes*, 39, 613, 1990.

59. Williams, S. K., Howarth, N. L., Devenny, J. J., Britensky, N. W., Structural and functional consequences of increased tubulin glycosylation in diabetes mellitus, *Proc. Natl. Acad. Sci. U.S.A.*, 72, 6546, 1982.

60. Brownlee, M., Advanced protein glycosylation in diabetes and aging, *Annu. Rev. Med.*, 46, 223, 1995.

61. Chakrabarti, S., Zhang, W-X, Sima, A. A. F., Optic neuropathy in the diabetic BB rat, *Adv. Exp. Biol. Med.*, 291, 257, 1991a.

62. Kamijo, M., Cherian, P. V., Sima, A. A. F., The preventive effects of aldose reductase inhibition on diabetic optic neuropathy in the BB/W rat, *Diabetologia*, 36, 893, 1993.

63. Kappelle, A. C., Bravenboer, B., Traber, J., Erkelens, D. W., Gispen, W. H., The Ca^{2+} antagonist nimodipine counteracts the onset of an experimental neuropathy in streptozotocin induced diabetic rats, *Neurosci. Res. Commun.*, 10, 95, 1992.

64. Kim, J., Rushovich, E. H., Thomas, T. P., Ueda, T., Agranoff, B. W., Greene, D. A., Diminished specific activity of cytosolic protein kinase C in sciatic nerve of streptozotocin-induced diabetic rats and its correction by dietary myo-inositol supplementation, *Diabetes*, 40, 545, 1991.

65. Low, P. A., Nicander, K. K., Tritschler, H. J., The roles of oxidative stress and antioxidant treatment in experimental diabetic neuropathy, *Diabetes*, 46 (Suppl. 2), 538, 1997.

66. Miwa, I., Hirano, M., Kanbara, M., Okuda, J., In vivo activities of aldose reductase inhibitors having a 1-(arylsulfanyl) hydantoin structure, *Biochem. Pharmacol.*, 40, 303, 1990.
67. Yue, D. K., Hanwell, M. A., Satchell, P. M., Turtle, J. R., The effect of aldose reductase inhibition on motor nerve conduction velocity in diabetic rats, *Diabetes*, 31, 789, 1982.
68. Price, D. E., Airey, C. M., Alani, S. M., Wales, J. K., Effect of aldose reductase inhibition on nerve conduction velocity and resistance to ischemic conduction block in experimental diabetes, *Diabetes*, 37, 969, 1988.
69. Yoshida, T., Nishioka, H., Yoshioka, K., Nakano, K., Kondo, M., Terashima, H., Effect of aldose reductase inhibitor ONO 2235 on reduced sympathetic nervous system activity and peripheral nerve disorders in STZ induced diabetic rats, *Diabetes*, 36, 6, 1987.
70. Carrington, A. L., Ettlinger, C. B., Calcutt, N. A., Tomlinson, D. R., Aldose reductase inhibition with imirestat — effects on impulse conduction and insulin-stimulation of Na^+/K^+-adenosine triphosphatase activity in sciatic nerves of streptozotocin-diabetic rats, *Diabetologia*, 34, 397, 1991.
71. Kikkawa, R., Hatanaka, I., Yasuda, H., Kabayashi, N., Shigeta, Y., Terashima, H., Morimura, T., Tsuboshima, M., Effect of a new aldose reductase inhibitor, (E)-3-carboxymethyl-5-[(2E)-methyl-3-phenlypropenylidene] rhodanine (ONO-2235) on peripheral nerve disorders in streptozotocin-diabetic rats, *Diabetologia*, 24, 290, 1983.
72. Cameron, N. E., Leonard, M. B., Ross, I. S., Whiting, P. H., The effects of sorbinil on peripheral nerve conduction velocity, polyol concentrations and morphology in the streptozotocin-diabetic rat, *Diabetologia*, 29, 168, 1986.
73. Kato, K., Nakayama, K., Ohta, M., Murakami, N., Murakami, K., Mizota, M., Miwa, I., Okuda, J., Effects of novel aldose reductase inhibitors, M16209 and M16287, on streptozotocin-induced diabetic neuropathy in rats, *Eur. J. Pharmacol.*, 193, 185, 1991.
74. Nishikawa, M., Yoshida, K., Okamoto, M., Itoh, Y., Kohsaka, M., Studies on WF 3681, a novel aldose reductase inhibitor. IV. Effect of FR-62765, a derivative of WF-3681, on the diabetic neuropathy in rats, *J. Antibiot.*, 44, 441, 1991.
75. Ao, S., Shingu, Y., Kikuchi, C., Takano, Y., Nomura, K., Fujiwara, T., Ohkubo, Y., Notsu, Y., Yamaguchi, I., Characterization of a novel aldose reductase inhibitor, FR74366, and its effects on diabetic cataract and neuropathy in the rat, *Metabolism*, 40, 77, 1991.
76. Kikkawa, R., Hatanaka, I., Yasuda, H., Kobayash, N., Shigeta, Y., Prevention of peripheral nerve dysfunction by an aldose reductase inhibitor in streptozotocin-diabetic rats, *Metabolism*, 33, 212, 1984.
77. Hirata, Y., Okada, K., Relation of Na^+, K^+-ATPase to delayed motor nerve conduction velocity: effect of aldose reductase inhibitor, AND-138, on NA^+, K^+-ATPase activity, *Metabolism*, 39, 563, 1990.
78. Hirata, Y., Fujimori, S., Okada, K., Effect of a new aldose reductase inhibitor, 9'-chloro-2', 3'-dihydrospro [pyrralidine-3,6' (5'H)-pyrrolo [1,2,3-de] [1,4]benzoxazine]-2,5,5'-trione (AND-138), on delayed motor nerve conduction velocity in streptozotocin-diabetic rats, *Metabolism*, 37, 159, 1988.
79. Stribling, D., Mirrlees, D. J., Harrison, H. E., Earl, D. C., Properties of ICI 128, 436, a novel aldose reductase inhibitor, and its effects on diabetic complications in the rat, *Metabolism*, 34, 336, 1985.
80. Cameron, N. E., Cotter, M. A., Robertson, S., The effect of aldose reductase inhibition on the pattern of nerve conduction deficits in diabetic rats, *Q. J. Exp. Physiol.*, 74, 917, 1989.
81. Tomlinson, D. R., Holmes, P. R., Mayer, J. H., Reversal, by treatment with an aldose reductase inhibitor, of impaired axonal transport and motor nerve conduction velocity in experimental diabetes mellitus, *Neurosci. Lett.*, 31, 189, 1982.
82. Hotta, N., Kakuta, H., Fukasawa, H., Kimura, M., Koh, N., Iida, M., Terashima, H., Morimura, T., Sakamoto, N., Effects of a fructose-rich diet and the aldose reductase inhibitor, ONO-2235, on the development of diabetic neuropathy in streptozotocin-treated rats, *Diabetologia*, 28, 176, 1985.
83. Schmidt, R. E., Plurad, S. B., Coleman, B. D., Williamson, J. R., Tilton, R. G., Effects of sorbinil, dietary myo-inositol supplementation, and insulin on resolution of neuroaxonal dystrophy in mesenteric nerves, *Diabetes*, 40, 574, 1991.

84. Schmidt, R. E., Plurad, S. B., Sherman, W. R., Williamson, J. R., Tilton, R. G., Effects of aldose reductase inhibitor sorbinil on neuroaxonal dystrophy and levels of myo-inositol and sorbitol in sympathetic autonomic ganglia of streptozocin-induced diabetic rats, *Diabetes*, 38, 569, 1989.

85. Dahlin, L. B., Archer, D. R., McLean, W. G., Treatment with an aldose reductase inhibitor can reduce the susceptibility of fast axonal transport following nerve compression in the streptozotocin-diabetic rat, *Diabetologia*, 30, 414, 1987.

86. Willars, G. B., Tomlinson, D. R., Robinson, J. P., Studies of sorbinil on axonal transport in streptozotocin-diabetic rats, *Metabolism*, 35 (Suppl.1), 66, 1986.

87. Noda, K., Umeda, F., One, H., Hisatomi, A., Chijiwa, Y., Nawata, H., Iayashi, H., Decreased VIP content in peripheral nerve from streptozocin-induced diabetic rats, *Diabetes*, 39, 608, 1990.

88. Carsten, R. E., Whalen, L. R., Ishii, D. N., Impairment of spinal cord conduction velocity in diabetic rats, *Diabetes*, 38, 730, 1989.

89. Mayer, J. H., Tomlinson, D. R., Axonal transport of cholinergic transmitter enzymes in vagus and sciatic nerves of rats with acute experimental diabetes mellitus; correlation with motor nerve conduction velocity and effects of insulin, *Neuroscience*, 9, 951, 1983.

90. Schofield, G. G., Furman, B. L., Marshall, I. G., The effect of acute alloxan diabetes on the sensitivity of the rat skeletal neuromuscular junction to drugs, *Acta Diabetol. Lat.*, 15, 287, 1978.

91. Sahgal, U. K. Roy, S., Ahuja, M. M., Singh, N., Diabetic neuropathy: an experimental study in alloxanised rats, with special reference to insulin therapy, *Acta Diabetol. Lat.*, 9, 983, 1972.

92. Jaramillo, J., Simard-Duquesne, N., Dvornik, D., Resistance of the diabetic rat nerve to ischemic inactivation, *Can. J. Physiol. Pharmacol.*, 63, 773, 1985.

93. Monckton, G., Pehowich, E., The effects of intermittent insulin therapy on the autonomic neuropathy in the streptozotocin diabetic rat, *Can. J. Neurol. Sci.*, 9, 79, 1982.

94. Fink, D. J., Purkiss, D., Mata, M., Alteration in retrograde axonal transport in streptozocin-induced diabetic rats, *Diabetes*, 36, 996, 1987.

95. Macioce, P., Filliattreau, G., Figliomeni, B., Hassig, R., Thiery, J., Di Giamberardini, L., Slow axonal transport impairment of coskeletal proteins in streptozocin-induced diabetic neuropathy, *J. Neurochem.*, 53, 1261, 1989.

96. McCallum, K. N., Sharma, A. K., Blanchard, D. S., Stribling, D., Mirrlees, D. J., Duguid, I. G., Thoms, P. K., The effect of continuous subcutaneous insulin infusion therapy on morphological and biochemical abnormalities of peripheral nerves in experimental diabetes, *J. Neurol. Sci.*, 74, 55, 1986.

97. Lowitt, S., Malone, J. E., Solem, A., Kosthals, A., Acetyl-carnitine improves neuronal function in streptozotocin (ST2) diabetic rats, *Diabetes*, 39, 155A, 1990.

98. Pacifici, L., Bellucci, A., Pioveasan, P., Maaccari, F., Gorio, A., Ramaci, M. T., Counteraction on experimentally induced diabetic neuropathy by levocarnitine actyl, *Int. J. Clin. Pharm. Res.*, 12, 231, 1992.

99. Spuler, M., Dimpfel, W., Tullner, H. U., Ganglioside therapy in experimental diabetic neuropathy, *Arzneim. Forsch.*, 38, 881, 1988.

100. Calcutt, N. A., Tomlinson, D. R., Willars, G. B., Ganglioside treatment of diabetic rats; effects on nerve adenosine triphosphatase activity and motor nerve conduction velocity, *Life Sci.*, 42, 1515, 1988.

101. Calcutt, N. A. Tomlinson, D. R., Willars, G. B., Ganglioside treatment of streptozotocin- diabetic rats prevents defective axonal transport of 6-phosphofructokinase activity, *J. Neurochem.*, 50, 1478, 1988.

102. Gorio, A., Aporti, F., Di Gregorio, F., Schiavinato, A., Siliprandi, R., Vitadello, M., Ganglioside treatment of genetic and alloxan-induced diabetic neuropathy, *Adv. Exp. Med. Biol.*, 174, 549, 1984.

103. Marini, P., Vitadello, M., Bianchi, R., Triban, C., Gorio, A., Impaired axonal transport of acetylcholinesterase in the sciatic nerve of alloxan-diabetic rats: effect of ganglioside treatment, *Diabetologia*, 29, 254, 1986.

104. Paro, M., Prosdocimi, M., Zhang, W.-X., Sutherland, G., Sima, A. A. F., Autonomic neuropathology in the BB-rat: alterations in bladder function, *Diabetes*, 38, 1023, 1989.

105. Antonella, S., Annarosa, M., Alfredo, G., Quantitative analysis of myelin and axolemma particle distribution in C578BL/Ks diabetic mice and the effects of ganglioside treatment, *J. Neurol. Sci.*, 69, 301, 1985.

106. Paro, M., Prosdocimi, M., Sima, A. A., Gangliosides improve urinary bladder dysfunction in experimental diabetic autonomic neuropathy, *Pharmacol. Res.*, 22 (Suppl. 3), 125, 1990.

107. Italiano, G., Magri, V., Paro, M., Prosdocimi, M., Diabetic autonomic neuropathy and bladder function: pharmacological use of gangliosides and insulin, *Funct. Neurol.*, 5, 203, 1990.

108. Triban, C., Guidolin, D., Fabris, M., Marini, P., Schiavinato, A., Dona, M., Bortolami, M. C., Di Giamberardino, L., Fiori, M. G., Ganglioside treatment and improved axonal regeneration capacity in experimental diabetic neuropathy, *Diabetes*, 38, 1012, 1989.

109. Yasuda, H., Sonobe, M., Yamash, M., Terado, M., Hatanaka, I., Huitian, Z., Shigeta, Y., Effect of prostaglandin E1 analog TFC612 on diabetic neuropathy in streptozotocin-induced diabetic rats: comparison with aldose reductase inhibitor ONO 2235, *Diabetes*, 38, 832, 1989.

110. Suzuki, K., Saito, N., Sakata, Y., Toyota, T., Goto, Y., A new prostaglandin E1 analogue (TFC-612) improves the reduction in motor nerve conduction velocity in spontaneously diabetic GK (Goto-Kakizaki) rats, *Prostaglandins*, 40, 463, 1990.

111. Yasuda, H., Sonobe, M., Hatanaka, I., Yamashita, M., Miyamoto, Y., Terada, M., Amenomori, M., Kikkawa, R., Shigeta, Y., Motoyama, Y., Saito, N., A new prostaglandin EI analogue (TFC-612) prevents a decrease in motor nerve conduction velocity in streptozocin-diabetic rats, *Biochem. Biophys. Res. Commun*, 150, 225, 1988.

112. Kim, J., Kyriazi, H., Greene, D. A., Normalization of Na,K-ATPase activity in isolated membrane fraction from sciatic nerves of streptozotocin-induced diabetic rats by dietary myo-inositol supplementation *in vivo* or protein kinase C agonists *in vitro*, *Diabetes*, 40, 558, 1991.

113. Cameron, N. E., Cotter, M. A., Robertson, S., Essential fatty acid diet supplementation: effects on peripheral nerve and skeletal muscle function and capillarization in streptozocin-induced diabetic rats, *Diabetes*, 40, 532, 1991.

114. Tomlinson, D. R., Robinson, J. P., Compton, A. M., Keen, P., Essential fatty acid treatment — effects on nerve conduction, polyol pathway and axonal transport in streptozotocin diabetic rats, *Diabetologia*, 32, 655, 1989.

115. Julu, P. O., Essential fatty acids prevent slowed nerve conduction in streptozotocin diabetic rats, *J. Diabetic Complications*, 2, 185, 1988.

116. Van der Zee, C. E., Van der Hoop, R. G., Gispen, W. H., Beneficial effect of Org 2766 in treatment of peripheral neuropathy in streptozotocin-induced diabetic rats, *Diabetes*, 38, 225, 1989.

117. Van der Zee, C. E., Van den Buuse, M., Gispen, W. H., Beneficial effect of an ACTH (4-9) analog on peripheral neuropathy and blood pressure response to tyramine in streptozocin diabetic rats, *Eur. J. Pharmacol.*, 177, 211, 1990.

118. Kihara, M., Schmelzer, J. D., Paduslo, J. F., Curran, G. L., Nickander, K. K., Low, P. A., Aminoguanidine effects on nerve blood flow, vascular permeability, electrophysiology, and oxygen free radicals, *Proc. Natl. Acad. Sci. U.S.A.*, 88, 6107, 1991.

119. Isaka, M., Okuda, Y., Bannai, C., Yamashita, K., Effect of aminoguanidine (AG) on myelinated and unmyelinated nerve conduction velocities (NCV) of streptozotocin (STZ) diabetic rats (Abstract), *Diabetes*, 40 (Suppl. 1), 124A, 1991.

120. Yagihashi, S., Kamijo, M., Baba, M., Yagihashi, N., Nagai, K., Effect of aminoguanidine on functional and structural abnormalities in peripheral nerve of STZ induced diabetic rats, *Diabetes*, 41, 47, 1992.

121. Sima, A. A. F., Chakrabarti, S., Long term suppression of postprandial hyperglycemia with acarbose retards development of neuropathies in the BB-rat, *Diabetologia*, 35, 325, 1992.

122. Iwata, N., Matsumura, M., Sakai, Y., Effects of vitamin B complex in functional changes of the peripheral nerves of alloxan-induced diabetic rats, *Nippon Yakurigaku Zasshi*, 75, 9, 1979.

123. Yagihashi, S., Tokui, A., Kashamura, H., Takagi, S., Imamura, K., *In vivo* effect of methylcobalamin on the peripheral nerve structure in streptozotocin diabetic rats, *Horm. Metab. Res.*, 14, 10, 1982.

124. Sakitama, K., Saito, K., Aikawa, M., Nago, M., Ishikawa, M., Effect of vitamin B mixture on neuropathy in streptozotocin-induced diabetic rats, *J. Nutr. Sci. Vitaminol.* (Tokyo), 35, 95, 1989.

125. Sonobe, M., Yasuda, H., Hatanaka, I., Teradi, M., Yamashita, M., Kikkawa, R., Shigeta, Y., Methylcobalamin improves nerve conduction in streptozotocin-diabetic rats without affecting sorbitol and myo-inositol contents of sciatic nerve, *Horm. Metab. Res.*, 20, 717, 1988.

126. Low, P. A., Tuck, R. R., Dyck, P. J., Schmelzer, J. D., Yao, J. K., Prevention of some electrophysiologic and biochemical abnormalities with oxygen supplementation in experimental diabetic neuropathy, *Proc. Natl. Acad. Sci. U.S.A.*, 81, 6894, 1984.
127. Low, P. A., Schmelzer, J. D., Ward, K. K., Curran, G. L., Poduslo, J. F., Effect of hyperbaric oxygenation on normal and chronic streptozotocin diabetic peripheral nerves, *Exp. Neurol.*, 99, 201, 1988.
128. Watanabe, K., Molecular biological study on pathogenesis of diabetic neuropathy: alterations in mRNA expression of aldose reductase and axonal cytoskeletal protein, *Hirosaki Med. J.*, 45, S196, 1993.
129. Mohiuddin, L., Fernyhough, P., Tomlinson, D. R., Reduced levels of mRNA encoding endoskeletal and growth-associated proteins in sensory ganglia in experimental diabetes, *Diabetes*, 44, 25, 1995.
130. McEwen, T. A. J., Sima, A. A. F., Autonomic neuropathy in the BB-rat assessment by an improved method for measuring heart rate variability, *Diabetes*, 36, 251, 1987.
131. Paro, M., Prosdocimi, M., Fiori, M. G., Sima, A. A. F., Autonomic innervation of the bladder in two models of experimental diabetes in the rat: function abnormalities, structural alterations and effects of ganglioside administration, *Urodinamica*, 1, 161, 1991.
132. Paro, M., Prosdocimi, M., Experimental diabetes in the rat: alterations in the vesical function, *J. Auton. Nerv. Syst.*, 21, 59, 1987.
133. Low, P. A., Lagerlund, T. D., McManis, P. G., Nerve blood flow and oxygen delivery in normal, diabetic and ischemic neuropathy, *Int. Rev. Neurobiol.*, 31, 355, 1989.
134. Tuck, R. R., Schmelzer, J. D., Low, P. A., Endoneural blood flow and oxygen tension in the sciatic nerves of rats with experimental diabetic neuropathy, *Brain*, 107, 935, 1984.
135. Cameron, N. E., Cotter, M. A., Ferguson, K., Robertson, S., Radcliffe, M. A., Effects of chronic α-adrenergic receptor blockade on peripheral nerve conduction, hypoxic resistance, polyols, Na-K ATPase activity and vascular supply in streptozocin-diabetic rats, *Diabetes*, 40, 1652, 1991.
136. Cameron, N. E., Cotter, M. A., Robertson, S., Angiotensin converting enzyme inhibition prevents development of muscle and nerve dysfunction and stimulated angiogenesis in streptozotocin-diabetic rats, *Diabetologia*, 35, 12, 1992.
137. Robertson, S., Cameron, N. E., Cotter, M. A., The effect of the calcium antagonist nifedipine on somatic nerve function in streptozotocin-diabetic rats, *Diabetologia*, 35, 1113, 1992.
138. Cameron, N. E., Cotter, M. A., Dines, K. C., Maxifield, E. K., Pharmacological manipulation of vascular endothelial function in nondiabetic and streptozotocin-diabetic rats: effects on nerve conduction, hypoxic resistance and endothelial capillarization, *Diabetologia*, 36, 516, 1993.
139. Cameron, N. E., Dines, K. C., Cotter, M. A., The potential contribution of endothelin-1 to neurovascular abnormalities in streptozotocin diabetic rats, *Diabetologia*, 37, 1209, 1994.
140. Cameron, N. E., Cotter, M. A., Effects of chronic treatment with a nitric oxide donor on nerve conduction abnormalities and endoneural blood flow in streptozotocin diabetic rats, *Diabetologia*, 37, 1209, 1994.
141. Williamson, J. R., Chang, K., Frangos, M., Hasan, K. S., Ido, Y., Kawamura, T., Nyengaard, J. R., Van Den Enden, M., Kilo, C., Rilton, R. G., Perspectives in diabetes. Hyperglycemic pseudohypoxia and diabetic complications, *Diabetes*, 42, 801, 1993.
142. Cameron, N. E., Cotter, M. A., Low, P. A., Nerve blood flow in early experimental diabetes in rats: relation to conduction deficits, *Am. J. Physiol.*, 261, E1, 1991.
143. Tilton, R. G., Chang, K., Pugliese, G., Eades, D. M., Province, M. A., Sherman, W. R., Kilo, C., Williamson, J. R., Prevention of hemodynamic and vascular albumin filtration changes in diabetic rats by aldose reductase inhibitors, *Diabetes*, 38, 1258, 1989.
144. Wolf, B. A., Williamson, J. R., Eason, R. A., Chang, K., Sherman, W. R., Turk, J., Diacylglycerol accumulation and microvascular abnormalities induced by elevated glucose levels, *J. Clin. Invest.*, 87, 31, 1990.
145. Pugliese, G., Tilton, R. G., Speedy, A., Santarelli, E., Eades, D. M., Province, M. A., Kilo, C., Sherman, W. R., Williamson, J. R., Modulation of haemodynamic and vascular filtration changes in diabetic rats by dietary myo-inositol, *Diabetes*, 39, 312, 1990.
146. Hotta, N., Kakuta, H., Fukusawa, H., Koh, N., Sakakibara, F., Komori, H., Sakamoto, N., Effect of niceritrol on streptozotocin induced diabetic neuropathy in rats, *Diabetes*, 41, 587, 1992.

147. Low, P. A., Nickander, K. K., Oxygen free radical effects in sciatic nerve in experimental diabetes, *Diabetes*, 40, 873, 1991.
148. Calcutt, N. A., Mizisin, A. P., Kalichman, M. W., Aldose reductase inhibition, Doppler flux and conduction in diabetic rat nerve, *Eur. J. Pharmacol.*, 251, 27, 1994.
149. Cotter, M. A., Dines, K. C., Cameron, N. E., Prevention and reversal of nerve dysfunction in streptozotocin-diabetic rats by treatment with the prostacyclin analog iloprotst, *Naunyn-Schmeidebergs Arch. Pharmacol.*, 347, 534, 1993.
150. Cameron, N. E., Cotter, M. A., Robertson, S., Rapid reversal of a motor nerve conduction deficit in streptozotocin-diabetic rats by the angiotensin converting enzyme inhibitor lisinopril, *Acta Diabetol.*, 30, 46, 1993.
151. Moore, S. A., Peterson, R. G., Felten, D. L., Cartwright, T. R., O'Conner, B. L., Reduced sensory and motor conduction velocity in 25-week-old diabetic C57BL/Ks(db/db) mice, *Exp. Neurol.*, 70, 548, 1980.
152. Robertson, D. M., Sima, A. A. F., Diabetic neuropathy in the mutant mouse [C57/BL/Ks(db/db)]: a morphometric study, *Diabetes*, 29, 60, 1980.
153. Sima, A. A. F., Robertson, D. A., Peripheral neuropathy in mutant diabetic mouse [C57BL/Ks(db/db)], *Acta Neuropathol.*, 44, 189, 1978.
154. Hanker, J. S., Ambrose, W. W., Yates, P. E., Koch, G. G., Carson, K. A., Peripheral neuropathy in mouse hereditary diabetes mellitus. I. Comparison of neurologic, histologic and morphometric parameters with dystonic mice, *Acta Neuropathol.*, 51, 145, 1980.
155. Carson, K. A., Bossen, E. H., Hanker, J. S., Peripheral neuropathy in mouse hereditary diabetes mellitus. II. Ultrastructural correlates of degenerative and regenerative changes, *Neuropathol. Appl. Neurobiol.*, 6, 361, 1980.
156. Sharma, A. K., Thoma, P. K., Gabriel, G., Stolinski, C., Dockery, P., Hollins, G. W., Peripheral nerve abnormalities in the diabetic mutant mouse, *Diabetes*, 32, 1152, 1983.
157. Bianchi, R., Marelli, C., Marini, P., Fabris, M., Triban, C., Fiori, M. G., Diabetic neuropathy in db/db mice develops independently of changes in ATPase and aldose reductase, *Diabetologia*, 33, 131, 1990.
158. Yagihashi, S., Tonosaki, A., Yamada, K.-I., Kakizaki, M., Goto, Y., Peripheral neuropathy in selectively-inbred spontaneously diabetic rats: electrophysiological, morphometrical and freeze-replica studies, *Tohoku J. Exp. Med.*, 138, 39, 1982.
159. Sharma, A. K., Thomas, P. K., Baker, R. W. R., Peripheral nerve abnormalities related to galactose administration in rats, *J. Neurol. Neurosurg. Psychiatry*, 39, 794, 1976.
160. Nukada, H., Dyck, P. J., Low, P. A., Lais, A. C., Sparks, M. F., Axonal caliber and neurofilaments are proportionally decreased in galactose neuropathy, *J. Neuropathol. Exp. Neurol.*, 45, 140, 1986.
161. Diabetes Control and Complications Trial Research Group, The effect of intensive treatment of diabetes on the development of long-term complications in insulin-dependent diabetes mellitus, *N. Engl. J. Med.*, 329, 977, 1993.
162. Santiago, J. V., Lessons from the diabetes control and complication trial, *Diabetes*, 42, 1549, 1993.
163. Gabbay, K. H., The polyol pathway and the complications of diabetes, *N. Engl. J. Med.*, 288, 831, 1976.
164. Greene, D. A., Lattimer, S. A., Sima, A. A. F., Sorbitol, phosphoinositides and sodium- potassium ATPase in the pathogenesis of diabetic complications, *N. Engl. J. Med.*, 316, 599, 1987.
165. Kador, P. F., Kinoshita, J. H., Role of aldose reductase in the development of diabetes associated complications, *Am. J. Med.*, 79 (Suppl. 5A), 8, 1985.
166. Kinoshita, J. H., Nishimura, C., The involvement of aldose reductase in diabetic complications, *Diabetes Metab. Rev.*, 4, 323, 1988.
167. Chakrabarti, S., Sima, A. A. F., Nakajima, T., Yagihashi, S., Greene, D. A., Aldose reductase in the BB-rat: isolation, immunological identification and localization in the retina and peripheral nerve, *Diabetologia*, 30, 244, 1987.
168. Ghahay, A., Murphy, L. J., Chakrabarti, S., Sima, A. A. F., Effects of insulin and statil treatment on aldose reductase expression in diabetic rats, *Diabetes*, 40, 1931, 1991.
169. Bagnasco, S., Balaban, R., Fales, H. M., Yang, Y.-M., Burg, M., Predominant osmotically active organic solutes in rat and rabbit, *J. Biol. Chem.*, 261, 5872, 1986.

170. Nishimura, C., Lou, M. F., Kinoshita, J. G., Depletion of myo-inositol and amino acids in galactosemic neuropathy, *J. Neurochem.*, 49, 290, 1987.

171. Stevens, M. J., Lattimer, S. A., Kamijo, M., Van Huysen, C., Sima, A. A. F., Greene, D. A., Osmotically-induced nerve taurine depletion and the compatible osmolyte hypothesis in experimental diabetic neuropathy in the rat, *Diabetologia*, 36, 608, 1993.

172. Greene, D. A., Sima, A. A. F., Stevens, M. J., Feldman, E. L., Lattimer, S. A., Complications: neuropathy, pathogenetic consideration, *Diabetes Care*, 15, 1903, 1992.

173. Greene, D. A., Lattimer, S. A., Altered sorbitol and myo-inositol metabolism as the basis for defective proteins kinase C and (Na$^+$, K$^+$)-ATPase regulation in diabetic neuropathy, *Ann. N.Y. Acad. Sci.*, 488, 334, 1986.

174. Greene, D. A., Lattimer, S. A., Action of sorbinil in diabetic peripheral nerve: relationship of polyol (sorbitol) pathway inhibition to a myo-inositol-mediated defect in Na$^+$-K$^+$-ATPase activity, *Diabetes*, 33, 712, 1984.

175. Greene, D. A., Lattimer, S. A., Carroll, P. B., Fernstrom, J. D., Finegold, D. N., A defect in sodium-dependent aminoacid uptake in diabetic rabbit peripheral nerve: correction by an aldose reductase inhibitor or myo-inositol administration, *J. Clin. Invest.*, 85, 1657, 1990.

176. Greene, D. A., Mackway, A. M., Decreased myo-inositol content and Na$^+$-K$^+$-ATPase activity in superior cervical ganglion of STZ diabetic rat and prevention by aldose reductase inhibition, *Diabetes*, 35, 1106, 1986.

177. Greene, D. A. Lattimer, S. A., Impaired rat sciatic nerve sodium-potassium adenosine trisphosphatase in acute streptozotocin diabetes and its correction by dietary myo-inositol supplementation, *J. Clin. Invest.*, 72, 1058, 1983.

178. Simpson, C. M. F., Hawthorne, J. N., Reduced Na$^+$-K$^+$ ATPase activity in peripheral nerve of streptozotocin-diabetic rats: a role for protein kinase C? *Diabetologia*, 31,

179. Cameron, N. E., Cotter, M. A., Dines, K. C., Maxfield, E. K., Carey, F., Mirrlees, D., Aldose reductase inhibition, nerve perfusion, oxygenation and function in streptozotocin-diabetic rats: dose–response considerations and independence from a myo-inositol mechanism, *Diabetologia*, 37, 651, 1994.

180. Jefferys, J. R. G., Palmano, K. P. Sharma, A. K., Thomas, P. K., Influence of dietary myo-inositol on nerve conduction and phospholipid in normal and diabetic rats, *J. Neurol. Neurosurg. Psychiatry*, 41, 333, 1978.

181. Yagihashi, S., Watanabe, K., Feedback inhibition of aldose reductase expression in the peripheral nerve of chronically streptozotocin diabetic rats, *Diabetes*, 41 (Suppl. 1), 141A, 1992.

182. Calcutt, N. A., Tomlison, D. R., Briswas, S., Coexistence of nerve conduction deficit with increased Na$^+$-K$^+$-ATPase activity in galactose fed mice: implication for polyol pathway and diabetic neuropathy, *Diabetes*, 39, 663, 1990.

183. Lampourne, J. E., Tomlison, D. R., Broron, A. M., Willars, G. B., Opposite effects of diabetes and galactosemia on adenosine triphosphatase activity in rat nervous tissue, *Diabetologia*, 30, 360, 1987.

184. Peiper, G. M., Gross, G. J., Oxygen free radical abolish endothelin dependent relaxation in diabetic rat aorta, *Am. J. Physiol*, 255, H825, 1988.

185. Cameron, N. E., Cotter, M. A., Impaired contraction and relaxation in aorta from streptozotocin-diabetic rats: role of polyol pathway, *Diabetologia*, 35, 1011, 1992.

186. Stevens, M. J., Dananberg, J., Feldman, E. L., Lattimer, S. A., Kamijo, M., Thomas, T. P., The linked roles of nitric oxide, aldose reductase, and (Na$^+$-K$^+$)-ATPase in the slowing of nerve conduction in the streptozotocin diabetic rat, *J. Clin. Invest.*, 94, 853, 1994.

187. Pugliese, G., Tilton, R. G., Williamson, J. R., Glucose-induced metabolic imbalances in the pathogenesis of diabetic vascular disease, *Diabetes Metab. Rev.*, 7, 35, 1991.

188. Corr, P. B., Gross, R. W., Sobel, B. E., Amphipathie metabolites and membrane dysfunction in ischemic myocardium, *Circ. Res.*, 55, 135, 1984.

189. Tahiliani, A. G., McNeill J. H., Diabetes induced abnormalities in the myocardium, *Life Sci.*, 38, 959, 1986.

190. Feuvray, D., Idell-Wenger, J. A., Nedy, J. R., Effects of ischemia on rat myocardial function and metabolism in diabetes, *Circ. Res.*, 44, 322, 1979.

191. Wand, K. K., Low, P. A. Schmelzer, J. D., Zochodne, D. W., Prostacyclin and noradrenaline in peripheral nerve of chronic experimental diabetes in rat, *Brain*, 112, 197, 1989.
192. Brownlee, M., Cerami, A., Vlassara, H., Advanced glycosylation end products in tissue end products in tissue and the biochemical basis of diabetic complications, *N. Engl. J. Med.*, 318, 1315, 1988.
193. Vlassara, H., Recent progress in advanced glycation end products and diabetic complications, *Diabetes*, 46 (Suppl. 2), 519, 1997.
194. Suarez, G., Non enzymatic browning of proteins and the sorbitol pathway, *Prog. Clin. Biol. Res.*, 304, 141, 1989.
195. Vlassara, H., Bucala, R., Striker, L., Pathogenetic effects of advanced glycosylation: Biochemical, biologic and clinical implication for diabetes and aging, *J. Lab. Invest.*, 70, 138, 1994.
196. Vlassara, H., Brownlee, M., Cerami, A., Nonenzymatic glycosylation of peripheral nerve protein in diabetes mellitus, *Proc. Natl. Acad. Sci. U.S.A.*, 78, 5190, 1981.
197. Vlassara, H., Brownlee, M., Cerami, A., Excessive nonenzymatic glycosylation of peripheral and central nervous system myelin components in diabetic rats, *Diabetes*, 32, 670, 1983.
198. Monnier, V. M., Koh, R., Cerami, A., Accelerated age-related browning of human collagen in diabetes mellitus, *Proc. Natl. Acad. Sci. U.S.A.*, 81, 583, 1984
199. Williams, S. K., Howarth, N. L., Devenny, J. J., Bitensky, M. W., Structural and functional consequences of increased tubulin glycosylation in diabetes mellitus, *Proc. Natl. Acad. Sci. USA*, 79, 6546, 1982.
200. Cullum, N. A., Mahon, J., Stringer, K., McLean, W. G., Glycation of rat sciatic nerve tubulin in experimental diabetes mellitus, *Diabetologia*, 34, 387, 1991.
201. Cameron, N. E., Cotter, M. A., Dines, K. C., Love, A., Effects of aminogunidine on peripheral nerve function and polyol pathway metabolites in streptozotocin diabetic rats, *Diabetologia*, 35, 946, 1992.
202. Zhu, X., Eichberg, J., 1,2-Diacylglycerol content and its arachidonyl-containing molecular species are reduced in sciatic nerve from streptozotocin-induced diabetic rats, *J. Neurochem*, 55, 1087, 1990.
203. Hermenegildo, C., Felipo, V., Minana, M.D., Romero, F. J., Grisolia, S., Sustained recovery of Na+/K+-ATPase activity in sciatic nerve of diabetic mice by administration of H7 or callphostin C, inhibitors of protein kinase C, *Diabetes*, 42, 257, 1993.
204. Martelli, E., Orafalian, Z., Kiolo, C., Corr, P. B., Williamson, J. R., Neural dysfunction and metabolic imbalances in diabetic rats: prevention by acetyl-ʟ-carnitine, *Diabetes*, 43, 1469, 1994.
205. King, G. L., Oliver, F. J., Inoguchi, T., Shiba, T., Banskota, N. K., Abnormalities of the vascular endothelium in diabetes, in *Diabetes Annual*, Marshall, S. M., Home, P. D., Alberti, K. G. M. M., Krall, L. P., Eds., Elsevier, Amsterdam, 1993, 107-126.
206. Hellweg, R., Hartung, H. D., Endogenous levels of nerve growth factor (NGF) are altered in experimental diabetes mellitus: a possible role for NGF in the pathogenesis of diabetic neuropathy, *J. Neurosci. Res.*, 26, 258, 1990.
207. Hellweg, R., Wohrle, M., Hartung, H. D., Strack, H., Hock, C., Federlin, K., Diabetes mellitus-associated decrease in nerve growth factor levels is reversed by allogenic pancreatic islet transplantation, *Neurosci. Lett.*, 125, 1, 1991.
208. Kasayama, S., Oka, T., Impaired production of nerve growth factor in the submandibular gland of diabetic mice, *Am. J. Physiol.*, 257, E400, 1989.
209. Jakobsen, J., Brimijoin, S., Skau, K., Sidepius, P., Wells, D., Retrograde axonal transport of transmitter enzymes, fucose-labelled protein, and nerve growth factor in streptozotocin-diabetic rats, *Diabetes*, 30, 797, 1981.
210. Tomlinson, D. R., Fernyhough, P., Diemel, L. T., Role of neurotrophins in diabetic neuropathy and treatment with nerve growth factors, *Diabetes*, 40 (Suppl. 2), S82, 1997.
211. Maeda, K., Fernyhough, P., Tomlinson, D. R., Regenerating sensory neurons of diabetic rats express reduced levels of mRNA for GAP-43, gamma-preprotachykinin and the nerve growth factor receptors, trkA and p75[NGFR], *Mol. Brain Res.*, 37, 166, 1996.
212. Robinson, J. P. Willars, G. B., Tomlinson, D. R., Keen, P., Axonal transport and tissue contents of substance P in rats with long-term streptozotocin-diabetes: effects of the aldose reductase inhibitor "statil," *Brain Res.*, 426, 339, 1987.

213. Tomlinson, D. R., Robinson, J. P. Willars, G. B., Keen, P., Deficient axonal transport of substance P in streptozocin-induced diabetic rats: effects of sorbinil and insulin, *Diabetes*, 37, 488, 1988.

214. Diemel, L. T., Stevens, E. J., Willars, G. B., Tomlinson, D. R., Depletion of substance P and calcitonin gene-related peptide in sciatic nerve of rats with experimental diabetes: effects of insulin and aldose reductase inhibition, *Neurosci. Lett.*, 137, 253, 1992.

215. Hanaoka, Y., Ohi, T., Furukawa, S., Furukawa, Y., Hayashi, K., Matukura, S., Effect of 4-methylcatechol on sciatic nerve growth factor level and motor nerve conduction velocity in experimental diabetic neuropathic process in rats, *Exp. Neurol.*, 115, 292, 1992.

216. Apfel, S. C., Arezzo, J. C., Brownlee, M., Federoff, H., Kessler, J. A., Nerve growth factor administration protects against experimental diabetic sensory neuropathy, *Brain Res.*, 634, 7, 1994.

217. Ekstrom, A. R. Kanje, M., Skottner, A., Nerve regeneration and serum levels of insulin-like growth factor-1 in rats with streptozotocin-induced insulin deficiency, *Brain Res.*, 496, 141, 1989.

218. Yang, H., Scheff, A. J., Schalch, D. S., Effects of streptozotocin-induced diabetes mellitus on growth and hepatic insulin-like growth factor 1 gene expression in the rat, *Metabolism*, 39, 295, 1990.

219. Graubert, M. D., Goldstein, S., Phillips, L. S., Nutrition and somatomedin: XXVII. Total and free IGF-1 and IGF binding proteins in rats with streptozocin-induced diabetes, *Diabetes*, 40, 959, 1991.

220. Bornfeldt, K. E., Arnqvist, J. H., Enberg, B., Matthews, L. S., Norstedt, G., Regulation of insulin-like growth factor-1 and growth hormone receptor gene expression by diabetes and nutritional state in rat tissues, *J. Endocrinol.*, 122, 651, 1989.

221. Frank, L. L., Diabetes mellitus in the texts of old Hindu medicine (Charaka, Susruta, Vagbhata), *Am. J. Gastroenterol.*, 27, 76, 1957.

222. Frank, R. N., On the pathogenesis of diabetic retinopathy: a 1990 update, *Ophthalmology*, 98, 586, 1991.

223. Klein, R., Klein, B. E. K., Moss, S. E., Davis, M. D., Demet, D. L., Glycosylated hemoglobin predicts the incidence and progression of diabetic retinopathy, *JAMA*, 260, 2864, 1988.

224. Blom, M. L., Green, W. R., Schalbat, A. P., Diabetic retinopathy: a review, *Del. Med. J.*, 66, 379, 1994.

225. Ceriello, A., Coagulation activation in diabetes mellitus: the role of hyperglycemia and therapeutic prospects, *Diabetologia*, 36, 1119, 1993.

226. Collier, A., Rumley, A. G., Paterson, J. R., Leach, J. P., Lowe, G. D. O., Small, M., Free radical activity and hemostatic factors in NIDDM patients with and without microalbuminurea, *Diabetes*, 41, 909, 1992.

227. Ceriello, A., Marchi, E., Palazzini, E., Quartraro, A., Giuglianno, D., Low molecular weight heparin restores antithrombin III activity from hyperglycemia induced alterations, *Diabetes Metab.*, 16, 86, 1990.

228. Ceriello, A., Giugliano, D., Quartraro, A., Dellorusso, P., Torella, R., Blood glucose may condition factor VII levels in diabetic and normal subjects, *Diabetologia*, 31, 889, 1988.

229. Coller, B. S., Frank, R. S., Milton, R. C., Granlick, H. R. Plasma cofactors of platelet function: correlation with diabetic retinopathy and hemoglobin A1a-c, *Ann. Int. Med.*, 88, 311, 1992.

230. Osterman, H., Vandeloo, J., Factors of the hemostatic system of the diabetic patients. A survey of controlled studies, *Hemostasis*, 16, 386, 1986.

231. Fukui, M., Nakamura, T., Ebihara, I., Shirato, I., Tomino, Y., Koide, H., ECM gene expression and its modulation by insulin in diabetic rats, *Diabetes*, 4, 1520, 1992.

232. Porta, M., Endothelium: the main actor in the remodelling of the retinal microvasculature in diabetes, *Diabetologia*, 39, 739, 1996.

233. Aiello, L. P., Avery, R. L., Arigg, P. G., Keyt, B. A., Jampel, H. D., Shah, S. T., Pasquale, L. R., Thiene, H., Iwamoto, M. A., Park, J. E., Nguyen, J. E., Aiello, L. M., Ferrara, N., King, G. L., Vascular endothelial growth factor in ocular fluid of patients with diabetic retinopathy and other retinal disorder, *N. Engl. J. Med.*, 331, 1480, 1994.

234. Aiello, L. P., Bursell, S-E., Clermont, A., Duh, E., Ishii, H., Takagi, C., Mori, F., Ciulla, T. A., Ways, K., Jirousek, M., Smith, L. E. H., King, G. L., Vascular endothelial growth factor-induced retinal permeability is mediated by protein kinase C *in vivo* and suppressed by an orally effective β-isoform-selective inhibitor, *Diabetes*, 46, 1473, 1997.

235. Forrester, J. V., Knott, R. M., McIntosh, L. C., Pathogenesis of proliferative diabetic retinopathy and maculopathy, in *The Diabetes Annual*, Marshall, S. M., Home, P. D., Alberti, K. G. M. M., and Krall, L. P., Eds., Elsevier, Amsterdam, 1993, 178-191.

236. Pfeiffer, A., Spranger, J., Meyer-Schwickerath, R., Schatz, H., Growth factor alterations in advanced diabetic retinopathy: a possible role of blood retina barrier breakdown, *Diabetes*, 46 (Suppl. 2), S82, 1997.

237. Engerman, R. L., Kern, T. S., Retinopathy in animal models of diabetes, *Diabetes Metab. Rev.*, 11, 109, 1995.

238. Engerman, R. L., Bloodworth, J. M. B., Jr., Experimental diabetic retinopathy in dogs, *Arch. Ophthalmol.*, 73, 205, 1965.

239. Engerman, R. L., Bloodworth, J. M. B., Jr., Nelson, S., Relationship of microvascular disease in diabetes to metabolic control, *Diabetes*, 26, 760, 1977.

240. Engerman, R. L., Kern, T. S., Progression of incipient diabetic retinopathy during good glycemic control, *Diabetes*, 36, 808, 1987.

241. Gardiner, T. A., Stitt, A. W., Anderson, H. R., Archer, D. B., Selective loss of vascular smooth muscle cells in the retinal microcirculation of diabetic dogs, *Br. J. Ophthalmol.*, 78, 54, 1994.

242. Engerman, R. L., Kern, T. S., Aldose reductase inhibition fails to prevent retinopathy in diabetic and galactosemic dogs, *Diabetes*, 42, 820, 1993.

243. Kern, T. S., Engerman, R. L., Vascular lesions in diabetes are distributed non-uniformly within the retina, *Exp. Eye Res.*, 60(5), 545, 1995.

244. Sousula, L., Beaumont, P., Hollows, F. C., Jonson, K. M., Dilatation and endothelial cell proliferation of retinal capillaries in streptozotocin diabetic rats: quantitative electron microscopy, *Invest. Ophthalmol.*, 11, 926, 1972.

245. Babel, J., Luenberger, P., A long term study on the ocular lesions in the streptozotocin rat, *Albrecht von Graefes Arch. Klin. Exp. Ophthalmol.*, 18, 191, 1974.

246. Studer, P. P., Muller, W. A., Reynold, A. E., Alteration of retinal capillaries by long term streptozotocin diabetes, in *Current Topics in Diabetes Research. Abstracts of 9th Congress of I.D.F. New Delhi*, 1976.

247. Sharma, N. K., Gardiner, T. A., Archer, D. B., A morphological and autoradiographic study of cell death and regeneration in the retinal microvasculature of normal and diabetic rats, *Am. J. Ophthalmol.*, 100, 51, 1985.

248. Chakrabarti, S., Tze, W. J., Tai, J., Sima, A. A. F., Prevention of diabetic retinal capillary pericyte degeneration and loss in by pancreatic islet allograft, *Curr. Eye Res.*, 6, 649, 1987.

249. Sima, A. A. F., Chakrabarti, S., Tze, W. J., Tai, J., Pancreatic islet allograft prevents basement membrane thickening in diabetic retina, *Diabetologia*, 31, 175, 1988.

250. Krupin, T., Waltman, S. R., Scharp, D. W., Oestrich, C., Fieldman, S. L., Becker, B., Ballinger, W. F., Lacy, P. E., Ocular fluorophotometry in streptozotocin diabetes mellitus in the rat: effect of pancreatic islet isograft, *Invest. Ophthalmol. Vis. Sci.*, 18, 1185, 1979.

251. Grimes, P. A., Laties, A. M., Early morphological alteration of the pigment epithelium in the streptozotocin induced diabetes: increased surface area of basal cell membrane, *Exp. Eye Res.*, 30, 631, 1980.

252. Kernal, A., Arnqvist, H., Effect of insulin treatment on the blood retinal barrier in the rats with streptozotocin induced diabetes, *Arch. Ophthalmol.*, 101, 968, 1983.

253. Stitt, A. W., Li, Y. M., Gardiner, T. A., Vlassara, H., A progressive intracellular AGE accumulation in association with pericyte loss has recently been demonstrated in STZ rats, *Diabetes*. 45 (Suppl. 2), 15A, 1996.

254. Hammes, H. P., Ali, S. S., Uhlmann, M., Weiss, A., Federlin, K., Geisen, K., Brownlee, M., Aminoguanidine does not inhibit the initial phase of experimental diabetic retinopathy in rats, *Diabetologia*, 38(3), 269, 1995.

255. Hammes, H. P., Martin, S., Federlin, K., Geisen, K., Brownlee, M., Aminoguanidine treatment inhibits the development of experimental diabetic retinopathy in rats, *Proc. Natl. Acad. Sci. U.S.A.*, 88, 11555, 1991.

256. Blair, N. P., Tso, M. O. M., Dodge, J. T., Pathologic studies of the blood retinal barrier in the spontaneously diabetic BB-rat, *Invest. Ophthalmol. Vis. Sci.*, 25, 302, 1984.

257. Sima, A. A. F., Chakrabarti, S., Garcia-Salinas, R., Basu, P. K., The BB rat — an authentic model of human diabetic retinopathy, *Curr. Eye Res.*, 4, 1087, 1985.

258. Chakrabarti, S., Prashar, S., Sima, A. A. F., Augmented polyol pathway activity and retinal pigment epithelial permeability in the diabetic BB-rat, *Diabetes Res. Clin. Pract.*, 8, 1, 1990.

259. Heegaard, S., Structure of the vitreoretinal border region in spontaneously diabetic BB-rats. *Acta Ophthalmol.*, 71, 637, 1993.

260. Chakrabarti, S., Sima, A. A. F., Effect of aldose reductase inhibition and insulin treatment on retinal capillary basement membrane thickening in BB-rat, *Diabetes*, 38, 1181, 1989.

261. Chakrabarti, S., Cherian, V., Sima, A. A. F., The effect of acarbose on diabetes and age related basement membrane thickening in retinal capillaries of the BB/W rat, *Diabetes Res. Clin. Pract.*, 20, 123, 1993.

262. Chakrabarti, S., Sima, A. A. F., The effect of myo-inositol treatment on basement membrane thickening in the retina of BB/W rat, *Diabetes Res. Clin. Pract.*, 16, 13, 1992.

263. Toussaint, D., Lesions retiniennes au cours de diabete alloxanique chez le rat, *Bull. Soc. Belge Ophthalmol.*, 143, 648, 1966.

264. Orloff, M., Lee, S., Charters, A., Granbort, D. E., Storock, G., Knox, D., Long term studies of pancreas transplantation in experimental diabetes mellitus, *Ann. Surg.*, 182, 198, 1975.

265. Musacchio, I., Palermo, N., Rodriguez, R., Microaneurysms in the retina of diabetic rats, *Lancet*, 1, 146, 1964.

266. Agarwal, P., Agarwal, L., Tandon, H., Experimental diabetic retinopathy in albino rats, *Orient. Arch. Ophthalmol.*, 4, 68, 1966.

267. Gibbs, G., Wilson, R., Ho, C. K., Experimental diabetes in monkey, *Proc. 2nd Int. Cong. Primates*, 3, 169, 1969.

268. Bresnick, G. H., Engerman, R., Davis, M. D., deVanecia, G., Myers, F. L., Patterns of ischemia in diabetic retinopathy, *Trans. Am. Acad. Ophthalmol. Otolaryngol.*, 81, 694, 1976.

269. Laver, N., Robison, W. G., Jr., Hansen, B. C., Spontaneously diabetic monkeys as a model for diabetic retinopathy, ARVO Abstract. *Invest. Ophthalmol. Vis. Sci.*, 35 (Suppl.), 1733, 1994.

270. Yokote, M., Retinal and renal microangiopathy in carp with spontaneous diabetes mellitus, *Adv. Metab. Disord.*, Suppl. 2, 399, 1993.

271. Engerman, R. L., Kern, T. S., Experimental galactosemia produces diabetic-like retinopathy, *Diabetes*, 33, 97, 1984.

272. Kern, T. S., Engerman, R. L., Galactose-induced retinal microangiopathy in rats, *Invest. Ophthalmol. Vis. Sci.*, 36, 490, 1994.

273. Kador, P. F., Takahashi, Y., Sato, S., Wyman, M., Amelioration of diabetes-like retinal changes in galactose-fed dogs, *Prev. Med.*, 23(5), 717, 1994.

274. Kador, P. F., Akagi, Y., Takahashi, Y., Ikebe, H., Wyman, M., Kinoshita, J. H., Prevention of retinal vessel changes associated with diabetic retinopathy in galactose-fed dogs by aldose reductase inhibitors, *Arch. Ophthalmol.*, 108, 1301, 1990.

275. Frank, R. N., Keirn, R. J., Kennedy, A., Frank, K. W., Galactose-induced retinal capillary basement membrane thickening: prevention by sorbinil, *Invest. Ophthalmol. Vis. Sci.*, 24, 1519, 1983.

276. Robison, W. G., Jr., Kador, P. F., Kinoshita, J. H. Retinal capillaries: basement membrane thickening by galactosemia prevented with aldose reductase inhibitor, *Science*, 221, 1177, 1983.

277. Robison, W. G., Jr, Nagata, M., Laver, N., Hohman, T. C., Kinoshita, J. H., Diabetic-like retinopathy in rats prevented with an aldose reductase inhibitor, *Invest. Ophthalmol. Vis. Sci.*, 30, 2285, 1989.

278. Robinson, G. W., Jr, Tillis, T. N., Laver, N., Kinoshita, J. H., Diabetes related histopathologies of rat retina prevented with an aldose reductase inhibitor, *Exp. Eye Res.*, 50, 355, 1990.

279. Shiba, T., Bursell, S. E., Clermont, A., Sportsman, R., Heath, W., King, G. L., Protein kinase C (PKC) activation is a causal factor for the alteration of retinal blood flow in diabetes of short duration, *Invest. Ophthalmol. Vis. Sci.*, Suppl., 32, 785, 1991.

280. Tilton, R. G., Chang, K., Allison, W., Williamson, J. R., Comparable diabetes induced increases in retinal blood flow assessed with conventional vs. molecular (^{3}H- Desmethylimiprimine) microspheres, *Invest. Ophthalmol. Vis. Sci (suppl).*, 33, 1048, 1992.

281. Cringle, S. J., Yu, D. Y., Alder, V. A, Su, E. N., Retinal blood flow by hydrogen clearance polarography in the streptozotocin-induced diabetic rat, *Invest. Ophthalmol. Vis. Sci.*, 34, 1716, 1993.

282. Tilton, R. G., Chang, K., Nyengaard, J. R., Van den Enden, M., Ido, Y., Williamson, J. R., Inhibition of sorbitol dehydrogenase. Effects on vascular and neural dysfunction in strepto-zocin-induced diabetic rats, *Diabetes*, 44, 234, 1995.

283. Tilton, R. G., Chang, K., Hasan, K. S., Smith, S. R., Petrash, J. M., Misko, T. P., Moore, W. M., Currie, M. G., Corbett, J. A., McDaniel, M. L., Williamson, J. R., Prevention of diabetic vascular dysfunction by guanidine. Inhibition of nitric oxide synthase vs. advanced glycation end-product formation, *Diabetes*, 42(2), 221, 1993.

284. Tilton, R. G., Change, K., Pugliese, G., Eades, D. M., Province, M. A., Sherman, W. R., Kilo, C., Williamson, J. R., Prevention of haemodynamic and vascular albumin filtration changes in diabetic rats by aldose reductase inhibitors, *Diabetes*, 38, 1258, 1989.

285. Hasan, K. S., Chang, K., Allison, W., Faller, A., Santiago, J. V., Tilton, R. G., Williamson, J. R. Glucose-induced increases in ocular blood flow are prevented by aminoguanidine and L-NMMA, inhibitors of nitric oxide synthase, *Invest. Ophthalmol. Vis. Sci.*, Suppl., 34, 1127, 1993.

286. Williamson, J. R., Chang, K., Allison, W. S., Tilton, R. G., Orfalian, Z., Arrigoni-Martelli, E., Acetyl-L-carnitine, but not L-carnitine attenuates diabetes-induced increases in vascular ^{131}I-BSA clearance, *Invest. Ophthalmol. Vis. Sci.*, 32, 1029, 1991.

287. Kunisaki, M., Bursell, S. E., Clermont, A. C., Ishii, H., Ballas, L. M., Kirousek, M. R., Umeda, F., Nawata, H., King, G. L., Vitamin E prevents diabetes-induced abnormal retinal blood flow via the diacylglycerol-protein kinase C pathway, *Am. J. Physiol.*, 269(2 Pt 1), E239, 1995.

288. Clermont, A. C., Brittis, M., Shiba, T., McGovern, T., King, G. L., Bursell, S. E., Normalization of retinal blood flow in diabetic rats with primary intervention using insulin pumps, *Invest. Ophthalmol. Vis. Sci.*, 35(3), 981, 1994.

289. Ishii, H., Kirousek, M. R., Koya, D., Takagi, C., Xia, P., Clermont, A., Bursell, S. E., Kern, T. S., Ballas, L. M., Heath, W. F., Stram, L. E., Feener, E. P., King, G. L., Amelioration of vascular dysfunctions in diabetic rats by an oral PKC β-inhibitor, *Science*, 272, 728, 1996.

290. Williamson, J. R., Chang, K., Rowold, E., Marvel, J., Tomlison, M., Sherman, W. R., Tilton, R. G., Kilo, C., Sorbinil prevents diabetes induced increased vascular permeability but does not alter collagen cross linking, *Diabetes*, 34, 1460, 1985.

291. Sakai, H., Tani, Y., Shirasawa, E., Shirao, Y., Kawasaki, K., Development of electroretinographic alterations in streptozotocin-induced diabetes in rats, *Ophthalmic Res.*, 27, 57, 1995.

292. Segawa, M., Hirata, Y., Fujimori, S., Kada, K., The development of electroretinogram abnor-malities and possible roles of polyol pathway activity in diabetic hyperglycemia and galac-tosemia, *Metabolism*, 37, 454, 1988.

293. MacGregor, L. C., Matchinsky, F. M., Treatment with an aldose reductase inhibitor or with myo-inositol arrests deterioration of electroretinogram of diabetic rats, *J. Clin Invest.*, 76, 887, 1985.

294. Akagi, Y., Hirofumi, T., Millen, J., Kador, P. F., Kinoshita, J. H., Aldose reductase localization in dog retinal mural cells, *Curr. Eye Res.*, 5, 883, 1986.

295. Kern, T. S., Engerman, R. L., Hexitol production by canine retinal microvessels, *Invest. Oph-thalmol. Vis. Sci.*, 26, 382, 1985.

296. Ludvigson, M. A., Sorenson, R. L., Immunohistochemical localization of aldose reductase. II. Rat eye and kidney, *Diabetes*, 29, 450, 1980.

297. Lee, T-S, Saltsman, K. A., Ohashi, H., King, G. L., Activation of protein kinase C by elevation of glucose concentration: proposal for a mechanism for the development of diabetic vascular complication, *Proc. Natl. Acad. Sci. U.S.A.*, 86, 5141, 1989.

298. Inoguchi, T., Battan, R., Handler, E., Sportsman, J. R., Heath, W., King, G. L., Preferential activation of protein kinase C isoform βII and diacylglycerol levels in the aorta and heart of diabetic rats, *Proc. Natl. Acad. Sci. U.S.A.*, 89, 11059, 1992.

299. Kowluru, R. A., Jirousek, M. R., Engerman, R. L., Kern, T. S., In the STZ rat PKC and Na/K ATPase alteration was prevented by specific B-II PKC inhibitor, *Diabetes*, 45 (Suppl. 2), 16A, 1996.

300. Xia, P., Inoguchi, T., Kern, T. S., Engerman, R. I., Oates, P. J., King, G. L., Characterization of the mechanism for the chronic activation of DAG–PKC pathway in diabetes and hypergalac-tosemia, *Diabetes*, 43, 1122, 1994.

301. Kern, T. S., Kowluru, R. A., Engerman, R. L., Abnormalities of retinal metabolism in diabetes or galactosemia: ATPases and glutathione, *Invest. Ophthalmol. Vis. Sci.*, 35(7), 2962, 1994.

302. Porte, D., Jr., Schwartz, M. W., Diabetes complications: why is glucose potentially toxic? *Science*, 272, 699, 1996.

303. Esposito, C., Gerlach, H., Brett, J., Endothelial receptor mediated binding of glucose modified albumin is associated with increased monolayer permeability and modulation of cell surface coagulant properties, *J. Exp. Med.*, 170, 1387, 1992.

304. Nawroth, P. P., Stern, D., Bierhaus, A., AGE-Albumin stimulierte Endothelzellen — ein in Vitro Modell diabetischer Spätschäden, *Diabetes Stoffwechs*, 1 (Suppl. 1), 153A, 1992.

305. Haitoglou, C. S., Tsilibary, E. C., Brownlee, M., Charnois, A. S., Altered cellular interaction between endothelial cells and nonenzymatically glucosylated laminin/Type IV collagen, *J. Biol. Chem.*, 267, 12404, 1992.

306. Rubanyi, G. M., Polokoff, M. A., Endothelins: molecular biology, biochemistry, pharmacology, physiology and pathophysiology, *Pharmacol. Rev.*, 46, 325, 1994.

307. Lin, U. W., Duh, E., Jian, Z., ET-1 expression have been demonstrated in the retina and heart of STZ diabetic rats, *Diabetes*, 45 (Suppl.), 48A, 1996.

308. Chakrabarti, S., Sima, A. A. F., Endothelin-1 and endothelin-3 like immunoreactivity in the eyes of normal and diabetic BB/W-rats, *Diabetes Res. Clin. Pract.*, 37, 109, 1997.

309. Lowe, W. L., Jr., Florkiewicz, R. Z., Yorek, M. A., Spanheimer, R. G., Albrecht, B. N., Regulation of growth factor mRNA levels in the eyes of diabetic rats, *Metabolism*, 44, 1038, 1995.

310. Sharp, P. S., The role of growth factors in the development of diabetic retinopathy, *Metabolism*, 44(10) (Suppl. 4), 72, 1995.

311. Pfeiffer, A., Spranger, J., Meyer-Schwickerath, R., Schatz, H., Growth factor alterations in advanced diabetic retinpathy: a possible role of blood retina barrier breakdown, *Diabetes*, 46 (Suppl. 2), S26, 1997.

312. Sorbinil Retinopathy Trial Research Group, A randomized trial of sorbinil, an aldose reductase inhibitor, in diabetic retinopathy, *Arch. Ophthalmol.*, 108, 1229, 1990.

313. Pfeifer, M. A., Schumer, M. P., Gelber, D. A., Aldose reductase inhibitors: The end of an era or the need for different trial designs? *Diabetes*, 46 (Suppl. 2), S82, 1997.

314. Yamaoka, T., Nishimura, C., Yamash, K., Itakura, M., Yamada, T., Fujimoto, J., Kokai, Y., Acute onset of diabetic pathological changes in transgen'c mice with human aldose reductase cDNA, *Diabetologia*, 38, 255, 1995.

315. Cagliero, E., Roth, T., Roy, S., Maiello, M., Lorenzi, M., Expression of genes related to the extracellular matrix in human endothelial cells: differential modulation by elevated glucose concentrations, phorbol ester, and cAMP, *J. Biol. Chem.*, 266, 14244, 1991.

316. Chojkier, M., Houglum, K., Solis-Herruzo, J., Brenner, D. A., Stimulation of collagen gene expression by ascorbic acid in cultured human fibroblasts: A role for lipid peroxidation? *J. Biol. Chem.*, 264, 16957, 1989.

317. Kreisberg, J. I., Biology of disease: hyperglycemia and microangiopathy. Direct regulation by glucose of microvascular cells, *Lab. Invest.*, 67, 416, 1992.

318. Nakamura, T., Ebihara, I., Fukui, M., Tomino, Y., Koida, H., Effect of a specific endothelin-A receptor antagonist on mRNA levels for extracellular matrix components and growth factors in diabetic glomeruli, *Diabetes*, 44, 895, 1995.

319. Roy, S., Lorenzi, M., Early biosynthetic changes in the diabetic like retinopathy of galactose fed rats, *Diabetologia*, 39, 735, 1996.

320. Aiello, L. P., Robinson, G. S., Lin, Y. W., Nishio, Y., King, G. L., Identification of multiple genes in bovine retinal pericytes altered by exposure to elevated levels of glucose by using mRNA differential display, *Proc. Natl. Acad. Sci. U.S.A.*, 91, 6231, 1994.

321. Roy, S., Cagliero, S., Lorenzi, M., Fibronectin overexpression in retinal microvessels of diabetic patients, *Invest. Ophthalmol. Vis. Sci.*, 37, 258, 1996.

322. Roy, S., Maiello, M., Lorenzi, M., Increased expression of basement membrane collagen in human diabetic retinopathy, *J. Clin. Invest.*, 93, 438, 1996.

323. Mandarino, L. J., Sundarraj, N., Finlayson, J., Hassell, J. R., Regulation of fibronectin and laminin synthesis by retinal capillary endothelial cells pericytes *in vitro*, *Exp. Eye Res.*, 57, 609, 1983.

324. Yagihashi, S., Yamagishi, S., Wada, R., Aizawa, S., Nishimura, C., Kokai, Y., Enhancement of neuropathic changes in human aldose reductase transgenic mouse rendered diabetic by streptozotocin, *Diabetes*, 43 (Suppl. 1), 108A, 1994.

7

Vascular Reactivity in Streptozotocin-Induced Diabetes

Ramaswamy Subramanian and Kathleen M. MacLeod

CONTENTS

7.1 Introduction

Abnormalities in vascular reactivity have been implicated as potential contributors to cardiovascular complications of diabetes mellitus. For instance, an association between altered vascular reactivity to neurotransmitters and/or circulating hormones, such as noradrenaline (NA) and angiotensin II, and peripheral vascular disease, such as hypertension, has been suggested in patients with diabetes mellitus.[1] However, efforts to investigate this further in animal models of diabetes, in particular in the streptozotocin (STZ) diabetic rat, have provided conflicting observations (see References 2 and 3 for reviews). Despite the existence of extensive literature on altered vascular reactivity in this model, no consistent picture has emerged, and the exact mechanisms underlying alterations that are reported are not fully understood. In this chapter, the aim is to highlight some of the controversies surrounding the question of changes in the reactivity of vasculature from STZ diabetic rats, and address some of the current issues that remain unresolved.

It should be noted from the outset that at least some of the contradictory observations concerning vascular reactivity in STZ diabetic rats may arise from differences in experimental approaches, including such factors as the dose and route of administration of STZ. This laboratory routinely uses 60 to 65 mg/kg STZ, a dose that has been demonstrated to be maximal with regard to production of hyperglycemia in rats.[4] Although this dose of STZ or one close to it (55 to 75 mg/kg) has been used in many other studies, doses ranging from a low of 35 mg/kg[5] to a high of 80 to 85 mg/kg have also been employed.[6-8] While intravenous injection (usually into the lateral tail vein) is a routinely used method of administration of STZ, a large number of studies have employed the intraperitoneal route of administration to induce diabetes. These differences could have resulted in diabetes of differing severity, which could influence the nature and extent of the changes in reactivity observed. Unfortunately, no method for determining the severity of the diabetic state in studies of vascular reactivity has been routinely employed; although blood glucose levels prior to sacrifice are usually reported, this parameter is subject to wide fluctuations depending on when the blood samples were taken in relation to food intake.

Another area of difference between studies is in the strain and gender of rats studied. Although male Wistar rats have been used routinely in this and other laboratories, male Sprague-Dawley rats are also commonly employed, and female Wistar, female Sprague-Dawley, male Wistar-Kyoto, male Lewis, female CSE, and male Holtzman albino rats have all been used.[9-17] In considering gender differences, it should be borne in mind that female rats are thought to be more resistant to the adverse effects of STZ-induced diabetes than male rats.[18,19] In addition, different strains of rat may be more or less susceptible to either the diabetogenic effects of STZ or the consequences of the diabetes induced, although this has not been systematically investigated.

Finally, it is important to note that studies of vascular reactivity in experimental diabetes have been conducted in a wide variety of different arteries and vascular beds, from rats with diabetes of widely varying duration, from acute (1 to 7 days to 6 weeks) to chronic (10 to 14 weeks to 1 year). There is evidence to indicate that the effect of diabetes on vascular reactivity differs in different vessels and at different durations of diabetes.[10] Therefore, the following sections summarize the studies of vascular reactivity according to vessel type and size (aortae, mesenteric, renal, and caudal arteries, and perfused hindquarters) at different durations of diabetes.

7.2 Functional Alterations in the Vasculature in STZ-Induced Diabetes

7.2.1 Agonist-Stimulated Contractile Responses

7.2.1.1 Aortae

There are a large number of reports of the effects of both acute and chronic STZ-induced diabetes on the reactivity of the aorta to vasoconstrictors. Although there is not complete agreement among studies, the majority report that contractile responses to NA and other agents, including phenylephrine (PE), 5-hydroxytryptamine (5-HT), and KCl, are not altered in this vessel within the first 7 to 21 days after STZ injection.[10,17,20,21] In contrast, Fulton et al.[22] found that maximum responses of aortae to endothelin-1 (ET-1) and KCl, but not to NA, were significantly diminished 2 weeks after STZ injection. One obvious difference between these studies is that Fulton and colleagues placed their aortic rings under a resting tension of 10 g, which they calculated to be a close approximation of the aortic wall tension *in vivo*. In most investigations a resting tension of 1 to 2 g is used; in this laboratory, it was determined that a resting tension of 2 g results in the optimum developed tension of both control and diabetic aortae to NA.[23] In another early study, it was reported that by 2 weeks after induction of diabetes, aortae were less responsive to both PE and KCl.[24] The diminished maximum responsiveness was not accompanied by a change in sensitivity (expressed as the pD2 or $-\log ED_{50}$) to PE, and persisted throughout the 12-week observation period. However, there were a number of experimental differences between that investigation[24] and others conducted at the same duration of diabetes which makes comparison among them difficult.

Studies that have examined the reactivity of aortae at durations of diabetes longer than 3 weeks have reported widely varying results. As early as 4 to 5 weeks after STZ injection, it was reported that aortae had a greater maximum contractile response to NA than control rats.[17] Similarly, in another investigation conducted 4 weeks after diabetes induction, aortae were more responsive to NA, PE, and KCl.[25] The increased responsiveness in the latter study was not accompanied by a change in sensitivity to the vasoconstrictors. In contrast, no change in sensitivity or responsiveness of aortae to NA or PE was detected 4 weeks after injection of STZ in yet another study.[26] Furthermore, we have not been able to detect any change in either sensitivity or maximum response of aortae to NA even 6 weeks after induction of diabetes (unpublished observations). These differences obtained in the same arterial preparation are not due to differences in the strain of rats used, or in the dose or route of administration of STZ, and are difficult to explain.

A number of studies have also been conducted in aortae from rats made diabetic 2 months previously, but again the results are not consistent. For instance, maximum contractile responses of aortae from diabetic rats to NA, 5-HT, and KCl were found to be significantly reduced, even when responses were normalized for the markedly smaller wet weight of the diabetic arteries in one investigation.[27] In contrast, maximum contractile responses of diabetic aortae to KCl were diminished, but those to PE were unaltered and the sensitivity to this agonist was increased in another study, while a significant decrease in sensitivity to NA, with no change in maximal response to this agonist or in sensitivity or responsiveness to PE, was detected in diabetic aortae in a third study.[26,28] In contrast, No change in sensitivity or maximum response to NA[29] and increased maximum contractile responses to both NA and KCl[30] were also reported in aortae from 2-month diabetic rats. Again, the reason for these widely varying results is not clear. In one study,[27] rats were fasted for 24 h prior to STZ injection, a procedure which may have increased the susceptibility of the animals to the diabetogenic effects of STZ (see Reference 31 and Chapter 1). The diminished contractile responsiveness of the aortae in that investigation could be related to a greater severity of diabetes in these animals. Beyond that, however, there are no obvious differences between these studies that could account for the variable results obtained.

There seems to be fairly general consensus that contractile responses of aortae from rats with diabetes of longer duration (from 3 to 12 months) to NA are enhanced, although there is no agreement regarding either the specificity of this effect or the underlying mechanisms. Studies from the authors' laboratory have consistently demonstrated an increase in maximum response to NA of aortae from male rats with chronic (12 to

16 weeks) STZ-induced diabetes.[23,32-37] This is associated with either a small increase or no change in the sensitivity to this agonist.[23,35,37] Maximum contractile responses of aortae to other α-adrenoceptor agonists, including methoxamine (in the presence of endothelium) and clonidine (in endothelium-denuded arteries) are also enhanced, although no change in sensitivity or maximum responsiveness of diabetic aortae to KCl can be detected.[23,32,35-37] Other investigators have also reported that maximum contractile responses of aortae from 10- to 12-week diabetic rats to NA are enhanced, with either an increase or no change in sensitivity to the agonist.[22,26,38-42] However, when contractile responses of diabetic aortae to KCl were determined, they were found to be increased in two studies, but to be impaired in a third.[39,41,42] In addition, although the authors found that contractile responsiveness to PE was also enhanced in 3-month diabetic rat aortae, this has not been seen in other investigations, although an increase in sensitivity with no effect on the maximum contractile response to PE was demonstrated in 13- to 15-week and 52-week diabetic rat aortae.[12,26,36,38,39,43]

There is general agreement that the major subtype of receptor mediating contractile responses of aortae from nondiabetic rats to NA and other α-adrenceptor agonists is the α1-receptor (see Reference 36 for a review). In light of this, it is interesting that enhanced contractile responses of aortae from 10- to 12-week diabetic rats to NA and clonidine were suggested to be due to increased activity of α2-adrenoceptors.[39] However, in this laboratory, the increased contractile responsiveness of 12- to 14-week diabetic aortae to NA, methoxamine, and clonidine was found to be mediated by stimulation of α1-adrenoceptors, based on pA2 values calculated for prazosin and yohimbine, antagonists that exhibit selectivity for α1- and α2-adrenoceptors, respectively.[36]

The influence of the endothelium on contractile responses of aortae from rats with chronic diabetes to α-agonists has also been controversial. Basal release of endothelium-derived relaxing factors has been demonstrated to attenuate contractile responses of rat aortae to α-adrenoceptor stimulation, leading investigators to hypothesize that enhanced contractile responses to NA could be secondary to decreased release of these factors in diabetic arteries.[44] If that were the case, then removal of the endothelium would be predicted to result in increases in contractile responses of control aortae to levels similar to those attained in diabetic aortae, and abolition of differences between them. In fact, the authors found that endothelium removal resulted in enhancement of maximum contractile responses of aortae from control, but not 12- to 14-week diabetic rats to NA and methoxamine.[37] However, concentration–response curves to these agonists were shifted to the same extent to the left on removal of endothelium from both diabetic and control aortae, and the sensitivity of the endothelium-denuded diabetic aortae remained significantly greater than control.[37] In addition, no response of either control or diabetic aortae to clonidine could be detected in the presence of endothelium. However, following endothelium removal, contractile responses of diabetic aortae to this agonist were significantly greater than control.[37] These data led to the suggestion that the enhanced contractile responses of diabetic aortae to α-adrenoceptor stimulation are not the result of a decrease in release of endothelium-derived relaxing factors. In agreement with these results, in other studies the enhanced sensitivity of diabetic aortae to PE was not dependent on the presence of endothelium, while enhanced contractile responses of diabetic aortae to NA were detected in endothelium-denuded aortae from 10- to 12-week diabetic rats.[12,41,42] However, in contrast, Chang and Stevens[43] reported that endothelium removal abolished the difference in sensitivity to PE between control and 52-week diabetic rat aortae.[43]

There is little information on the effect of chronic diabetes on vasoconstrictors other than α-adrenoceptor agonists. However, maximal contractile responses of aortae from 8- to 12-week diabetic rats to 5-HT were reported to be enhanced,[45] and the authors have observed that contractile responses of aortae from 12- to 14-week diabetic rats to the

G protein activator sodium fluoride (NaF) are also enhanced to an extent similar to the NA response.[46] This suggests that the enhanced reactivity is not selective for a particular receptor, but may be related to activation of a common postreceptor event. On the other hand, the lack of enhancement of contractile responses to K^+ depolarization at the same time suggests that there is no generalized increase in the contractility of aortae, due to a change in the structure of the artery or in the contractile proteins.

It is worth noting that the majority of the studies described above were conducted in aortae from male rats. Very little attention has been paid to the possibility that there could be gender differences in the effect of STZ-induced diabetes on vascular reactivity. However, the changes in contractile responses to agonists observed by the authors in diabetic male rat arteries vary considerably from those that had been detected in an early study conducted on diabetic female rat aortae. For instance, in contrast to the increased maximum contractile responses to NA and 5-HT detected in aortae from 12- to 14-week diabetic male rats, contractile responses to 5-HT were unchanged, while the sensitivity but not the maximum response to NA was significantly increased in aortae from female rats with diabetes of 14 weeks duration compared with their age- and gender-matched controls.[10]

Treatment with insulin has been demonstrated to prevent the onset of exaggerated responses to NA and to reverse the increased responsiveness to vasoactive agonists once it is established.[23] This suggests that the altered responsiveness detected in aortae from rats with diabetes of 12- to 14-weeks duration is a result of the diabetic state, rather than due to a direct toxic effect of STZ. However, as mentioned earlier, there is no general consensus regarding the underlying cause, and mechanism(s) for the enhancement have not been fully elucidated. Some of the possible mechanisms suggested to be involved include enhanced metabolism of phosphoinositides resulting in elevated IP_3 and diacylglycerol (DAG) levels, increased activation of protein kinase C (PKC), and increased influx of extracellular Ca^{2+} and/or mobilization of intracellular Ca^{2+}. These mechanisms will be discussed later in this chapter. In addition, although hyperglycemia has been implicated as the potential underlying cause for the aberrant responses of diabetic blood vessels, the lack of association between elevated glucose and altered contractile responses demonstrated in some studies does not support this hypothesis. The influence of hyperglycemia on contractile responses to vasoactive agonists will also be discussed in a later section.

7.2.1.2 Mesenteric Arteries

The effects of diabetes induced by STZ on the reactivity of various parts of the mesenteric vascular bed, from the largest artery, the superior mesenteric artery, through third-order mesenteric artery branches to the whole perfused mesenteric bed, have been investigated. A number of studies, including the authors', have demonstrated that the sensitivity and/or maximum responsiveness of isolated superior mesenteric arteries from rats with 12- to 14-week STZ-induced diabetes to α-adrenoceptor stimulation are enhanced.[23,32,35,37,47,48] Similarly, an increase in sensitivity and maximum response of mesenteric arteries from rats with diabetes of 42 weeks duration to NA has also been reported.[49] In contrast, no change in contractile response of isolated superior mesenteric artery to NA 2 weeks after STZ administration was found in another investigation.[50] Clearly, the short duration of diabetes in the latter study may be the reason for this observation.

The receptors mediating enhanced contractile responses to NA in superior mesenteric artery from diabetic rats have been characterized pharmacologically, through calculation of pA2 values for selective antagonists.[36,51] As the authors found in aortae, contractile responses of mesenteric arteries from both control and diabetic rats to NA, methoxamine and clonidine appear to arise from stimulation of α1-adrenoceptors.[36,51] However, although the authors observed that maximum contractile responses of mesenteric arteries from 12- to

14-week diabetic rats to NaF were also enhanced, responses of diabetic mesenteric arteries to K^+ depolarization were not significantly different from control.[23,32,46] In contrast, others have reported a nonspecific increase in contractile responsiveness of this artery to any procedure that results in activation of membrane Ca^{2+} channels.[47,51] This discrepancy does not seem to be attributable to any known differences in the experimental procedures employed and remains unexplained.

Studies on the reactivity of mesenteric resistance arteries from diabetic rats to α-adreno-ceptor stimulation have reported varying results. For instance, a decrease in sensitivity with no change in maximum response to NA was found 7 to 9 days after STZ injection.[50] On the other hand, Taylor et al.[52] were unable to detect a difference in response of mesen-teric resistance arteries to PE 3 weeks after STZ injection, although they observed an increase in sensitivity to NA after 5 to 6 weeks of diabetes and an increase in maximum response with no change in sensitivity to NA after 8 to 10 weeks of diabetes.[9,16,52] In contrast to the latter results, Wang et al.[53] were unable to detect a change in reactivity of mesenteric arterioles to PE after either 4 or 8 weeks of diabetes.[53] However, in addition to differences in duration of diabetes, there were differences in the strain and gender of the rats used and in the dose and route of administration of STZ in these studies, which renders it difficult to make comparisons between them.

The limited number of studies that have been conducted in the perfused mesenteric bed have also given rise to inconsistent results. An increase in sensitivity of the perfused mesenteric bed to NA was found 2 to 10 weeks after STZ injection, with no correlation between the NA pD2 value and the duration of diabetes in one investigation.[54] In contrast, a decrease or no change in reactivity to NA, measured as the change in perfusion pressure to intraluminal application of the agonist, was observed in 8-week diabetic perfused mesenteric vascular bed, while no change in reactivity to NA was detected in the mesen-teric vascular bed from rats with a longer duration of diabetes (12 to 17 weeks).[5,8,55] A variety of differences among the studies, including the use of a low dose of STZ, overnight fasting of the rats prior to STZ injection, induction of diabetes in adult rats, and the use of female rats, limits comparison of results among them.[5,8,54,55]

The contribution of endothelial dysfunction to the altered responses of superior mesen-teric artery and mesenteric resistance arteries to vasoconstrictors has been examined in a number of studies. In one, responses to NA and other α-agonists remained elevated in superior mesenteric arteries from rats with 10 to 12 weeks of diabetes following endothe-lium removal.[51] In the authors' investigation, removing the endothelium abolished the difference in maximum response to both NA and methoxamine between mesenteric arter-ies from control and 12- to 14-week diabetic rats.[37] However, as seen in aortae, it was also found that the sensitivities to NA and methoxamine were increased to the same extent in mesenteric arteries from both control and diabetic rats following endothelium removal, while the maximum response to clonidine was significantly greater in diabetic than control endothelium-denuded mesenteric arteries.[37] More recently, the authors observed that con-tractile responses of superior mesenteric arteries from control and diabetic rats to NaF were not altered by endothelium removal and that the maximum contractile response of diabetic arteries to NaF remained significantly greater than control in the absence of a functional endothelium.[46] In contrast, it was reported that pre-treatment with the nitric oxide synthase (NOS) inhibitor, N^G-nitro-L-arginine methyl ester (L-NAME) resulted in increased sensitivity of mesenteric resistance arteries from control but not 5- to 6-week diabetic rats to NA, and abolished the difference between them, suggesting that the enhanced sensitivity of the diabetic mesenteric resistance arteries to NA was the result of defective release of nitric oxide (NO).[16] However, this same group reported that at a later time point (8- to 10-weeks), contractile responses of mesenteric resistance arteries from diabetic rats to NA were still increased in the presence of L-NAME.[9] Therefore, overall these data suggest that the enhanced contractile responsiveness of both large and small mesenteric arteries from rats with diabetes of longer than 8 weeks duration to α-adrenoceptor stimulation are not the result of defective release of endothelial-derived relaxing factors.

The effects of insulin treatment on altered responsiveness of mesenteric arteries to vasoconstrictors have not been consistent in different studies. In acute (7 to 9 days) diabetes, insulin treatment failed to prevent the decrease in sensitivity of isolated mesenteric resistance arteries to NA.[50] In this situation, the impaired sensitivity to NA was proposed to be mediated by an increase in osmolality due to elevated glucose.[50] In another investigation, treatment of 8- to 10-week diabetic rats with a dose of insulin that elevated insulin levels well above those in control rats failed to prevent the enhanced maximum response of mesenteric resistance arteries to NA.[9] The authors of that study proposed that hyperinsulinemia might be exerting an effect on the contractility of the diabetic arteries.[9] On the other hand, treatment of rats with insulin for 12 weeks after STZ injection resulted in enhancement of the maximum responses of mesenteric resistance arteries to NA compared with responses of arteries from both control and untreated diabetic rats.[56] Since this was not seen in diabetic rats following islet transplantation, it also might be due to an effect of hyperinsulinemia, although this cannot be evaluated since insulin levels were not reported.[56] In contrast to the results obtained in mesenteric resistance arteries, in the authors' studies, insulin treatment both prevented the enhanced responsiveness of 12- to 14-week diabetic superior mesenteric arteries to NA, and reversed it once established.[23] This is consistent with the increased maximum response to NA being a consequence of the diabetic state, rather than due to a direct toxic effect of STZ on the artery.

7.2.1.3 Caudal Artery

There are few studies of diabetes-induced vascular dysfunction in the caudal artery, and as in other arteries, the results of these studies are not consistent. Both the sensitivities and maximum contractile responses of strips of caudal artery to NA and methoxamine were reported to be enhanced 4 weeks after induction of diabetes.[57] This is in agreement with the finding that the sensitivity and responsiveness of rings of caudal artery from 12- to 14-week diabetic rats to NA were increased.[58] In contrast, no difference in contractile response to NA was observed in caudal artery rings from 8-week diabetic rats compared with control.[59] In both studies in which NA responsiveness and sensitivity was increased, contractile responses of K^+-depolarized diabetic vessels to increasing extracellular calcium were not altered compared with control, indicating that the enhanced NA responsiveness is not the result of a generalized increase in contractility or a structural change in the artery.[57,58] However, as in aortae and mesenteric artery, maximum contractile responses of caudal artery from 12- to 14-week diabetic rats to the G protein activator, NaF, were also enhanced, suggesting that there is increased activation of postreceptor events in diabetic caudal arteries.[46]

It had been proposed that the altered reactivity of arteries from diabetic rats might result from autonomic neuropathy, which is known to be a common complication of diabetes. However, the authors could detect no signs of autonomic neuropathy in the caudal artery after 12- to 14-weeks of diabetes.[58] Contractile responses of diabetic caudal arteries to the indirect acting sympathomimetic agent tyramine were enhanced to the same extent as the NA response, while pretreatment with hydrocortisone, timolol, and desipramine increased the contractile responses of both control and diabetic caudal arteries to NA to the same extent.[58] These results were not consistent with those of Hart et al.,[59] who reported that contractile responses to tyramine and the content of NA were diminished, while the accumulation of NA metabolites was increased in caudal arteries from 8-week diabetic rats, suggesting that their animals had, in fact, developed autonomic neuropathy.[59] The only notable difference between the study of Hart et al. and the author's study was the strain of animal used, this being Sprague-Dawley in the former and Wistar in the latter investigation.[58,59] It is possible that diabetic neuropathy develops only in some strains of diabetic rats, or requires some as yet unknown conditions to develop. Alternatively, it is possible that the effects of autonomic neuropathy are more prominent at earlier stages of the disease.

The contribution of altered endothelial function to enhanced contractile responses of caudal arteries from diabetic rats to NA has not been extensively examined. However, the authors found that the exaggerated response to NA occurred in caudal arteries lacking a functional endothelium, suggesting that it is not the result of decreased release of endothelium-derived relaxing factors.[58]

7.2.1.4   Renal Artery

Nephropathy, associated with changes in the structure and function of the renal vasculature represents a major long-term complication of diabetes. As a result, the function of renal arteries and arterioles, particularly with respect to the endothelium, has been investigated in several studies. The renal artery itself has been reported to respond to NA with an increase in maximum responsiveness but no change in sensitivity 8 weeks after induction of diabetes.[60] An increase in responsiveness of the diabetic arteries to K^+-depolarization was also detected in the same investigation, indicating that the enhanced contractility was not limited to receptor-mediated events.[60] On the other hand, the sensitivities (expressed as the concentration of agonist required to reduce the lumen diameter by 40 to 50%) of small renal arteries to NA were reported to be increased 6 weeks, but to be similar to control 16 and 24 weeks, after onset of diabetes.[14] However, it is not clear from the report that the sensitivities of the arteries from diabetic animals were compared with those of the appropriate age-matched control animals, so it is difficult to estimate the significance of the findings.[14] Finally, an increase in both the sensitivity and responsiveness of the perfused kidney to NA was detected 12 days after STZ injection, suggesting an early increase in the reactivity of the resistance vessels of the kidney to this agonist.[6] Taken together, the results of these studies suggest that the reactivity of renal arteries to NA is increased relatively soon after the onset of diabetes. Whether this enhancement is related to endothelial dysfunction and decreased release of endothelium-derived relaxing factors is not entirely clear. Although the status of the renal artery endothelium was not mentioned in the report of Inazu et al.,[60] in the perfused rat kidney the vasodilatory effect of Ach was reported to be enhanced.[6] Although the latter observation is consistent with increased release of endothelium-derived relaxing factors in response to Ach, whether basal release of these substances is altered in the diabetic preparation was not investigated. In addition, whether the increased responsiveness of the renal vasculature to NA is sustained in diabetes of longer duration remains to be investigated.

7.2.1.5   Perfused Hindquarters

A very limited number of studies of vascular reactivity have been performed in the perfused rat hindquarters, a skeletal muscle vascular bed. In one investigation, the time dependence of the change in reactivity of Tyrode-perfused hindquarters from diabetic and control rats was followed over a period of 1 to 12 weeks.[61] Both the sensitivity and responsiveness of this preparation to NA were found to increase within 1 week after STZ injection, and remained elevated throughout the 12-week experimental period.[61] In contrast, in another study, the responsiveness of the blood-perfused hindquarters from 6 week diabetic rats to ET-1 was unchanged, while that to 5-HT was decreased compared with that of age-matched control animals.[62] It is not clear whether the difference in results between the two studies is due to differences in the effects of physiological solution vs. blood on hindquarter reactivity or to different effects of diabetes on responses to agonists acting at distinct receptors. However, this preparation should form the basis for further investigation both because it is an important contributor to vascular resistance and because it represents a model of skeletal muscle vasculature, which may be affected differently by diabetes than the more commonly investigated visceral vascular beds and large arteries.

7.2.2 Endothelium-Dependent and -Independent Relaxation

7.2.2.1 Aortae

It should come as no surprise that there is a lack of consensus on the effects of STZ-induced diabetes on endothelium-dependent relaxant responses of aortae to vasodilators, given the variability in reports of its effects on contractile responses of this preparation to agonists. A number of studies have indicated impaired responsiveness and/or sensitivity of aortae from rats with acute and chronic diabetes to Ach.[13,21,25,28,29,40,43,63-67] However, others have not detected any impairment of endothelium-dependent relaxation of aortae to Ach in diabetes of similar duration.[7,12,20,27,37,68] In some studies in which impaired relaxant responses to Ach were detected, responses to other endothelium-dependent vasodilators were also measured. Whereas endothelium-dependent relaxation of aortae to histamine was reported in one study to be impaired at 8 to 12 weeks of diabetes, in another no change in histamine-induced relaxation at 4 and 12 weeks of diabetes was observed.[66,67] Endothelium-dependent relaxation of diabetic aortae in response to A23187 and to ADP were also reported to be impaired.[40,64]

Regardless of whether or not endothelium-dependent relaxation was found to be defective, there is general agreement that endothelium-independent relaxation to nitroglycerin (GTN) and/or sodium nitroprusside (SNP) is not altered in aortae from rats with either acute or chronic diabetes.[12,20,28,29,40,65,67,68] This suggests that the pathways coupling elevated cGMP levels with relaxation in vascular smooth muscle cells are intact in diabetic aortae.

It is not clear why impairment of endothelium-dependent relaxation in aortae has been observed in some studies and not in others. There are no obvious systematic differences in experimental procedures employed that could give rise to this discrepancy, and for the present it remains unexplained. However, studies that have been directed toward determining the cause of impaired relaxation, where it has been shown to occur, have suggested some possibilities which will be discussed in a later section.

7.2.2.2 Mesenteric Arteries

There are only a limited number of reports on the effect of diabetes on endothelium-dependent and -independent relaxant responses of the superior mesenteric artery. The authors found no significant difference in either the sensitivity or the maximum response of mesenteric arteries from 12- to 14-week diabetic rats to Ach, despite the greater contractile response of the diabetic arteries to NA.[37] In contrast, Fukao et al.[69] more recently reported that the endothelium-dependent relaxation of the superior mesenteric artery from 8- to 12-week diabetic rats to Ach was diminished, and that this was related at least in part to defective release of endothelium-dependent hyperpolarizing factor (EDHF) in the diabetic arteries.[69]

detected 2 days after STZ injection, but cytosolic Ca^{2+} was significantly elevated by 7 days and remained elevated 14 days after induction of diabetes. This was associated with a decrease in Na^+-K^+-ATPase activity detected in crude membranes prepared from intact aortae, and it was suggested that the low Na^+-K^+-ATPase activity might be the driving force for the increased cytosolic Ca^{2+} levels.[88] However, whether or not this abnormality persists in diabetes of longer duration or is associated with the enhanced contractile response to NA is not clear.

Renal afferent arterioles in blood-perfused juxtamedullary nephrons from 2-week diabetic rats exhibited a decrease in vasoconstrictor response to high K^+ compared with arterioles from control rats.[89] In separate experiments, the increase in intracellular Ca^{2+} produced by high K^+ was also found to be depressed in fura 2–loaded isolated afferent arterioles incubated in Ringer's solution containing 20 mM glucose. However, this depression was reversed by exposing the arterioles for a short time to Ringer's solution containing 5 mM glucose.[89] Incubation of arterioles from control rats in the presence of 20 mM glucose, even for as long as 2 to 3 h, had no effect on the K^+-evoked increased in intracellular Ca^{2+}. These data were interpreted to suggest that in the hyperfiltration stage of diabetes, a hyperglycemia-induced impairment in Ca^{2+} influx though voltage-dependent Ca^{2+} channels occurs in renal afferent arterioles, and contributes to afferent vasodilation. It is not clear whether or not this effect persists in diabetes of longer duration.

An abnormality in the NA-stimulated Ca^{2+} signaling pathway has been suggested by Tam et al.[90] to be a potential mechanism for increased responsiveness to vasoactive agonists in caudal artery from 12- and 16-week diabetic rats. Basal intracellular Ca^{2+} levels measured with fura 2 in isolated single caudal artery vascular smooth muscle cells (VSMC) from control and diabetic rats were not significantly different, and both control and diabetic VSMC responded to NA with an initial transient calcium peak followed by a lower sustained response. The sensitivity (pD2 value) of the initial transient response to NA was significantly greater, but the maximum response was less, in diabetic VSMC than in control. The authors of the study suggested that increased release of Ca^{2+} from intracellular stores in response to NA-stimulated increases in IP_3 production in the diabetic VSMC might lead to a larger Ca^{2+} transient at lower concentrations of NA, but a lower one at higher doses due to saturation of IP_3 receptors.[90] It is not clear whether the abnormal Ca^{2+} responses were accompanied by altered contractile responses of the diabetic VSMC to NA, since the latter were not reported in this investigation.

The preliminary evidence supports the possibility that both basal and stimulated increases in intracellular Ca^{2+} levels may be altered, at least under some circumstances, in diabetic arteries, although it is clear that much remains to be learned about the precise role of Ca^{2+} in mediating altered reactivity to vasoconstrictors. Studies in which changes in both tension and intracellular Ca^{2+} levels are measured in the same preparations would be very useful in defining the contribution of Ca^{2+} to the altered contractile responses of arteries from diabetic rats to agonists.

7.3.3   Cyclic GMP

Cyclic GMP is believed to be responsible for mediating the relaxant responses of vascular smooth muscle to endothelial NO released tonically in the absence of vasodilators, and in response to receptor stimulation (see Reference 44 for a review). It follows that tonic release of NO from the endothelium of rat arteries can be monitored by measuring basal cGMP levels in these arteries. In an investigation from this laboratory, no significant difference in cGMP levels in endothelium-intact aortae from 12- to 14-week diabetic rats compared with control was detected, while removal of the endothelium resulted in a decrease in cGMP levels of both control and diabetic aortae to the same extent.[37] In contrast, a marked and significant decrease in basal cGMP levels was detected in 8- to 10-week endothelium-intact diabetic aortae compared with control by another group.[91] The only difference of note in experimental procedures between the two studies was the duration of diabetes, leading to the possibility that the basal release of NO is diminished at 8 weeks of diabetes but has returned to normal 1 month later. However, it is impossible to rule out other factors that may have contributed to a difference in results between the two studies. Interestingly, in a later investigation from the same laboratory, cGMP levels in the effluent of the perfused mesenteric bed from 10-week diabetic rats were not significantly different from control, suggesting that basal release of NO may not be altered in this preparation at this stage of diabetes.[92]

As might be expected, studies in which cGMP levels in the presence of Ach have been measured in diabetic arteries demonstrate that changes in levels of this cyclic nucleotide parallel relaxation responses to Ach. For instance, this laboratory observed no significant differences in Ach-induced relaxation or elevation of cGMP levels between control and diabetic aortae from 12- to 14-week diabetic rats.[37] On the other hand, impaired relaxation to Ach was associated with impaired Ach-induced elevation of cGMP levels in aortae from rats with diabetes of 8 to 10 weeks duration.[91,93] Similarly, impaired relaxation of the perfused mesenteric bed to Ach was associated with diminished cGMP levels in the effluent of this preparation from 10-week diabetic rats.[92]

It is interesting to speculate why defective endothelium-dependent relaxation and cGMP elevation are observed in diabetic arteries in some studies but not in others. Comparison of experimental protocols indicates considerable variations, such as in the dose of STZ used to induce diabetes, the type and concentration of agonists used to precontract the vessels, and the strain of rat used, but none which could be clearly related to the different results obtained. The possible factors contributing to defective endothelium-dependent relaxation in diabetic arteries when it has been detected have been quite extensively investigated. The results of these investigations are summarized below.

7.4 Endothelial Dysfunction in Diabetes

Alterations in the NO pathway giving rise to impaired relaxation appear to arise at the level of the endothelium, since relaxation in response to endothelium-independent cGMP-elevating agents is largely preserved in diabetic arteries. Defective production and release of NO and/or its increased breakdown, occurring independently or at the same time, have been proposed to contribute to altered relaxation. It is possible that more than one mechanism is involved in diabetes-induced endothelial dysfunction and that different mechanisms predominate at different durations of diabetes, although evidence for this speculation is lacking. In addition, hyperglycemia has been proposed to be the major underlying cause of impaired endothelium-dependent relaxation, through a variety of different mechanisms. However, in all studies of endothelial function in STZ-induced diabetes, arteries would have been exposed to relatively severe hyperglycemia *in vivo*, yet endothelial dysfunction *in vitro* is observed in only some cases. This suggests that exposure to chronic hyperglycemia alone is not sufficient to induce persistent impairment of endothelium-dependent relaxation.

7.4.1   Nitric Oxide Production and Release

The authors are not aware of any studies that have directly measured the release of NO from the endothelium of diabetic arteries. However, pharmacological investigations have suggested that the production of NO in response to Ach may be reduced under some circumstances in arteries from diabetic rats. Impaired relaxation of aortae from rats with diabetes of both 8 and 12 weeks duration to Ach was detected in one such study.[15] Treatment of 8-week diabetic aortae with either L-arginine, or an analog of the NOS cofactor, tetrahydrobiopterin, *in vitro*, improved Ach-induced relaxation, suggesting that lack of substrate or cofactor for NOS may have been the cause of impaired relaxation.[15,29,93] However, pretreatment with L-arginine failed to reverse the impaired relaxation of aortae from 12-week diabetic rats to Ach, suggesting that a different mechanism may be responsible for the defective response to Ach at this later time.[15] Furthermore, investigators in another study were unable to reverse the defective relaxation of 2-month diabetic aortae to Ach by incubating the arteries in the presence of L-arginine (although at a threefold lower concentration than that used in Reference 15).[28]

Increased, rather than decreased, release of NO by arteries from diabetic rats has also been proposed to occur, although in some cases this was associated with increased destruction of NO, and impaired relaxation. For instance, relaxation of NA-contracted rings of aortae from 8- to 10-week diabetic rats in the presence of the free-radical scavenger superoxide dismutase (SOD) was significantly greater than control.[94] Since this relaxation was sensitive to L-NMMA and endothelium removal, it was suggested to result from NO release, the action of which is normally masked by its increased breakdown by free radicals.[94] The relaxant response of renal arteries from 6-week diabetic rats to Ach was enhanced in the presence of the free-radical scavenger 1,3–dimethyl thiourea (DMTU), and a prostaglandin H_2/thromboxane A_2 antagonist.[14] The investigators proposed that increased release of NO in response to Ach was masked by increased free-radical and prostaglandin endoperoxide production in the diabetic renal arteries.[14] The release of NO in response to Ach also appeared to be enhanced in mesenteric resistance arteries from 6-week diabetic rats, since relaxation of arteries to this agonist were enhanced compared with control.[56] However, the response to Ach was no longer different from control in 12-week diabetic mesenteric resistance arteries, suggesting that either NO release had returned to normal or was being offset by increased breakdown at this later time point.[56] Similarly, enhanced relaxation to Ach in renal artery from 12-day diabetic rats was detected, suggesting that at this early time there is increased NO production, which is not opposed by other factors which limit its action.[6]

Overall, changes in the release of NO do not appear routinely in arteries from diabetic rats and, when detected, are not always in the same direction. Therefore, it seems unlikely that they contribute to a large extent to defective endothelium-dependent responses in diabetic arteries. Other mechanisms, such as increased free radical–mediated destruction of NO, may play a more important role in this process.

7.4.2   Nitric Oxide Breakdown

7.4.2.1   Increased Oxidative Stress

There is mounting evidence that increased production of free radicals leads to the inactivation of NO in diabetic aortae in those studies in which defective endothelium-dependent relaxation to Ach has been demonstrated to occur.[15,21,28,65,68] The ability of free radical scavengers to protect against the impairment of endothelium-dependent relaxation in response to Ach has already been mentioned in the previous section. This has been confirmed in a number of other investigations in aortae from diabetic rats.[25,28,40,95,96] In addition, elevated levels of superoxide anion and lipid peroxidation in diabetic aortae have also been detected.[25] There is little information regarding the involvement of free radicals in the impairment of endothelium-dependent relaxant responses in arteries other than the aortae from diabetic rats. However, both SOD and DMTU significantly improved Ach-induced relaxation in mesenteric arteries while DMTU had the same effect in renal arteries from 6-week diabetic rats.[14,70] These data suggest that free radical–mediated NO destruction may be a common mechanism of endothelial dysfunction in diabetic arteries.

Diabetes-induced increases in free radical production have been proposed to arise by several different mechanisms, which may not be mutually exclusive. One mechanism was proposed by the same group that observed reversal of impaired Ach-induced relaxation of 8-week diabetic aorta with L-arginine and tetrahydrobiopterin.[15,93] These investigators also found that low doses of SOD and the hyroxyl radical scavenger, catalase, together improved the relaxant response of 8-week diabetic aortae to Ach.[96] They reconciled their disparate observations by proposing that reduced intracellular levels of L-arginine and tetrahydrobiopterin result not only in reduced NO production but in NOS synthase acting as an NADPH oxidase and enhancing the production of H_2O_2 and superoxide anion. Thus, at this stage, both a decrease in NO synthesis and accumulation of free radicals, which in turn may cause cellular damage and inactivate NO, were suggested to occur.

7.4.2.2 Polyol Pathway

Hyperglycemia stimulates the polyol pathway through increased activity of aldose reductase, leading to conversion of glucose to sorbitol and then to fructose (see Reference 97 for a review). Increased aldose reductase activity is associated with increased utilization of NADPH, which has been suggested to result in cellular depletion of this cofactor. Since NADPH is also a co-factor for NOS and for glutathione reductase, reduced production of both NO and glutathione could result, the latter leading to oxidative stress and increased destruction of NO.[64] A role for this pathway in defective endothelium-dependent relaxation was suggested by the observation that treatment of diabetic rats with an aldose reductase inhibitor (ARI) resulted in preservation of Ach-induced relaxation of 3-month diabetic rat aortae, which was impaired in diabetic rats not treated with the ARI.[64] However, in another investigation, treatment of diabetic rats with an ARI failed to prevent the decrease in sensitivity of mesenteric resistance vessels from diabetic rats to Ach.[54] It is possible that different mechanisms may contribute to endothelial dysfunction in aortae and mesenteric arteries from diabetic rats, and that the aldose reductase pathway may be more prominent in aortae that mesenteric artery.

7.4.2.3 Advanced Glycation End Products

Long-term exposure of plasma and cell membrane proteins to hyperglycemia leads to the accumulation of advanced glycosylation end products (AGE), due to nonenzymatic glycation between glucose and the amino groups of proteins (see Reference 97 for a review). AGEs have been suggested to quench endothelial-derived NO and to lead to the production of free radicals, both of which may impair relaxation to Ach. Treatment of 2-month diabetic rats with aminoguanidine, an inhibitor of advanced glycosylation reactions, and the free radical scavengers, butylated hydroxy toluene (BHT), and *n*-acetylcysteine prevented the impaired relaxation of aortae to Ach, suggesting a role for AGEs in endothelial dysfunction.[28] However, since AGEs take days to weeks to accumulate, this mechanism most likely contributes to chronic hyperglycemia-induced endothelial dysfunction.

The question of why defective endothelium-dependent vasodilation and cGMP elevation in response to Ach are observed in diabetic arteries in some studies but not in others
remains unanswered. However, should increased oxidative stress prove to be the cause
of endothelial dysfunction in diabetic arteries, the possibility that oxidative stress was
more severe in some studies than in others, due to additional factors such as differences
in environment or diet, should be considered. That different degrees of oxidative stress
could be present is suggested by variations in the degree to which endothelium-dependent
relaxation to Ach was attenuated in diabetic aortae in different studies, although in each
case the attenuation was totally prevented by treatment with free radical–scavenging
agents.[28,42]

7.5 Summary and Conclusions

The foregoing discussion makes it abundantly clear that many questions about the
vascular consequences of STZ-induced diabetes remain unanswered. Although many
studies have demonstrated altered contractile responses of large conductance and smaller
resistance vessels in both acute and chronic STZ diabetes, the inconsistencies in these
findings make it extremely difficult to establish the exact nature and direction of the
changes with increasing duration of the disease. In addition, while it appears that the
altered responsiveness of arteries isolated from STZ diabetic rats to vasoconstrictors and
endothelium-dependent vasodilators is a consequence of the diabetic state, the specific
contribution(s) of the metabolic alterations associated with this condition to the altered
reactivity is not yet known.

It seems to have been relatively well established that contractile responses of large
arteries (aortae, mesenteric and caudal) from rats with STZ-induced diabetes of 10 weeks
or longer duration are enhanced compared with those of age-matched control animals,
and that this enhancement is not secondary to decreased release of endothelium-derived
relaxing factors. However, while some studies, including those from this laboratory, suggest that the increased reactivity is due to alterations in signaling events downstream from
G protein–coupled receptors, other studies have suggested that there is a more generalized
increase in responsiveness to any procedure that activates membrane Ca^{2+} channels. This
discrepancy remains to be resolved. In addition, more studies need to be conducted on
resistance vessels from rats with chronic diabetes, to confirm whether or not the increased
reactivity detected in large arteries is also observed in smaller arteries that have a greater
impact on peripheral resistance.

It is clear that hyperglycemia has been strongly implicated as the underlying factor
responsible for impaired relaxation to endothelium-dependent vasodilators in diabetic
arteries. However, studies from this laboratory and others did not detect evidence of
impaired endothelial function in arteries from rats with chronic diabetes, despite the
presence of prolonged and severe hyperglycemia. Other factors must therefore contribute to endothelial dysfunction in those studies in which it has been detected. Much
attention over the past decade has been focused on hyperglycemia-induced free radical–initiated oxidative stress and its role in diabetes-induced endothelial dysfunction.
However, it should be noted that most of the reported studies were performed in arteries
from rats with relatively short-term diabetes, while the long-term role of free radicals
in chronic diabetes remains to be investigated. In addition, most of the studies investigating the effects of free radicals on vascular reactivity have been conducted in aortae,
while the nature of changes associated with free radical–mediated oxidative stress in

smaller arteries has not yet been determined. Last, most of the studies have focused on changes in the release and action of NO in diabetic arteries, and it is not clear whether or not the release or the levels of other endogenous substances such as prostanoids are altered in diabetes.

Hyperglycemia has been implicated as the factor underlying an increase in PKC activity and in expression of specific PKC isoforms detected in aortae from acutely diabetic rats. However, many of the biochemical studies in this area have either been performed independently of functional studies or in isolated VSMC, which makes extrapolation of their observations to the function of intact arteries difficult. It would be useful to investigate both the functional and biochemical changes in peripheral arteries in diabetes in the same study under similar experimental conditions, to circumvent the influence of extraneous factors such as the age and gender of animals, dose of STZ, and duration and severity of diabetes. Using this approach, the authors have shown increased phosphoinositide turnover in association with enhanced contractile responses of arteries from rats with chronic diabetes to NA, and have implicated increased activation of PKC as playing a major role in the enhanced responsiveness. Further investigation is required to determine if there is a link between hyperglycemia-induced increases in PKC activity and the increased response to NA in arteries from rats with chronic diabetes.

In conclusion, alterations in vascular reactivity have been detected in both short-term and long-term STZ-induced diabetes. However, the precise nature and mechanism(s) underlying the altered responses of both conductance vessels and resistance arteries remain to be elucidated. In addition, the variable results reported by different laboratories, particularly with regard to the acute changes in reactivity detected within the first 1 to 2 months after induction of diabetes, may limit the usefulness of the STZ diabetic rat model to the study of the chronic vascular changes occurring in diabetes of longer duration.

Acknowledgments

The authors wish to acknowledge Heart and Stroke Foundation of B.C. & Yukon and the Medical Research Council of Canada for providing support of their research in the form of operating grants.

References

1. Christlieb, A. R., Tonka, H. V., and Solano, A., Vascular reactivity to angiotensin II and to norepinephrine in diabetic subjects, *Diabetes*, 25, 268, 1976.
2. Ozturk, Y., Melih Altan, V., and Yildizoglu-ari, N., Effects of experimental diabetes and insulin on smooth muscle functions, *Pharmacol. Rev.*, 48(1), 69, 1996.
3. Tomlinson, K. C., Gardiner, S. C., Hebden, R. A., and Bennett, T., Functional consequences of streptozotocin-induced diabetes mellitus with particular reference to the cardiovascular system, *Pharmacol. Rev.*, 44(1), 103, 1992.
4. Junod, A., Lambert, A. E., Stauffacher, W., and Renold, A. E., Diabetogenic action of streptozotocin: relationship of dose to metabolic response, *J. Clin. Invest.*, 48, 2129, 1969.
5. Furman, B. L. and Sneddon, P., Endothelium-dependent vasodilator responses of the isolated mesenteric bed are preserved in long term streptozotocin diabetic rats, *Eur. J. Pharmacol.*, 232, 29, 1993.

6. Bhardwaj, R. and Moore, P. K., Increased vasodilator response to acetylcholine of renal blood vessels from diabetic rats, *J. Pharm. Pharmacol.*, 40, 739, 1988.
7. Wakabayashi, I., Hatake, K., Kimura, N., Kakishita, E., and Nagai, K., Modulation of vascular tonus by the endothelium in experimental diabetes, *Life Sci.*, 40, 643, 1987.
8. Longhurst, P. A. and Head, R. J., Responses of the isolated perfused mesenteric vasculature from diabetic rats: the significance of appropriate control tissues, *J. Pharmacol. Exp. Ther.*, 235(1), 45, 1985.
9. Taylor, P. D., Oon, B. B., Thomas, C. R., and Poston, L., Prevention by insulin treatment of endothelial dysfunction but not enhanced noradrenaline-induced contractility in mesenteric resistance arteries from streptozotocin-induced diabetic rats, *Br. J. Pharmacol.*, 111, 35, 1994.
10. MacLeod, K. M. and McNeill, J. H., The influence of chronic experimental diabetes on contractile responses of rat isolated blood vessels, *Can. J. Physiol. Pharmacol*, 63, 52, 1985.
11. Fujii, K., Soma, M., Huang, Y. S., Manku, M. S., and Horrobin, D. F., Increased release of prostaglandins from the mesenteric vascular bed of diabetic animals: the effects of glucose and insulin, *Prostaglandins Leukotrienes Med.*, 24(2-3), 151, 1986.
12. Murray, P., Pitt, B., and Webb, R. C., Ramipril prevents hypersensitivity to phenylephrine in aorta from streptozotocin-induced diabetic rats, *Diabetologia*, 37, 664, 1994.
13. Shimizu, K., Muramatsu, M., Kakegawa, Y., Asano, H., Toki, Y., Miyazaki, Y., Okumura, K., Hashimoto, H., and Ito, T., Role of prostaglandin H2 as an endothelium-derived contracting factor in diabetic state, *Diabetes*, 42, 1246, 1993.
14. Dai, F.-X., Diederich, A., Skopec, J., and Diederich, D., Diabetes-induced endothelial dysfunction in streptozotocin-treated rats: role of prostaglandin endoperoxides and free radicals, *J. Am. Soc. Nephrol.*, 4, 1327, 1993.
15. Pieper, G. M., Jordan, M., Adams, M. B., and Roza, A. M., Restoration of vascular endothelial function in diabetes, *Diabetes Res. Clin. Pract.*, 31 Suppl, S157, 1996.
16. Taylor, P. D., McCarthy, A. L., Thomas, C. R., and Poston, L., Endothelium-dependent relaxation and noradrenaline sensitivity in mesenteric resistance arteries of streptozotocin-induced diabetic rats, *Br. J. Pharmacol.*, 107, 393, 1992.
17. Owen, M. P. and Carrier, G. O., Calcium dependence of norepinephrine-induced vascular contraction in experimental diabetes, *J. Pharmacol. Exp. Ther.*, 212(7), 253, 1980.
18. Rodrigues, B. and McNeill, J. H., Comparison of cardiac function in male and female diabetic rats, *Gen. Pharmacol.*, 18(4), 421, 1987.
19. Rossini, A. A., Williams, R. M., Appel, M. C., and Like, A. A., Sex differences in the multiple-dose streptozotocin model of diabetes, *Endocrinol.*, 103(4), 1518, 1978.
20. Mulhern, M. and Docherty, J. R., Effects of experimental diabetes on the responsiveness of rat aorta, *Br. J. Pharmacol.*, 97, 1007, 1989.
21. Sikorski, B. W., Hodgson, W. C., and King, R. G., Effects of hemoglobin and *N*-nitro-L-arginine on constrictor and dilator responses of aortic rings from streptozotocin diabetic rats, *Eur. J. Pharmacol.*, 242, 275, 1993.
22. Fulton, D. J. R., Hodgson, W. C., Sikorski, W. B., and King, R. G., Attenuated responses to endothelin 1, KCl and CaCl2, but not noradrenaline of aortae from rats with streptozotocin-induced diabetes mellitus, *Br. J. Pharmacol.*, 104, 928, 1991.
23. MacLeod, K. M., The effect of insulin treatment on changes in vascular reactivity in chronic, experimental diabetes, *Diabetes*, 34, 1160, 1985.
24. Pfaffman, M. A., Ball, C. R., Darby, A., and Hilman, R., Insulin reversal of diabetes-induced inhibition of vascular contractility in the rat, *Am. J. Physiol.*, 242, (*Heart Circ. Physiol.* 11), H490, 1982.
25. Chang, K. C., Chung, S. Y., Chong, W. S., Suh, J. S., Kim, S. H., Noh, H. K., Seong, B. W., Ko, H. J., and Chun, K. W., Possible superoxide radical-induced alteration of vascular reactivity in aortas from streptozotocin-treated rats, *J. Pharmacol. Exp. Ther.*, 266(2), 992, 1993.
26. Wong, K. K. and Tzeng, S. F., Norepinephrine-induced contractile responses in isolated rat aortae from different duration of diabetes, *Artery*, 19(1), 1, 1992.
27. Head, R. J., Longhurst, P. A., Panek, R. L., and Stitzel, R. E., A contrasting effect of the diabetic state upon the contractile responses of aortic preparations from the rat and rabbit, *Br. J. Pharmacol.*, 91, 275, 1987.

28. Archibald, V., Cotter, M. A., Keegan, A., and Cameron, N. E., Contraction and relaxation of aortas from diabetic rats: effects of chronic antioxidant and aminoguanidine treatments, *Naunyn Schmiedeberg's Arch. Pharmacol.*, 353, 584, 1996.

29. Pieper, G. M., Acute amelioration of diabetic endothelial dysfunction with a derivative of the nitric oxide synthase cofactor, tetrahydrobiopterin, *J. Cardiovasc. Pharmacol.*, 29, 8, 1997.

30. Karasu, C., Ozansoy, G., Bozkurt, O., Erdogan, D., and Omeroglu, S., Antioxidant and triglyceride–lowering effects of vitamin E associated with the prevention of abnormalities in the reactivity and morphology of aorta from streptozotocin-diabetic rats, *Metabolism*, 46(8), 872, 1997.

31. Wright J. R. Jr., and Lacy, P. E., Synergistic effects of adjuvants, endotoxin and fasting on induction of diabetes with multiple low doses of streptozotocin in rats, *Diabetes*, 37, 112, 1988.

32. Abebe, W., Harris, K. H., and MacLeod, K. M., Role of extracellular Ca^{2+} in the selective enhancement of contractile responses of arteries from diabetic rats to noradrenaline, *Can. J. Physiol. Pharmacol.*, 72, 1544, 1994.

33. Abebe, W. and MacLeod, K. M., Influence of diabetes on norepinephrine-induced inositol 1,4,5-trisphosphate levels in rat aorta, *Life Sci.*, 49(13), PL85, 1991.

34. Abebe, W. and MacLeod, K. M., Enhanced arterial contractility to noradrenaline in diabetic rats is associated with increased phosphoinositide metabolism, *Can. J. Physiol. Pharmacol.*, 69, 355, 1991.

35. Abebe, W. and MacLeod, K. M., Protein kinase C–mediated contractile responses of arteries from diabetic rats, *Br. J. Pharmacol.*, 101, 465, 1990.

36. Abebe, W., Harris, K. H., and MacLeod, K. M., Enhanced contractile responses of arteries from diabetic rats to α_1-adrenoceptor stimulation in the absence and presence of extracellular calcium, *J. Cardiovasc. Pharmacol.*, 16, 239, 1990.

37. Harris, K. H. and MacLeod, K. M., Influence of the endothelium on contractile responses of arteries from diabetic rats, *Eur. J. Pharmacol.*, 153, 55, 1988.

38. Scarborough, N. L. and Carrier, G. O., Increased α_2-adrenoceptor mediated vascular contraction in diabetic rats, *J. Auton. Pharmac.*, 3, 177, 1983.

39. Scarborough, N. L. and Carrier, G. O., Nifedipine and alpha adrenoceptors in rat aorta. II. Role of extracellular calcium in enhanced alpha$_2$-adrenoceptor-mediated contractions in diabetes, *J. Pharmacol. Exp. Ther.*, 231(3), 603, 1984.

40. Pieper, G. M. and Gross, G. J., Oxygen free radicals abolish endothelium-dependent relaxation in diabetic rat aorta, *Am. J. Physiol.*, 255 (*Heart Circ. Physiol.* 24), H825, 1988.

41. Ozcelikay, A. T., Pekiner, C., Ari, N., Ozturk, Y., Ozuari, A., and Altan, V. M., The effect of vanadyl treatment on vascular responsiveness of streptozotocin-diabetic rat, *Diabetologia*, 37, 572, 1994.

42. Hattori, Y., Kawasaki, H., Fukao, M., Gando, S., Akaishi, Y., and Kanno, M., Diminishment of contractions associated with depolarization-evoked activation of Ca^{2+} channels in diabetic rat aorta, *J. Vasc. Res.*, 33, 454, 1996.

43. Chang, K. S. K. and Stevens, W. C., Endothelium-dependent increase in vascular sensitivity to phenylephrine in long term streptozotocin diabetic rat aorta, *Br. J. Pharmacol.*, 107, 983, 1992.

44. MacLeod, K. M., Ng, D. D., Harris, K. H., and Diamond, J., Evidence that cGMP is the mediator of endothelium-dependent inhibition of contractile responses of rat arteries to alpha-adrenoceptor stimulation, *Mol. Pharmacol.*, 32(1), 59, 1987.

45. Hattori, Y., Kawasaki, H., Kanno, M., and Fukao, M., Enhanced 5-HT$_2$ receptor mediated contractions in diabetic rat aorta: participation of Ca^{2+} channels associated with protein kinase C activity, *J. Vasc. Res.*, 32(4), 220, 1995.

46. Weber, L. P., Chow, W. L., Abebe, W., and MacLeod, K. M., Enhanced contractile responses of arteries from streptozotocin diabetic rats to sodium fluoride, *Br. J. Pharmacol.*, 118(1), 115, 1996.

47. Agrawal, D. K. and McNeill, J. H., Vascular responses to agonists in rat mesenteric artery from diabetic rats, *Can. J. Physiol. Pharmacol.*, 65, 1484, 1987.

48. White, R. E. and Carrier, G. O., Vascular contractions induced by activation of membrane calcium ion channels is enhanced in streptozotocin–diabetes, *J. Pharmacol. Exp. Ther.*, 253(3), 1057, 1990.

49. Jackson, C. V. and Carrier, G. O., Supersensitivity of isolated mesenteric arteries to noradrenaline in the long-term experimental diabetic rat, *J. Auton. Pharmac.*, 1, 399, 1981.

50. Nielsen, H., Bonnema, S. J., and Flyvberg, A., Effects of diabetes, insulin treatment and osmolality on contractility of isolated rat resistance arteries, *Pharmacol. Toxicol.*, 77, 209, 1995.
51. White, R. E. and Carrier, G. O., Enhanced vascular α-adrenergic neuroeffector system in diabetes: importance of calcium, *Am. J. Physiol.*, 255 (*Heart Circ. Physiol.* 24), 1036, 1988.
52. Taylor, P. D., Graves, J. E., and Poston, L. D., Selective impairment of acetylcholine-mediated endothelium-dependent relaxation in isolated resistance arteries of the streptozotocin-induced diabetic rat, *Clin. Sci.*, 88, 519, 1995.
53. Wang, S. P., West, M. W., Dresner, L. S., Fleishhacker, J. F., Distant, D. A., Mueller, C. M., and Wait, R. B., Effects of diabetes and uremia on mesenteric vascular reactivity, *Surgery*, 120, 328, 1996.
54. Taylor, P. D., Wickenden, A. D., Mirrlees, D. J., and Poston, L., Endothelial function in the isolated perfused mesentery and aortae of rats with streptozotocin-induced diabetes, *Br. J. Pharmacol.*, 111, 42, 1994.
55. Ralevic, V., Belai, A., and Burnstock, G., Effects of streptozotocin-diabetes on sympathetic nerve, endothelial and smooth muscle function in the rat mesenteric arterial bed, *Eur. J. Pharmacol.*, 286, 193, 1995.
56. Heygate, K. M., Davies, J., Holmes, M., James, R. F. L., and Thurston, H., The effect of insulin treatment and of islet transplantation on the resistance artery function in the STZ-induced diabetic rat, *Br. J. Pharmacol.*, 119, 495, 1996.
57. Ramanadham, S., Lyness, W. H., and Tenner, Jr., T. E., Alterations in aortic and tail artery reactivity to agonists after streptozotocin treatment, *Can. J. Physiol. Pharmacol.*, 62, 418, 1984.
58. Weber, L. P. and MacLeod, K. M., Contractile responses of caudal arteries from diabetic rats to adrenergic nerve stimulation, *J. Vasc. Res.*, 31, 25, 1994.
59. Hart, J. L., Freas, W., McKenzie, J. E., and Muldoon, S. M., Adrenergic nerve function and contractile activity of the caudal artery of the streptozotocin diabetic rat, *J. Auton. Nerv. Syst.*, 25, 49, 1988.
60. Inazu, M., Sakai, Y., and Homma, I., Contractile responses and calcium mobilization in renal arteries of diabetic rats, *Eur. J. Pharmacol.*, 203, 79, 1991.
61. Friedman, J. J., Vascular sensitivity and reactivity to norepinephrine in diabetes mellitus, *Am. J. Physiol.*, 256, (*Heart Circ. Physiol.* 25), H1134, 1989.
62. James, G. M. and Hodgson, W. C., Attenuated 5-HT2 receptor-mediated responses in hindquarters of diabetic rats, *Eur. J. Pharmacol.*, 294, 109, 1995.
63. Otter, D. J. and Chess-Williams, R., The effects of aldose reductase inhibition with ponalrestat on changes in vascular function in streptozotocin diabetic rats, *Br. J. Pharmacol.*, 113, 576, 1994.
64. Cameron, N. E. and Cotter, M. A., Impaired contraction and relaxation in aorta from streptozotocin diabetic rats: role of polyol pathway, *Diabetologia*, 35, 1011, 1992.
65. Endo, K., Abiru, T., Machida, H., Kasuya, Y., and Kamata, K., Endothelium-derived hyperpolarizing factor does not contribute to the decrease in endothelium-dependent relaxation in the aorta of streptozotocin-induced diabetic rats, *Gen. Pharmacol.*, 26(1), 149, 1995.
66. Orie, N. N., Aloamaka, C. P., and Iyawe, V. I., Duration-dependent attenuation of acetylcholine but not the histamine-induced relaxation of the aorta in diabetes mellitus, *Gen. Pharmacol.*, 24(2), 329, 1993.
67. Oyama, Y., Kawasaki, H., Hattori, Y., and Kanno, M., Attenuation of endothelium-dependent relaxation in aorta from diabetic rats, *Eur. J. Pharmacol.*, 131, 75, 1986.
68. Hattori, Y., Kawasaki, H., Abe, K., and Kanno, M., Superoxide dismutase recovers altered endothelium-dependent relaxation in diabetic rat aorta, *Am. J. Physiol.*, 261, (*Heart Circ. Physiol.* 30), H1086, 1991.
69. Fukao, M., Hattori, Y., Kanno, M., Sakuma, I., and Kitabatake, A., Alterations in endothelium-dependent hyperpolarization and relaxation in mesenteric arteries from streptozotocin-induced diabetic rats, *Br. J. Pharmacol.*, 121(7), 1383, 1997.
70. Diederich, D., Skopec, J., Diederich, A., and Dai, F.-X., Endothelial dysfunction in mesenteric resistance arteries of diabetic rats: role of free radicals, *Am. J. Physiol.*, 266 (*Heart Circ. Physiol.* 35), H1153, 1994.
71. Ralevic, V., Belai, A., and Burnstock, G., Impaired sensory-motor nerve function in the isolated mesenteric arterial bed of streptozotocin-diabetic and ganglioside-treated streptozotocin diabetic rats, *Br. J. Pharmacol.*, 110, 1105, 1993.

72. Wang, Y. -X., Brooks, D. P., and Edwards, R. M., Attenuated glomerular cGMP production and renal vasodilation in streptozotocin-induced diabetic rats, *Am. J. Physiol.*, 264 (*Regulatory Integrative Comp. Physiol.* 33), R952, 1993.

73. Legan, E., Effects of streptozotocin-induced hyperglycemia on agonist-stimulated phosphatidylinositol turnover in rat aorta, *Life Sci.*, 45, 371, 1989.

74. Abebe, W. and MacLeod, K. M., Augmented inositol phosphate production in mesenteric arteries from diabetic rats, *Eur. J. Pharmacol.*, 225, 29, 1992.

75. Okumura, K., Nishiura, T., Awaji, Y., Kondo, J., Hashimoto, H., and Ito, T., 1,2-Diacylglycerol content and its fatty acid composition in thoracic aorta of diabetic rats, *Diabetes*, 40, 820, 1991.

76. King, G. L., Ishii, H., and Koya, D., Diabetic vascular dysfunctions: a model of excessive activation of protein kinase C, *Kidney Int.*, 52 (Suppl. 60), S77, 1997.

77. Kunisaki, M., Fumio, U., Nawata, H., and King, G. L., Vitamin E normalizes diacylglycerol-protein kinase C activation induced by hyperglycemia in rat vascular tissues, *Diabetes*, 45 (Suppl. 3), S117, 1996.

78. Inoguchi, T., Battan, R., Handler, E., Sportsman, R. J., Heath, W., and King, G. L., Preferential elevation of protein kinase C isoform βII and diacylglycerol levels in the aorta and heart of diabetic rats: differential reversibility to glycemic control by islet cell transplantation, *Proc. Natl. Acad. Sci. U.S.A.*, 89, 11059, 1992.

79. Inoguchi, T., Xia, P., Kunisaki, M., Higashi, S., Feener, E. P., and King, G. L., Insulin's effect on protein kinase C and diacylglycerol induced by diabetes and glucose in vascular tissues, *Am. J. Physiol.*, 267 (*Endocrinol. Metab.* 30), E369, 1994.

80. Williams, B. and Schrier, R. W., Characterization of glucose-induced *in situ* protein kinase C activity in cultured vascular smooth muscle cells, *Diabetes*, 41(11), 1464, 1992.

81. Nishizuka, Y., Intracellular signaling by hydrolysis of phospholipids and activation of protein kinase C, *Science*, 258(5082), 607, 1992.

82. Shiba, T., Inoguchi, T., Sportsman, J. R., Heath, W. F., Bursell, S., and King, G. L., Correlation of diacylglycerol level and protein kinase C activity in rat retina to retinal circulation, *Am. J. Physiol.*, 265 (5 Pt. 1), E783, 1993.

83. Birch, K. A., Heath, W. F., Hermeling, R. N., Johnston, C. M., Stramm, L., Dell, C., Smith, C., Williamson, J. R., and Reifel-Miller, A., LY290181, an inhibitor of diabetes-induced vascular dysfunction, blocks protein kinase C–stimulated transcriptional activation through inhibition of transcription factor binding to a phorbol response element, *Diabetes*, 45(5), 642, 1996.

84. Bohr, D. F., Vascular smooth muscle: dual effect of calcium, *Science*, 139, 597, 1963.

85. Berridge, M. J. and Irvine, R. F., Inositol triphosphate: a novel second messenger in cellular signal transduction, *Nature* (London), 312, 315, 1984.

86. Rinaldi, G. J. and Cingolani, H. E., Effect of diabetes on fast response to norepinephrine in rat aorta, *Diabetes*, 41, 30, 1992.

87. Hattori, Y., Kawasaki, H., Kanno, M., Gando, S., and Fukao, M., Attenuated contractile response of diabetic aorta to caffeine but not to noradrenaline in Ca^{2+}-free medium, *Eur. J. Pharmacol.*, 256(2), 215, 1994.

88. Ohara, T., Sussman, K. E., and Draznin, B., Effect of diabetes on cytosolic free Ca^{2+} and Na^+, K^+ ATPase in rat aorta, *Diabetes*, 40, 1560, 1991.

89. Carmines, P. K., Ohishi, K., and Ikenaga, H., Functional impairment of renal afferent arteriolar voltage-gated calcium channels in rats with diabetes mellitus, *J. Clin. Invest.*, 98, 2564, 1996.

90. Tam, E. S. L., Ferguson, D. G., Bielefeld, D. R., Lorenz, J. N., Cohen, R. M., and Pun, R. Y. K., Norepinephrine-mediated calcium signaling is altered in vascular smooth muscle of diabetic rat, *Cell. Calcium*, 21(2), 143, 1997.

91. Kamata, K., Miyata, N., and Kasuya, Y., Impairment of endothelium-dependent relaxation and changes in levels of cyclic GMP in aorta from streptozotocin-induced diabetic rats, *Br. J. Pharmacol.*, 97(2), 614, 1989.

92. Abiru, T., Watanabe, Y., Kamata, K., and Kasuya, Y., Changes in endothelium-dependent relaxation and levels of cyclic nucleotides in the perfused mesenteric arterial bed from streptozotocin-induced diabetic rats, *Life Sci.*, 53, PL7, 1993.

93. Pieper, G. M. and Dodlinger, L. A., Plasma and vascular tissue arginine are decreased in diabetes: acute arginine supplementation restores endothelium-dependent relaxation by augmenting cGMP production, *J. Pharmacol. Exp. Ther.*, 283(2), 684, 1997.

94. Langenstroer, P. and Pieper, G. M., Regulation of spontaneous EDRF release in diabetic rat aorta by oxygen free radicals, *Am. J. Physiol.*, 263 (1 Pt 2), H257, 1992.
95. Pieper, G. M., Langenstroer, P., and Gross, G. J., Hydroxyl radicals mediate injury to endothelium-dependent relaxation in diabetic rat, *Mol. Cell. Biochem.*, 122, 139, 1993.
96. Pieper, G. M., Langenstroer, P., and Siebeneich, W., Diabetic-induced endothelial dysfunction in rat aorta: role of hydroxyl radicals, *Cardiovasc. Res.*, 34, 145, 1997.
97. Cohen, R. A., Dysfunction of vascular endothelium in diabetes mellitus, *Circulation*, 87 (Suppl. V), V67, 1993.

8

Cardiovascular Function in the Intact, Streptozotocin-Treated Rat

R. Anthony Hebden

CONTENTS

8.1 Introduction

Diabetes mellitus is a disorder of metabolism that, in its fully developed form, is characterized by fasting hyperglycemia, polydipsia, glycosuria, and polyuria. Mortality from cardiovascular disease in patients with diabetes is more than twice that of the general population.[1] Consequently, there has been much interest in the etiology of cardiovascular disorders associated with this disease.

The streptozotocin (STZ)-injected rat displays many of the features seen in humans with diabetes including fasting hyperglycemia, polydipsia, glycosuria, and polyuria.[2] Since rats injected with STZ do not require insulin to survive, it is probably more accurate to describe them as models of hypoinsulinemia rather than of insulin-dependent diabetes mellitus. Despite this, the STZ-treated rat is considered to be an extremely useful model of human diabetes mellitus.

The following is an overview of the effects that STZ administration has upon integrated cardiovascular function in the intact rat. In the majority of studies cited, experiments were performed within weeks of STZ administration. Therefore, while rats injected with STZ rapidly develop the secondary complications associated with diabetes mellitus, it is more appropriate to consider these studies as an investigation of acute insulin deficiency. This does not negate their value, however, as they provide invaluable information regarding the underlying pathophysiological changes that may lead to the development of long-term complications of diabetes mellitus.

8.2   Integrated Cardiovascular Function

8.2.1   Heart Rate

A resting bradycardia is routinely observed in STZ-treated rats.[3-18] The bradycardia occurs rapidly after injection of STZ and has been reported as early as 4 days[14] and 5 days[19] following STZ administration.

The mechanism behind the reduction in resting heart rate remains to be elucidated. It may occur as a consequence of increased vagal activity and/or decreased sympathetic drive. However, Hebden et al.[10] observed a significantly larger fall in heart rate in STZ-treated rats compared with saline-treated controls following administration of the ganglion blocker pentolinium, despite the fact that the former were already bradycardic compared with the controls. This observation suggests that sympathetic drive to the heart was enhanced in the animals treated with STZ. Furthermore, the finding of a significantly greater reduction in heart rate following pentolinium would also appear to rule out the possibility that the bradycardia was a consequence of enhanced vagal drive. However, since atropine was not given to these animals, this cannot be categorically stated.[10]

It is apparent from several studies that the intrinsic heart rate of the STZ-treated animal is reduced. For example, Maeda et al.[19] reported that intrinsic heart rate obtained after atropine and propranolol blockade was significantly lower in rats injected 5 days earlier with STZ compared with control rats. Furthermore, Hebden et al.[10,11] observed that resting heart rate was significantly lower in ganglion-blocked rats injected with STZ 3 weeks earlier, compared with ganglion-blocked, control animals. Consistent with these *in vivo* studies, the intrinsic rate of spontaneously beating atria[20] and whole hearts[21] from STZ-treated rats have been observed to be significantly lower than their respective controls.

A discussion on the mechanism(s) responsible for this intrinsic bradycardia is beyond the scope of the current section and the reader is referred to the excellent review by Tomlinson et al.[22] Interestingly, however, it was recently reported by Shah et al.[17] that the bradycardia observed in STZ-treated rats was prevented by daily oral administration of the calcium channel blocker nifedipine. This is unlikely to be a direct cardiac effect as nifedipine acts on vascular smooth muscle and has minimal effect on cardiac calcium channels. Consistent with this supposition is the observation that nifedipine reversed not only the STZ induced bradycardia, but also STZ-induced hypothyroidism,[17] suggesting that the intrinsic bradycardia was a function of the hypothyroid status of the STZ-treated rats. Support for this theory is provided by the observation that hearts from hypothyroid rats have similar depressed myofibrillar ATPase activity and shift in myosin isoenzyme distribution to that seen in STZ-treated rats[23] and that both of these biochemical changes can be reversed in STZ-treated rats by thyroid hormone replacement therapy.[24] While the above is very intriguing, it may be misleading to use the results of Shah et al.[17] to define a causal relationship between the resting bradycardia and hypothyroid state of the STZ-treated rat. That is, Shah et al.[17] found STZ-treated rats to be hypertensive, and it is possible that under these conditions, bradycardia will be an inevitable baroreflex response, which will be corrected by treatment with the antihypertensive agent nifedipine, irrespective of the latters effect of the latter on thyroid status.

8.2.2 Blood Pressure

A number of researchers have found that rats become hypertensive following STZ administration.[4,17,25-34] However, blood pressure has also been found to be reduced[3,5,8,10-12,14-16,18,19,35-40] or unchanged[13,41-44] by STZ administration.

The reason for these disparate findings is not immediately obvious. While it is not due to the dosage of STZ given nor the time following STZ administration that blood pressure was measured, there is good evidence that it may be methodological in origin. That is, in all but three[4,34,45] of the studies reported above that have found STZ-treated rats to be hypertensive, blood pressure was measured indirectly with a tail cuff plethysmograph. However, both Kohler et al.[35] and Kusaka et al.[46] found that conscious, STZ-treated rats exhibited systolic hypertension when blood pressure was measured indirectly using tail cuff plethysmography, but were normotensive when blood pressure was measured intra-arterially. This lead Kusaka et al.[46] to conclude that "the existence of so-called STZ hypertension in the rat is suspicious." Furthermore, both Tomlinson et al.[37] and Katovitch et al.[40] have reported that conscious rats were normotensive when blood pressure was measured with a tail cuff, but were hypotensive when blood pressure was measured directly.

It has been suggested that morphological changes in the tails of the STZ-treated rats can account for the spurious hypertension observed in these animals.[12] However, it does not explain the STZ induced hypertension reported by Bunag et al.,[4] Norton et al.,[34] and Hayashi et al.,[45] since these investigators used an intra-arterial catheter to monitor blood pressure. In the study of Bunag et al.[4] diastolic pressure was increased without any increase in systolic or mean blood pressure, while in the study of Hayashi et al.[45] mean blood pressure was increased with no reported values for systolic and diastolic blood pressure. This led Tomlinson et al.[22] to comment that there have been no reported cases of systolic hypertension from intra-arterial recordings in STZ-treated rats. Consistent with this comment is the study by Norton et al.,[34] who observed that mean arterial pressure was elevated but did not comment on intra-arterial systolic or diastolic pressures.

General consensus would appear to support the proposition that blood pressure is reduced in STZ-treated rats. If this is indeed the case, then what is the mechanism responsible for this? In the conscious rat, the peripheral regulation of arterial blood pressure is primarily attributable to the activity of the autonomic nervous system. However, in certain pathophysiological states one cannot rule out a possible role for vasopressin (AVP) and the renin–angiotensin system. For example, there is evidence that both are important mediators of blood pressure recovery following hypotensive hemorrhage.[47,48] Furthermore, converting enzyme inhibitors have proved to be extremely efficacious in treating hypertension in rats,[31,34,49] clearly indicating a role for the renin–angiotensin system in this state.

Therefore, it is necessary to look not only at the autonomic nervous system of STZ-treated rats, but also the status of AVP and the renin–angiotensin system to elucidate any abnormalities that may exist in blood pressure maintenance in these animals.

8.2.2.1 Autonomic Nervous System

A thorough review is beyond the scope of this chapter, and thus the following discussion will be limited to only the most salient findings to date. Those readers who wish to investigate this topic in detail are referred to the excellent review by Tomlinson et al.[22]

In 1980, Monckton and Pehowich[50] reported degenerative changes in the autonomic nervous system of Wistar rats as early as 24 h after STZ administration, with widespread degeneration of ganglionic tissue occurring between 3 days and 6 weeks. In contrast to this, Schmidt and Scharp[51] found no evidence of autonomic neuropathy in Wistar-Lewis rats 3.5 months after STZ treatment. This difference may have been due to the fact that Monckton and Pehowich[50] used a dose of STZ (80 mg/kg) that causes a more severe diabetes, characterized by rapid onset of ketoacidosis and an increased mortality rate. It is also possible that the difference was a result of the different strain of rats used. Consistent with this is the finding of mesenteric axonopathy in Sprague-Dawley rats, injected 1.5 to 3 months earlier with STZ.[52] Interestingly, in the same study, Schmidt et al.[52] found no evidence of neuropathy in the spleen, bladder, vas deferens, or iris of rats treated 4 to 12 months earlier with STZ, suggesting that the structural changes may be highly specific.

Although there is good evidence supporting the development of neuropathy following long-term hyperglycemia,[53,54] the actual time frame of onset is still unknown. It is tempting to ignore the results of Monckton and Pehowich[50] and assume that data from experiments investigating the cardiovascular function of rats with short-term diabetes (less than 10 weeks following STZ administration, for example) can be interpreted without having to account for autonomic neuropathy. However, this is probably unrealistic, as Lund et al.[55] reported morphological changes within the cardiac parasympathetic nerves of rats injected with STZ 8 weeks earlier. Therefore, all investigators utilizing STZ-injected rats need to be aware of the potential for neuropathy as a confounding factor when interpreting data.

A plausible mechanism for the development of neuropathy in STZ-treated rats has been advanced and is described here. Nerve trunks contain the enzymes aldose reductase (which converts glucose to sorbitol) and sorbitol dehydrogenase (which converts sorbitol to fructose). This chain of reactions is known as the sorbitol pathway.[56] In the presence of hyperglycemia, an augmentation of flux through the sorbitol pathway would lead to neural accumulation of sorbitol and fructose, generating an osmotic fluid shift, which would in turn cause edema and subsequent neural degeneration. This mechanism, called the *osmotic hypothesis*, has been gaining in popularity since first being proposed.[57] The exact site of edema is unknown, although both the Schwann cell[58] and the endoneurial space[59] have been suggested. Consistent with the osmotic hypothesis, Schmidt et al.[60] observed increased sorbitol levels in superior cervical, superior mesenteric, and coeliac ganglia from STZ-treated rats. Furthermore, in the same study, it was found that aldose reductase inhibition reduced, but did not normalize, axonal dystrophy in superior mesenteric ganglia from STZ-treated rats.[60] In a later study, Schmidt et al.[61] reported that aldose reductase inhibition, initiated several months after STZ treatment, was able to prevent further structural changes in mesenteric nerves.

An understanding of the potentially myriad effects of autonomic neuropathy on cardiovascular function in STZ-treated rats currently exists at a somewhat rudimentary level. This is not altogether surprising, as separating out abnormalities in function due to neuropathy from those that are due to alterations in other systems is extremely difficult. For example, the observation of an impaired cardiovascular response to an acute cold wind stress in STZ-treated rats[62] may be due to autonomic neuropathy, although it might also be explained by a reduction in β-receptor sensitivity. Similarly, the finding of impaired baroreflex and chemoreflex responsiveness in STZ-treated rats has been attributed to autonomic dysfunction,[18,55] but whether this is due to neuropathy, or some other mechanism, is not obvious.

Contractile response to electrical field stimulation has been shown to be reduced in caudal arteries of rats treated 8 weeks earlier with STZ.[63] Sato et al.[64] found that left atria isolated from STZ-treated rats showed a greater attenuation of contractile response to transmural stimulation than to norepinephrine, implying that norepinephrine release during nerve stimulation may be reduced. Interestingly, Hashimoto et al.[65] demonstrated that treatment with an aldose reductase inhibitor gave rise to an improvement in cardiac responsiveness to transmural nerve stimulation in STZ-treated rats and suggested that aldose reductase was having a beneficial effect on cardiac neuropathy.

A number of other experiments, involving STZ-treated rats, also indicate the presence of neuropathy. For example, Fushima et al.,[66] were unable to demonstrate an increase in plasma norepinephrine concentration in response to blood withdrawal, while Chang et al.[67] reported that rats developed persistent diarrhea within 4 to 5 months of STZ administration.

In summary, there is clear evidence indicating autonomic neuropathy in STZ-treated rats, although time of onset remains to be clearly delineated. While there is also evidence indicating that neuropathy may impact upon cardiovascular regulation, much research is required to separate those changes in function that can be ascribed to neuropathy from those due to other causes.

8.2.2.2   *Vasopressin*

It has been found that plasma AVP levels are elevated, in rats, 3 days,[68] 2 weeks,[69] and 6 weeks[70] following STZ administration. This elevation would appear to be due to increased release from the posterior pituitary, rather than reduced clearance as Van Itallie and Fernstrom[70] found there to be a significant reduction in the level of AVP in the posterior pituitaries of STZ-treated rats. Furthermore, both Loesch et al.[71] and Dheen et al.[72] reported hypertrophy of the paraventricular and supraoptic nuclei of STZ-treated rats, consistent with hyperactivity, while Fernstrom et al.[73] reported that AVP synthesis was increased in the hypothalami of STZ-treated rats.

The elevation in circulating AVP levels observed in STZ-treated rats would appear to be closely associated with the hypoinsulinemic condition of these animal, as Vokes and Robertson[68] reported that insulin administration caused a rapid reduction in plasma AVP levels. However, the exact mechanism by which hypoinsulinemia increases release of AVP from the posterior pituitary remains to be elucidated.

Plasma osmolality, the primary determinant of AVP release,[74] is known to be significantly elevated in STZ-treated rats.[2] However, this hyperosmolality is largely due to an increase in plasma glucose, which is known to act as an ineffective osmole when used to stimulate AVP release.[75] Furthermore, plasma sodium levels are reduced following STZ.[2] While it is possible that the osmoreceptor may be more sensitive to plasma sodium in the diabetic condition, experiments that have investigated the relationship between sodium administration and AVP release have been unable to corroborate this hypothesis, either in STZ-treated rats[70,76,77] or in patients with diabetes mellitus.[78]

Studies in patients with diabetes suggest a second possibility, namely, that glucose uptake by osmoreceptor neurons is insulin dependent. Vokes and Robertson[68] reported that, in patients with poorly controlled insulin-dependent diabetes mellitus, administration of hypertonic glucose led to an increase in plasma AVP levels without altering other known osmotic or hemodynamic stimuli. This phenomenon was not observed under insulin-replete conditions,[79] suggesting that glucose may become an effective stimulus for AVP release during insulin deficiency.

A reduction in plasma volume is also a stimulus for AVP release. Rats develop an osmotic diuresis within 24 h of STZ administration, and, since the increase in fluid intake at this time is less than the urine output, these animals are in a negative water balance.[2] It is likely, therefore, that both cellular dehydration and extracellular fluid volume depletion are responsible for initiating the observed polydipsia. Within 12 days of STZ injection, rats reach a new steady state where the difference between fluid intake and urine output is not consistently different from that seen in control rats.[2] Therefore, when reporting blood or plasma volumes, the time following STZ administration must be considered.

Katayama and Lee[28] reported that the plasma volume of rats was significantly reduced 7 days after STZ administration. However, at 21 days after STZ administration, when rats are in a new steady state for fluid balance, plasma volume was normal when expressed in absolute terms and elevated when expressed as a function of body weight.[80] A similar volume expansion in blood volume, when expressed as a function of body weight, was also observed 6 weeks following STZ administration.[36] Interpretation of blood and plasma volume data is complicated by the nature of body weight loss and change in body composition following STZ treatment. The diabetic animals are invariably lighter than their controls,[2] and display an almost complete loss of white adipose tissue,[81] as well as some loss of lean body tissue.[82] Thus expressing blood or plasma volume as a function of body weight may be misleading. In an attempt to overcome this problem, Carbonell et al.[9] measured blood volume in rats injected 12 weeks earlier with STZ and compared these results to age-matched and weight-matched (younger) controls. It was found that volume in the STZ-treated rats was reduced when compared with age-matched controls, but expanded when compared with weight-matched controls.

From the above discussion, it is clear that there is little evidence to support the hypothesis that AVP is elevated in STZ-treated rats as a result of a contraction of blood volume. Whether these animals are actually volume expanded is open to debate. Measurement of right atrial pressure would suggest that STZ-treated rats may, in fact, be normovolemic.[36]

The effect of an increase in circulating AVP on cardiovascular function in STZ-treated rats is not fully understood. Administration of a V1-receptor antagonist has been shown to be without effect on blood pressure in these animals.[10] However, it has also been found that STZ-treated rats have an impaired AVP-mediated recovery in blood pressure following ganglion blockade.[10] The mechanism for this is not fully understood, although it may be due to the reduced vascular sensitivity to AVP seen in STZ-treated animals.[11] Consistent with this is the finding of V1-receptor and V2-receptor downregulation,[69] as well as a reduction in hepatic V1-receptor mRNA transcription[83] in STZ-treated rats.

It is possible that blood pressure may not be a sensitive enough variable to monitor when attempting to determine the role of AVP in cardiovascular function. That is, a lack of change in blood pressure following administration of an AVP antagonist does not necessarily indicate that AVP is not involved in cardiovascular regulation. For example, Kuznetsova et al.[84] administered a combined V1/V2-receptor antagonist to conscious STZ-treated rats and found that, while blood pressure remained unchanged, there was a significant increase in total peripheral resistance and a significant reduction in cardiac index, stroke volume, and blood flow to the skin, skeletal muscle, stomach, small intestine, and kidneys. Clearly, more studies like that of Kuznetsova et al.[84] are required if the role of AVP in cardiovascular regulation in the STZ-treated rat is to be delineated.

In summary, AVP levels have been shown to be elevated in STZ-treated rats, although the mechanism(s) responsible remain to be elucidated. While there is evidence indicating that the role of AVP in cardiovascular regulation is modified following STZ administration, this area is poorly understood and much research remains to be done in conscious, STZ-treated rats.

8.2.2.3 Renin–Angiotensin System

Plasma renin activity (PRA) has been shown to be significantly reduced following STZ administration,[26,27,85-87] and is probably due, at least in part, to the observed reduction in plasma renin concentration.[86,88] The mechanism responsible for the reduced plasma renin concentration has not yet been clearly defined, although it is possible that it may be due to hyalinization of the afferent arteriole, adjacent to the juxtaglomerular apparatus, acting as a barrier to renin release.[89,90] Another possibility is that the hyporeninemia is caused by the reduction in endogenous renal prostaglandin production seen in STZ-treated rats since both prostacyclin and prostaglandin E_2 are known stimuli of renin release.[26,28]

The reduction in plasma renin concentration is unlikely to be due to a reduction in renal synthesis, since renal renin stores have been found to be unchanged[26,91] following STZ administration. Furthermore, while one study has reported renal renin mRNA levels to be reduced in the STZ-treated rat,[87] two other studies found renin mRNA levels to be normal following STZ.[91,92]

The effect of STZ administration upon other components of the renin–angiotensin system is less obvious. For example, plasma angiotensinogen concentration has been found to be normal[87] or reduced,[93] although the finding of a reduction in hepatic, renal, and adrenal angiotensinogen mRNA level is consistent with the latter.[91,92] Circulating angiotensin II (AII) levels have also been found to be normal[94] or reduced[85] following administration of STZ. Recently, Brown et al.[93] reported that AII receptor density was increased in the left ventricle, liver, and adrenal gland of STZ-treated rats, while renal receptor density was significantly reduced. Consistent with this latter finding, Kalyinyak et al.[92] found glomerular AII receptor number to be decreased in STZ-treated rats.

Administration of STZ is associated with an elevation in circulating levels of angiotensin-converting enzyme (ACE).[30,95] The mechanism responsible for this phenomenon remains to be elucidated. It may reflect damage to the vascular endothelium,[96,97] and/or an increase in tissue ACE synthesis spilling into the circulation. The potential effect of enhanced metabolism of bradykinin, as a consequence of increased ACE activity, on cardiovascular function, remains to be determined.

The effect of the changes described above on cardiovascular function in the STZ-treated rat is not fully understood. Hebden et al.[10] found that administration of captopril was without immediate effect on the blood pressure of Wistar rats treated 3 weeks earlier with STZ. However, after 1 h of administration, blood pressure was significantly reduced in the STZ-treated rats, but unaltered in control animals.[10] While the mechanism for this is not known, one might speculate that it may have been due to inhibition of tissue ACE activity leading to a reduction in bradykinin metabolism. Tomlinson et al.[37] found that captopril caused a modest hypotension in control and STZ-treated Brattleboro and Long Evans rats, indicating that blood pressure was not differentially dependent on the renin–angiotensin system in any of these groups. This difference in outcome between these two studies may be attributable to the different strain of rat used.

Chronic daily treatment with ACE inhibitors has been found to prevent or reverse the increase in blood pressure seen in STZ-treated rats by some investigators.[31,98] However, since these studies measured blood pressure indirectly, it is unclear whether the STZ-treated rats in these studies were indeed hypertensive.

Finally, it has been shown that STZ-treated rats have impaired AII-mediated blood pressure recovery following ganglion blockade.[10,37] This could be due to impaired release of renin, a reduction in synthesis of AII or reduced vascular sensitivity to AII.

In summary, there is a great deal of evidence to suggest that the renin–angiotensin system is modified following STZ administration. While preliminary data would indicate that the role of the renin–angiotensin system in cardiovascular regulation is also modified, this is yet unproved and consequently much research remains to be performed utilizing the conscious, STZ-treated rat.

8.2.3   Baroreflex Function

The pulse interval response to a drug-induced increase in arterial pressure, as a measure of cardiac baroreflex sensitivity, was first described by Smyth et al.[99] using human subjects. The bradycardia observed in response to an elevation in arterial pressure has been shown in humans,[100] rabbits,[101] and rats[102] to be almost completely vagal in origin. These findings are consistent with those of Chang and Lund[8] who reported that in STZ-treated rats, the bradycardia observed in response to phenylephrine administration was abolished by the muscarinic receptor antagonist atropine.

Although cardiac baroreflex responsiveness has been found to be unaltered[19] or reduced[18] in STZ-treated rats in response to phenylephrine, the majority of investigators have found cardiac baroreflex sensitivity to be elevated in STZ-treated rats in response to a challenge with a pressor agent. For example, Bunag et al.[4] observed a significantly enhanced baroreflex response in urethane-anesthetized STZ-treated rats given either norepinephrine or AVP as the pressor agent. Jackson and Carrier[5] observed enhanced baroreflex sensitivities in conscious, STZ-treated rats in response to the pressor agents norepinephrine and AII, while Dowell et al.[103] reported similar findings in pentobarbital anesthetized rats when the pressor agent was isoproterenol. Furthermore, Tomlinson et al.[104] found an increased baroreflex response in STZ-treated rats in response to the α-1 adrenoceptor agonist methoxamine.

The findings of Tomlinson et al.[104] are consistent with those of Hebden et al.[11] who reported that conscious STZ-treated rats demonstrated an enhanced baroreflex response to methoxamine. However, Hebden et al.[11] also reported that the baroreflex response to both AII and AVP was normal in these animals, findings which contradict those of Bunag et al.[4] with regard to AVP, and Jackson and Carrier[5] with regard to AII. The reason for the observed differences is unknown. While an argument can be made for questioning the validity of baroreflex measurements taken from anesthetized animals,[4] Jackson and Carrier[5] used conscious rats. Of particular interest was the pressor response seen in the STZ-treated animals following administration of the ganglionic antagonist pentolinium.[11] Simplistically, following removal of the efferent limb of the baroreflex with this compound, the pressor effects of exogenous agonists should give a direct measure of vascular sensitivity, and the difference in the magnitude of the pressor response between the blocked and unblocked states a measure of the degree of baroreflex buffering in the intact animal. Following blockade of the ganglia it was observed that while the pressor responsiveness was significantly increased (as one might expect) in the control animals in response to AII and AVP, there was significantly reduced potentiation in the pressor response to AII and AVP in the STZ-treated animals. These data are consistent with the hypothesis that the bradycardia seen in the STZ-treated rat in response to these pressor agents is either not involved or its involvement is reduced in baroreflex buffering in the intact state. That is, in these animals, a fall in heart rate may not translate into a reduction in cardiac output.[11]

Of particular interest is the study of Chang and Lund[8] who measured cardiac baroreflex sensitivity to phenylephrine in rats at different times following STZ administration. It was found that cardiac baroreflex sensitivity was increased in the STZ-treated animals at 12 weeks and at 24 weeks, but by 48 weeks it was significantly reduced. This led the authors to suggest that the fall in baroreflex responsiveness may have been caused by parasympathetic neuropathy, although morphological studies were not performed to confirm this. Furthermore, 59% of all animals injected with STZ were dead at 48 weeks, leading to a possible bias in the data collected.[8]

In summary, the effect of STZ administration upon baroreflex function in the rat is poorly understood, mainly as a result of the plethora of contradictory data that has been generated thus far. This lack of consistency can primarily be attributed to the different methodologies employed. That is, these studies have investigated the effects of various pressor agents on the blood pressure of conscious or anesthetized animals at different times following STZ administration. Furthermore, few researchers have attempted to determine the presence or absence of neuropathy in their experimental animals. Finally, it is critical that the vascular responsiveness of these animals also be determined in the absence of baroreflex buffering to separate out those effects that are due to a change in vascular sensitivity from those that are due to alterations in another section of the baroreflex loop.

8.2.4 Vascular Responsiveness

A number of studies have investigated vascular sensitivity in vessels taken from STZ-treated rats. While these studies have provided a great deal of valuable information, there are limitations associated with extrapolation of the data to the whole animal. That is, the vessels being studied are invariably arteries, which are not true resistance vessels, they have no innervation, there is an absence of blood in contact with the endothelium, and manipulation of the tissue can lead to damage, or even removal, of the endothelial layer. Measuring vascular sensitivity in the intact animal is clearly more physiologically valid.

However, the very factors that ensure the physiological validity of such a model can, in themselves, confound data interpretation. For example, it cannot be assumed that an equivalent elevation in blood pressure in control and STZ-treated rats following administration of a pressor agent is supportive of the hypothesis that sensitivity of this tissue is unaltered by the diabetic state. It is equally possible that pressor sensitivity of the tissue is altered but is masked by a change in baroreflex sensitivity in the STZ-treated animals. Therefore, it is necessary to measure baroreflex sensitivity to be able to interpret data obtained *in vivo*. This can be achieved most easily by measuring pressor responsiveness in the intact state and following removal of the efferent limb of the baroreflex. The latter is achieved by either ganglion blockade or by pithing the animal.

Because of the complexity associated with controlling, or at least taking into account, numerous variables, it is not altogether surprising that few investigators choose to measure vascular sensitivity in intact, STZ-treated animals. Consequently, there is a paucity of data in this area.

A reduction in pressor responsiveness to norepinephrine has been seen in intact, conscious, STZ-treated rats,[5,16,45] in ganglion-blocked, conscious, STZ-treated rats[5] and in pithed, STZ-treated rats.[105] Pressor responsiveness to α-1 agonism has also been found to be reduced in intact and ganglion-blocked, STZ-treated rats[11] as well as in pithed, STZ-treated rats.[106] Pressor responsiveness to the α-2 agonists UK-14,304 and B-HT933 was found to be normal in pithed STZ-treated rats in one study,[107] but reduced in another.[106] The reason for the difference in results with regard to α-2 agonism is not readily apparent. It may be due to the different strain of rats used or the length of time following STZ administration that the studies were performed. That is, Heijnis et al.[107] studied pithed, Wistar rats 3 months following induction of diabetes, whereas Beenen et al.[106] studied pithed, WKY rats 2 months after induction of diabetes.

Pressor responsiveness to AII has been shown to be reduced in intact,[5] ganglion-blocked,[11] and pithed[106] STZ-treated rats. A similar reduction in responsiveness has been observed in intact,[4] and ganglion-blocked[11] STZ-treated rats in response to the AVP.

Studies have also investigated the effect of STZ treatment on the response to depressor agents. Responsiveness to acetylcholine has been shown to be attenuated in intact[16] and pithed[108] STZ-treated rats. In an elegant study by Lash and Bohlen,[109] it was reported that the vasodilator response was reduced in the intestinal arterioles of STZ-treated rats following iontophoretic application of acetylcholine. In contrast to the above, Kiff et al.[110] did not observe any difference in the depressor response to acetycholine between control and diabetic rats.

Depressor responsiveness to isoproterenol has been found to be normal[16] or reduced[111] in intact, STZ-treated rats, while the vasodepressor response to hydralazine and verapamil has been found to be normal in intact, STZ-treated rats.[16] Caution must be exercised in interpretation of these findings, however, as in these studies the potential for differential baroreflex buffering between control and diabetic animals was not investigated.

In summary, the above describes a somewhat confusing and often contradictory picture of the effect of STZ on vascular sensitivity in the whole animal. Factors responsible for this situation include the length of time following STZ injection, the different strains used, and the potential for alterations in baroreflex buffering that went uninvestigated. While these are important issues, there is a fundamental question that must be addressed before considering any of these confounding factors. That is, is there any value or relevance to measuring vascular responsiveness as a change in blood pressure in STZ-treated animals? It is reasonable to speculate that blood pressure alone may not be a sensitive measure of integrated cardiovascular function and, instead, should be monitored along with cardiac output and regional blood flow.

8.3   Cardiomyopathy

In 1972, Rubler et al.[112] proposed the existence of a diabetic cardiomyopathy (based upon post-mortem findings) in four adults with diabetes mellitus and congestive heart failure, in the absence of valvular, congenital, or hypertensive heart disease or significant coronary atherosclerosis. Since that time, it has become increasingly evident that diabetes mellitus is associated with a specific cardiomyopathy, the pathogenesis of which is poorly understood.[113]

To elucidate the underlying cause of diabetic cardiomyopathy, a number of studies have been carried out using rats injected with STZ. For example, in a study by Penpargkul et al.,[114] hearts taken from rats administered with STZ 8 weeks previously exhibited a significant reduction in peak left ventricular systolic pressure and rate of left ventricular pressure development (+dP/dt) and decline (–dP/dt). Furthermore, in a study carried out using isolated left ventricular papillary muscle taken from rats injected with STZ 5 weeks previously, Fein et al.[115] reported that both the velocity of shortening and rate of relaxation were significantly reduced compared with normal papillary muscle.

A depression in cardiac function in rats following STZ administration has been confirmed by numerous researchers using both isolated cardiac tissue and isolated, perfused hearts.[116,117] It has been found that this reduction in function can be reversed[118] or prevented[118,119] by insulin treatment.

There is also evidence of cardiomyopathy in conscious STZ-treated rats. For example, Carbonell et al.[9] reported that rats injected 12 weeks previously with STZ demonstrated a decrease in peak left ventricular contractility and relaxation (peak ±dP/dt). Litwin et al.,[120] found there to be a significant decrease in resting left ventricular systolic pressure, developed pressure and peak left ventricular contractility (+dP/dt), and a significant increase in left ventricular end-diastolic pressure and the time constant of left-ventricular relaxation in conscious rats injected with STZ 26 days earlier. All of the abnormalities described by Litwin et al.[120] were reversed by insulin administration. In contrast to the above studies, Schenk et al.[44] reported that peak left ventricular systolic pressure and peak left ventricular contractility and relaxation (±dP/dt) were normal in conscious rats treated

6 weeks previously. Interestingly, these same parameters were significantly reduced in STZ-treated rats made hypertensive by administration of DOCA, when compared with DOCA-treated control animals.[44] The reason for the disparity between these studies is not readily apparent, although it may be due to the latter using Sprague-Dawley rats, a strain that has been shown to have a slower rate of development of diabetes-induced myocardial dysfunction compared with other strains.[121] In a recent study, Sevak and Goyal[98] found that STZ administration caused a reduction in left ventricular developed pressure which was not further aggravated by DOCA administration. Furthermore, treatment of both STZ and STZ DOCA rats with the converting enzyme inhibitor lisinopril was associated with an improvement in left ventricular developed pressure.[98]

Recently, Ueno et al.[39] reported that chronic administration of the stable prostacyclin analog, beraprost, to STZ-treated rats was associated with a normalization of the elevation in left ventricular end-diastolic pressure, ST/R ratio, and plasma CK levels observed in the untreated diabetic animals. While these findings are very interesting, the mechanism behind the beneficial effect of beraprost on these parameters remains unknown.

A decrease in cardiac compliance (i.e., stiffer myocardium) is believed to be responsible for the alteration in diastolic function seen in the diabetic rat.[122] However, the mechanism responsible for the reduced compliance remains to be elucidated. Recently, Norton et al.[34] reported that the intact STZ-treated rat exhibited a decrease in left ventricular compliance that was not associated with an increase in myocardial collagen content, although there was a measured increase in the formation of advanced glycosylation end products (AGEs) of myocardial collagen. Treatment with aminoguanidine, an agent that decreases the formation of collagen cross-linkages produced by the formation of AGEs, prevented the decrease in diastolic function seen in the STZ-treated rats. The converting enzyme, captopril, reduced blood pressure but failed to decrease myocardial stiffness, suggesting that the decrease in compliance is not due to an increase in afterload or a direct effect of the renin–angiotensin system.[34]

In summary, data from *in vivo* studies clearly support the conclusion from earlier *in vitro* studies that STZ administration is associated with a specific cardiomyopathy, similar to that described in humans with diabetes. Since it would appear to be an invaluable model of human diabetic cardiomyopathy, researchers attempting to elucidate the mechanism(s) responsible for this condition should continue to utilize the STZ-injected rat.

8.4 Conclusion

There is now overwhelming evidence that STZ administration is associated with a small, but significant reduction in blood pressure, a resting bradycardia, and the development of a specific cardiomyopathy. There is also good evidence that baroreflex function is altered following STZ, although much research remains to be done before the nature of this alteration is fully understood and the underlying mechanism elucidated.

There are clearly two confounding factors associated with all experiments that utilize STZ-treated rats, namely, length of time following STZ administration and strain of rat used. Since a number of pathophysiological changes that occur following STZ administration appear to be time dependent, and since different strains of rat appear to have different degrees of susceptibility to these changes, it is crucial that investigators, using this model of diabetes, clearly identify the rationale for their experimental methodology.

The study of integrated cardiovascular function in the intact, STZ-treated rat is still in its infancy. For example, little is known regarding the direct or indirect effect(s) of hypoinsulinemia on the central nervous system. Furthermore, although information is available regarding how STZ alters factors, such as the renin–angiotensin system, that are known to be involved in cardiovascular regulation, an understanding of how these alterations impact upon integrated cardiovascular function is lacking. With recent developments in technology, it is now possible to perform these experiments. Therefore, in the upcoming years the understanding of integrated cardiovascular function in STZ-treated rats will advance significantly, and it is hoped that this, in turn, will ultimately lead to improved treatments and outcomes for individuals with diabetes mellitus.

References

1. Garcia, M.J., McNamara, P.M., Gordon, T., and Kannell, W.B., Morbidity and mortality in diabetics in the Framingham population: sixteen year follow-up study. *Diabetes* 23, 105-111, 1974.
2. Hebden, R.A., Gardiner, S.M., Bennett, T., and MacDonald, I.A., The influence of streptozotocin-induced diabetes mellitus on fluid and electrolyte handling in rats. *Clin. Sci.* 70, 111-117, 1986.
3. Pfaffman, M.A., The effects of streptozotocin-induced diabetes and insulin treatment on the cardiovascular system of the rat. *Res. Commun. Chem. Pathol. Pharmacol.* 28, 27-41, 1980.
4. Bunag, R.D., Tomita, T., and Sasaki, S., Streptozotocin diabetic rats are hypertensive despite reduced hypothalamic responsiveness. *Hypertension* 4, 556-565, 1982.
5. Jackson, C.V. and Carrier, G.O., Influence of short-term experimental diabetes on blood pressure and heart rate in response to norepinephrine and angiotensin II in the conscious rat. *J. Cardiovasc. Pharmacol.* 5, 260-265, 1983.
6. Seager, M.J., Singal, P.K., Orchard, R., Pierce, G.N., and Dhalla, N.S., Cardiac cell damage: a primary myocardial disease in streptozotocin-induced chronic diabetes. *Br. J. Exp. Pharmacol.* 65, 613-623, 1984.
7. Charocopos, F. and Gavras, H., Cardiovascular effects of dobutamine and converting enzyme inhibition in rats with diabetic ketoacidosis. *Pharmacology* 30, 65-70, 1985.
8. Chang, K.S.K. and Lund, D.D., Alterations in the baroreceptor reflex control of heart rate in streptozotocin diabetic rats. *J. Mol. Cell. Cardiol.* 18, 617-624, 1986.
9. Carbonell, L.F., Salom, M.G., Garcia-Estan, J., Salazar, F.J., Ubeda, M., and Quesada, T., Hemodynamic alterations in chronically conscious unrestrained diabetic rats. *Am. J. Physiol.* 252, H900-H905, 1987.
10. Hebden, R.A., Bennnett, T., and Gardiner, S.M., Abnormal blood pressure recovery during ganglion blockade in diabetic rats. *Am. J. Physiol.* 252, R102-R108, 1987.
11. Hebden, R.A., Bennett, T., and Gardiner, S.M., Pressor sensitivities to vasopressin, angiotensin II or methoxamine in diabetic rats. *Am. J. Physiol.* 253, R726-R734, 1987.
12. Kusaka, M., Kishi, K., and Sokabe, H., Does so-called streptozotocin hypertension exist in rats? *Hypertension* 10, 517-521, 1987.
13. Akiyama, N., Okumura, K., Watanabe, Y., Hashimoto, H., Ito, T., Ogawa, K., and Satake, T., Altered acetylcholine and norepinephrine concentrations in diabetic rat hearts: role of parasympathetic nervous system in diabetic cardiomyopathy. *Diabetes* 38, 231-236, 1989.
14. Tomlinson, K.C., Gardiner, S.M., and Bennett, T., Diabetes mellitus in Brattleboro rats: cardiovascular, fluid and electrolyte status. *Am. J. Physiol.* 256, R1279-R1285, 1989.
15. Yamamoto, J. and Nakai, M., Coronary hemodynamics in diabetic spontaneously hypertensive rats. *Clin. Exp. Hypertens.* 12, 325-342, 1990.
16. Yu, Z. and McNeill, J.H., Blood pressure and heart rate response to vasoactive agents in conscious diabetic rats. *Can. J. Physiol. Pharmacol.* 70, 1542-1548, 1992.
17. Shah, T.S., Satia, M.C., Gandhi, T.P., Bangaru, R.A., and Goyal, R.K., Effects of chronic nifedipine treatment on streptozotocin-induced diabetic rats. *J. Cardiovasc. Pharmacol.* 26, 6-12, 1995.

18. Dall'Ago, P., Fernandes, T.G., Machado, U.F., Bello, A.A., and Irigoyen, M. C., Baroreflex and chemoreflex dysfunction in streptozotocin-diabetic rats. *Braz. J. Med. Biol. Res.* 30, 119-124, 1997.

19. Maeda, C.Y., Fernandes, T.G., Timm, H.B., and Irigoyen, M.C., Autonomic dysfunction in short-term experimental diabetes. *Hypertension* 26, 1100-1104, 1995.

20. Yu, Z. and McNeill, J.H., Altered inotropic responses in diabetic cardiomyopathy and hypertensive-diabetic cardiomyopathy. *J. Pharmacol. Exp. Ther.* 257, 64-71, 1991.

21. Li, X., Tanz, R.D., and Chang, K.S.K., Effect of age and methacholine on the rate and coronary flow of isolated hearts of diabetic rats. *Br. J. Pharmacol.* 97, 1209-1217, 1989.

22. Tomlinson, K.C., Gardiner, S.M., Hebden, R.A., and Bennett, T., Functional consequences of streptozotocin-induced diabetes mellitus, with particular reference to the cardiovascular system. *Pharmacol. Rev.* 44, 103-150, 1992.

23. Yazaki, Y. and Raben, M.S., Effect of the thyroid state on the enzymatic characteristics of cardiac myosin. *Circ. Res.* 208-215, 1975.

24. Dillman, W.H., Influence of thyroid hormone administration on myosin ATPase activity and myosin isoenzyme distribution in the hearts of diabetic rats. *Metabolism* 31, 199-204, 1982.

25. Kawashima, H., Igarashi, T., Nakajima, Y., Akiyama, Y., Usuki, K., and Ohtake, S., Chronic hypertension induced by streptozotocin in rats. *Naunyn Schmiedebergs Arch. Pharmacol.* 305, 123-126, 1978.

26. Funakawa, S., Okahara, T., Imanashi, M., Komori, T., Yamamoto, K., and Tochino, Y., Renin-angiotensin system and prostacyclin biosynthesis in steptozotocin diabetic rats. *Eur. J. Pharmacol.* 94, 27-33, 1983.

27. Hayashi, M., Kitajima, W., and Saruta, T., Aldosterone responses to angiotensin II, adrenocorticotropin and potassium in chronic experimental diabetes mellitus in rats. *Endocrinology* 115, 2205-2209, 1984.

28. Katayama, S. and Lee, J.B., Hypertension in experimental diabetes mellitus. Renin-prostaglandin interaction. *Hypertension* 7, 554-561, 1985.

29. Rodrigues, B., Goyal, R.K., and McNeill, J.H., Effects of hydralazine on streptozotocin-induced diabetic rats: prevention of hyperlipidemia and improvement in cardiac function. *J. Pharmacol. Exp. Ther.* 237, 292-299, 1986.

30. Hartmann, J.F., Szemplinski, M., Hayes, N.S., Keegan, M.E., and Slater, E.E., Effects of the angiotensin converting enzyme inhibitor, lisinopril, on normal and diabetic rats. *J. Hypertens.* 6, 677-683, 1988.

31. Ramos, O.L., Diabetes mellitus and hypertension: state of the art lecture. *Hypertension* 11 (Suppl. I), I-14-I-18, 1988.

32. Fein, F.S., Miller, B., Flores, M., and Morton, E., Myocardial adaption to chronic propranolol therapy in diabetic rats. *J. Cardiovasc. Pharmacol.* 17, 846-853, 1991.

33. Takeda, Y., Miyamori, I., Yoneda, T., and Takeda, R., Production of endothelin-1 from the mesenteric arteries of streptozotocin-induced diabetic rats. *Life Sci.* 48, 2553-2556, 1991.

34. Norton, G.R., Candy, G., and Woodiwiss, A.J., Aminoguanidine prevents the decreased myocardial compliance produced by streptozotocin-induced diabetes mellitus in rats. *Circulation* 93, 1905-1912, 1996.

35. Kohler, L., Boillat, N., Luthi, P., Atkinson, J., and Peters-Haefeli, L., Influence of streptozotocin-induced diabetes on blood pressure and on renin formation and release. *Naunyn Schmiedebergs Arch. Pharmacol.* 313, 257-261, 1980.

36. Hebden, R.A., Todd, M.E., and McNeill, J.H., Relationship between atrial granularity and release of ANF in rats with diabetes mellitus. *Am. J. Physiol.* 257, R932-R938, 1989.

37. Tomlinson, K.C., Gardiner, S.M., and Bennett, T., Blood pressure in streptozotocin-treated Brattleboro and Long-Evans rats. *Am. J. Physiol.* 258, R852-R859, 1990.

38. Litwin, S.E., Raya, T.E., Daugherty, S., and Goldman, S., Peripheral circulatory control of cardiac output in diabetic rats. *Am. J. Physiol.* 261, H836-H842, 1991.

39. Ueno, Y., Koike, H., and Nishio, S., Beneficial effects of Beraprost Sodium, a stable prostacyclin analogue, in diabetic cardiomyopathy. *J. Cardiovasc. Pharmacol.* 26, 603-607, 1995.

40. Katovitch, M.J., Hanley, K., Strubbe, G., and Wright, B.E., Effects of streptozotocin-induced diabetes and insulin treatment on blood pressure in the male rat. *Proc. Soc. Exp. Biol. Med.* 208, 300-306, 1995.

41. Rodgers, R.L., Depressor effect of diabetes in the spontaneously hypertensive rat: associated changes in heart performance. *Can. J. Physiol. Pharmacol.* 64, 1177-1184, 1986.
42. Yamamoto, J., Blood pressure and metabolic effects of streptozotocin in Wistar- Kyoto and spontaneously hypertensive rats. *Clin. Exp. Hypertens.* 10, 1065-1083, 1988.
43. Kiff, R.J., Gardiner, S.M., Compton, A.M., and Bennett, T., The effects of endothelin-1 and NG-nitro-L-arginine methyl ester on regional haemodynamics in conscious rats with sreptozotocin-induced diabetes mellitus. *Br. J. Pharmacol.* 103, 1321-1326, 1991.
44. Schenk, J., Hebden, R.A., Dai, S., and McNeill, J.H., Integrated cardiovascular function in the conscious streptozotocin-diabetic deoxycorticosterone-acetate-hypertensive rat. *Pharmacology* 48, 211-215, 1994.
45. Hayashi, M., Senba, S., Saito, I., Kitajima, W., and Saruta, T., Changes in blood pressure, urinary kallikrein and urinary protaglandin E_2 in rats with streptozotocin-induced diabetes. *Naunyn Schmiederbergs Arch. Pharmacol.* 322, 290-294, 1983.
46. Kusaka, M., Kishi, K., Sokabe, H., Miyazawa, A., and Yagi, S., Renal lesions of streptozotocin-induced diabetes mellitus in spontaneously hypertensive rats. *Jpn. Heart J.* 26, 681-685, 1985.
47. Zerbe, R.L., Bayorh, M.A., and Feuerstein, G., Vasopressin: an essential pressor factor for blood pressure recovery following hemorrhage. *Peptides* 3, 509-514, 1982.
48. Zerbe, R.L., Feuerstein, G., Meyer, D.K., and Kopin, I.J., Cardiovascular, sympathetic and renin–angiotensin system responses to hemorrhage in vasopressin-deficient rats. *Endocrinology* 111, 608-613, 1982.
49. Sato, T., Nara, Y., Kato, Y., and Yamori, Y., Effect of antihypertensive treatment with alacepril on insulin resistance in diabetic spontaneously hypertensive rats. *Metab. Clin. Exp.* 45(4), 457-462, 1996.
50. Monckton, G. and Pehowich, E., Autonomic neuropathy in the streptozotocin diabetic rat. *Can. J. Neurol. Sci.* 7, 135-142, 1980.
51. Schmidt, R.E. and Scharp, D.W., Axonal dystrophy in experimental diabetic autonomic neuropathy. *Diabetes* 31, 761-770, 1982.
52. Schmidt, R.E., Plurad, S.B., and Modert, C.W., Experimental diabetic autonomic neuropathy characterization in streptozotocin-diabetic Sprague-Dawley rats. *Lab. Invest.* 49, 538-552, 1983.
53. Kniel, P.C., Junker, U., Perrin, I.V., Bestetti, G.E., and Rossi, G.L., Varied effects of experimental diabetes on the autonomic nervous system of the rat. *Lab. Invest.* 54, 523-530, 1986.
54. Schmidt, R.E. and Plurad, S.B., Ultrastructural and biochemical characterization of autonomic neuropathy in rats with chronic streptozotocin diabetes. *J. Neuropathol. Exp. Neurol.* 45, 525-544, 1986.
55. Lund, D.D., Subieta, A.R., Pardini, B.J., and Chang, K.S., Alterations in cardiac parasympathetic indices in STZ induced diabetic rats. *Diabetes* 41, 160-166, 1992.
56. Gabbay, K.H., Merola, L.O., and Field, R.A., Sorbitol pathway: presence in nerve and cord with substrate accumulation in diabetes. *Science* 151, 209-210, 1966.
57. Gabbay, K.H., The sorbitol pathway and the complications of diabetes. *N. Engl. J. Med.* 288, 831-836, 1973.
58. Clements, R.S., Peripheral nerve biochemistry in diabetes. *Clin. Physiol.* 5 (Suppl. 5), 19-22, 1985.
59. Tomlinson, D.R. and Mayer, J.H., Defects of axonal transport in diabetes mellitus — a possible contribution to the aetiology of diabetic neuropathy. *J. Autonom. Pharmacol.* 4, 59-72, 1984.
60. Schmidt, R.E., Plurad, S.B., Sherman, W.R., Williamson, J.R., and Tilton, R.G., Effects of aldose reductase inhibitor sorbinil on neuroaxonal dystrophy and levels of myo-inositol and sorbitol in sympathetic autonomic ganglia of streptozotocin-induced diabetic rats. *Diabetes* 38, 569-579, 1989.
61. Schmidt, R.E., Plurad, S.B., Coleman, B.D., Williamson, J.R., and Tilton, R.G., Effects of sorbinil, dietary myo-inositol supplementation and insulin on resolution of neuroaxonal dystrophy in mesenteric nerves of streptozotocin-induced diabetic rats. *Diabetes* 40, 574-582, 1991.
62. Kilgour, R.D. and Williams, P.A., Impaired cardiovascular responsiveness to an acute cold wind stress in streptozotocin-diabetic rats. *Comp. Biochem. Physiol.* 107, 537-543, 1994.
63. Hart, J.L., Freas, W., McKenzie, J.E., and Muldoon, S.M., Adrenergic nerve function and contractile activity of the caudal artery of the streptozotocin diabetic rat. *J. Auton. Nerv. Syst.* 25, 49-57, 1988.

64. Sato, N., Hashimoto, H., Takiguchi, Y., and Nakashima, M., Altered responsiveness to sympathetic nerve stimulation and agonists of isolated left atria of diabetic rats: no evidence for involvement of hypothyroidism. *J. Pharmacol. Exp. Ther.* 248, 367-371, 1989.

65. Hashimoto, H., Satoh, N., Takiguchi, Y., and Nakashima, M., Effects of an aldose reductase inhibitor, ONO-2235, insulin and their combination on the altered responsiveness to nerve stimulation and agonists of the isolated atria of diabetic rats. *J. Pharmacol. Exp. Ther.* 253, 552-557, 1990.

66. Fushima, H., Inoue, T., Kishino, B., Nishikawa, M., Tochino, M., Funakawa, S., Yamatodani, A., and Wada, H., Abnormalities in plasma catecholamine response and tissue catecholamine accumulation in streptozotocin diabetic rats: a possible role for diabetic neuropathy. *Life. Sci.* 35, 1077-1081, 1984.

67. Chang, E.B., Bergenstal, R.M., and Field, M., Diarrhea in streptozotocin-treated rats. Loss of adrenergic regulation of intestinal fluid and electrolyte transport. *J. Clin. Invest.* 75, 1666-1670, 1985.

68. Vokes, T. and Robertson, G.L., Effect of insulin on the osmoregulation of thirst and vasopressin, in *Vasopressin*. Schrier, R.W., Ed., Raven Press, New York, 1985, 271-279.

69. Trinder, D., Phillips, P.A., Stephenson, J.M., Risvanis, J., Aminian, A., Adam, W., Cooper, M., and Johnston, C.I., Vasopressin V1 and V2 receptors in diabetes mellitus. *Am. J. Physiol.* 266, E217-E223, 1994.

70. Van Itallie, C.M. and Fernstrom, J.D., Osmolal effects on vasopressin secretion in the streptozotocin-diabetic rat. *Am. J. Physiol.* 242, E411-E417, 1982.

71. Loesch, A., Lincoln, J., and Burnstock, G., The hypothalamo-neurohypophysial system in streptozotocin-diabetic rats: ultrastructural and immunocytochemical evidence for alterations of oxytocin- and vasopressin-containing neuronal profiles. *Acta Neuropathol.* 75, 391-401, 1988.

72. Dheen, S.T., Tay, S.S., and Wong, W.C., Arginine vasopressin- and oxytocin-like immunoreactive neurons in the hypothalamic paraventricular and supraoptic nuclei of streptozotocin-induced diabetic rats. *Arch. Histol. Cytol.* 57, 461-472, 1994.

73. Fernstrom, J.D., Fernstrom, M.H., and Kwok, R.P., *In vivo* somatostatin, vasopressin and oxytocin synthesis in diabetic rat hypothalamus. *Am. J. Physiol.* 258, E661-E666, 1990.

74. Robertson, G.L., The regulation of vasopressin function in health and disease. *Recent Prog. Horm. Res.* 33, 333-385, 1977.

75. Zerbe, R.L. and Robertson, G.L., Osmoregulation of thirst and vasopressin secretion in human subjects: effect of various solutes. *Am. J. Physiol.* 244, E607-E614, 1983.

76. Charlton, J.A., Thompson, C.J., Palmer, J.M., Thornton, S., and Baylis, P.H., Osmoregulation of vasopressin secretion in the insulin-withdrawn streptozotocin-treated diabetic rat. *J. Endocrinol.* 123, 413-419, 1989.

77. Akaishi, T. and Homma, S., Baroreceptor control of vasopressin-producing cells in streptozotocin diabetic rats. *Brain Res. Bull.* 31, 719-722, 1992.

78. Iwasaki, Y., Kondo, K., Murase, T., Hasegawa, H., and Oiso, Y., Osmoregulation of plasma vaspressin in diabetes mellitus with sustained hyperglycemia. *J. Neuroendocrinol.* 8, 755-760, 1996.

79. Vokes, T., Aycinena, P.R., and Robertson, G.L., Effect of insulin on osmoregulation of vasopressin. *Am. J. Physiol.* 252, E538-E548, 1987.

80. Hebden, R.A., Bennett, T., and Gardiner, S.M., Blood pressure recovery following haemorrhage in rats with streptozotocin-induced diabetes mellitus. *Circ. Shock.* 26, 321-330, 1988.

81. Geloen, A., Roy, P.E., and Bukowiecki, L.J., Regression of white adipose tissue in diabetic rats. *Am. J. Physiol.* 257, E547-E553, 1989.

82. Pillion, D.J., Jenkins, R.L., Atchinson, J.A., Stockard, C.R., Clements, R.S., and Grizzle, W.E., Paradoxical organ-specific adaptions to streptozotocin diabetes mellitus in adult rats. *Am. J. Physiol.* 254, E749-E755, 1988.

83. Phillips, P.A., Risvanis, J., Hutchins, A.M., Burrell, L.M., MacGregor, D., Gundlach, A.L., and Johnston, C.I., Down-regulation of vasopressin V1a receptor mRNA in diabetes mellitus in the rat. *Clin Sci.* 88, 671-674, 1995.

84. Kuznetsova, L.V., Medvedeva, N.A., and Medvedeva, O.S., Hemodynamic changes in waking rats with acute streptozotocin diabetes after administration of the combined V2/V1 vasopressin antagonist. *Biul. Eksp. Biol. Med.* 115, 594-596, 1993.

85. Kigoshi, T., Imaizuma, N., Azukizawa, S., Yamamoto, I., Uchida, K., Konishi, F., and Morimoto, S., Effects of angiotensin II, adrenocorticotropin, and potassium on aldosterone production in adrenal zona glomerulosa cells from streptozotocin-induced diabetic rats. *Endocrinology* 118, 183-188, 1986.

86. Ubeda, M., Hernandez, I., Fenoy, F., and Quesada, T., Vascular and adrenal renin-like activity in chronically diabetic rats. *Hypertension* 11, 339-343, 1988.

87. Cassis, L.A., Downregulation of the renin–angiotensin in streptozotocin-diabetic rats. *Am. J. Physiol.* 262, E105-E109, 1992.

88. Ballerman, B.J., Skorecki, K.L., and Brenner, B.M., Reduced glomerular angiotensin II receptor density in early untreated diabetes mellitus in the rat. *Am. J. Physiol.* 247, F110-F116, 1984.

89. Christlieb, A.R., Renin-angiotensin aldosterone system in diabetes mellitus. *Diabetes* 25, (Suppl. 2), 820-825, 1976.

90. Nakamura, R., Saruta, T., Yamagami, K., Saito, I., Kondo, K., and Matsuki, S., Renin and the juxtaglomerular apparatus in diabetic nephropathy. *J. Am. Geriatr. Soc.* 26, 17-21, 1978.

91. Correa-Rotter, R., Hostetter, T.H., and Rosenberg, M.E., Renin and angiotensinogen gene expression in experimental diabetes mellitus. *Kidney Int.* 41, 796-804, 1992.

92. Kalinyak, J.E., Sechi, L.A., Griffin, C.A., Don, B.R., Tavangar, K., Kraemer, F.B., Hoffman, A.R., and Schambelan, M., The renin–angiotensin system in streptozotocin-induced diabetes mellitus in the rat. *J. Am. Soc. Nephrol.* 4, 1337-1345, 1993.

93. Brown, L., Wall, D., Marchant, C., and Sernia, C., Tissue-specific changes in angiotensin II receptors in streptozotocin-diabetic rats. *J. Endocrinol.* 154, 355-362, 1997.

94. Vallon, V., Wead, L.M., and Blantz, R.C., Renal hemodynamics and plasma and kidney angiotensin II in established diabetes mellitus in rats: effect of sodium and salt restriction. *J. Am. Soc. Nephrol.* 5, 1761-1767, 1995.

95. Valentovic, M.A., Elliot, C.W., and Bell, J.G., The effect of streptozotocin-induced diabetes and insulin treatment on angiotensin converting enzyme activity. *Res. Commun. Chem. Pathol. Pharmacol.* 58, 27-39, 1987.

96. Porta, M., La Selva, M., Molinatti, P., and Molinatti, G.M., Endothelial cell function in diabetic microangiopathy. *Diabetologia* 30, 601-609, 1987.

97. Matucci-Cerinic, M., Jaffa, A., and Kahaleh, B., Angiotensin converting enzyme: an *in vivo* and *in vitro* marker of endothelial injury. *J. Lab. Clin. Invest.* 120, 428-433, 1992.

98. Sevak A.R. and Goyal, R.K., Effects of chronic treatment with lisinopril on cardiovascular complications in streptozotocin diabetic and DOCA hypertensive rats. *Pharmacol. Res.* 34, 201-209, 1996.

99. Smyth, H.S., Sleight, P., and Pickering, G.W., Reflex regulation of arterial pressure during sleep in man. A quantitative method of assessing baroreflex sensitivity. *Circ. Res.* 24, 109-121, 1969.

100. Pickering, T.G., Gribben, B., and Sleight, P., Comparison of the reflex heart rate response to rising and falling arterial pressure in man. *Cardiovasc. Res.* 6, 277-283, 1972.

101. Weinstock, M. and Rosin, A.J., Relative contributions of vagal and cardiac sympathetic nerves to the reflex bradycardia induced by a pressor stimulus in the conscious rabbit: comparison of steady state and ramp methods. *Clin. Exp. Pharmacol. Physiol.* 11, 133-141, 1984.

102. Coleman, T.G., Arterial baroreflex control of heart rate in the conscious rat. *Am. J. Physiol.* 238, H515-H520, 1980.

103. Dowell, R.T., Atkins, F.L., and Love, S., Integrative nature and time course of cardiovascular alterations in the diabetic rat. *J. Cardiovasc. Pharmacol.* 8, 406-413, 1986.

104. Tomlinson, K.C., Gardiner, S.M., and Bennett, T., Central effects of angiotensins I and II in conscious streptozotocin-treated rats. *Am. J. Physiol.* 258, R1147-R1156, 1990.

105. Lucas, P.D., Effects of streptozotocin-induced diabetes and noradrenaline infusion on cardiac output and its regional distribution in pithed rats. *Diabetologia* 28, 108-112, 1985.

106. Beenen, O.H., Mathy, M.J., Pfaffendorf, M., and van Zwieten, P.A., Influence of nifedipine on pressor responses induced by different alpha-adrenoceptor agonists and angiotensin II in pithed diabetic hypertensive rats. *J. Hypertension* 14, 847-853, 1996.

107. Heijnis, J.B., Mathy, M.J., Pfaffendorf, M., and van Zwieten, P.A., Differential effects of alpha-1 and alpha-2 adrenoceptor agonists on peripheral vasoconstriction in pithed diabetic rats. *J. Cardiovasc. Pharmacol.* 20, 554-558, 1992.

108. Foy, J.M. and Lucas, P.D., Effect of experimental diabetes, food deprivation and genetic obesity on the sensitivity of pithed rats to autonomic agents. *Br. J. Pharmacol.* 57, 229-234, 1976.
109. Lash, J.M. and Bohlen, H.G., Structural and functional origins of suppressed acetylcholine vasodilation in diabetic rat intestinal arterioles. *Circ. Res.* 69, 1259-1268, 1991.
110. Kiff, R.J., Gardiner, S.M., Compton, A.M., and Bennett, T., Selective impairment of hindquarters vasodilator responses to bradykinin in conscious Wistar rats with streptozotocin-induced diabetes mellitus. *Br. J. Pharmacol.* 103, 1357-1362, 1991.
111. Jobidon, C., Nadeau, A., Tancrede, G., and Rousseau-Migneron, S., Diminished hypotensive response to isoproterenol in streptozotocin diabetic rats. *Gen. Pharmacol.* 20, 39-46, 1989.
112. Rubler, S., Dlugash, J., Yuceoglu, Y.Z., Kumral, T., Branwood, A.W., and Grishman, A., New type of cardiomyopathy associated with diabetic glomerulosclerosis. *Am. J. Cardiol.* 30, 595-602, 1972.
113. Fein, F.S. and Sonnenblick, E.H., Diabetic cardiomyopathy. *Prog. Cardiovasc. Dis.* 27, 255-270, 1985.
114. Penpargkul, S., Schaible, T., Yipintsoi, T., and Scheuer, J., The effect of diabetes on performance and metabolism of rat hearts. *Circ. Res.* 47, 911-921, 1980.
115. Fein, F.S., Kornstein, L.B., Strobeck, J.E., Capasso, J.M., and Sonnenblick, E.H., Altered myocardial mechanics in diabetic rats. *Circ. Res.* 47, 922-933, 1980.
116. McNeill, J.H., Endocrine dysfunction and cardiac performance. *Can. J. Physiol. Pharmacol.* 63, 1-8, 1985.
117. Tahiliani, A.G. and McNeill, J.H., Diabetes induced abnormalities in the myocardium. *Life Sci.* 38, 959-974, 1986.
118. Tahiliani, A.G., Vadlamudi, R.V.S.V., and McNeill, J.H., Prevention and reversal of altered myocardial function in diabetic rats by insulin treatment. *Can. J. Physiol. Pharmacol.* 61, 516-523, 1983.
119. Fein, F.S., Malhotra, A., Miller-Green, B., Scheuer, J., and Sonnenblick, E.H., Altered myocardial mechanics in diabetic rats. *Am. J. Physiol.* 247, H817-H823, 1984.
120. Litwin, S.E., Raya, T.E., Anderson, P.G., Daugherty, S., and Goldman, S., Abnormal cardiac function in the streptozotocin-diabetic rat. Changes in active and passive properties of the left ventricle. *J. Clin. Invest.* 86, 481-488, 1990.
121. Dai, S. and McNeill, J.H., Myocardial performance of STZ diabetic DOCA-hypertensive rats. *Am. J. Physiol.* 263, H1798-H1805, 1992.
122. Schaffer, S.W., Mozzaffari, M.S., Artman, M., and Wilson, G.L., Basis for myocardial mechanical defects associated with noninsulin-dependent diabetes. *Am. J. Physiol.* 256, E25-E30, 1989.

9

Treatment and Pharmacological Interventions in Streptozotocin Diabetes

Mary L. Battell, Brian Rodrigues, Violet G. Yuen, and John H. McNeill

CONTENTS

9.1 Introduction

The pathological changes produced by streptozotocin (STZ) diabetes are outlined in the various chapters of this volume. Various treatments to reverse or prevent these changes have been studied including the most obvious one, insulin. In some cases, a number of parameters have been studied; in others, only blood glucose has been examined. It should also be noted that many treatment studies have been carried out for relatively brief periods of time. In the case of some treatments, there have been excellent recent reviews published and only a brief discussion is required here. Other topics that have not been reviewed are discussed more extensively.

9.2   Insulin

Treatment of STZ diabetic rats with Protamine Zinc Insulin at a dose of about 9 U/kg/day for 4 to 6 weeks subcutaneously has been shown to decrease blood glucose in a number of studies.[1-4] In these studies, insulin treatment lowered the elevated levels of food and water intake, blood glucose, triglycerides, cholesterol, and HbA_{1c} to control or close to control levels.[3] The best results were obtained when the dose was carefully adjusted to each animal since there were varying requirements among the STZ diabetic rats. Cardiac dysfunction was returned to normal in STZ diabetic rats treated with insulin for 4 weeks following 6 weeks of diabetes[5] but not following 6 months of diabetes.[2]

Impairment of cardiac sarcoplasmic reticulum function and impairments in various membrane enzymes were also prevented by insulin treatment in STZ diabetic rats.[1,3] Treatment of STZ diabetic rats with insulin for 3 months prevented glycosuria and reduced, but did not totally eliminate, histological changes in rat heart.[6] Implantation of osmotic minipumps filled with concentrated regular insulin resulted in 7 out of 20 STZ diabetic rats attaining adequate levels of blood glucose for up to 35 days. There was again considerable variation among the animals and some were hyper- and some hypoglycemic in this study.[7] Using regular beef/pork insulin, 15 to 17 U/kg/day in STZ diabetic rats produced euglycemia, while regular human insulin required a dose of 22 to 24 U/kg/day (unpublished observations[8]). A similar difference was noted using intermediate-acting insulin.

9.3   Vanadium

Vanadium compounds are the most-studied substances for the long-term treatment of STZ diabetes. Vanadium exhibits insulin-mimetic effects particularly *in vitro* and insulin-enhancing, and possibly insulin-mimetic effects in the STZ diabetic rat. The subject has been reviewed extensively,[9-12] most recently by Verma et al.[13] Heyliger et al.[14] were the first to demonstrate an effect of vanadium *in vivo* in the diabetic rat. In that study, 6-week STZ diabetic rats were treated with sodium orthovanadate over a 4-week period. Plasma glucose was returned to euglycemic levels, but plasma insulin values were not increased. The decrease in heart function that normally occurred in STZ diabetic rats was prevented by the vanadate treatment. The dose of vanadate used in this study was about 100 mg/kg/day given in the drinking water, and, in most of the studies using vanadium compounds, the drugs have been given in a similar manner. The original observation of Heyliger et al.[14] has been confirmed many times with both vanadate[15] and vanadyl[16] forms of vanadium. More recently, organic vanadium compounds, most notably, bis(maltolato)oxovanadium(IV) (BMOV), have also been shown to be effective.[17-19] BMOV is two to three times more potent than vanadyl sulfate on a molar basis when given either orally or parenterally.[19] Other organic vanadium compounds shown to have antidiabetic actions in STZ diabetic rats include vanadyl-cysteine methyl ester, vanadyl-oxalate, -malonate, -salicylaldehyde, -(+)tartarate,[20] -methylpicolinate,[21] as well as coordination complexes with maltol or kojic acid.[22] A different class of compounds, the peroxovanadium compounds, has also been shown to reduce blood glucose levels in nondiabetic Sprague-Dawley rats and in diabetic BB rats[23] as well as in STZ diabetic rats.[24] These compounds are effective at very low doses (700 µg vanadium/kg body weight) following a single i.p. administration with blood glucose values in the STZ diabetic rats returning to preadministration levels by 48 h.[24]

Elevated blood lipids are lowered to normal levels by vanadium treatment[18,25] and long-term studies of up to 1 year have shown a prevention of secondary complications such as cataracts,[18,26,27] and cardiac[25,28] and renal dysfunction.[29] Early reports of vanadium toxicity appear to be exaggerated (see Thompson et al.[30] for review) and STZ animals can be maintained for up to a year without apparent toxicity.[26,29,31-33] Vanadium does appear to suppress appetite in control animals, which generally show a decreased weight gain during chronic vanadium treatment. Suppression of appetite is difficult to ascertain in the treated diabetic animals since correction of the diabetic state will reduce the elevated food intake in these animals. It should be noted that when vanadium salts are given in the drinking water some animals may refuse to drink, particularly at concentrations of compounds greater than 1 mg/ml. If an STZ diabetic animal does not drink, dehydration and death will rapidly result. In such cases removal of the vanadium solution and substitution of water as the drinking solution prevents the adverse effects from occurring. Vanadium can then be reintroduced at a lower concentration and the concentration gradually increased over several days.[30]

Chronic administration of vanadyl sulfate to STZ rats for several weeks followed by withdrawal can result in long-term euglycemia long after the treatment has stopped.[25,34] The mechanism of this effect is not known, but it has been shown to depend on the insulin values in the diabetic animals. Persistent euglycemia is more likely to occur in STZ diabetic animals with higher insulin values even when these values are still markedly less than normal.[34] The mechanism of most vanadium compounds in enhancing the effects of insulin appears to be due to phosphatase inhibition at points distal to the insulin receptor (reviewed by Verma et al.[13]), but the peroxovanadium compounds also have a direct effect on the insulin receptor.[35]

The therapeutic potential of the vanadium compounds for treatment of diabetes in humans has been indicated in the small clinical trials, which have been done using metavanadate[36] and vanadyl sulfate[37-39] where positive effects on carbohydrate and lipid metabolism during the 2 to 3 week trials were seen. In one study, the positive effects were still present out to 2 weeks following cessation of treatment.[37]

Another insulin-enhancing agent, the biguanide compound metformin, which is used to treat noninsulin-dependent diabetes in humans is also effective in the STZ diabetic rat. Treatment for 8 weeks reduced glucose and triglyceride levels and prevented the onset of cardiac dysfunction.[40]

9.4 Other Trace Metals in Diabetic Rats

9.4.1 Selenium

Along with vanadium and other metals, selenium has been reported to have insulin-like effects. The insulin-like effects of selenium were first reported *in vitro* by Ezaki,[41] using isolated rat adipocytes. Stimulation of glucose transport activity by translocation of glucose transporters, stimulation of cAMP phosphodiesterase activity and stimulation of ribosomal S6 protein phosphorylation were all reported in this study. Tyrosyl phosphorylations of 210-, 170-, 120-, 95-, 70-, and 60-kDa proteins but, significantly, not the insulin receptor were all shown. More recently, MAP kinase and S6 kinase activity were shown to be stimulated in rat adipocytes following preincubation with both vanadium and selenium.[42]

In vivo insulin-like effects of selenate were reported in 1991 by McNeill et al.[43] using STZ diabetic Wistar rats. The rats were treated with sodium selenate, administered i.p. daily for 8 weeks at doses ranging from 10 to 15 μmoles/kg. The selenium-treated diabetic rats had partially improved blood glucose levels without an increase in plasma insulin levels. Food and fluid intakes, which were elevated in the diabetic rats, were partially restored to normal due to the treatment. In addition to the improvement in plasma glucose levels, improvements in integrated glucose response to both oral and i.v. administration of glucose were seen when selenate (16.5 μmol/kg) was administered orally.[44] Battell et al.[45] reported that selenate administered i.p. was able to improve heart function in STZ diabetic rats.

Glucose-lowering effects of selenium have also been reported in pancreatectomized rats[46] and male Swiss albino mice made diabetic with STZ.[47] The insulin levels in the diabetic rats treated with selenate were not increased relative to the untreated diabetic rats,[43-46] and insulin levels were reduced in the nondiabetic rats treated with selenate in the absence of any change in glucose levels,[43,45] suggesting increased insulin sensitivity. In the study by Ghosh et al.[47] treatment with selenium prior to administration of STZ preserved the insulin-producing ability of the β-cells as indicated by insulin levels that were not different from control.[47]

In addition to its possible role as an insulin mimetic, selenium is an essential trace metal. It is present in glutathione peroxidase,[48] which forms part of the system for dealing with free radicals. Since increased oxidative stress is reported in diabetes[49,50] selenium may play a role in response to this stress. Plasma selenium concentrations have been reported to be increased in STZ diabetic rats[51] and diabetic children[52] which may be reflective of an increased need. The apparent elevations of rat plasma selenium occurred along with alterations in the activities of the enzymes of the antioxidant defense system, particularly the selenium-dependent glutathione peroxidase.[48]

9.4.2   Lithium

Lithium has been shown to have effects on glucose metabolism in rats made diabetic by pancreatectomy or alloxan. Lithium carbonate (0.3 mg/ml) was administered in the drinking water 3 to 4 weeks following 90% removal of the pancreas.[53] Pancreatectomy results in plasma glucose levels of 21.3 mM (fed) and 7.3 (fasted) compared to 8.4 mM (fed) and 5.6 (fasted) in the sham-operated controls. Lithium treatment for 2 weeks normalized fasting plasma glucose, partially normalized fed glucose, reversed the drop in whole body glucose uptake, and increased muscle glycogenic rates to values that were greater than control. This study also showed an increase in insulin sensitivity in the control rats as indicated by higher muscle glycogenic rates, and increased whole body glucose uptake in rats with reduced plasma insulin levels. Treatment with lithium carbonate in the drinking water also resulted in a significant drop in blood glucose levels in alloxan diabetic rats.[54] In this study, treatment with lithium did not change the insulin levels.

In contrast to the reports that lithium lowers blood glucose in diabetic rats following 2 weeks of oral treatment,[53-55] intravenous infusion of 4 meq/kg lithium chloride resulted in a rise in plasma glucose at 60 min in both nondiabetic and STZ diabetic rats.[56] Plasma glucose returned close to the preinfusion levels by 2 h. In another report, a single i.v. administration of lithium (1 meq/kg) 30 min prior to an i.v. administration of glucose resulted in significantly higher glucose levels and, more importantly, lower plasma insulin levels over the 30-min period of observation.[57] These results are in direct conflict with the observation that chronic administration of lithium can lower glucose levels in diabetic rats.[53-55] Interestingly, the rise in glucose levels in both diabetic and nondiabetic rats following acute administration of lithium[56,57] has also been reported with selenium. A single i.p. administration of sodium selenate to nondiabetic rats resulted in an increase in plasma glucose,[58] whereas chronic oral or i.p. administration[43-46] lowered plasma glucose in diabetic rats.

9.4.3 Zinc

Single administration of zinc to diabetic rats has been reported to both increase[59] and decrease[60] blood glucose. Etzel and Cousins[59] administered 25 μmol of zinc i.p. to STZ diabetic rats and demonstrated that serum glucose increased from 30 to 34 mM in the zinc-treated rats 1 h following zinc administration. Similar results were also shown in nondiabetic rats. In the study by Shisheva et al.[60] diabetic rats received 100 mg/kg $ZnCl_2$ i.p. or 210 mg/kg $ZnCl_2$ by oral gavage. Following both methods of administration, blood glucose levels dropped; i.p. administration dropped levels within 2 to 3 h. This glucose-lowering effect was sustained for 6 to 10 h. In this study, no change in blood glucose was seen when $ZnCl_2$ was similarly administered to nondiabetic rats.

The level of zinc in diabetic animals is of interest since it has been reported that humans with Type I diabetes have a significantly lower level of plasma zinc and higher urinary loss of zinc[61] but with no difference in the muscle level.[61] In 6-month diabetic rats,[62] plasma zinc levels were not different compared with control rats, but urine, erythrocyte, and lymphocyte levels per cell were all higher compared with control. Diabetic liver and femur had higher levels of zinc per gram dry weight of tissue, whereas diabetic muscle had a lower level and there was no difference in kidney. In a shorter duration study (28 days), increased levels of zinc in liver, but also in kidney were shown in STZ diabetic rats.[63] The question of zinc absorption and retention has been examined in a study using ^{65}Zn; this study also manipulated diet so that the effect of diabetes-induced hyperphagia could be separated out, and the ratio of three important trace metals, zinc, iron, and copper, were the same.[64] Male nondiabetic and diabetic Long-Evans rats were divided into groups on diets containing low (10 ppm) or high (20 ppm) levels of zinc and low or high levels of protein. The levels of zinc or protein in the diet had no effect on serum glucose levels or on food intake in diabetic rats. At termination (28 days of diabetes) the zinc content in the kidney was significantly higher in the diabetics than in the controls. The zinc intake of the diabetic rats was about twofold greater than that of the control rats, reflecting a greater food intake. The actual zinc absorption (in mg Zn/4 days) was greater in the diabetic rats, but this was more than compensated for by an almost tenfold higher zinc urinary excretion.[64]

9.4.4 Magnesium, Molybdate, and Tungstate

Magnesium levels in diabetic rat plasma, liver, and kidney were found to be lower than control.[65] Magnesium sulfate supplementation (2.5 mM in drinking water), initiated 7 days after induction of diabetes and continued for 10 weeks,[65] returned liver and kidney levels to normal and resulted in a slight elevation of plasma levels. This supplementation had no effect on plasma glucose levels in either control or diabetic rats, but did partially improve the response to an oral glucose load in the diabetic rats. The depressed heart function in the diabetic animals was unaffected by treatment.

Molybdate has been demonstrated to have effects similar to vanadium and selenium in partially correcting the symptoms of diabetes in STZ diabetic rats.[66] Thus, sodium molybdate when administered in drinking water (0.4 to 0.5 g/l) and in food (0.75 to 1.25 g/kg) normalized plasma glucose levels by the end of the 8-week treatment period. Food and fluid intake, and glucosuria were significantly improved by this treatment, as was glucose tolerance in response to an oral or intravenous glucose load. These improvements in glucose metabolism occurred in the absence of any changes in plasma insulin or improved insulin output during the oral or intravenous glucose challenge tests. Plasma urea (an indicator of kidney function) and plasma AST and ALT (indicators of liver function) were elevated in the diabetic rats. These parameters were partially normalized by the treatment. Permolybdate and pertungstate have also shown to lower blood glucose in STZ diabetic rats when administered as a single i.p. dose of 0.1 mol/kg with the maximum effect seen at 6 to 8 h.[67]

9.5   Chromium and Its Role in Diabetes

There is an extensive history concerning the possible involvement of chromium in diabetes. Chromium deficiency is thought to contribute to the development of diabetes, and supplementation with chromium is widely used as a treatment for diabetes. This use continues even though there is much debate about its usefulness. Chromium first became important when it was found to be part of "glucose tolerance factor" (GTF), a factor that was isolated from various sources including yeast, but which for many years was refractory to analysis of the component that contributed to the improvement in glucose tolerance.[68,69]

Because of the controversy about the role of chromium, one would have expected that extensive studies would have been done in animal models of diabetes. Unfortunately, the studies to date using chromium are limited. Rats made diabetic with STZ received GTF (partially purified from yeast), in an amount of either 12.5 ng Cr or 5 ng Cr, injected i.v.[70] Blood glucose levels fell in diabetic rats that had received GTF with the lowest values seen at 4 to 6 h. By 24 h, glucose values were still reduced in some of the rats. The higher dose of Cr resulted in a more rapid drop in blood glucose, but the lowest level recorded was the same for both doses.

The most-compelling evidence for an effect of chromium in diabetic rats came with studies using stroke-prone spontaneously hypertensive rats (SHRSP) and Wistar Kyoto (WKY) rats made diabetic with STZ.[71] Chromium was administered to diabetic and non-diabetic rats of both strains by a daily i.p. injection of 20 μg/kg body weight over a 4-week period. Changes in glucose tolerance were assessed with an i.p. glucose tolerance test using 2 g glucose per kg body weight. Administration of chromium to both diabetic SHRSP and WKY rats, significantly decreased the area under the glucose curve even though the output of insulin remained depressed. The area under the glucose curve was also reduced in the nondiabetic SHRSP and WKY rats and this occurred in the presence of a reduced insulin release suggestive of an improvement in insulin sensitivity.

9.6 Vitamin C

9.6.1 Introduction

The study of vitamin C (ascorbic acid) in STZ diabetic animals is of importance because people with diabetes may have a deficiency of ascorbic acid even when intake levels are normal. Ascorbic acid is involved in the tissue response to oxidative stress so that treatment may help in preventing the onset of the complications of diabetes, several of which may be due, in part, to oxidative stress. Numerous studies have demonstrated that patients with both Type I and Type II diabetes have lower ascorbate levels than controls.[72-74] It should be noted that some tissues concentrate ascorbic acid to levels that are higher than what is found in the plasma, and, hence, tissue ascorbic acid levels may show differences not found in the plasma.[75] The lower levels of ascorbic acid found in plasma and tissue of patients with diabetes could be related to changes in ascorbic acid transport. Ascorbic acid and glucose compete for the same glucose transport system, as does dehydroascorbic acid, the oxidation product of ascorbic acid. In granulocytes it has been shown *in vitro* that, at glucose concentrations that are typical of diabetic hyperglycemia (14 mM), competitive inhibition of ascorbic acid uptake by glucose occurs.[76] Additionally, Stankova,[72] have reported that in diabetic granulocytes maximal velocity of transport of dehydroascorbate, 2-deoxyglucose, and 3-O-methylglucose are decreased to the same extent suggesting a decrease in numbers of glucose transporters.

Supplementation with ascorbic acid has been reported to have beneficial effects, mainly in patients with NIDDM. Thus, in a group of elderly patients with NIDDM, 2 × 500 mg ascorbic acid per day for 4 months resulted in an improvement in whole-body glucose disposal, a decrease in plasma insulin levels, as well as an improvement in the levels of cholesterol and triglycerides.[77] There was no change in the plasma glucose levels in this group of patients. Eriksson and Kohvakka[78] examined the effect of 2 g of ascorbic acid per day on 29 subjects with IDDM and found no differences in body mass index, glycosylated hemoglobin, blood glucose, cholesterol, HDL-cholesterol, or triglycerides. However, this same study, using 27 subjects with NIDDM, showed a decrease in glycosylated hemoglobin, blood glucose, cholesterol, and triglycerides.

9.6.2 Levels of Vitamin C in Experimental Models of Diabetes

A deficiency of ascorbic acid would seem less likely in diabetic rats than in humans as rats can synthesize ascorbic acid. However, several studies have reported that levels in diabetic rats are significantly reduced. Diabetic female Wistar rats had a lower plasma ascorbic acid level than that of control rats, 4 weeks after diabetes induction.[74,79] Young et al.[80] also found that the levels of plasma ascorbic acid and its principal metabolite, dehydroascorbate, were significantly lower in diabetic rats. In other studies, no differences were found in the levels of ascorbic acid in the plasma of rats made diabetic with STZ.[73,81,82] It is notable that in the studies cited, there is little agreement on the levels of ascorbic acid in the blood of rats with normal values stated ranging from 48 to 128 mol/l while diabetic values ranged from 18 to 95 mmol/l. It may be coincidental that studies that specified that precautions were taken to prevent the oxidation of ascorbic acid are also the studies that reported significant differences between diabetic and control animals. As in humans, particular tissues may show significant differences in levels of ascorbic acid. This has been reported in kidney[83,84] and liver[84] of diabetic rats.

9.6.3   Vitamin C Treatment in STZ Diabetic Rats

9.6.3.1   *Direct Effects on the Diabetic State*

Whether or not ascorbic acid is deficient in diabetes, treatment with ascorbic acid could have direct effects on the diabetic status of an animal or could result in an improvement in the complications seen with STZ. Ascorbic acid in the drinking water (150 to 200 mg/kg/day) had no effect on the high glucose levels of diabetic rats.[85,86] However, treatment of diabetic rats with ascorbate at a dose of about 1 g/kg/day did result in modest, but significant improvements in plasma glucose, and glycated albumin and hemoglobin. Gembal et al.[87] have also reported that administration of ascorbic acid (1 g/l in drinking water) resulted in an improvement in glycosylated hemoglobin levels as early as 1 month after treatment, while improvements in fructosamine levels were seen by 3 months. In this study, no effects were seen on the level of plasma glucose. With high doses of vitamin C,[82] a reduction in plasma glucose from 29.9 ± 0.5 in the untreated diabetic rats to 22.3 ± 2.4 mmol/l in the vitamin C–treated rats was observed. Moreover, glycosylated hemoglobin and plasma triglycerides and ketones were all reduced by the treatment. These studies suggest that it is possible to improve the diabetic status of STZ diabetic rats with ascorbic acid, provided that the dose is high enough.

Several authors have demonstrated improvements in plasma lipid levels following administration of vitamin C. Young et al.[80] reported that treatment of diabetic rats with 1 g/l of ascorbic acid lowered the elevated cholesterol levels. Using 1 or 2 g/l ascorbic acid in the drinking water of STZ diabetic rats, Dai and McNeill[88] were able to show a lowering of plasma triglyceride and cholesterol levels in a dose-dependent manner. Free fatty acid (FFA) levels in the plasma were also reduced by the treatment to values that were not significantly different from controls.

9.6.3.2   *Effects on the Complications of Diabetes*

Of greater importance than the direct effects on the diabetic state are the reports of improvements in the complications of diabetes that have been reported following administration of ascorbic acid. The diabetic cardiomyopathy seen in STZ diabetic rats, as measured by decreased left ventricular developed pressure and positive and negative rates of pressure change, was remarkably improved by treatment with ascorbic acid.[88] The authors suggested that the mechanism of this improvement could be an increase in carnitine concentration and/or a decrease in sorbitol accumulation in the myocardium. Nerve conduction velocity in sciatic nerve was improved by about 36%, as was sciatic nerve endoneurial blood flow by a dose of 150 mg/kg per day ascorbic acid.[85] Jones and Hothersall[86] studied two processes thought to be intimately involved in the production of cataracts: the formation of advanced glycation end products and indicators of oxidation in proteins in the lenses of diabetic rats. The rat model was studied at 21 days after the initiation of diabetes, a point at which perturbations of lens metabolism have occurred but cataracts have not yet formed. Some of the indicators of protein oxidation were improved by the ascorbate supplementation, whereas others were unchanged compared with the untreated diabetic rats. The formation of advanced glycation end products was prevented by the treatment. Young et al.[80] have reported that plasma and erythrocyte malondialdehyde, urinary malondialdehyde excretion, and plasma-conjugated dienes, all of which were elevated in STZ diabetic rats were not improved by treatment with 1 g/l ascorbate in the drinking water. The ascorbic acid treatment did result in a modest improvement in the levels of glycated albumin and glycosylated hemoglobin. This effect might be secondary to the somewhat reduced levels of plasma glucose in the treated rats.

In conclusion, several factors should be considered when studying ascorbic acid metabolism in the STZ diabetic rat. Rats can synthesize ascorbic acid, which likely leads to some discrepant results when comparing with human diabetes. Ascorbic acid, at least *in vitro*, has been shown to contribute to recycling of α-tocopherol,[89] so that there is some potential that the effects attributed to ascorbic acid may be related to α-tocopherol metabolism. As ascorbic acid is highly concentrated in certain tissues, lack of an effect on, for example, measures of oxidative stress in plasma, may not indicate the lack of an effect in tissues where the complications of diabetes take place. For readers to evaluate studies, the dose of treatment should be stated and the presence or absence of ascorbic acid in the diet should be specified. Studies where more than one dose has been used are more convincing with respect to the effect or lack of effect of treatment with ascorbic acid on any parameter.

9.7 Vitamin E in Streptozotocin Diabetic Rats

Lipid peroxide levels in serum, as measured by thiobarbituric acid reactive substances (TBARS) are known to increase in diabetes.[90-93] Lipid peroxide may accelerate alterations in collagen. Serum TBARS and collagen-linked fluorescence were shown to be increased in STZ diabetic rats.[94] Vitamin E (α-tocopherol) acts as an antioxidant and may be able to prevent the changes that are associated with increased oxidative stress in diabetes. Aoki et al.[94] showed that serum TBARS were normalized in STZ diabetic rats when fed a vitamin E–supplemented diet containing 50 IU (≈50 mg) per 100 g of diet (the control diet contained 2 IU vitamin E per 100 g diet.) After 4 weeks of treatment, TBA reactants, which were significantly elevated in the diabetic rats, were normalized. Although the collagen-linked fluorescence in the diabetic rats was not corrected by the treatment, the increased thermal rupture time of the collagen fibers was corrected by vitamin E. The elevated level of glycated hemoglobin in the diabetic rats was not corrected by the tocopherol treatment and may have been a result of very high fasting glucose levels (more than 20 mmol/l) in the rats in this study. It should be noted that the serum tocopherol levels were higher in the diabetic rats, even without supplementation, possibly because of the increased food intake that occurs during diabetes. Increased levels of plasma α-tocopherol in unsupplemented diabetic rats were also reported by Nickander et al.[95] Studies by Keegan et al.[96] and Rösen et al.[97] have detailed improvements in relaxation in rat aorta[96] and heart[97] following treatment with a 1% dietary supplement or an approximately fourfold increase in the level of vitamin E in the diet. Maximum acetylcholine-induced relaxation of phenylephrine precontracted aortas was 75% in the vitamin E–treated group compared with only 60% in the untreated group following 2 months of diabetes.[96] Vitamin E treatment had no effect on blood glucose or weight loss due to the diabetic state.[96] Rösen et al.[97] showed that the 5-hydroxytryptamine-stimulated endothelium-dependent increase in coronary flow in isolated perfused hearts is progressively impaired by diabetes. This impairment was further exacerbated by a vitamin E–deficient diet but was prevented by vitamin E supplementation, which also preserved the structure of the myocardium. Vitamin E supplementation has also been shown to prevent diabetes-induced abnormalities in rat retinal blood flow.[98]

In pregnant rats, Sivan et al.[99] described improvements in neural tube defect and resorption rates in rats treated with vitamin E and then made diabetic on day 6 of gestation. In another study on diabetes-induced teratogenic effects,[100] female rats were first made diabetic, mated, and then treated with vitamin E. The treatment in this case reduced the rate of embryo malformations, and increased their size and maturation, but did not improve the rate of resorptions.

In contrast to the above studies that report either positive or no effects of vitamin E treatment, a study by Trachtman et al.[101] suggests that considerable caution should be used. They supplemented STZ diabetic rats with a vitamin E–containing diet (10 IU compared with the normal diet of 3 IU/100 mg diet) and continued the treatment for 50 weeks. The vitamin E treatment resulted in a significant mortality (84%) by 6 months and exacerbation of nephropathy. The primary difference in the studies reporting positive effects and the study by Trachtman and co-workers is the length of the treatment.

In summary, none of the studies using vitamin E demonstrated an effect on plasma glucose levels. When using vitamin E, it is useful to analyze both plasma and tissue α-tocopherol levels in the groups studied, both to determine the efficacy of the supplementation and to determine the "normal" levels in diabetic and in nondiabetic animals. Administration has most commonly been via diet[94,97,101] but also by i.p. injection[96,98] and by oral gavage.[99,100]

9.8   Interventions that Affect Lipid Metabolism

9.8.1   Carnitine

For fatty acids to be oxidized, they must be transported across the inner mitochondrial membrane. Carnitine acts as a cofactor, allowing acyl groups to be shuttled between intramitochondrial and extramitochondrial pools of CoA, and hence adequate levels are required for energy production. Carnitine is also capable of storing, transporting, and excreting potentially toxic acyl compounds, by facilitating their conversion to acyl carnitines, when the metabolic system malfunctions or is overloaded. Unlike the corresponding acyl CoA, acyl carnitines can diffuse out of the cell into the bloodstream. Urinary clearances for the potentially toxic acylcarnitines are 10- to 20-fold higher than for free carnitine; therefore, excess amounts of serum acylcarnitine can be rapidly eliminated by the kidneys.

When the carnitine level in tissues is increased, the preexisting acetyl CoA is transformed into acetyl carnitine which can then (1) remain as a storage depot, (2) be converted into fatty acid or cholesterol, or (3) cross the mitochondrial membrane back to the cytosol and from there into the circulation to be eventually excreted in the urine. An important consequence of this effect of carnitine is that it serves as a buffer of the metabolically critical acetyl CoA pool and hence decreases the intramitochondrial acetyl CoA/CoA ratio. As acetyl CoA, by activating pyruvate dehydrogenase kinase, inactivates pyruvate dehydrogenase, a decrease in this ratio results in a subsequent increase in the oxidative utilization of glucose. In addition, as the rate of oxidation of pyruvate is increased, this metabolite is diverted from its reduction to lactate to its oxidation to acetyl CoA.

As carnitine plays such an important role in myocardial substrate utilization in the control heart, a cardiac sensitivity to depletion of carnitine (as seen during diabetes) is understandable. Lack of sufficient carnitine may be a factor responsible for inadequate entry of long-chain fatty acids into the mitochondrial matrix and hence an impaired utilization. This leads to an accumulation within the plasma or cytosol of FFA and/or a number of intermediates involved in FFA oxidation (e.g., acyl CoA) which, if sufficiently large, may disrupt myocardial cell function.

It is thus evident that adequate levels of carnitine are required for normal FFA and energy metabolism in heart muscle, and that changes in the levels of carnitine may affect energy production and muscle performance. Carnitine was administered to rats from the onset of diabetes to see whether or not this intervention could replenish total myocardial carnitine levels and possibly prevent the depression in heart after chronic diabetes. L-Carnitine treatment of diabetic rats significantly increased myocardial carnitine levels, reduced plasma glucose and triglycerides, and significantly improved diabetic cardiac performance.[102]

9.8.2 Hydralazine

Hydralazine, a vasodilator used for the treatment of hypertension and congestive heart failure, has one unusual property, and that is its ability to lower blood lipids. In STZ diabetic rats, hydralazine had triglyceride-lowering properties and was capable of preventing the cardiodepressant effect of diabetes. The improvement in cardiac function by hydralazine could not be explained on the basis of its direct actions on the heart.[103] While hydralazine was capable of preventing the cardiac dysfunction that occurs in STZ diabetic rats,[103] other lipid-lowering agents (prazosin, clofibrate, and others) failed to protect against cardiac dysfunction.[104]

The reason triglyceride levels are decreased in the hydralazine-treated diabetic rats, even when they lack insulin is unclear. It could be speculated that hydralazine, like insulin, inhibits adipose tissue lipolysis. To determine if the mechanism of action of hydralazine as a lipid-lowering agent occurred at the site of adipose tissue, the *in vitro* effects of hydralazine were tested in adipose tissue from control and diabetic rats. The results indicated that hydralazine had no effect on the basal release of glycerol from adipose tissue, which remained elevated in the diabetic rats.[104] Another possible explanation for the decrease in plasma lipids is that the metabolic changes observed in untreated diabetes are, in many respects, similar to those produced by the infusion of catecholamines. Indeed, isoproterenol, used as the lipolytic stimulus, increases glycerol output from both control and diabetic adipose tissue. Thus, the absence of elevated plasma lipids in the hydralazine-treated diabetic rats could be due to a direct effect of hydralazine on the action of cate-cholamines. However, it has been reported that hydralazine does not reduce the isoprot-erenol-induced glycerol release at any concentration, in control and diabetic rats.[104] It could hence be concluded that the triglyceride-lowering effect of hydralazine does not occur at the site of the adipose tissue. Whether hydralazine may directly influence the rate of lipid or lipoprotein biosynthesis in the liver is as yet unknown. However, the liver is the major site of metabolism of hydralazine, and it is possible that a relationship exists between the metabolism of hydralazine and hepatic lipid synthesis.

9.9 Agents That Prevent Development of STZ-Induced Diabetes

9.9.1 Nicotinamide and Other Poly(ADP-Ribose) Synthetase Inhibitors

Very early in the history of the use of STZ to induce diabetes, it was reported that diabetes induction could be prevented by administration of nicotinamide.[105] Junod et al.[106] showed that the effectiveness of protection of nicotinamide against the development of diabetes depended on the dose of nicotinamide and the interval between injection of nicotinamide and that of STZ. Some degree of protection was provided when the nicotinamide was injected up to 6 h in advance of STZ. With a dose range between 125 and 500 mg/kg nicotinamide, a complete protection against the diabetogenic effects of STZ was observed. In these studies, nicotinamide was administered either 10 min or 2 h prior to STZ. Yamamoto et al.[107,108] established that part of the mechanism of diabetes induction by both STZ and alloxan was that these compounds caused DNA strand breaks to activate nuclear poly(ADP-ribose) synthetase, thereby depleting cellular NAD levels and inhibiting proinsulin synthesis. Thus, poly(ADP-ribose) synthetase inhibitors such as nicotinamide and 3-aminobenzamide could prevent the onset of diabetes.[109,110] This ability of nicotinamide to prevent the onset of diabetes has been exploited in studies where nicotinamide was used to distinguish between the effects of STZ per se and the effects of the ensuing diabetes.[111,112] Nicotinamide has also been used in combination with STZ to produce a very mild form of diabetes such that the rats are not hyperphagic, glycosuric, or polyuric, but have increased levels of hemoglobin A_1, reduced insulin response to an i.v. glucose challenge, and slight elevations of plasma glucose.[113] Another aspect of the interaction of nicotinamide and STZ is shown in the report by Rakieten et al.,[114] who noted an increasing number of pancreatic islet cell tumors in rats treated with STZ plus nicotinamide over a 14 to 18 month period. Dixit et al.[115] transplanted such tumors under the kidney capsule of Fisher inbred severely diabetic rats and reported a complete amelioration of the diabetic state in about 60% of the animals.

9.9.2   Other Agents

Nickel chloride was shown to prevent the diabetogenic effects of STZ in an experiment where rats were made diabetic with a single injection of 100 mg/kg STZ s.c.[116] Plasma insulin levels were reduced by about 25% in the STZ-injected rats compared with controls, and the levels were normal in the rats pretreated with $NiCl_2$ (10 mg/kg s.c.). STZ-injected rats had normal levels of superoxide dismutase (SOD) in erythrocytes but reduced levels of both SOD and copper in the pancreas at 72 h after injection of STZ. The nickel-pretreated STZ-injected rats had elevated erythrocyte SOD, normalized pancreas SOD, and elevated pancreas copper. The authors suggested that the mechanism of the preventative effect was related to a nickel-induced elevation in SOD that might be related to changes in copper levels. $NiCl_2$ was also shown to prevent diabetes induction by 100 mg/kg alloxan.[117,118] It would have been useful if the authors had extended these studies to times greater than 72 h.

Zinc injected 12 h prior to the injection of 60 mg/kg STZ has been shown to significantly reduce the plasma glucose levels measured at 3 to 6 weeks after diabetes induction.[119] The authors used zinc several hours prior to the STZ injection to induce the synthesis of metallothionein which had been shown to be an oxygen free radical scavenger.[120] Zinc, manganese, chromium, and cobalt have also been shown to prevent hyperglycemia at 24 h following injection of 150 mg/kg alloxan.[121] All metals were used as chlorides at a dose of 1 mg/kg i.v. administered immediately before and 15 min after alloxan. Histological examination of the pancreas indicated that zinc protected the β-cells but this was not seen with manganese, chromium, or cobalt.

In a study of STZ induced diabetes in mice, sodium selenite, administered orally at a dose of 0.01 μg/mouse, beginning 7 days prior to injection of 55 mg/kg STZ i.p., prevented the elevation of plasma glucose levels at 6 weeks following diabetes induction.[47] The plasma insulin level of the selenite-treated STZ-injected rats was maintained at normal levels.

9.10   Deoxycorticosterone Acetate

Since diabetes frequently occurs along with hypertension, several models combining the two conditions have been developed. In fact, it was thought that STZ induced diabetes in rats was automatically accompanied by hypertension.[122,123] This was subsequently shown to be a result of the method of measurement of blood pressure.[124,125] Deoxycorticosterone acetate (DOCA) along with sodium chloride was reported to produce malignant hypertension in chicks.[126] Sasaki and Buñag[127] combined hypertension with diabetes by implanting silicon rubber molds containing 50 mg/kg DOCA in Sprague-Dawley rats. After 1 week, the left kidney was removed from the rats, and the rats were given 0.9% saline to drink in place of water. At about 7 weeks of age, diabetes was induced with 50 mg/kg STZ; 4 weeks after implantation of DOCA, blood pressure was elevated to about 160 mmHg. Hebden et al.[128] reasoned that in hypertensive patients with diabetes, hypertension more commonly develops subsequently to diabetes. Thus, these authors induced diabetes in Wistar rats with 55 mg/kg STZ; after diabetes had been confirmed, 25 mg/kg DOCA was injected into the rats and they were started on saline (0.9%) instead of water. The DOCA injections were repeated twice weekly throughout the study. By 6 weeks, the systolic/diastolic blood pressures, measured by a catheter into the abdominal aorta, were 188/131 for the control-hypertensive and 189/138 for the diabetic-hypertensive groups. These authors reported that the DOCA-hypertension-producing treatment resulted in a somewhat reduced plasma glucose levels in the diabetic-hypertensive group (14.1 mM glucose diabetic-hypertensive compared with 22.4 mM diabetic). This partial amelioration of the hyperglycemia was not accompanied by an increase in plasma insulin, nor was there an improvement in the plasma lipid levels in the diabetic-hypertensive group. In fact, levels of triglycerides, phospholipids, and cholesterol in the diabetic-hypertensive group were significantly greater than all the other groups. Atherosclerotic changes were seen in the blood vessels from both the control-hypertensive and diabetic-hypertensive groups. A subsequent study by the same group[129] confirmed the findings that plasma triglyceride and cholesterol were elevated in diabetic-hypertensive rats compared with diabetic, control, or control-hypertensive groups. After 6 weeks of hypertensive diabetes, the animals had a glucose tolerance that was improved compared with that of the diabetic group, but was still worse than the control groups. In addition, the control animals rendered hypertensive with the DOCA treatment released less insulin following an oral glucose challenge than the control animals that were normotensive. The improvement in the plasma glucose levels of STZ diabetic DOCA-hypertensive rats compared with STZ diabetic rats has not always been seen. Tilton et al.[130] found no difference in plasma glucose levels following 1, 2, or 3 months of DOCA-hypertension STZ diabetes compared with STZ diabetes alone in male Sprague-Dawley rats made diabetic with 60 mg/kg STZ. The only obvious difference in the methodology compared with the studies where plasma glucose levels were reduced by the treatment[128,129,131] was the use of nephrectomy in the latter study. The authors of the studies where DOCA-hypertension combined with STZ diabetes partially ameliorated the hyperglycemia[128,129,131] suggest that the DOCA treatment may improve insulin sensitivity. That insulin sensitivity is improved is suggested by the fact that the release of insulin during an oral glucose tolerance test was reduced in the DOCA-treated nondiabetic rats.[131] However, no mechanism for the improvement in insulin sensitivity was suggested.

9.11   Herbal Medicines

Many countries, especially in the developing world, have a long history of the use of herbal remedies in diabetes and many other diseases and many schools of medicine or pharmacy offer courses in pharmacognosy. Active research programs continue to be carried out. Thus, STZ diabetic rats have been used extensively in the testing of these medicines. STZ diabetic mice and rabbits and the same species made diabetic with alloxan have been used, as well. It is not possible to discuss the entire literature within this chapter, so the discussion will focus on a few selected studies. Glombitza et al.[132] studied the butanol extract of *Zizyphus spina-christi* and a saponin glycoside isolated from the butanol extract. Male albino rats were made diabetic with STZ, then treated with the butanol extract or the saponin glycoside, administered orally for 1 or 4 weeks. Nondiabetic animals, treated similarly, showed no changes in plasma glucose or insulin at either 1 or 4 weeks, while both the butanol extract and, to a much smaller extent, the saponin glycoside isolated from it were able to reduce blood glucose from about 11.8 mM to about 7.1 mM or to 10.6 mM, respectively. A modest increase in insulin levels was seen in the diabetic rats treated with the butanol extract at 4 weeks. While the decrease in blood glucose with the saponin glycoside was modest, an oral glucose tolerance test at 4 weeks also indicated that both extracts resulted in an improvement in glucose tolerance. El-Fiky et al.[133] studied the acute effects of *Luffy aegyptiaca* (seeds) and *Carissa edulis* (leaves) extracts on male albino rats made diabetic with 40 mg/kg STZ. Only rats with moderate hyperglycemia (10 to 13 mM glucose) were used in the experiment. Extracts of the two plants were dissolved in dimethylsulfoxide and administered to the rats by oral gavage. Blood glucose levels were taken prior to the administration and out to 3 h past administration of the compounds and were compared with the glucose levels in rats receiving metformin. *L. aegyptiaca* and *C. edulis* decreased the blood glucose to about 7.4 and 8.9 mM, respectively, while 500 mg/kg metformin reduced blood glucose levels to about 6.9 mM. STZ diabetic rats were also used to test *Myrcia Uniflora* extracts in a 3-week treatment period.[134] The extracts were administered by oral gavage twice daily beginning 2 to 3 days after STZ administration. Blood glucose levels were reduced within 2 weeks of treatment from levels of about 34 mM to about 30 mM. Fluid intake, urine volume, and urine glucose content were all reduced by the treatment. The treatment had no effect on pancreatic insulin content at termination of the experiment, nor on plasma insulin levels. Al-Awadi et al.[135] investigated the effects of a mixture of nigella sativa, myrrh, gum arabic, gum asafoetida, and aloe, boiled in water for 10 min. The authors state that this is a mixture in common use among Kuwaitis with diabetes. Diabetes was induced in male Wistar rats with 60 mg/kg STZ, following which the rats received daily insulin injections for 7 days before the 1 week treatment with the plant extract. Fasting blood glucose in the diabetic rats was reduced from about 16 mM to about 9 mM by the treatment, and fasting blood glucose was also slightly reduced in the nondiabetic rats. The sum of the fasting, 1-h, and 2-h glucose values following an oral glucose challenge was reduced from 58.6 to 44.5 mM. The extract had no effect on serum insulin levels during the glucose tolerance test nor was the intestinal absorption of glucose altered by the treatment. *Eugenia jambolana*, a subtropical fruit in India prescribed by Indian Ayurvedic Vaidas to people with diabetes as both a fruit pickle and as a seed powder was assessed in STZ diabetic rabbits.[136] The jambolan seed powder reduced mean blood sugars in the rabbits to values similar to that seen with phenformin administration. Serum cholesterol, FFAs, and triglyceride levels were all reduced to normal by both the jambolan seed and the phenformin treatment. In all, 11 different plants[137] were administered to STZ diabetic mice in food (6.25% by weight of diet) and in drinking water prior to induction of diabetes and continued for 30 days following induction of diabetes. Agrimony, alfalfa, coriander, eucalyptus, and juniper all lowered mean values for basal plasma glucose in the diabetic mice but had no effect on normal mice, whereas blackberry, celandine, garlic, lady's mantle, lily of the valley, and licorice had no effects on either diabetic or normal mice.

9.12 Conclusion

This chapter has looked at many of the therapeutic interventions for diabetes that have been examined in STZ diabetic rats. The list of cited agents is by no means exhaustive. This model is useful for examining acute effects following single administrations of an agent as well as chronic effects. Chronic treatment has some times been as short as a few days, but has also been carried out for a year or longer. Some of the treatments examined are normal human nutrients, for example, the vitamins and trace elements. In these cases, several studies have attempted to examine whether a deficiency occurs in diabetes and the effect of supplementation to correct that deficiency. However, there is no clear-cut difference between supplementation and pharmacological intervention.

Several of the complications of diabetes occur in STZ diabetic rats and treatment interventions can be focused on particular organs, such as the eye. STZ diabetes can also be combined with other conditions that occur frequently in humans with diabetes, especially hypertension. In these cases treatment interventions can be examined for their effects on both conditions.

Although the STZ diabetic rat is a highly useful model, investigators must be aware of its limitations. Most usually, the dose of STZ to induce diabetes is such that there are residual functioning β-cells in the pancreas, allowing the animal to survive without exogenous insulin (see Chapter 1). Thus, the STZ diabetic rat is a model of hypoinsulinemic diabetes rather than a model of completely insulin-dependent diabetes. The residual insulin-secreting capacity is an advantage in that the animals are easier to maintain than completely insulin-dependent animals.

Acknowledgments

The studies described in the chapter from the authors' laboratory were supported by operating grants from the Medical Research Council of Canada, the Heart and Stroke Foundation of B. C. and Yukon, and the Canadian Diabetes Association (J. H. McNeill) and the Canadian Diabetes Association (B. Rodrigues). The financial support of the Canadian Diabetes Association (scholarship to B. Rodrigues) is gratefully acknowledged; as well as the secretarial assistance of Sylvia Chan.

References

1. Lopaschuk, G. D., Tahiliani, A., Vadlamudi, R. V. S. V., and McNeill, J. H., Cardiac sarcoplasmic reticulum function in insulin- or carnitine-treated diabetic rats, *Am. J. Physiol.*, 245, H969, 1983.
2. Tahiliani, A., Lopaschuk, G. D., and McNeill, J. H., Effect of insulin treatment on long-term diabetes-induced alteration of myocardial function, *Gen. Pharmacol.*, 15, 545, 1984.
3. Bhimji, S., Godin, D. V., and McNeill, J. H., Insulin reversal of biochemical changes in hearts from diabetic rats, *Am. J. Physiol.*, 251, H670, 1986.
4. Cam, M. C., Cros, G. H., Serrano, J.-J., Lazaro, R., and McNeill, J. H., *In vivo* antidiabetic actions of Naglivan, an organic vanadyl compound in streptozotocin-induced diabetes, *Diabetes Res. Clin. Pract.*, 20, 111, 1993.
5. Tahiliani, A., Vadlamudi, R. V. S. V., and McNeill, J. H., Prevention and reversal of altered myocardial function in diabetic rats by insulin treatment, *Can. J. Physiol. Pharmacol.*, 61, 516, 1983.
6. McGrath, G. M. and McNeill, J. H., Cardiac ultrastructural changes in streptozotocin-induced diabetic rats: effects of insulin treatment, *Can. J. Cardiol.*, 2, 164, 1986.
7. Lopaschuk, G. D., Tahiliani, A., and McNeill, J. H., Continuous long-term insulin delivery in diabetic rats utilizing implanted osmotic minipumps, *J. Pharmacol. Meth.*, 9, 71, 1983.
8. Rodrigues, B., personal communication, 1998.
9. Brichard, S. M., Lederer, J., and Henquin, J. C., The insulin-like properties of vanadium: a curiosity or a perspective for the treatment of diabetes? *Diabete Metab.*, 17, 435, 1991.
10. Cros, G., Mongold, J.-J., Serrano, J.-J., Ramanadhum, and McNeill, J. H., Effects of vanadyl derivatives on animal models of diabetes, *Mol. Cell. Biochem.*, 109, 163, 1992.
11. Orvig, C., Thompson, K. H., Battell, M., and McNeill, J. H., Vanadium compounds as insulin mimics, in *Metal Ions in Biological Systems*, Vol. 31, Sigel, H. and Sigel, A., Eds., Marcel Dekker, Basel, 1995, Chap. 17.
12. Brichard, S. M. and Henquin, J. C., The role of vanadium in the treatment of diabetes, *Trends Pharmacol. Sci.*, 16, 265, 1995.
13. Verma, S., Cam, M. C., and McNeill I. H., Nutritional factors that can favorably influence the glucose/insulin system: vanadium, *J. Am. Coll. Nutr.*, 1, 11, 1998.
14. Heyliger, C. E., Tahiliani, A. G., and McNeill, J. H., Effect of vanadate on elevated blood glucose and depressed cardiac performance of diabetic rats, *Science*, 227, 1474, 1985.
15. Meyerovitch, J., Farfel, Z., Sack, J., and Shechter, Y., Oral administration of vanadate normalizes blood glucose levels in streptozotocin-treated rats, *J. Biol. Chem.*, 262, 6658, 1987.
16. Ramanadhum, S., Cros, G. H., Mongold, J.-J., Serrano, J.-J., and McNeill, J. H., Enhanced *in vivo* sensitivity of vanadyl treated diabetic rats to insulin, *Can. J. Physiol. Pharmacol.*, 68, 486, 1990.
17. McNeill, J. H., Yuen, V. G., Hoveyda, H. R., and Orvig, C., Bis(maltolato)oxovanadium(IV) is a potent insulin mimic, *J. Med. Chem.*, 35, 1489, 1992.
18. Yuen, V. G., Orvig, C., and McNeill, J. H., Glucose lowering effects of a new organic vanadium complex, bis(maltolato)oxovanadium(IV), *Can. J. Physiol. Pharmacol.*, 71, 263, 1993.
19. Yuen, V. G., Orvig, C., and McNeill, J. H., Comparison of the glucose-lowering properties of vanadyl sulfate and bis(maltolato)oxovanadium(IV) following acute and chronic administration, *Can. J. Physiol. Pharmacol.*, 73, 55, 1995.
20. Sakurai, H., Tsuchiya, K., Nukatsuka, M., Kawada, J., Ishikawa, S., Yoshida, H., and Komatsu, M., Insulin-mimetic action of vanadyl complexes, *J. Clin. Biochem. Nutr.*, 8, 193, 1990.
21. Fujimoto, S., Fujii, K., Yasui, H., Matsushita, R., Takada, J., and Sakurai, H., Long-term acting and orally active vanadyl-methylpicolinate complex with hypoglycemic activity in streptozotocin-induced diabetic rats, *J. Clin. Biochem. Nutr.*, 23, 113, 1997.
22. Yuen, V. G., Caravan, P., Gelmini, L., Glover, N., McNeill, J. H., Setyawati, I. A., Zhou, Y., and Orvig, C., Glucose lowering properties of vanadium compounds: comparison of coordination complexes with maltol or kojic acid as ligands, *J. Inorg. Biochem.*, 68, 109, 1997.

23. Yale, J.-F., Lachance, D., Bevan, A. P., Vigeant, C., Shaver, A., and Posner, B. I., Hypoglycemic effects of peroxovanadium compounds in Sprague-Dawley and diabetic BB rats, *Diabetes*, 44, 1274, 1995.

24. Shisheva, A., Ikonomov, O., and Shechter, Y., The protein tyrosine phosphatase inhibitor, pervanadate, is a powerful antidiabetic agent in streptozotocin-treated diabetic rats, *Endocrinology*, 134, 507, 1994.

25. Ramanadhum, S., Brownsey, R. W., Cros, G. H., Mongold, J.-J., and McNeill, J. H., Sustained prevention of myocardial abnormalities in diabetic rats following withdrawal from oral vanadyl treatment, *Metabolism*, 38, 1022, 1989.

26. Dai, S., Thompson, K. H., and McNeill, J. H., One-year treatment of streptozotocin-induced diabetic rats with vanadyl sulfate, *Pharmacol. Toxicol.*, 74, 101, 1994.

27. Ugazio, G., Bosia, S., Burdino, E., and Grignolo, F., Amelioration of diabetes and cataract by Na$_3$VO$_4$ plus U-83836E in streptozotocin treated rats, *Res. Commun. Mol. Pathol. Pharmacol.*, 85, 313 1994.

28. Yuen, V. G., Orvig, C., Thompson, K. H., and McNeill, J. H., Improvement in cardiac dysfunction in streptozotocin-induced diabetic rats following chronic oral administration of bis(maltolato)oxovanadium(IV), *Can. J. Physiol. Pharmacol.*, 71, 270, 1993.

29. Dai, S., Thompson, K. H., Vera, E., and McNeill, J. H., Toxicity studies on one-year treatment of nondiabetic and streptozotocin diabetic rats with vanadyl sulfate, *Pharmacol. Toxicol.*, 75, 265, 1994.

30. Thompson, K. H., Battell, M. L., and McNeill, J. H., Toxicology of vanadium in mammals, in *Vanadium in the Environment*, Vol. 31, Nriagu, Ed., John Wiley & Sons, New York, 1998, 21.

31. Dai, S., Yuen, V. G., Orvig, C., and McNeill, J. H., Prevention of diabetes-induced pathology in STZ diabetic rats by bis(maltolato)oxovanadium(IV), *Pharmacol. Commun.* 3, 311, 1993.

32. Dai, S. and McNeill, J. H., One-year treatment of nondiabetic and streptozotocin-diabetic rats with vanadyl sulfate did not alter blood pressure or haematological indices, *Pharmacol. Toxicol.*, 74, 110, 1994.

33. Dai, S., Vera, E., and McNeill, J. H., Lack of haematological effect of oral vanadium treatment in rats, *Pharmacol. Toxicol.*, 76, 263, 1995.

34. Cam, M. C., Faun, J., and McNeill, J. H., Concentration-dependent glucose lowering effects of vanadyl are maintained following treatment withdrawal in streptozotocin diabetic rats, *Metabolism*, 44, 332, 1995.

35. Bevan, A. P., Drake, P. G., Yale, J.-F., Shaver, A., and Posner, B. I., Peroxovanadium compounds: biological actions and mechanism of insulin-mimesis, *Mol. Cell. Biochem.*, 153, 49, 1995.

36. Goldfine, A. B., Simonson, D. C., Folli, F., Patti, M.-E., and Kahn, C. R., Metabolic effects of sodium metavanadate in humans with insulin-dependent and noninsulin-dependent diabetes mellitus *in vivo* and *in vitro* studies, *J. Clin. Endocrinol. Metab.*, 80, 3311, 1995.

37. Cohen, N., Halberstam, M., Shlimovich, P., Chang, C. J., Shamoon, H., and Rossetti, L., Oral vanadyl sulfate improves hepatic and peripheral insulin sensitivity in patients with noninsulin-dependent diabetes mellitus, *J. Clin. Invest.*, 95, 2501, 1995.

38. Halberstam, M., Cohen, N., Shlimovich, P., Rossetti, L., and Shamoon, H., Oral vanadyl sulfate improves insulin sensitivity in NIDDM but not in obese nondiabetic subjects, *Diabetes*, 45, 659, 1996.

39. Boden, G., Chen, X., Ruiz, J., van Rossum, G. D. V., and Turco, S., Effects of vanadyl sulfate on carbohydrate and lipid metabolism in patients with noninsulin-dependent diabetes mellitus, *Metabolism*, 45, 1130, 1996.

40. Verma, S. and McNeill, J. H., Metformin improves cardiac function in isolated streptozotocin diabetic rat hearts, *Am. J. Physiol.*, 266, H714, 1994.

41. Ezaki, O., The insulin like effects of selenate in rat adipocytes, *J. Biol. Chem.*, 265, 1124, 1990.

42. Hei, Y. J., Farabahkshian, S., Chen, X., Battell, M. L., and McNeill, J. H., Stimulation of MAP kinase and S6 kinase by vanadium and selenium in rat adipocytes, *Mol. Cell. Biochem.*, 178, 367, 1998.

43. McNeill, J. H., Delgatty, H. L. M., and Battell, M. L., Insulin-like effects of sodium selenate in streptozotocin-induced diabetes in rats, *Diabetes*, 40, 1675, 1991.

44. Becker, D. J., Reul, B., Ozcelikay, A. T., Buchet, J. P., Henquin, J.-C., and Brichard, S. M., Oral selenate improves glucose homeostasis and partly reverses abnormal expression of liver glycolytic and gluconeogenic enzymes in diabetic rats, *Diabetologia*, 39, 3, 1996.
45. Battell, M. L., Delgatty, H. M. L., and McNeill, J. H., Sodium selenate corrects glucose tolerance and heart function in STZ diabetic rats, *Mol. Cell. Biochem.*, 179, 27, 1998.
46. Iizuki, Y., Sakurai, E., and Hikichi, N., Effects of selenium on the serum glucose and insulin levels in diabetic rats, *Nippon Yakurigaku Zasshi Folia Pharmacol. Jpn.*, 100, 151, 1992.
47. Ghosh, R., Mukherjee, B., and Chatterjee, M., A novel effect of selenium on streptozotocin-induced diabetic mice, *Diabetes Res.*, 25, 165, 1994.
48. Rotruck, J. T., Pope, A. L., Ganther, H. E., Swanson, A. B., Hafeman, D. G., and Hoekstra, W. G., Selenium: biochemical role as a component of glutathione peroxidase, *Science*, 179, 588, 1973.
49. Oberley, L. W., Free radicals and diabetes, *Free Radical Biol. Med.*, 5, 113, 1988.
50. Baynes, J. W., Perspectives in diabetes, role of oxidative stress in development of complications in diabetes, *Diabetes*, 40, 405, 1991.
51. Dohi, T., Kawamura, K., Morita, K., Okamoto, H., and Tsujimoto, A., Alterations of plasma selenium concentrations and the activities of tissue peroxide metabolism enzymes in streptozotocin-induced diabetic rats, *Horm. Metab. Res.*, 20, 671, 1988.
52. Gebre-Medhin, M., Ewald, U., Plantin, L., and Tuvemo, T., Elevated serum selenium in diabetic children, *Acta Paediatr. Scand.*, 73, 109, 1984.
53. Rossetti, L., Normalization of insulin sensitivity with lithium in diabetic rats, *Diabetes*, 38, 648, 1989.
54. Srivastava, P., Saxena, A. K., Kale, R. K., and Baquer, N. Z., Insulin-like effects of lithium and vanadate on the altered antioxidant status of diabetic rats, *Res. Commun. Chem. Pathol. Pharmacol.*, 80, 283, 1993.
55. Rossetti, L., Giaccari, A., Klein-Robbenhaar, E., and Vogel, L. R., Insulinomimetic properties of trace elements and characterization of their *in vivo* mode of action, *Diabetes*, 39, 1243, 1990.
56. Hermida, O. G., Fontela, T., Ghiglione, M., and Uttenthal, L. O., Effect of lithium on plasma glucose, insulin, and glucagon in normal and streptozotocin-diabetic rats: role of glucagon in the hyperglycaemic response, *Br. J. Pharmacol.*, 111, 861, 1994.
57. Shah, J. H. and Pishdad, G., The effect of lithium on glucose- and tolbutamide-induced insulin release and glucose tolerance in the intact rat, *Endocrinology*, 107, 1300, 1980.
58. Potmis, R. A., Nonavinakere, V. K., Rasekh, H. R., and Early, J. L., II, Effect of selenium on plasma ACTH, β-endorphin, corticosterone, and glucose in rats: influence of adrenal enucleation and metyrapone pretreatment, *Toxicology*, 79, 1, 1993.
59. Etzel, K. R. and Cousins, R. J., Hyperglycemic action of zinc in rats, *J. Nutr.*, 113, 1657, 1983.
60. Shisheva, A., Gefel, D., and Shechter, Y., Insulinlike effects of zinc ion *in vitro* and *in vivo*. Preferential effects on desensitized adipocytes and induction of normoglycemia in streptozotocin-induced rats, *Diabetes*, 41, 982, 1992.
61. Sjogren, A., Edvinson, L., Floren, C. H., and Abdulla, M., Zinc and copper in striated muscle and body fluids from subjects with diabetes mellitus Type 1, *Nutr. Res.*, 6, 147, 1986.
62. Raz, A. and Havivi, E., Influence of chronic diabetes on tissue and blood cells status of zinc, copper, and chromium in the rat, *Diabetes Res.*, 7, 19, 1988.
63. Failla, M. L. and Kiser, R. A., Hepatic and renal metabolism of copper and zinc in the diabetic rat, *Am. J. Physiol.*, 244, E115, 1983.
64. Johnson, W. T. and Canfield, W. K., Intestinal absorption and excretion of zinc in streptozotocin-diabetic rats as affected by dietary zinc and protein, *J. Nutr.*, 115, 1217, 1985.
65. Thompson. K. H., Mehr-Rahimi, B., and McNeill, J. H., Magnesium supplementation of STZ diabetic rats. Lack of effect on diabetic cardiomyopathy, *Magnesium Bull.*, 16, 4, 1994.
66. Özcelikay, A. T., Becker, D. J., Ongemba, L. N., Pottier, A.-M., Henquin, J.-C., and Brichard, S. M., Improvement of glucose and lipid metabolism in diabetic rats treated with molybdate, *Am. J. Physiol.*, 270, E344, 1996.
67. Li, J., Elberg, G., Gefel, D., and Shechter, Y., Permolybdate and pertungstate — potent stimulators of insulin effects in rat adipocytes: mechanism of action, *Biochemistry*, 34, 6218, 1995.
68. Wallach, S., Clinical and biochemical aspects of chromium deficiency, *J. Am. Coll. Nutr.*, 4, 107, 1985.

69. Mertz, W., Chromium in human nutrition: a review, *J. Nutr.*, 123, 626, 1993.
70. Mirsky, N., Glucose tolerance factor reduces blood glucose and free fatty acids levels in diabetic rats, *J. Inorg. Biochem.*, 49, 123, 1993.
71. Yoshimoto, S., Sakamoto, K., Wakabayashi, I., and Masui, H., Effect of chromium administration on glucose tolerance in stroke prone spontaneously hypertensive rats with streptozotocin-induced diabetes, *Metabolism*, 41, 636, 1992.
72. Stankova, L., Riddle, M., Larned, J., Burry, K., Menashe, D., Hart, J., and Bigley, R., Plasma ascorbate and blood cell dehydroascorbate transport in patients with diabetes mellitus, *Metab. Clin. Exp.*, 33, 347, 1984.
73. Som, S., Basu, S., Mukherjee, D., Deb, S., Roy Choudhury, P., Mukherjee, S., Chatterjee, S. N., and Chatterjee, I. B., Ascorbic acid metabolism in diabetes mellitus, *Metabolism*, 30, 572, 1981.
74. Yue, D. K., McLennan, S., McGill, M., Fisher, E., Heffernan, S., Capogreco, C., and Turtle, J. R., Abnormalities of ascorbic acid metabolism and diabetic control: differences between diabetic patients and diabetic rats, *Diabetes Res. Clin. Pract.*, 9, 239, 1990.
75. Cunningham, J. J., Ellis, S. L., McVeigh, K. L., Levine, R. E., and Calles-Escandon, J., Reduced mononuclear leukocyte ascorbic acid content in adults with insulin-dependent diabetes mellitus consuming adequate dietary vitamin C, *Metab. Clin. Exp.*, 40, 146, 1991.
76. Moser, U., Uptake of ascorbic acid by leukocytes, *Ann. N.Y. Acad. Sci.*, 498, 200, 1987.
77. Paolisso, G., Balbi, V., Volpe, C., Varricchio, G., Gambardella, A., Saccomanno, F., Ammendola, S., Varricchio, A., and D'Onofrio, F., Metabolic benefits deriving from chronic vitamin C supplementation in aged noninsulin dependent diabetics, *J. Am. Coll. Nutr.*, 14, 387, 1995.
78. Eriksson, J. and Kohvakka, A., Magnesium and ascorbic acid supplementation in diabetes mellitus, *Ann. Nutr. Metab.*, 39, 217, 1995.
79. Yue, D. K., McLennan, S., Fisher, E., Heffernan, S., Capogreco, C., Ross, G. R., and Turtle, J. R., Ascorbic acid metabolism and polyol pathway in diabetes, *Diabetes*, 38, 257, 1989.
80. Young, I. S., Tate, S., Lightbody, J. H., McMaster, D., and Trimble, E. R., The effects of desferrioxamine and ascorbate on oxidative stress in the streptozotocin diabetic rat, *Free Radical Biol. Med.*, 18, 833, 1995.
81. Kowluru, R. A., Kern, T. S., Engerman, R. L., and Armstrong, D., Abnormalities of retinal metabolism in diabetes or experimental galactosemia. III. Effects of antioxidants, *Diabetes*, 45, 1233, 1996.
82. Clarke, J., Snelling, J., Ioannides, C., Flatt, P. R., and Barnett, C. R., Effect of vitamin C supplementation on hepatic cytochrome P450 mixed-function oxidase activity in streptozotocin-diabetic rats, *Toxicol. Lett.*, 89, 249, 1996.
83. Mekinová, D., Chorváthová, V., Volkovová, K., Staruchová, M., Grancicová, E., Klvanová, J., and Ondreicka, R., Effect of intake of exogenous vitamin C, E, and β-carotene on the antioxidative status in kidneys of rats with streptozotocin-induced diabetes, *Nahrung*, 39, 257, 1995.
84. Yew, M. S., Effect of streptozotocin diabetes on tissue ascorbic acid and dehydroascorbic acid, *Horm. Metab. Res.*, 15, 158, 1983.
85. Cotter, M. A., Love, A., Watt, M. J., Cameron, N. E., and Dines, K. C., Effects of natural free radical scavengers on peripheral nerve and neurovascular function in diabetic rats, *Diabetologia*, 38, 1285, 1995.
86. Jones, R. H. V. and Hothersall, J. S., The effects of diabetes and dietary ascorbate supplementation on the oxidative modification of rat lens β_L crystallin, *Biochem. Med. Metab. Biol.*, 50, 197, 1993.
87. Gembal, M., Druzynska, J., Kowalczyk, M., Przepiera, Cybal, M., Arendarczyk, W., Wojcikowski, Cz., The effect of ascorbic acid on protein glycation in streptozotocin-diabetic rats, *Diabetologia*, 37, 731, 1994.
88. Dai, S. and McNeill. J. H., Ascorbic acid supplementation prevents hyperlipidemia and improves myocardial performance in streptozotocin diabetic rats, *Diabetes Res. Clin. Pract.*, 27, 11, 1995.
89. Niki, E., Interaction of ascorbate and α-tocopherol, *Ann. N.Y. Acad. Sci.*, 498, 186, 1987.
90. Nishigaki, I., Hagihara, M., Tsunekawa, H., Maseki, M., and Yagi, K., Lipid peroxide levels of serum lipoprotein fractions of diabetic patients, *Biochem. Med.*, 25, 373, 1981.

91. Jennings, P. E., Jones, A. F., Florkowski, C. M., Lunec, J., and Barnett, A. H., Increased diene conjugates in diabetic subjects with microangiopathy, *Diabetic Med.*, 4, 452, 1987.

92. Hiramatsu, K., and Arimori, S., Increased superoxide production by mononuclear cells of patients with hypertriglyceridemia and diabetes, *Diabetes*, 37, 832, 1988.

93. Velaquez, E., Winocour, P. H., Kesteven, P., Alberti, K. G., and Laker, M. F., Relation of lipid peroxides to macrovascular disease in Type II diabetes, *Diabetes Med.*, 8, 752, 1991.

94. Aoki, Y., Yanagisawa, Y., Yazaki, K., Oguchi, H., Kiyosawa, K., and Furuta, S., Protective effect of vitamin E supplementation on increased thermal stability of collagen in diabetic rats, *Diabetologia*, 35, 913, 1992.

95. Nickander, K., Schmelzer, J. D., Rohwer, D. A., and Low, P. A., Effect of α-tocopherol deficiency on indices of oxidative stress in normal and diabetic peripheral nerve, *J. Neurol. Sci.*, 126, 5, 1994.

96. Keegan, A., Walbank, H., Cotter, M. A., and Cameron, N. E., Chronic vitamin E treatment prevents defective endothelium-dependent relaxation in diabetic rat aorta, *Diabetologia*, 38, 1475, 1995.

97. Rösen, P., Ballhausen, T., Bloch, W., and Addicks, K., Endothelial relaxation is disturbed by oxidative stress in the diabetic rat heart: influence of tocopherol as antioxidant, *Diabetologia*, 38, 1157, 1995.

98. Kunisaki, M., Bursell, S.-E., Clermont, A. C., Ishii, H., Balas, L. M., Jirousek, M. R., Umeda, F., Nawata, H., and King, G. L., Vitamin E prevents diabetes-induced abnormal retinal blood flow via the diacylglycerol-protein kinase C pathway, *Am. J. Physiol.*, 269, E239, 1995.

99. Sivan, E., Reece, E. A., Wu, Y.-K., Homko, C. J., Polansky, M., and Borenstein, M., Dietary vitamin E prophylaxis and diabetic embryopathy: morphologic and biochemical analysis, *Am. J. Obstet. Gynecol.*, 175, 793, 1996.

100. Viana, M., Herrera, E., and Bonet, B., Teratogenic effects of diabetes mellitus in the rat. Prevention by vitamin E, *Diabetologia*, 39, 1041, 1996.

101. Trachtman, H., Futterweit, S., Maesaka, J., Ma, C., Valderrama, E., Fuchs, A., Tarectecan, A. A., Rao, P. S., Sturman, J. A., Boles, T. H., Fu, M.-X., and Baynes, J., Taurine ameliorates chronic streptozotocin-induced diabetic nephropathy in rats, *Am. J. Physiol.*, 269, F429, 1995.

102. Rodrigues, B., Xiang, H., and McNeill, J. H., Effect of L-carnitine treatment on lipid metabolism and cardiac performance in chronically diabetic rats, *Diabetes*, 37, 1358, 1988.

103. Rodrigues, B., Goyal, R. K., and McNeill, J. H., Effects of hydralazine on streptozotocin-induced diabetic rats: prevention of hyperlipidemia and improvement in cardiac function, *J. Pharmacol. Exp. Ther.*, 237, 292, 1986.

104. Rodrigues, B., Grassby, P. F., Battell, M. L., Lee, S. Y. N., and McNeill, J. H., Hypertriglyceridemia in experimental diabetes: relationship to cardiac dysfunction, *Can. J. Physiol. Pharmacol.*, 72, 447, 1994.

105. Schein, P. S., Cooney, D. A., and Vernon, M. L., The use of nicotinamide to modify the toxicity of streptozotocin diabetes without loss of antitumor activity, *Cancer Res.*, 27, 2324, 1967.

106. Junod, A., Lambert, A. E., Stauffacher, W., and Renold, A. E., Diabetogenic action of streptozotocin: relationship of dose to metabolic response, *J. Clin. Invest.*, 48, 2129, 1969.

107. Yamamoto, H., Uchigata, Y., and Okamoto, H., Streptozotocin and alloxan induce DNA strand breaks and poly(ADP-ribose) synthetase in pancreatic islets, *Nature*, 294, 284, 1981.

108. Yamamoto, H., Uchigata, Y., and Okamoto, H., DNA strand breaks in pancreatic islets by *in vivo* administration of alloxan or streptozotocin, *Biochem. Biophys. Res. Commun.*, 103, 1014, 1981.

109. Uchigata, Y., Yamamoto, H., Kawamura, A., and Okamoto, H., Protection by superoxide dismutase, catalase, and poly(ADP-ribose) inhibitors against alloxan- and streptozotocin-induced islet DNA strand breaks and against the inhibition of proinsulin synthesis, *J. Biol. Chem.*, 257, 6084, 1982.

110. Uchigata, Y., Yamamoto, H., Nagai, H., and Okamoto, H., Effect of poly(ADP-ribose) synthetase inhibitor administration to rats before and after injection of alloxan and streptozotocin on islet proinsulin synthesis, *Diabetes*, 32, 316, 1983.

111. Barnett, C. R., Gibson, G. G., Wolf, R., and Flatt, P. R., Induction of cytochrome P450III and P450IV family of proteins in streptozotocin-induced diabetes, *Biochem. J.*, 268, 765, 1990.

112. Ballmann, M. and Conlon, J. M., Changes in the somatostatin, substance P and vasoactive intestinal polypeptide content of the gastrointestinal tract following streptozotocin-induced diabetes in the rat, *Diabetologia*, 28, 355, 1985.

113. Pugliese, G., Tilton, R. G., Speedy, A., Chang, K., Santarelli, E., Province, M. A., Eades, D., Sherman, W. R., and Williamson, J. R., Effects of very mild vs. overt diabetes on vascular haemodynamics and barrier function in rats, *Diabetologia*, 32, 845, 1989.

114. Rakieten, N., Gordon, B. S., Beaty, A., Cooney, D. A., Davis, R. D., and Schein, P. S., Pancreatic islet cell tumors produced by combined action of streptozotocin and nicotinamide, *Proc. Soc. Exp. Biol. Med.*, 137, 280, 1971.

115. Dixit, P. K., Bauer, E., Younoszai, R., and Hegre, O., Reversal of diabetes by the isotransplantation of nicotinamide-streptozotocin-induced islet adenoma in rats, *Transplantation*, 33, 163, 1982.

116. Novelli, E. L. B. and Rodrigues, N. L., Effect of nickel chloride on streptozotocin diabetes in rats, *Can. J. Physiol. Pharmacol.*, 66, 663, 1988.

117. Novelli, E. L. B., Rodrigues, N. L., and Ribas, B. O., Nickel chloride protection against alloxan- and streptozotocin-induced diabetes, *Braz. J. Med. Biol. Res.*, 21, 129, 1988.

118. Novelli, E. L. B., Rodrigues, N. L., and Ribas, B. O., Nickel chloride and diabetes II. Calcium, zinc, phosphorus and iron determinations in alloxan diabetic and in rats treated by nickel chloride injections, *Bol. Estud. Med. Biol. Mex.*, 35, 221, 1987.

119. Yang, J. and Cherian, M. G., Protective effects of metallothionein on streptozotocin-induced diabetes in rats, *Life Sci.*, 55, 43, 1994.

120. Thornalley, P. J. and Vasak., M., Possible role for metallothionein in protection against radiation-induced oxidative stress. Kinetics and mechanism of its reaction with superoxide and hydroxyl radicals, *Biochem. Biophys. Acta*, 827, 36, 1985.

121. Mikhail, T. H. and Awadallah, R., The effect of ATP and certain trace elements on the induction of experimental diabetes, *Z. Ernährungswiss*, 16, 176, 1977.

122. Buñag, R. D., Tomita, T., and Sasaki, S., Streptozotocin diabetic rats are hypertensive despite reduced hypothalamic responsiveness, *Hypertension Dallas*, 4, 556, 1982.

123. Kawashima, H., Igarashi, T., Nakajima, Y., Akiyama, Y., Usuki, K., and Ohtake, S., Chronic hypertension induced by streptozotocin in rats, *Naunyn Schmiedebergs Arch. Pharmacol.*, 305, 123, 1978.

124. Kusaka, M., Kishi, K., and Sokabe, H., Does so called streptozotocin hypertension exist in rats? *Hypertension Dallas*, 10, 417, 1987.

125. Jackson, C. V. and Carrier, G. O., Influence of short-term experimental diabetes on blood pressure and heart rate response to norepinephrine and angiotensin II in the conscious rat, *J. Cardiovasc. Pharmacol.*, 5, 260, 1983.

126. Selye, H., Hall, C. E., and Rowley, E. M., Malignant hypertension produced by treatment with desoxycorticosterone acetate and sodium chloride, *Can. Med. Assoc. J.*, 49, 88, 1943.

127. Sasaki, S. and Buñag, R. D., Hypothalamic responsiveness in DOCA hypertensive rats augmented by streptozotocin-induced diabetes, *J. Cardiovasc. Pharmacol.*, 4, 1042, 1982.

128. Hebden, R. A., Todd, M. E., Tang, C., Gowen, B., and McNeill, J. H., Association of DOCA hypertension with induction of atherosclerosis in rats with short term diabetes mellitus, *Am. J. Physiol.*, 258, R1042, 1990.

129. Dai, S., Fraser, H., and McNeill, J. H., Effects of deoxycorticosterone acetate on glucose metabolism in nondiabetic and streptozotocin-diabetic rats, *Can. J. Physiol. Pharmacol.*, 70, 1468, 1992.

130. Tilton, R. G., Pugliese, G., Faller, A. M., LaRose, L. S., Province, M. A., and Williamson, J. R., Interactions between hypertension and diabetes on vascular function and structure in rats, *J. Diabetes Comp.*, 6, 187, 1992.

131. Dai, S. and McNeill, J. H., Myocardial performance of STZ diabetic DOCA-hypertensive rats, *Am. J. Physiol.*, 263, H1798, 1992.

132. Glombitza, K.-W., Mahran, G. H., Mirhom, Y. W., Michel, K. G., and Motawi, T. K., Hypoglycemic and antihyperglycemic effects of *Zizyphus spina-christi* in rats, *Planta Med.*, 60, 244, 1994.

133. El-Fiky, F. K., Abou-Karam, M. A., and Afify, E. A., Effect of *Luffy aegyptiaca* (seeds) and *Carissa edulis* (leaves) extracts on blood glucose level of normal and streptozotocin diabetic rats, *J. Ethnopharmacol.*, 50, 43, 1996.

134. Pepato, M. T., Oliveira, J. R., Kettelhut, I. C., and Migliorini, R. H., Assessment of the antidiabetic activity of *Myrcia uniflora* extracts in streptozotocin diabetic rats, *Diabetes Res.*, 22, 49, 1993.
135. Al-Awadi, F. M., Khattar, M. A., and Gumaa, K. A., On the mechanism of the hypoglycemic effect of a plant extract, *Diabetologia*, 28, 432, 1985.
136. Kedar, P. and Chakrabarti, C. H., Effects of jambolan seed treatment on blood sugar, lipids and urea in streptozotocin induced diabetes in rabbits, *Ind. J. Physiol. Pharmacol.*, 27, 135, 1983.
137. Swanston-Flatt, S. K., Day, C., Bailey, C. J., and Flatt, P. R., Traditional plant treatments for diabetes. Studies in normal and streptozotocin diabetic mice, *Diabetologia*, 33, 462, 1990.

Section II

Other Experimental Models
of Diabetes

10

Other Models of Type I Diabetes

Mary L. Battell, Violet G. Yuen, Subodh Verma, and John H. McNeill

CONTENTS

10.1 Introduction

In this chapter the chemical and surgical induction of Type I diabetes models other than streptozotocin (STZ) diabetes will be discussed along with some comparisons to the more commonly used STZ diabetic model. The mechanism by which alloxan induces diabetes is considered, followed by a discussion of the nature of the diabetic state in rabbits where alloxan is widely used to study the long-term complications of diabetes. Alloxan is used to induce diabetes in numerous species, and the advantages and disadvantages as compared with STZ are discussed. Pancreatectomy is also used in a wide variety of species. This model is favoured in studies of pancreas and islet cell transplantation. Some of its advantages compared with chemical induction of diabetes are discussed. Dexamethasone can be used to induce models of both insulin-dependent and noninsulin-dependent diabetes. When investigators have wanted a model in which the mechanism of induction of diabetes includes, at least partly, the immune response that occurs in IDDM in humans, STZ combined with complete Freund's adjuvant has been used. The models discussed in this chapter are used to a lesser extent than STZ diabetes but are still very important.

10.2   Alloxan-Induced Diabetes

10.2.1   Mechanism of Induction of Diabetes by Alloxan

The mechanism by which alloxan results in diabetes in susceptible species has not been entirely clarified. It has been shown that alloxan has several effects on the β-cells of the pancreas, and it is likely that some combination of these effects results in the destruction of β-cells by alloxan. Reviews by Malaisse[1] and Lenzen and Panten[2] present two different proposals to explain the mechanism. Alloxan is a highly reactive molecule that is readily reduced to dialuric acid,[3] which is then auto-oxidized back to alloxan resulting in the production of H_2O_2, O_2, O_2^-, and hydroxy radical.[4] Alloxan has been shown to induce DNA strand breaks in isolated islets[5] and in islets following *in vivo* administration of alloxan.[6] More recent work has shown that the DNA fragmentation is mediated by H_2O_2.[7] The induction of DNA strand breaks activates nuclear poly(ADP-ribose) synthetase[5] resulting in depletion of cellular NAD levels.[5] Two factors appear to make the islet especially sensitive to the effects of alloxan; the first factor is that alloxan is rapidly taken up into islet cells,[8] and the second factor is the sensitivity of islets to peroxides.[9]

A second mechanism proposed for the diabetogenic effects of alloxan concerns its ability to react with protein sulfydryl (SH) groups. The proposed mechanism involves reaction of alloxan with the SH groups on glucokinase, a signal recognition enzyme in the pancreatic β-cell, which couples changes in blood glucose concentration to the rate of insulin secretion.[2,10,11] By this mechanism, inhibition of glucokinase and other SH-containing membrane proteins on the β-cell would eventually result in cell necrosis.[12,13] One of the effects of alloxan on the β-cell is the inhibition of glucose-stimulated insulin release,[14] and this is likely related to the inhibition of the glucokinase. As yet, however, there is no convincing evidence that the reaction of alloxan with protein SH groups would result in the cellular and nuclear necrosis that occur within minutes when alloxan induces diabetes in rabbits and other animals.[14,15]

A study of the effects of alloxan on glucose oxidation and viability of islets from humans, rats, and mice showed that there were major species differences in response to alloxan.[16] These species differences are further outlined below.

10.2.2   Alloxan-Induced Diabetes in Rabbits

Since the initial description in 1943 of alloxan-induced β-cell necrosis in rabbits,[17,18] this compound has continued to be used to induce experimental diabetes. This model produces typical signs of diabetes and characteristic long-term complications involving the eye,[19,20] heart,[21] cardiovascular system,[22] and kidney.[23] The major drawback of this model is the difficulty in determining a dose of alloxan that will produce sustained diabetes in rabbits without mortality. There is a great variation in the susceptibility of individual animals to alloxan, and mortality may occur because of the marked hypoglycemia that follows about 6 h after the injection of alloxan,[17,23] as well as because of the hyperglycemia that occurs in the week following injection of alloxan.[23] These problems continued to be reported with this model as late as 1987 when Zhao et al.[24] reported that doses of 60 to 100 mg/kg produced one of four responses; long-term hyperglycemia, temporary hyperglycemia, no hyperglycemia, or death. Remarkably, some rabbits were able to withstand repeated increasing doses of alloxan without development of hyperglycemia. Table 10.1 summarizes the results of various doses of alloxan used in the study by Zhao et al. and outlines two

TABLE 10.1

Results of Various Doses of Alloxan in Rabbits

Dose (mg/kg)	No. of Rabbits	Long-Term Hyperglycemia	Temporary Hyperglycemia	No Hyperglycemia	Death
1. Zhao et al.[24]					
60	3	1	2	0	0
75	2	0	0	0	2
90	6	0	0	0	6
100	2	2	0	0	0
60 + 60	4	0	2	2	0
Multiple	6	0	4	2	0
2. McDowell et al.[25]					
90 to 100	21	9	1	9	2
3. Ingerman-Wojenski et al.[26]					
150	55	31	0	5	19

Notes:

1. Zhao et al.[24] Responses reported by Zhao et al. to various doses of alloxan monohydrate prepared fresh in sterile saline administered via marginal ear vein over 5 min. Long-term hyperglycemia, >19.3 mM glucose; no hyperglycemia, <11 mM over 5 days. Rabbits were followed for 10 weeks.

2. McDowell et al.[25] Results of injection of alloxan injected i.v. The hyperglycemic group had a mean blood glucose of 20.9 ± 1.2 mM, and the animals that did not develop hyperglycemia had a mean blood glucose of 6.57 ± 0.3 mM. All animals received a 5% solution of dextrose in water to drink overnight and two injections of 5 ml of a 50% solution of dextrose s.c. Rabbits were used 24 weeks later.

3. Ingerman-Wojenski et al.[26] The rabbits that received alloxan were given 0.6% glucose in water for 24 h. Rabbits were used 5 or 9 weeks later.

important findings. First, there is no correlation between increasing doses of alloxan and percentage of animals exhibiting sustained diabetes. Second, higher doses are not necessarily associated with higher mortality. The authors suggest that larger rabbits may be more susceptible to mortality resulting from alloxan injection. Table 10.1 also lists the observations from two other key studies.[25,26] At a dose of 90 to 100 mg/kg, McDowell et al.[25] reported that 43% of the rabbits become hyperglycemic over the long term, 43% exhibited no hyperglycemia, and 10% died. Ingerman-Wojenski et al.[26] using a dose of 150 mg/kg, reported that 56% exhibited hyperglycemia, 9% had no hyperglycemia, while 35% died.

The typical blood glucose curves that follow injection of alloxan were described by Howell and Taylor.[27] Alloxan injection (160 mg/kg i.v.) is followed by an initial rise in blood glucose at 2 h, followed by a drop to a nadir of about 2.75 mM at 8 h, then an increase to 16.6 mM at 24 h. During the hypoglycemic phase, insulin levels were about 150% of the mean control values. To allow animals to survive the hyperglycemia which begins at about 24 h, many workers have administered insulin to yield models with varying degrees of severity of diabetes. For example, Pollack et al.[28] administered a very low dose of insulin (average 1.7 U) to one group, which resulted in a severely diabetic but nonketotic state, whereas a higher dose (11.8 U) resulted in a well-controlled state of diabetes. O'Meara et al.[29] also treated two groups, which they call well controlled (7.5 U insulin per day) and poorly controlled (4.5 U insulin per day). In some cases, small amounts of insulin were given to a few rabbits to allow the animals in question to gain weight while maintaining a hyperglycemic blood glucose level.[25]

TABLE 10.2

Alloxan Diabetes in Rabbits

Strain	Sex	Weight (kg)	Dose, i.v. (mg/kg)	Glucose (mmol)	Duration	Outcome	Ref.
New Zealand	M	2.5–3.3	140–150 over 7 min.	28.2–31.9	To 6 months	25% mortality	28
(Intervention: 1–2 U/day insulin starting 2–3 days after alloxan in almost all rabbits)							
New Zealand	F	1.8–2.5	150 over 15 min.	>13.8	10 weeks	20% not diabetic, 15% mortality	63
(Intervention: 5% sucrose instead of drinking water for 24 h.)							
New Zealand	M	3.0–4.0	140	>22	19 days	—	29
(Intervention: insulin)							
New Zealand	M	3.5–3.8	65	17–21	To 6 months	0% mortality	22
(Intervention: glucose i.p. 2 times)							
New Zealand	M	2.2–2.5	150	19.9	6 weeks	20% not diabetic	64
New Zealand	M	1.5–2.5	100	23.3	10–12 weeks	—	21
(Intervention: 20% glucose, s. c. 4 to 6 times, NaCl, i.v.)							
Japanese	M	3.5–4.0	120	—	120 days	15% mortality, 20% not diabetic	19
(Intervention: 30% glucose injected when needed)							
New Zealand	M	9 weeks	110	13.8–19.3	10 weeks	66% stable diabetes, 34% temporary	20
New Zealand	M	3.5–3.8	65	17	5 weeks	0% mortality	65
(Intervention: glucose i.p.)							

Some of the doses of alloxan used and the interventions used to prevent death due to hypoglycemia are summarized in Table 10.2. To counter hypoglycemia, most workers administer glucose. Sodium chloride has also been used to prevent dehydration.[21]

One of the main reasons for the continued use of alloxan in rabbits is the relative ineffectiveness of STZ in rabbits. It was initially reported that STZ was not effective in rabbits[30,31] even at doses of 200 mg/kg. By contrast, some authors have reported elevated blood glucose levels and characteristic islet cell alterations following doses of 300 mg/kg[32] and at doses of 150 mg/kg to rabbits previously rendered hypoglycemic with insulin.[33] A dose of 65 mg/kg STZ injected intravenously into 24-h fasted rabbits has also been reported to result in weight loss, hyperlipidemia, and elevation of blood glucose to 12.7 mM.[34]

10.2.3   Alloxan Diabetes in Other Species

Alloxan has been used in a wide variety of species for the induction of experimental models of diabetes mellitus. These species include rodents, such as the rat and mouse, dogs, cats, and nonhuman primates. The literature available for primates is extremely limited and will be discussed only briefly.

Alloxan has typically been administered by three main routes: intravenous, intraperitoneal, and subcutaneous. The solutions of alloxan are acidic in nature; therefore, the preferred route of administration in most species is intravenous.[35] The doses required for the induction of diabetes vary between species and route of administration. In rats, the dose of alloxan ranges from 50 to 300 mg/kg depending on the route of administration.[36]

The lower dose range is typically administered by intravenous injection, while the higher dose is used primarily for subcutaneous injection. The dose range for the pigeon, cats, dogs, and monkeys is 65 to 200 mg/kg by intravenous injection.[36] Alloxan was found to be ineffective as a diabetogenic agent in ducks.[36]

A comparison of STZ- and alloxan-induction of diabetes in rats shows that alloxan has been associated with significantly higher mortality than STZ.[37] These authors point out that STZ may induce a diabetic state that more closely resembles that observed in many humans in that human patients with diabetes exhibit hyperglycemia usually in the absence of ketone body formation.[37] Alloxan-induced diabetes in rats is associated with an increase in free fatty acid levels and ketone bodies not seen in STZ diabetic animals.[37] On the other hand, studies aimed at examining immunodeficiency in mice revealed that alloxan had no detrimental effects on the lymphoid cells necessary for normal immune response.[38] Both STZ and alloxan induce similar states of hyperglycemia and hyperlipidemia; however, the rate of reversal of the diabetic state in mice is greater with alloxan than with STZ suggesting a less stable form of the diabetic state.[38]

Both STZ and alloxan have been utilized for the induction of diabetes mellitus in nonhuman primates (monkeys and baboons).[39] Monkeys respond with varying degrees of diabetes to a single dose of either diabetogenic agent and will, with time, develop overt diabetes requiring insulin therapy. The development of secondary complications such as retinopathy appears to be more rapid with alloxan than STZ. The most recent report of the use of alloxan in monkeys was in 1982.[39]

10.3 Pancreatectomy

The induction of diabetes mellitus can be achieved through the surgical removal of all or part of the pancreas. In the partial pancreatectomy more than 90% of the organ must be removed to produce some form of diabetes.[36] Depending upon the amount of intact pancreatic cells, diabetes may range in duration from a few days to several months.[40] Total removal of the pancreas results in an insulin-dependent form of diabetes, and insulin therapy is required to maintain experimental animals. The portion of the pancreas usually left intact following a subtotal pancreatic resection is typically the anterior lobe or a portion thereof.[40]

One advantage of the chemical induction of diabetes mellitus with agents such as STZ and alloxan is the maintenance of pancreatic function in cells other than the β-cell. The surgical removal of the pancreas results in the removal of not only the β-cell and loss of insulin secretory function but also removal of both the α- and δ-cells and the loss of the counterregulatory hormones glucagon and somatostatin. In addition, there is a loss of the pancreatic enzymes necessary for proper digestion; therefore, the diet for pancreatectomized animals must be supplemented with these pancreatic enzymes.[31-44]

The effectiveness of the induction of diabetes mellitus following a pancreatectomy is dependent to a degree on the identification of the pancreas and the ability to identify and preserve adequate segments of the organ. In animal species such as dogs,[45] pigs,[44] and nonhuman primates[46-48] the pancreas is a discrete organ that is readily isolated and resected. This is not the case with rodents such as the rat where the pancreas is a very diffuse organ. The total resection of the pancreas in rats is very difficult to achieve, and the development and severity of the diabetic state appear to be strain specific.[40]

In the rhesus monkey (*Macaca mulatta*), experiments have compared the diabetic state in pancreatectomized monkeys with STZ-induced diabetic monkey. A total pancreatectomy resulted in 100% development of diabetes, whereas STZ at doses of 30 to 55 mg/kg by intravenous administration was effective in only 50% of animals.[47] A comparison of the animals that did become diabetic following STZ administration and those that had undergone total pancreatectomy demonstrated no differences in the hyperglycemic level (19 to 24 m*M*), the dose of insulin required for treatment (4 U/day), glycosylated hemoglobin levels, or blood pressure. There was, however, a difference in lipid response in the two methods of diabetes induction. While triglyceride levels were elevated in both conditions, there was no elevation in cholesterol levels following a total pancreatectomy. STZ-induced diabetic monkeys, on the other hand, demonstrated an increase in cataract formation not observed in pancreatectomized animals.[46,47,49]

In pigs, there are some differences seen in the diabetic state between pancreatectomized and STZ-induced diabetic states. Total pancreatectomy results in the development of an insulin-dependent diabetic state in pigs.[44] The dose of STZ given to achieve a similar diabetic condition is 150 mg/kg. While there is no difference in the hyperglycemia that results (12 to 15 mmol/l), the detectable insulin levels are much higher in the STZ diabetic animals (20 mU/ml) as compared with pancreatectomized pigs (5 mU/ml).[43,44] Doses of less than 85 mg/kg STZ in pigs produce a diabetic state that undergoes reversal in approximately 2 weeks, and doses of less than 35 mg/kg produce no detectable effects on glucose metabolism.[44]

Since the complete removal of the pancreas is difficult to achieve with the rat, most experiments with this model are done on the partially pancreatectomized animal. A method introduced in 1983 provided a technique for total pancreatectomy but also involved the removal of the spleen.[50] The removal of the pancreas results in a loss of glucose and nonglucose stimulated insulin secretion,[51] increased intestinal sucrase activity,[52] and decreased wound healing.[53] Reports on pancreatectomy in the dog are associated with a body of work on transplantation techniques.[54]

It should be noted that there is a body of work in which a combination of therapies is administered for the development of an experimental diabetic state. The use of pancreatectomy in combination with chemical agents, such as alloxan and streptozotocin,[45,55] produces a stable form of diabetes mellitus in animals such as cats and dogs that does not occur when each procedure is applied independently. The combination therapy reduces the organ damage associated with chemical induction and minimizes the interventions, such as enzyme supplementation, necessary to maintain a pancreatectomized animal.

10.4 Dexamethasone-Induced Diabetes Mellitus

Dexamethasone is a long-acting glucocorticoid that stimulates gluconeogenesis and insulin secretion and inhibits glucose uptake by the fat cells. Dexamethasone has been used to produce models of noninsulin-dependent diabetes and also, when used at higher doses or in combination with other methods, to produce a model of insulin-dependent diabetes. Treatment of rats with dexamethasone produces a noninsulin-dependent diabetes mellitus thought to be due to insulin resistance following glucocorticoid administration.[56] An insulin-dependent form of diabetes was produced when dexamethasone was administered at a dose of 2 to 5 mg/kg by intraperitoneal injection over a number of days. Administration has been given on a daily and twice daily basis. The success rate for development of hyperglycemia with dexamethasone alone was 25%.[56,57] Dexamethasone administration decreased glucose-stimulated insulin secretion and significantly reduced GLUT-2 levels in the β-cell.[57] In rats that have undergone a partial pancreatectomy (80%), the administration of a dose of dexamethasone four times lower is sufficient to induce a stable form of diabetes mellitus.[58] The therapeutic administration of corticosteroids in veterinary practice has resulted in the unintentional development of diabetes mellitus in dogs. It is speculated that, since this complication occurs in overweight animals of advanced age, these animals may be in an undiagnosed prediabetic state that is exacerbated by corticosteroid therapy.[59]

10.5   Streptozotocin Combined with Complete Freund's Adjuvant

Since development of insulin-dependent diabetes in humans is an immune-mediated response, attempts have been made to develop a model that involved an immune response. Ziegler et al.[60] administered complete Freund's adjuvant (CFA) to female 8-week-old Wistar rats followed 1 day later with 25 mg/kg STZ. The injections of CFA and STZ were repeated for two subsequent weeks. Rats that received STZ alone (25 mg/kg for 3 weeks) showed no increase in plasma glucose levels despite a 50% drop in plasma insulin and a 60% reduction in pancreatic insulin content at day 26. Rats receiving CFA alone showed no change in plasma glucose or insulin levels but did demonstrate a significant decrease in pancreatic insulin content (by 35%). Animals receiving both STZ and CFA had elevated glucose (28 mM) by day 22, with a simultaneous drop in plasma (63%) and pancreatic (94%) insulin. These authors also showed the generation of complement-dependent cytotoxic autoantibodies against islet cells in plasma samples from STZ-CFA-treated rats as measured by Cr^{51} release from prelabled islet cells. Kohnert et al.[61] showed that a single injection of CFA followed 24 h later by STZ (25 mg/kg) in male Lewis rats produced a 69% drop in pancreatic insulin content within 48 to 96 h while plasma glucose levels remained normal (7.6 mM). Neither CFA nor STZ alone had any effect on pancreatic insulin content. A second administration of the CFA–STZ combination 1 week later resulted in a further drop in pancreatic insulin content (to 8% of control levels) and an elevation in plasma glucose to 20 mM. Two injections of CFA resulted in a drop in pancreatic insulin content of 33% accompanied by a slight decrease in plasma glucose levels while two injections of STZ produced no change in these parameters. Each of CFA), incomplete Freund's adjuvant, *Mycobacterium butyricum* (a component of CFA), Listeria monocytogenes (another granuloma-inducing organism), or endotoxin administered 24 h prior to STZ (25 mg/kg) and then repeated in the three subsequent weeks all produced hyperglycemia.[62] Fasting for 48 h (24 h prior to and 24 h subsequent to the STZ injection) also produced hyperglycemia.[62] Neither four administrations of CFA nor of STZ alone resulted in persistent hyperglycemia. This model has been used primarily to clarify the process of β-cell destruction that occurs in Type I diabetes in humans.

10.6   Conclusions

No animal model of diabetes mellitus is a perfect model of the disease as it occurs in humans; hence, a wide variety of models continue to be employed. Surgical removal of the pancreas completely avoids cytotoxic effects on other tissues, which do occur with chemical induction. However, it results in the loss of other important cells in the pancreas

35. Wilson, G. L., Patton, N. J., McCord, J. M., Mullins, D. W., and Mossman, B. T., Mechanisms of streptozotocin- and alloxan-induced damage in rat B cells, *Diabetologia*, 27, 587, 1984.

36. Duff, G. L. and Murray, E. G. D., The pathology of the pancreas in experimental diabetes mellitus, *Am. J. Med. Sci.*, 210, 81, 1945.

37. Mansford, K. R. L. and Opie, L., Comparison of metabolic abnormalities in diabetes mellitus induced by streptozotocin or by alloxan, *Lancet*, 1, 670, 1968.

38. Gaulton, G. N., Schwartz, J. L., and Eardley, D. D., Assessment of the diabetogenic drugs alloxan and streptozotocin as models for the study of immune defects in diabetic mice, *Diabetologia*, 28, 769, 1985.

39. Howard, C. F., Nonhuman primates as models for the study of human diabetes mellitus, *Diabetes*, 31, 37, 1982.

40. Kaufmann, F. and Rodriguez, R. R., Subtotal pancreatectomy in five different rat strains: incidence and course of development of diabetes, *Diabetologia*, 27, 38, 1984.

41. Gabel, H., Bitter-Suermann, H., Henriksson, C., Save-Soderbergh, J,. Lundholm, K., and Brynger, H., Streptozotocin diabetes in juvenile pigs. Evaluation of an experimental model, *Horm. Metab. Res.*, 17, 275, 1985.

42. Karmann, H. and Mialhe, P., Progressive loss of sensitivity of the A cell to insulin in geese made diabetic by subtotal pancreatectomy, *Horm. Metab. Res.*, 14, 452, 1982.

43. Pattou, F., Kerr-Conte, J., Amrouni, H., Xia, Y., Lefebvre, A., Lefebvre, J., and Proye, C., Ultimate assessment of pig islet isolation by autotransplantation after pancreatectomy, *Transplant. Proc.*, 27, 3403, 1995.

44. Wilson, J. D., Dhall, D. P., Simeonovic, C. J., and Lafferty, K. J., Induction and management of diabetes mellitus in the pig, *Aust. J. Exp. Biol. Med. Sci.*, 64, 489, 1986.

45. Tschoepe, D., Job, F. P., Huebinger, A., Freytag, G., Torsello, G., Peter, B., and Gries, F. A., Combined subtotal pancreatectomy with selective streptozotocin infusion — a model for the induction of insulin deficiency in dogs, *Res. Exp. Med.*, 189, 141, 1989.

46. Jones, C. W., West, M. S., Hong, D. T., and Jonasson, O. Peripheral glomerular basement membrane thickness in the normal and diabetic monkey, *Lab. Invest.*, 51, 193, 1984.

47. Jonasson, O., Jones, C. W., Bauman, A., John E., Manaligod, J., and Tso, M. O. M., The pathophysiology of experimental insulin-deficient diabetes in the monkey, *Ann. Surg.*, 201, 27, 1985

48. Stout, L. C., Folse, D. S., Maier, J., Crosby, W. M., Kling, R., Williams, G. R., Price, W. E., Geyer, J. R., Padula, R., Whorton, E., and Kimmelstiel, P., Quantitative glomerular morphology of the normal and diabetic baboon kidney, *Diabetologia*, 29, 734, 1986.

49. Ericzon, B. G., Wijnen, R. M. H., Kubota, K., Bogaard, A. V. D., and Kootstra, G., Diabetes induction and pancreatic transplantation in the cynomolgus monkey: methodological considerations, *Transplant Int.*, 4, 103, 1991.

50. Houry, S. and Huguier, M., Total splenopancreatectomy in the rat, *Eur. Surg. Res.*, 15, 328, 1983.

51. Leahy, J. L., Bonner-Weir, S., and Weir, G. C.,. Abnormal glucose regulation of insulin secretion in models of reduced B-cell mass, *Diabetes*, 33, 667, 1984.

52. Takeguchi, T., Mori, K., Takano, S., and Akagi, M., Hyperglycemia induces intestinal sucrase activity in subtotally pancreatectomized rats, *Gastroenterol. Jpn.*, 20, 20, 1985.

53. Grandini, S. A., The effect of partial-pancreatectomy-induced diabetes on wound healing subsequent to tooth extraction, *Oral Surg.*, 45, 191, 1978.

54. Madureira, M. L. C., Adult pancreatic tissue fate after pancreatic fragment autotransplantation into the spleen of the pancreatectomized dog, *World J. Surg.*, 18, 259, 1994.

55. Reiser, H. J., Whitworth, U. G., Hatchell, D. L., Sutherland, F. S., Nanda, S., McAdoo, T., and Hardin, J. R., Experimental diabetes in cats induced by partial pancreatectomy alone or combined with local injection of alloxan, *Lab. Anim. Sci.*, 37, 449, 1987.

56. Ogawa, A., Johnson, J. H., Ohneda, M., McAllister, C. T., Inman, L., Alam, T., and Uner, R. H., Roles of insulin resistance and β-cell dysfunction in dexamethasone-induced diabetes, *J. Clin. Invest.*, 90, 497, 1992.

57. Takahashi, K., Suda, K., Lam, H.-C., Ghatei, M. A., and Bloom, S. R., Endothelin-like immunoreactivity in rat models of diabetes mellitus, *J. Endocrinol.*, 130, 123, 1990.

58. Bates, R. W. and Garrison, M. M., Synergism among growth hormone, ACTH, cortisol and dexamethasone in the hormonal induction of diabetes in rats and the diabetogenic effect of tolbutamide, *Endocrinology*, 93, 1109, 1973.

59. Jeffers, J. G., Shanley, K. J., and Schick, R. O., Diabetes mellitus induced in a dog after administration of corticosteroids and methylprednisolone pulse therapy, *J. Am. Vet. Med.*, 199, 77, 1991.

60. Ziegler, M., Ziegler, B., Hehmke, B., Dietz, H., Hildmann, W., and Kauert, C., Autoimmune response directed to pancreatic beta cells in rats induced by combined treatment with low doses of streptozotocin and complete Freund's adjuvant, *Biomed. Biochim. Acta*, 5, 675, 1984.

61. Kohnert, K.-D., Ziegler, B., Fält, K., Odselius, R., Ziegler, M., and Falkmer, S., Biochemical, immunohistochemical and ultrastructural studies of the alteration of pancreatic beta cells resulting from the combined effects of complete Freund's adjuvant and nondiabetogenic doses of streptozotocin, *Exp. Clin. Endocrinol.*, 89, 259, 1987.

62. Wright, J. R., Jr., and Lacy, P. E., Synergistic effects of adjuvants, endotoxin, and fasting on induction of diabetes with multiple low doses of streptozotocin in rats, *Diabetes*, 37, 112, 1988.

63. Nordestgaard, B. G. and Zilversmit, D. B., Hyperglycemia in normotriglyceridemic, hypercholesterolemic insulin-treated diabetic rabbits does not accelerate atherogenesis, *Atherosclerosis*, 72, 37, 1988.

64. Tesfamariam. B., Jakubowski, J. A., and Cohen, R. A., Contraction of diabetic rabbit aorta caused by endothelium-derived PGH_2-TxA_2, *Am. J. Physiol.*, 257, H1327, 1989.

65. Richardson, M., Hadcock, S. J., DeReske, M., and Cybulsky, M. I., Increased expression *in vivo* of VCAM-1 and E-selectin by the aortic endothelium of normolipemic and hyperlipemic diabetic rabbits, *Arteriosclerosis Thrombosis*, 14, 760, 1994.

11

The Neonatal STZ Model of Diabetes

Stephen W. Schaffer and Mahmood Mozaffari

CONTENTS

11.1 Determinants of Noninsulin-Dependent Diabetes in Humans

Noninsulin-dependent diabetes mellitus (NIDDM) is the most common form of diabetes in Western populations.[1] As its name implies, NIDDM is commonly controlled by noninsulin regimens, such as diet or oral hypoglycemic agents. Clinical onset of the disease is insidious and is genetically linked. A key question regarding NIDDM is whether the primary cause is a genetic defect in the insulin-secreting β-cells of the pancreas (insulin deficiency) or in the insulin-signaling pathway (insulin resistance). Clarification of this issue has been hampered by the inadequacy of available *in vivo* tests, as well as the complex interaction between insulin deficiency and insulin resistance.

It is generally accepted that both the amount of insulin secreted and the pattern of insulin secretion by the pancreas are abnormal in patients with overt NIDDM.[2] Normally, an abrupt rise in plasma glucose, the most important insulin secretagogue, leads to a

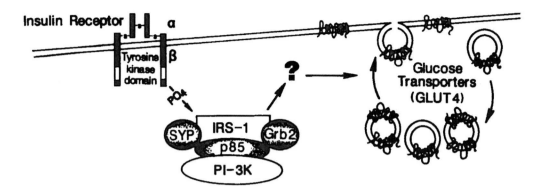

FIGURE 11.1

The insulin signal transduction pathway. The binding of insulin to its receptor activates a tyrosine protein kinase, which then phosphorylates several proteins, including IRS-1. The phosphorylated form of IRS-1 serves as a docking protein capable of binding several proteins, including phosphatidylinositol-3-kinase (PI-3 kinase). Once bound, PI-3 kinase is activated and through some unknown mechanism promotes the translocation of the glucose transporter, GLUT 4, to the cell surface. This cascade of reactions, which results in an acceleration in glucose transport, is defective in the noninsulin-dependent diabetic rat.

biphasic release in insulin from the pancreas. The rapid first phase of this process lasts for 1 to 3 min and is believed to play an important role in maintaining glucose tolerance. Since this rapid initial phase is virtually absent in the patients with NIDDM,[3] it is not surprising that patients with NIDDM is severely glucose intolerant. The slower-developing second phase is more prolonged and is largely dependent upon the extent and duration of the glucose elevation. The magnitude of phase 2 insulin secretion is often enhanced during the early stages of NIDDM. However, as the degree of hyperglycemia worsens, the β-cells slowly become desensitized to glucose, causing phase 2 insulin secretion to decline and the patient to become hypoinsulinemic.[4]

The recognition that NIDDM is a heterogenous disease suggests that multiple genes may contribute to the development of the insulin secretory defect. One such gene, glucokinase, was recently identified in an autosomal dominant form of NIDDM.[5] This mutation impairs insulin secretion by interfering with the glucose-sensing mechanism of the β-cell. Another gene implicated in the development of NIDDM is the ATP-dependent K$^+$ channel. Although this transporter is required for the induction of insulin secretion by most secretagogues, association between the polymorphism of this gene and NIDDM has not been consistently observed.[6] Also implicated in the development of NIDDM is a mutation in the insulin gene, which produces a defective form of insulin.[7]

Resistance to insulin action is also present in the majority of patients with NIDDM, including patients with borderline glucose intolerance and no evidence of insulin deficiency.[8,9] Most clinical and isolated human cell studies have focused on the inability of insulin to adequately promote glucose utilization by muscle, inhibit glucose production by liver, and reduce the rate of lipolysis in adipose tissue.[10-12] Based on these studies, investigators have concluded that both impaired insulin receptor function and a postreceptor defect contribute to the development of insulin resistance, although the latter appears more important. One postreceptor site that may contribute to insulin resistance is the phosphorylation of IRS-1 (insulin receptor substrate 1) by insulin receptor kinase. Since this reaction represents an early step in insulin signaling, it is linked to many actions of insulin (Figure 11.1). Therefore, it is significant that gene variants of both IRS-1 and insulin receptor kinase have been discovered in patients with NIDDM.[13,14] These mutations invariably reduce the degree of IRS-1 phosphorylation, causing inadequate docking and activation of other signaling proteins, ultimately leading to an impairment in insulin action.[15] The net result is that processes, such as insulin-induced activation of glucose metabolism, are impaired in patients with NIDDM, although impaired glucose metabolism can also be attributed to defects in hexokinase activity[16] or in the expression, translocation, and activity of insulin-sensitive glucose transporters.[17-19]

One reason that both insulin resistance and insulin deficiency occur simultaneously in most patients with NIDDM is that insulin deficiency acts through some undetermined mechanism to trigger insulin resistance.[20] Moreover, insulin resistance raises plasma glucose content, which in turn promotes downregulation in the amount of insulin released in response to glucose.[21,22] Because of these complex interactions, the primary cause of NIDDM at the molecular level has not been established.

11.2   Neonatal STZ Model of Noninsulin-Dependent Diabetes

Animal studies have been useful in exploring the molecular mechanisms underlying the development of NIDDM. An animal model that has been particularly useful in examining the importance of β-cell dysfunction in the development of NIDDM is the neonatal streptozotocin (STZ) rat. There have been numerous variations of this model, some that have profound effects on the severity of the diabetic condition. Nonetheless, all variations are based on the premise that neonatal rats treated with STZ (80 to 100 mg/kg) at birth (n0 STZ rats) or within the first 5 days following birth (n1–5 STZ rats) experience severe pancreatic β-cell destruction, accompanied by a decrease in pancreatic insulin stores and a rise in plasma glucose levels.[23,24] However, in contrast to adult rats treated with STZ, the β-cells of the treated neonates partially regenerate.[25] Following an initial spike in plasma glucose, the STZ-treated neonatal rat becomes normoglycemic by 3 weeks of age. In the next few weeks, the β-cell number increases, the extent depending upon both the age at which the animal is treated with STZ and the species of the treated rat.[23-27] The effect of treatment age on the outcome is extremely dramatic. While pancreatic insulin content is 90% depleted in 10-week-old n5 STZ Wistar rats (treated with STZ at 5 days of age), the insulin content of either the 10-week-old n0 STZ or the n2 STZ Wistar rat is 50%[23] (Figure 11.2). Yet, significant species differences are also observed in this model. While pancreatic insulin levels are similar in 10-week-old n2 STZ SHR and n5 STZ Wistar rats,[23,27] the magnitude of the STZ-induced decline in insulin levels is less in the n2 STZ Wistar Kyoto (WKY) rat than either the n2 STZ Wistar or the n2 STZ Sprague-Dawley rat.[24,27] Consequently, n5 STZ Wistar and n2 STZ SHR rats develop a more severe diabetic condition, characterized by overt hyperglycemia, severe hypoinsulinemia, and insulin resistance. The mildest form of diabetes occurs in the n2 STZ WKY rat.

The aging process also affects the diabetic state of the STZ-treated rat. Although 10-week-old n2 STZ Wistar rats exhibit normal nonfasting glucose and insulin levels, they are markedly glucose intolerant. However, these animals become progressively more glucose intolerant with age. By 6 months of age, a glucose challenge provokes a condition of severe hyperglycemia and hyperinsulinemia (Figure 11.3). Upon further aging, insulin secretion of the n2 STZ male Wistar rat is dramatically altered. Although not reflected in basal plasma insulin levels, this change in insulin secretion is detected as a severe impairment in the response to a glucose challenge. The aging process also affects the response of the nondiabetic control rat, which by 12 months of age begins to show signs of insulin resistance characterized by increased plasma insulin content but normal plasma glucose levels (see Figure 11.3). Thus, both basal plasma insulin levels and the rise in plasma insulin

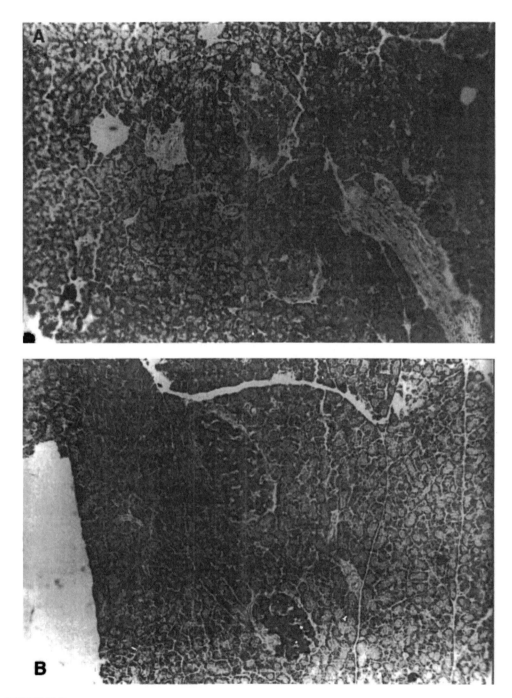

FIGURE 11.2
Effect of streptozotocin on the histology of the pancreas. β-cells from (**A**) noninsulin-dependent diabetic (n2 STZ) and (**B**) nondiabetic Wistar rats were stained using a peroxidase antiperoxidase technique with primary antibodies for insulin. The intensity of insulin staining is significantly reduced in the 6-month-old n2 STZ Wistar rat.

A

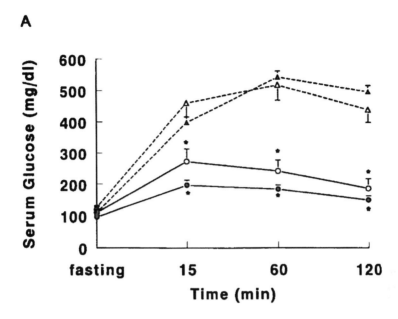

B

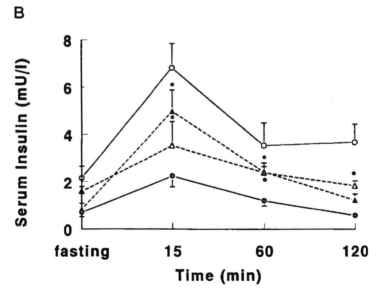

FIGURE 11.3
Effect of aging on serum glucose and insulin levels following a glucose challenge — 6 month (●,▲) and 14-month (○,△) nondiabetic (●,○) and noninsulin-dependent diabetic (▲,△) Wistar rats were fasted overnight before intraperitoneal administration of glucose (2 g/kg body wt). Shown are the changes in glucose (A) and insulin (B) levels following the glucose challenge. Values shown represent means ± S.E.M. of five rats. Asterisks denote significant difference from the nondiabetic control ($p < 0.05$). (Data were obtained from Schaffer and Wilson[28] and used with the permission of *Diabetologia*.)

in response to a glucose challenge are significantly greater in 12 month old nondiabetic rats than in either the 1-year-old diabetic or the 6-month-old nondiabetic rat.[28]

11.2.1 Pancreatic Insulin Secretion in the Neonatal STZ Model

The regulation of insulin secretion is extremely complex, involving numerous secretagogues and modulators. The most important controller of insulin secretion is glucose. The mechanism underlying glucose signaling involves its metabolism to generate ATP, which in turn promotes the closure of the ATP-dependent K^+ channel, resulting in depolarization of the β-cell. A voltage-dependent Ca^{2+} influx into the cell ensues, with the rise in $[Ca^{2+}]_i$ triggering insulin secretion.[29] This ATP-dependent mechanism is not unique to glucose because other metabolites, such as glyceraldehyde and mannose, also function as insulin secretagogues (Figure 11.4). Insulin secretion triggered by these metabolic secretagogues is generally defective in the neonatal NIDDM model.[30-32] Attempts to identify the site of this defect have led to the observation that the characteristic increase in $[Ca^{2+}]_i$ in response to glucose is clearly abnormal in the n0 STZ Wistar rat.[33] Yet, both the extent and pattern of insulin secretion induced by elevations in extracellular Ca^{2+} are normal, suggesting that an early step in the glucose-signaling pathway must be defective in the n0 STZ β-cell.[34] This defect may involve impaired citric acid cycle activity, which slows the rate of glucose oxidation and ATP generation.[32] Significantly, a metabolic defect has also been invoked to explain the hypersensitivity of n1 STZ β-cells to two nonglucose secretagogues, octanoate and glutamine. According to Grill et al.,[31] glucose metabolism is depressed in the n1 STZ β-cell; therefore, fatty acid metabolism is enhanced and assumes a more important role in regulating insulin secretion. A nutrient secretagogue, leucine, also experiences an exaggerated response in the diabetic rat.[30] However, its hypersensitivity can be traced to enhanced rates of leucine transamination rather than an interaction between glucose and leucine metabolism.

Another secretagogue, whose response is defective in the n2 STZ β-cell, is the amino acid arginine.[35] Interestingly, arginine does not function as a nutrient secretagogue, but instead acts by depolarizing the β-cell. Since insulin secretion, as well as the arginine-mediated elevation in $[Ca^{2+}]_i$, is enhanced in the n2 STZ β-cell, it suggests that the depolarization step is also defective in the n2 STZ β-cell.[33] Interestingly, treatment of the diabetic rat with insulin normalizes the response to arginine, supporting the notion that chronic hyperglycemia and/or hypoinsulinemia triggers the abnormal insulin response.

In contrast to most insulin secretagogues, the response to acute sulfonylurea exposure is identical in isolated pancreata from n0 STZ Wistar, n5 STZ Wistar, and nondiabetic control rats.[30,36] Since the sulfonylurea functions by inhibiting the ATP-dependent K^+ channel, the channel appears to be operating normally in the NIDDM rat. This may be a major reason for the improvement in the metabolic status of the n2 STZ rat treated chronically with a sulfonylurea.[37]

Agonists that trigger the activation of protein kinase A promote insulin secretion by elevating $[Ca^{2+}]_i$ and sensitizing the secretory machinery to Ca^{2+}.[29] Giroix et al.[30] found that isolated pancreata obtained from 3- to 5-month-old n0 STZ male Wistar rats exhibit enhanced responsiveness to the β-adrenergic agonist isoproterenol. Similarly, hypersensitivity to the phosphodiesterase inhibitor IBMX (3-isobutyl-1-methylxanthine) has been noted in pancreata obtained from n0 STZ Sprague-Dawley rats.[31] Thus, the Ca^{2+}-modulating actions of protein kinase A are abnormal in the diabetic β-cell.

11.2.2 Insulin Resistance in the Neonatal STZ Model

The insulin glucose clamp technique has commonly been used to evaluate insulin action *in vivo*. Based on this technique, Blondel et al.[23] found that whole-body glucose utilization

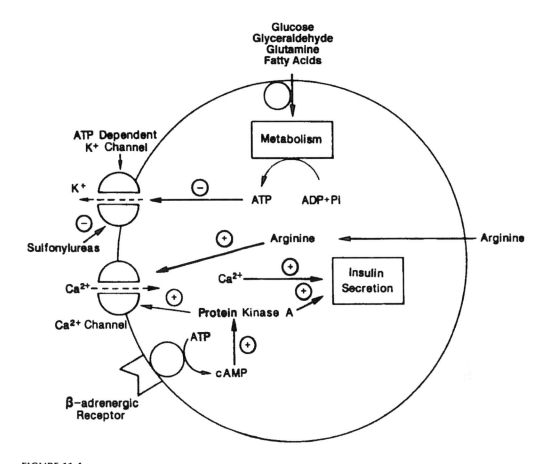

FIGURE 11.4
Mechanisms underlying the promotion of insulin secretion by various secretagogues. In the neonatal STZ rat, while insulin secretion induced by the most important secretagogue, glucose, is reduced, other metabolic secretagogues, such as fatty acids, glyceraldehyde, and glutamine, release more insulin. By comparison, non-metabolic insulin secretagogues exhibit either a normal response (sulfonylureas) or an exaggerated response (arginine) in the diabetic rat. The regulation of insulin secretion may also be abnormal, i.e., activators of protein kinase A promote greater insulin secretion in the diabetic rat.

was normal in the 10-week-old n2 STZ Wistar female rat, but was significantly reduced in the severely diabetic n5 STZ female Wistar rat. They also found that the n5 STZ, but not the n0 STZ rat, exhibited reduced suppression of hepatic glucose production by insulin. Somewhat unexpected was an observation made by the same group[38] that the n0 STZ rat exhibited a significant elevation in insulin sensitivity. Although the basis underlying this link between hypoinsulinemia and increased insulin sensitivity in the young, n0 STZ rat has not been established, alterations in insulin receptor function appear to have been ruled out as a cause.[39] A likely scenario is that an early step in the signal transduction pathway of insulin becomes defective, causing increased insulin sensitivity of several events, including glycogenesis, lipogenesis, glucose production, amino acid transport, and glucose oxidation.[38,39]

In contrast to the observed hypersensitivity to insulin in the n2 STZ female Wistar rat, n2 STZ male Wistar rats develop insulin resistance. By 8 weeks of age, insulin-mediated promotion of 3-O-methylglucose transport by adipocytes isolated from n2 STZ male Wistar rats is depressed over 50%.[40] Impairment in the ability of insulin to stimulate glucose metabolism in the heart of the n2 STZ male Wistar rat has also been described.[28]

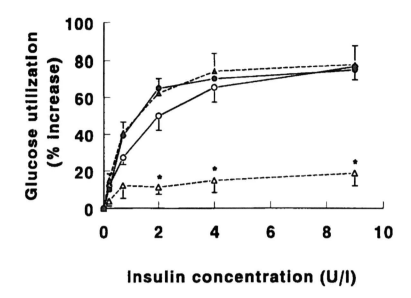

FIGURE 11.5

Development of insulin resistance in the noninsulin-dependent diabetic heart. Hearts from 6-month-old (●,▲) and 14-month-old (○,△) noninsulin-dependent diabetic (▲,△) and nondiabetic (●,○) Wistar rats were perfused with Krebs–Henseleit buffer containing 10 mM [3-³H]-glucose. The coronary effluent was collected and the rate of ³H-H$_2$O formation was determined. Shown is the percent change in glucose utilization following exposure to varying concentrations of insulin. Asterisks denote significant difference between the 14-month-old diabetic and its age-matched nondiabetic control ($p < 0.05$). No evidence of insulin resistance was apparent at 6 months of age; however, by 14 months of age the animal exhibits severe insulin resistance. (From Schaffer, S. W. and Wilson, G. L.,[28] *Diabetologia*, 36, 195, 1993. With permission.

Severe insulin resistance is also a characteristic of some insulin sensitive tissues of n2 STZ male Sprague-Dawley rats. Trent et al.[41] found that adipocytes prepared from 6-week-old n2 STZ male Sprague-Dawley rats exhibit a dramatic reduction in insulin-mediated acceleration of both glucose oxidation and lipogenesis. Moreover, insulin-mediated stimulation of insulin receptor tyrosine kinase and Ca^{2+},Mg^{2+}-ATPase activity of kidney basolateral membranes in 10-week-old n2 STZ Sprague-Dawley rats is suppressed.[42,43] Yet, in apparent contrast to n2 STZ adipocytes and kidneys, impaired insulin responsiveness is not detected in n2 STZ epitrochlearis muscle even though the basal rate of glucose transport and utilization is significantly depressed.[44] These data indicate that insulin resistance develops at different rates in various n2 STZ tissues. This conclusion is borne out by examining insulin responsiveness of cardiac muscle isolated from n2 STZ male Wistar rats.[28,45] At 4- to 6-months of age, the response of the diabetic and nondiabetic heart to insulin is identical (Figure 11.5). After 4 months, the metabolic status of the n2 STZ rat begins to deteriorate, with basal myocardial glucose utilization falling approximately 20% relative to the control. This situation worsens by 1 year of age, as the reduction in basal glucose utilization becomes more severe. Yet, insulin responsiveness in the n2 STZ heart only becomes significantly reduced between 12 and 16 months of age (see Figure 11.5). Thus, as the n2 STZ male Wistar rat ages, it not only becomes more glucose intolerant but also insulin resistant.

11.2.3   Defective Carbohydrate and Lipid Metabolism in the Neonatal STZ Rat

Maintenance of glucose homeostasis in the nondiabetic and diabetic rat largely depends upon the metabolism of glucose by the liver and muscle. Usually, increased rates of hepatic

TABLE 11.1

Effect of Noninsulin-Dependent Diabetes on Myocardial 3-*O*-Methylglucose Transport and Glucose Utilization

Condition	3-*O*-Methylglucose Transport (μmol/min/g dry wt)	Glucose Utilization (μmol/g dry wt/h)
Nondiabetic	2.52 ± 0.11	270 ± 21
Noninsulin-dependent diabetes	1.63 ± 0.14*	184 ± 20*

Note: Hearts from 12-month-old noninsulin-dependent diabetic (n2 STZ) and nondiabetic male Wistar rats were perfused with buffer containing either ^{14}C-3-*O*-methyl-D-glucose or [3-^{3}H]-glucose. Glucose utilization was determined from the rate of tritium release from [3-^{3}H]-glucose into water. The rate of 3-*O*-methylglucose transport was evaluated from the rate at which radioactive 3-*O*-methylglucose was washed out of the heart following exposure to a substrate-free buffer. Values shown represent means ± S.E.M. of four to five hearts. Asterisks denote significant difference from the nondiabetic control ($p < 0.05$). Both 3-*O*-methylglucose transport and glucose utilization were depressed approximately 35% in the diabetic heart relative to its age-matched nondiabetic control.

gluconeogenesis are considered one of the dominant mechanisms underlying the development of hyperglycemia in NIDDM.[46] However, this does not seem to be the case in the 2-month-old n0 STZ female Wistar rat, in which elevated rates of basal hepatic glucose output are balanced by the increased effectiveness of insulin in suppressing glucose output.[39] Thus, at 2 months of age, the observed glucose intolerance that develops in the n0 STZ rat seems to be caused primarily by reduced rates of peripheral glucose uptake. On the other hand, the elevated rate of gluconeogenesis is an important contributor to the severe hyperglycemic condition that develops in the n5 STZ rat.[23]

The defect in peripheral glucose uptake and metabolism has been the focus of several studies using perfused hearts isolated from the n2 STZ male Wistar rat. It has been documented that basal rates of glucose utilization are significantly reduced in diabetic hearts, a defect attributed to a combination of reduced glucose transport and impaired flux through the rate-limiting enzyme of glycolysis, phosphofructokinase.[47] The view that impaired glucose transport contributes to the observed reduction in glucose metabolism is supported by the observation that the degree of impairment in basal 3-*O*-methylglucose transport and glucose utilization of isolated diabetic and nondiabetic hearts are identical (Table 11.1). However, the contribution of impaired glucose uptake becomes minimal when the heart is exposed to saturating levels of insulin, which increases the intracellular glucose concentration well above the K_m for hexokinase. Thus, in the presence of insulin, phosphofructokinase appears to play the dominant role in determining the rate of glycolysis in the n2 STZ heart. This conclusion is also based on the crossover theorem, which assumes that when a rate-limiting enzyme causes a reduction in flux through a metabolic pathway, the concentration of its reactants rise and its products decline. Figure 11.6 shows a typical crossover plot comparing the levels of glycolytic intermediates in NIDDM and nondiabetic hearts. Since the concentration of glucose-6-phosphate is slightly elevated in the diabetic heart, whereas the concentration of fructose 1,6 bisphosphate is significantly reduced relative to the nondiabetic control, it follows that flux through glycolysis is limited by the activity of phosphofructokinase (see Figure 11.6). Since an identical pattern prevails in the absence and presence of insulin, phosphofructokinase is considered an important limiting enzyme for glycolysis in the n2 STZ heart.

In contrast to glucose metabolism, fatty acid metabolism of the n2 STZ heart is normal. Neither the rate of endogenous fatty acid oxidation nor the levels of long-chain fatty acyl esters (both carnitine and CoA) are altered by the NIDDM condition.[48] This is not surprising in light of evidence that the neonatal STZ model, in contrast to the adult STZ model, exhibits no significant alteration in plasma free fatty acid and triglyceride levels (Table 11.2).

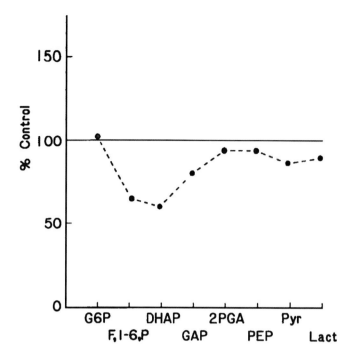

FIGURE 11.6

Effect of noninsulin-dependent diabetes on myocardial glycolytic intermediates. Hearts from n2 STZ (dashed line) and nondiabetic (solid line) Wistar rats were perfused with buffer containing 11 mM glucose. The data for the 12-month-old diabetic hearts are expressed as percent of the nondiabetic values. G-6-P, glucose-6-phosphate; F,1-6,P, fructose 1,6 bisphosphate; DHAP, dihydroxyacetate phosphate; GAP, glyceraldehyde 3-phosphate; 2PGA, 2-phosphoglyceric acid; PEP, phosphoenolpyruvate; Pyr, pyruvate; Lact, lactate. (From Schaffer, S. W. et al., *Diabetes*, 35, 593, 1986. With permission of the American Diabetes Association.)

TABLE 11.2

Effect of Noninsulin-Dependent Diabetes on Plasma Levels of Key Lipid Components

Substance	Nondiabetic	Noninsulin-Dependent Diabetic
Free fatty acids (μmol/l)	335 ± 24	337 ± 44
Triglycerides (mg %)	93 ± 28	60 ± 18
Cholesterol (mg %)	148 ± 14	141 ± 30

Note: Plasma from nonfasting, 6-month-old noninsulin-dependent diabetic (2n STZ) and nondiabetic male Wistar rats were analyzed for key lipid components. Although triglyceride levels tended to be elevated in the diabetic group, the difference was not statistically significant. Values shown represent means ± S.E.M. of four samples.

11.2.4   Complications Observed in the Neonatal STZ Rat

11.2.4.1   Contractile Defects of the Noninsulin-Dependent Diabetic Heart

Although diabetic cardiomyopathy develops slowly in the n2 STZ rat, its progression is similar to the development of other NIDDM-linked defects. The first signs of impaired contractile function are noted 8 months after administration of STZ.[45] However, by 12 to 14 months the abnormality develops into an overt cardiomyopathy, characterized by reduced rates of pressure development (+dP/dt) and relaxation (–dP/dt) and an impairment in maximal systolic pressure, cardiac work, and cardiac output (Table 11.3).

TABLE 11.3

Impaired Myocardial Contractile Function of the Noninsulin-Dependent Diabetic Rat

Parameter	Nondiabetic	Noninsulin-Dependent Diabetic
+dP/dt (cm H_2O/s)	2905 ± 162	2148 ± 135*
–dP/dt (cm H_2O/s)	2484 ± 195	1840 ± 130*
Left ventricular pressure (cm H_2O)	149 ± 3	136 ± 4*
Cardiac work (kg-mg/g dry wt/min)	0.31 ± 0.03	0.26 ± 0.02*
Cardiac output (ml/min)	69.9 ± 4.9	58.8 ± 4.1*

Note: Hearts from 12-month-old noninsulin-dependent diabetic (n2 STZ) and nondiabetic Wistar rats were perfused with Krebs–Henseleit buffer containing 11 mM glucose. Following stabilization for 15 min, several hemodynamic parameters were measured. Values shown are means ± S.E.M. of five to seven hearts. Asterisks denote significant difference from the age-matched nondiabetic control ($p < 0.05$).

These myocardial defects are manifest in n2 STZ hearts perfused under a wide range of conditions, including different substrates, various concentrations of Ca^{2+}, and saturating concentrations of insulin. Thus, the diabetic heart undergoes basic changes that preclude it from responding normally to acute changes in the composition of the perfusion medium.

One of the most dramatic abnormalities associated with the cardiomyopathy is a reduction in diastolic compliance, manifest as a leftward shift in the pressure–volume relationship of the isolated heart (Figure 11.7). This defect has been attributed to either the accumulation of glycoproteins in the interstitium or an elevation in intracellular Ca^{2+} levels.[48,49] The latter hypothesis is based on a recent study by Takamatsu and Wier,[50] who showed that Ca^{2+} overload promotes premature sarcoplasmic reticular Ca^{2+} release, which in turn initiates propagating zones of elevated $[Ca^{2+}]_i$ known as Ca^{2+} waves. These Ca^{2+} waves prevent the normal sequestration of Ca^{2+} by the sarcoplasmic reticulum, thereby interfering with normal diastolic function.[51]

Calcium overload may also contribute to impaired systolic function through several mechanisms. First, premature sarcoplasmic reticular Ca^{2+} release not only causes diastolic dysfunction, but also transiently depletes sarcoplasmic reticular Ca^{2+} stores, leading to impaired systolic function.[51] Second, Ca^{2+} overload appears to modulate the expression of certain muscle proteins. Of particular interest is the myosin V_1 to V_3 shift, which occurs in the n2 STZ heart and is thought to adversely affect muscle contraction.[52] Since this isozyme transition also occurs in the adult STZ-treated rat and is prevented by the administration of the Ca^{2+} antagonist, verapamil, it has been proposed that $[Ca^{2+}]_i$ regulates myosin isozyme content.[53] Third, Ca^{2+} overload decreases Ca^{2+} responsiveness of the muscle proteins.[54] This may occur because elevations in $[Ca^{2+}]_i$ activate specific protein kinase C isozymes, which in turn phosphorylate key muscle proteins, such as troponin T, troponin I, and C-protein. It has been shown that once phosphorylated, these muscle proteins are incapable of maintaining normal actomyosin Mg^{2+} ATPase activity,[55,56] which according to numerous studies leads to a reduction in muscle contraction. Although the status of actomyosin ATPase activity has not been measured in the n2 STZ heart, it is significant that myocardial protein kinase C_α activity is elevated, while protein phosphatase 1 activity is reduced in the NIDDM heart (Table 11.4).

11.2.4.1.1 *Basis for Impaired Ca^{2+} Handling in the n2 STZ Heart*

Maintenance of Ca^{2+} homeostasis by several key transporters is absolutely essential for normal contraction. Upon depolarization of the myocyte, a Ca^{2+} transient is generated, with the upstroke of the transient dominated by both Ca^{2+} influx via the L-type Ca^{2+} channel and release of Ca^{2+} from the sarcoplasmic reticulum. Some investigators believe that Ca^{2+} may also enter the cell via the Na^+–Ca^{2+} exchanger, with this source of Ca^{2+} assuming a more important role as the $[Na^+]_i$ increases. Decay of the Ca^{2+} transient involves the

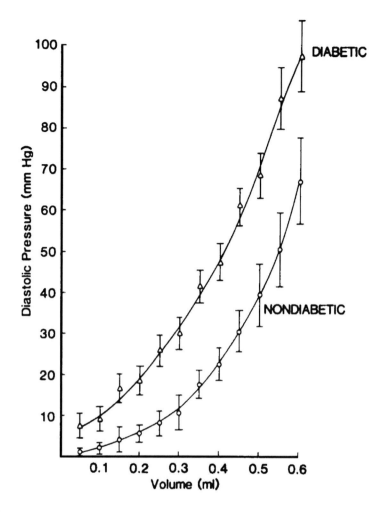

FIGURE 11.7
Effect of noninsulin-dependent diabetes on diastolic compliance. A deflated balloon was inserted into the myocardium of 12-month-old n2 STZ (Δ) and nondiabetic (O) male Wistar rats. After determining baseline pressure, 50 μl increments of saline were injected into the balloon and the pressure within the balloon measured. Values shown represent the means ± S.E.M. of 8 to 12 hearts. Diastolic pressure at all volumes were significantly elevated in the diabetic heart. (From Schaffer, S. W. et al., *Am. J. Physiol.*, 256, E25, 1989. With permission of the American Physiological Society.)

combined actions of the sarcoplasmic reticular Ca^{2+} pump and the sarcolemmal Na^+–Ca^{2+} exchanger. Nearly 65 to 90% of the Ca^{2+} decay process involves the pumping of Ca^{2+} into the sarcoplasmic reticular storage vesicles.[57] The Na^+–Ca^{2+} exchanger plays a minor role in Ca^{2+} decay, although it is the major mechanism for extrusion of Ca^{2+} from the myocyte. Therefore, an active Na^+–Ca^{2+} exchanger is essential for ensuring a balance between cellular Ca^{2+} influx and Ca^{2+} efflux.[58]

Calcium transport in the n2 STZ rat heart is dominated by the imbalance that develops between Ca^{2+} handling by the sarcoplasmic reticular Ca^{2+} pump and the Na^+–Ca^{2+} exchanger.[59,60] While sarcoplasmic reticular Ca^{2+} activity is only slightly depressed in the n2 STZ heart, the activity of the Na^+–Ca^{2+} exchanger is significantly reduced (Figure 11.8). This imbalance is made worse by the impairment in Na^+,K^+-ATPase activity, which elevates myocardial $[Na^+]_i$, further interfering with the ability of the Na^+–Ca^{2+} exchanger to extrude

TABLE 11.4

Effect of Noninsulin-Dependent Diabetes on the Activities of Sarcolemmal Protein Kinase C_α and Protein Phosphatase 1

Condition	Protein Kinase C_α Activity (nmol/mg/min)	Protein Phosphatase 1 Activity (pmol/mg/h)
Nondiabetic	0.48 ± 0.04	292.0 ± 29.6
Noninsulin-dependent diabetic	0.89 ± 0.18*	165.2 ± 24.4*

Note: Enriched sarcolemma was prepared from 12-month-old noninsulin-dependent diabetic (n2 STZ) and nondiabetic Wistar rats. Sarcolemmal protein phosphatase 1 activity (measured using phosphorylase a as a substrate) has been defined as inhibitor 2 sensitive protein phosphatase activity. For the measurement of protein kinase C_α activity, enriched sarcolemma was extracted with 1% Triton X-100 and the resulting extract subjected to DEAE cellulose and hydroxylapatite chromatography. Protein kinase C_α was the second peak to emerge from the hydroxylapatite column. Values shown represent the means ± S.E.M. of four preparations. Asterisks denote significant difference from the nondiabetic control ($p < 0.05$).

Ca^{2+} adequately from the myocyte.[59] Consequently, during diastole, unusually large amounts of Ca^{2+} are pumped into the sarcoplasmic reticular vesicles. As predicted on the basis of this scenario, the amount of Ca^{2+} released from the sarcoplasmic reticulum in response to caffeine is greater in the n2 STZ myocyte than the nondiabetic cell (Figure 11.9). Interestingly, this excessive accumulation of Ca^{2+} by the sarcoplasmic reticulium occurs without a change in the number of ryanodine receptors, suggesting that the defect resides with the Ca^{2+}-loading rather than the Ca^{2+}-releasing step. Another abnormality noted in the n2 STZ myocyte is the elevation in basal $[Ca^{2+}]_i$ (see Figure 11.9). This defect has been attributed to impaired Na^+–Ca^{2+} exchanger activity, coupled with a rise in $[Na^+]_i$.[59,60] Although the rise in $[Ca^{2+}]_i$ is insufficient to cause acute myocardial injury, it may be responsible for many of the chronic contractile defects noted in the NIDDM heart.

11.2.4.1.2 Contribution of Altered Phosphorylation Toward Impaired Contractile Function of the n2 STZ Heart

The signal transduction pathway of insulin involves a series of phosphorylation and dephosphorylation steps, which ultimately leads to a change in the phosphorylation state and function of specific target proteins (see Figure 11.1). Therefore, it is not surprising that the activity of several of the key protein kinases and phosphatases are affected by diabetes (see Table 11.4). Although a direct link has not yet been established between changes in the phosphorylation state of specific proteins and the development of contractile defects in the n2 STZ heart, the use of various agonists suggest that the two parameters are related. Of particular interest is the observation that the positive inotropic effect of the β-adrenergic agonist isoproterenol is significantly depressed in the n2 STZ heart (Figure 11.10). Since activation of protein kinase A is unaffected by the diabetic condition,[61] it is likely that the responsiveness of the target protein to the phosphorylation event must be defective in the n2 STZ heart. Whether the primary abnormality involves a Ca^{2+} transporter or a contractile protein still remains to be established.

Another agent, whose responsiveness is affected by diabetes, is the protein kinase C activator phorbol myristate acetate. At phorbol myristate acetate concentrations of either 10 or 100 nM, the drug-induced decline in contractile function occurs more rapidly in the diabetic heart than in the age matched nondiabetic heart (Figure 11.11). This difference in response to phorbol myristate acetate may arise because the activity of certain protein kinase C isozymes, such as protein kinase C_α, is elevated in the diabetic heart. According to this scenario, the diabetes-mediated elevation in protein kinase C activity causes a hypersensitive response to the actions of phorbol myristate acetate, leading to a greater

A

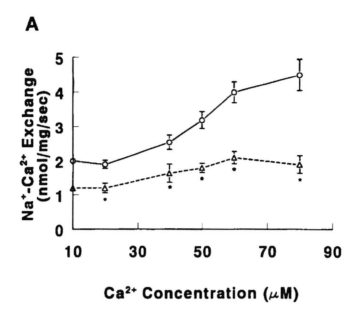

Ca²⁺ Concentration (μM)

B

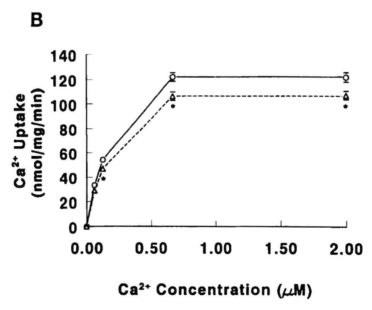

Ca²⁺ Concentration (μM)

FIGURE 11.8

Effect of noninsulin-dependent diabetes on calcium transport by the sarcolemmal Na^+–Ca^{2+} exchanger and the sarcoplasmic reticular Ca^{2+} pump. (**A**). Enriched sarcolemmal vesicles were loaded with buffer containing 140 mM NaCl. The exchange reaction was initiated by placing the vesicles in buffer containing varying concentrations of ^{45}Ca. Values shown represent means ± S.E.M. of five preparations. Asterisks denote significant difference between 12-month-old n2 STZ (Δ) and nondiabetic (O) hearts. (**B**). Enriched sarcoplasmic reticulum was prepared from n2 STZ (Δ) and nondiabetic (O) hearts. ATP-dependent Ca^{2+} uptake was determined over a free-Ca^{2+} concentration of 0.06 to 2.0 μM. Data represent means ± S.E.M. of five preparations. Asterisks denote significant difference between the diabetic and nondiabetic groups ($p < 0.05$).

reduction in actomyosin ATPase activity and a more severe alteration in Ca^{2+} movement.[55,56,62] At the present time, it is unclear whether or not this mechanism accounts for the hypersensitivity to phorbol myristate acetate in the n2 STZ heart. Nonetheless, the

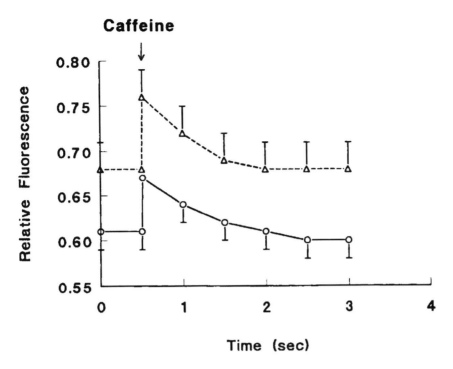

FIGURE 11.9

Effect of noninsulin-dependent diabetes on the caffeine-mediated Ca^{2+} transient. Cardiomyocytes were isolated from 12-month-old n2 STZ ($\triangle$) and nondiabetic (O) male Wistar rats. After loading the cells with fura-2 and establishing baseline fluorescence, the myocytes were exposed to 10 mM caffeine. The change in fura-2 fluorescence was then monitored as a function of time. The data are expressed as relative fluorescence of the fluorophore. Values shown represent means ± S.E.M. of four different experiments. $[Ca^{2+}]_i$ of the diabetic myocyte is significantly elevated relative to the nondiabetic ($p < 0.05$).

study reinforces the notion that the abnormal phosphorylation status is an important contributor to the development of the diabetic cardiomyopathy.

11.2.4.2 Renal Defects of the Noninsulin-Dependent Diabetic Rat

Despite the introduction of the neonatal STZ rat model over 20 years ago, relatively little information is available regarding the effects of NIDDM on the kidney of this model. Several early reports explored the effects of NIDDM on Ca^{2+} metabolism of the renal proximal tubule cell,[43,63] an important target site of insulin action. These studies demonstrated increased basal activity of the high-affinity Ca^{2+},Mg^{2+} ATPase of renal basolateral membranes prepared from 10-week-old n2 STZ rats. However, the normal stimulation in ATPase activity by insulin was virtually absent in the NIDDM kidney, although the responsiveness to parathyroid hormone and cyclic adenosine monophosphate was unaffected by the diabetic condition.[43] Despite these alterations in ATPase activity, renal function as indexed by creatinine clearance and 24-h urinary excretion of Ca^{2+} and phosphate was not affected in this model.[64] Moreover, neither fluid nor sodium excretion over a 24-h period was altered in the n2 STZ WKY rat.[65] In fact, nearly identical percentages of a total fluid and sodium load were excreted by the n2 STZ and nondiabetic WKY rat following an intravenous administration of a saline volume load (Figure 11.12). Consistent with these observations has been the demonstration that the activity of renal basolateral Na^+,K^+-ATPase, which is intimately involved in the regulation of renal fluid and sodium homeostasis, is similar between n2 STZ and nondiabetic rats.[66]

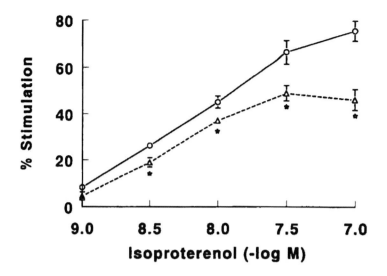

FIGURE 11.10

Effect of noninsulin-dependent diabetes on isoproterenol-mediated stimulation of myocardial contractility. Hearts from 12-month-old n2 STZ (△) and nondiabetic (○) male Wistar rats were perfused on a standard working heart apparatus. Isoproterenol was added stepwise to the perfusion buffer and changes in ventricular pressure rise measured with a Statham P23 Gb pressure transducer. The data are expressed as percent stimulation above basal levels and represent means ± S.E.M. of four to six hearts. Asterisks denote significant difference from the nondiabetic control ($p < 0.05$). At concentrations greater than 3 nM, isoproterenol increased contractility more in the nondiabetic. (From Schaffer, S. W. et al. *Am. J. Physiol.*, 260, C1165, 1991. With permission of the American Physiological Society.)

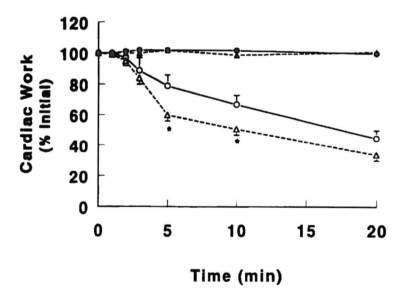

FIGURE 11.11

Effect of noninsulin-dependent diabetes on the negative inotropic effect of phorbol myristate acetate. Hearts from 12-month-old n2 STZ (▲,△) and nondiabetic (●,○) male Wistar rats were perfused with Krebs–Henseleit buffer containing 10 mM glucose. At time 0, either 10 nM phorbol myristate acetate (○,△) or the inactive phorbol ester, 4α-phorbol 12,13 didecanoate (●,▲) was added to the buffer and the change in both cardiac output and aortic pressure was monitored as a function of time. The data are expressed as percent of initial cardiac work (aortic pressure × cardiac output) and represent means ± S.E.M. of five hearts. Asterisks denote significant difference from the nondiabetic heart ($p < 0.05$). The rate of decline in cardiac work was greater in the diabetic heart.

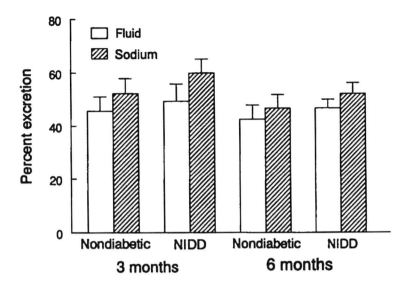

FIGURE 11.12
Effect of noninsulin-dependent diabetes (NIDD) on fluid and sodium excretion following a sodium load. At 3 and 6 months of age, n2 STZ and nondiabetic WKY rats were implanted with femoral vessels and bladder catheters. After 3 days, each rat was infused over a 30-min period with an isotonic saline solution equivalent to 5% of the animal's body weight. Urine was collected for 90 min and the excretion of fluid and sodium was determined as a percent of the total volume and sodium administered to each rat. The diabetic condition had no influence on either sodium or fluid excretion.

The lack of a significant impact of diabetes on kidney function of the 3- and 6-month-old WKY rat should be taken in the context of the mild, but progressive nature of the NIDDM condition in these rats. It is likely that, similar to cardiac complications, a longer duration of diabetes is required for manifestation of the diabetes-related functional alterations of the kidney. In accordance with this view, several modifications have been introduced to accelerate the onset of the diabetic nephropathy. In one such manipulation, it has been demonstrated that combining hypertension with neonatal STZ treatment accelerates the development of a nephropathy,[67,68] with the severity of the condition correlated with the degree of hyperglycemia.[68] However, this apparent link between the nephropathy and hyperglycemia needs to be further investigated since arterial pressure rises at an early age (6 to 12 weeks) in spontaneously hypertensive rats,[69] whereas the noninsulin-dependent diabetic condition progresses more slowly, implying that the nephropathy in the n2 STZ SHR may relate more to systemic hypertension than to the effects of NIDDM. This idea is supported by the observation that blood pressure is more elevated in the 3-month-old n2 STZ SHR than in the nondiabetic SHR.[70]

An alternative approach to unmasking diabetes-related renal functional alterations of the NIDDM rat involves surgical reduction of renal mass. Figure 11.13 shows that unilateral nephrectomy performed at 4 weeks of age results in a greater reduction in renal excretory responses to a saline volume load in the 3-month-old NIDDM rat than in its age-matched nondiabetic control. Consistent with the observed reduction in saline-stimulated diuresis and natriuresis in the nephrectomized NIDDM rat is a reduction in the baseline glomerular filtration rate (Figure 11.14). Moreover, following administration of a saline volume load, the glomerular filtration rate increases significantly more in the nephrectomized nondiabetic than in the nephrectomized NIDDM rat.[71] Although a reduction in renal mass results in both compensatory renal hypertrophy and major alterations in renal tubular transport and glomerular function,[72-74] the data suggest that in contrast

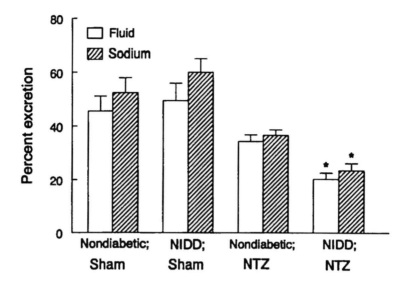

FIGURE 11.13

Effect of nephrectomy on sodium and fluid excretion of the nondiabetic and noninsulin-dependent diabetic (NIDD) WKY rat. At 4 weeks of age, all animals underwent either a right nephrectomy (NTZ) or a sham operation. To prepare for renal function studies, 3-month-old animals were implanted with femoral vessel and bladder catheters. After 3 days, each rat was infused over a 30-min period with an isotonic saline solution equivalent to 5% of the animal's body weight. Urine was collected for 90 min and the excretion of fluid and sodium was determined as a percent of the total volume and sodium administered to each rat. Unilateral nephrectomy caused a greater reduction in renal excretion of fluid and sodium in the diabetic than the nondiabetic rat. Asterisks denote significant difference from all other groups ($p < 0.05$). (From Mozaffari, M. S. et al.· *J. Pharmacol. Toxicol. Methods*, 37, 197, 1997. With permission.)

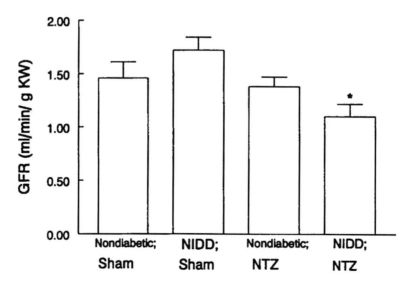

FIGURE 11.14

Effect of unilateral nephrectomy on the glomerular filtration rate of the noninsulin-dependent diabetic (NIDD) and nondiabetic WKY rat. Asterisks denote significant difference from all other groups ($p < 0.05$). The nephrectomized (NTZ) NIDD rat manifested a lower baseline glomerular filtration rate (GFR) than all other groups. (From Mozaffari, M. S. et al., *J. Pharmacol. Toxicol. Methods*, 37, 197, 1997. With permission.)

to the nephrectomized nondiabetic rat, the nephrectomized NIDDM rat is compromised in the manifestation of these compensatory changes. More importantly, it is possible that the inability to maintain sodium and fluid balance efficiently during the feeding cycle might leave the nephrectomized NIDDM rat in a state of volume and sodium retention for prolonged periods of time. This imbalance could become more prominent under dietary Na+ excess, which might trigger the development of elevated arterial pressure. In this regard, it is significant that patients with diabetes mellitus often experience difficulty in disposing of acute sodium loads.[75] According to Mbanaya et al.,[76] this effect may be more marked in patients with NIDDM and hypertension.

11.2.5 Modulation of the Metabolic Defects by Antihyperglycemic Agents

Oral hypoglycemic agents have been widely used in the treatment of noninsulin-dependent diabetes. Since the neonatal STZ rat is an established model of noninsulin-dependent diabetes, it is not surprising that it has been used to study the actions of various oral hypoglycemic agents. These studies have illustrated the utility of the neonatal STZ model in evaluating the hypoglycemic activity of new antihyperglycemic agents, such as linogliride fumarate[77] and KAD-1229.[78] The model has also been useful in contrasting the actions of the first- and second-generation sulfonylureas. However, complicating the interpretation of some of the data is the presence of both therapeutic "responders" and "nonresponders" in the same experimental population. According to Serradas et al.,[36] nonresponders tend to be more severely hyperglycemic than the responders, as evidenced by the presence of primarily nonresponders in the severely diabetic n5 STZ rat population and primarily responders among less severely diabetic n5 STZ rats. Also, milder forms of NIDDM, such as the n2 and n3-STZ Sprague-Dawley rat and the n2 STZ Wistar rat, respond favourably to sulfonylurea therapy.[36,37] Interestingly, the improvement in the metabolic state of the milder NIDDM rat following chronic sulfonylurea therapy is not always reflected in the glucose tolerance test. Schaffer et al.[37] found that chronic glipizide therapy improves insulin resistance in the heart of the n2 STZ Wistar rat without correcting the defect in glucose intolerance.

Studies designed to investigate the mechanism underlying the efficacy of sulfonylureas in the neonatal STZ rat have also been informative. One important finding is that the ability of the sulfonylureas to function as insulin secretagogues is identical in the nondiabetic and the diabetic rat, including both responders and nonresponders. Since only the responders show improvement in glucose tolerance following chronic sulfonylurea therapy, Serradas et al.[36] concluded that the sulfonylurea effect must be unrelated to acute release of insulin by the oral agent. Rather, the beneficial effects of antihyperglycemic therapy must be caused by the observed elevation in islet sensitivity to glucose and a postreceptor potentiation in insulin action. This scenario is attractive because it would explain both the improvement in glucose tolerance and the reduction in insulin resistance.

11.3 Comparison of Neonatal STZ Rat Model with Other Animal Models of Noninsulin-Dependent Diabetes

Several animal models of noninsulin-dependent diabetes have been developed. Although most of these models carry a genetic predisposition to develop noninsulin-dependent diabetes, the neonatal STZ rodent model is unique, depending on a chemical rather than

TABLE 11.5

Key Features of Noninsulin-Dependent Diabetic Animal Models

Property	Sand Rat	GK Rat	n2 STZ Rat
Body weight	↑	=	=
Insulin receptor number	↓	↓	↑
Receptor tyrosine kinase activity	↓	=	↑
Insulin sensitivity	↓	↓	↓
Rate of gluconeogenesis	↑	↑	↑
Pancreatic β-cell number	↓	↓	↓
Glucose-induced insulin secretion rate	↓	↓	↓

Note: Signs in the table indicate increases (↑), decreases (↓) or no change (=) in the key properties of three different animal models of noninsulin-dependent diabetes.

a genetic lesion. Because the chemical lesion in the neonatal STZ model is induced by STZ, a specific pancreatic toxin, the initial pathological lesion in the NIDDM model is restricted to the pancreas. By contrast, most genetic models are characterized by multiple lesions affecting numerous processes.

The most widely studied genetic model of insulin resistance and glucose intolerance is the obese Zucker rat. Although the Zucker rat has been described as a model of noninsulin-dependent diabetes, the rat is normoglycemic, indicating that it is a more appropriate model of obesity than diabetes.[79] For the same reason, the ob/ob mouse, the WKY rat group, the corpulent cp rat group, the KK mouse, and the NZO mouse, which have all been touted as NIDDM models, are more accurately classified as obesity models.[79] However, overt hyperglycemia does develop in several species with concomitant obesity, including the C57BKS db/db mouse, the sand rat (*Psammomys obesus*) and the Otsuka-Long-Evans-Tokushima Fatty rat. In these three NIDDM models, the initial lesion triggering the development of diabetes appears to be the appearance of the hyperinsulinemic state. It has been proposed that chronic exposure to elevated insulin levels induces pancreatic and extrapancreatic changes that adversely affect the ability of insulin to regulate glucose levels. One adverse consequence of hyperinsulinemia is its link to the downregulation of insulin receptor function, which in turn leads to insulin resistance. Another consequence of excessive insulin secretion is the "exhaustion" or deterioration of the β-cell, resulting in a decline in insulin secretion. In the C57BKS db/db mouse, a transition from a hyperinsulinemic–normoglycemic state to a severe hypoinsulinemic–hyperglycemic state occurs at about 2 to 4 months of age.[80] Although this transition is genetically predetermined, its severity is modulated by diet. Interestingly, diet is also an important determinant of diabetes in the sand rat. In fact, the decline in pancreatic β-cell function is only manifest after excessive food intake[79,81] (Table 11.5). In the Otsuka-Long-Evans-Tokushima Fatty rat, β-cell dysfunction also triggers onset of diabetes. However, the prevailing view is that a defect in the proliferative capacity of the β-cell plays a major role in the development of the diabetes.[82]

In addition to the genetically obese NIDDM models, two rodent models of nonobese, noninsulin-dependent diabetes have been described, the GK rat[83,84] and the BHE rat.[85] In both species, a decrease in β-cell mass precedes the onset of hyperglycemia (see Table 11.5). Despite the fall in β-cell number, insulin secretion is initially adequate and a normoglycemic state is maintained. However, the remaining β-cells subsequently undergo a sequence of changes, ultimately leading to impaired glucose-induced insulin secretion and the appearance of hyperglycemia and hypoinsulinemia. Although metabolic abnormalities, such as elevated rates of gluconeogenesis and impaired insulin responsiveness, have also been observed in these models, many of the metabolic changes do not precede the onset of hyperglycemia, suggesting that they are contributors to the severity of the glucose-intolerant state rather than initiators of the process.

The major advantage of the nonobese, genetic NIDDM models and the neonatal STZ rat model is the existence of NIDDM without the complicating influence of obesity. Although all of these models are capable of providing important information on the mechanisms underlying the development of NIDDM, the neonatal STZ model has been the most widely characterized. Thus, the neonatal model has been invaluable in studying the complications of NIDDM. Since pathophysiological changes are noted in the kidney, heart, and other tissues of the NIDDM rat, this model will continue to provide fertile ground for investigating the causes of diabetes-induced complications. It will also continue to provide valuable information on the efficacy of various antihyperglycemic agents.

Acknowledgments

This work is supported in part with grants from the American Heart Association (Southeast Affiliate).

References

1. Kahn, C.R., Weir, G.C., *Joslin's Diabetes Mellitus*, Lea & Febiger, Philadelphia, 1994, chap. 12.
2. Ward, W. K., Beard, J. C., Halter, J. B., Pfeifer, M. A., Porte D., Jr., Pathophysiology of insulin secretion in noninsulin-dependent diabetes mellitus, *Diabetes Care*, 7, 491, 1984.
3. Brunzell, J. D., Robertson, R. P., Lerner, R. L., Hazzard, W. R., Ensinck, J. W., Bierman, E. L., Porte, D., Jr., Relationships between fasting plasma glucose levels and insulin secretion during intravenous glucose tolerance tests, *J. Clin. Endocrinol. Metabol.*, 42, 222, 1976.
4. Robertson, R. P., Defective insulin secretion in NIDDM: Integral part of a multiplier hypothesis, *J. Cell. Biochem.*, 48, 227, 1992.
5. Stoffel, M., Froguel, P. H., Takeda, J., Zouali, H., Vionnet, N., Nishi, S., Weber, I. T., Harrison, R. W., Pilkis, S. J., Lesage, S., Vaxillaire, M., Velko, G., Sun, F., Iris, F., Passa, P. H., Cohen, D., Bell, G. I., Human glucose kinase gene: isolation, characterization, and identification of two missense mutations linked to early-onset noninsulin-dependent (type 2) diabetes mellitus, *Proc. Natl. Acad. Sci. U.S.A.*, 89, 7698, 1992.
6. Velho, G., Froguel, P. H., Genetic determinants of noninsulin-dependent diabetes mellitus: strategies and recent results, *Diabetes Metab.* (Paris), 23, 7, 1997.
7. Haneda, M., Polonsky, K. S., Bergenstal, R. M., Jaspan, J. B., Shoelan, S. E., Blix, P. M., Chan, S. J., Kwok, S. C. M., Wishner, W. B., Zeidler, A., Olefsky, J. M., Freidenberg, G., Tager, H. S., Steiner, D. F., Rubenstein, A. H., Familial hyperinsulinemia due to a structurally abnormal insulin: definition of an emerging new clinical syndrome, *N. Engl. J. Med.*, 310, 1288, 1984.
8. Reaven, G. M., Bernstein, R., Davis, B., Olefsky, J. M., Nonketotic diabetes mellitus: insulin deficiency or insulin resistance? *Am. J. Med.*, 60, 80, 1976.
9. Swislocki, A. L. M., Donner, C. C., Fraze, E., Chen, Y.-D. I., Reaven, G. M., Can insulin resistance exist as a primary defect in noninsulin-dependent diabetes mellitus? *J. Clin. Endocrinol. Metabol.*, 64, 778, 1987.
10. Caro, J. F., Dohm, L. G., Pories, W. J., Sinha, M. K., Cellular alterations in liver, skeletal muscle and adipose tissue responsible for insulin resistance in obesity and Type II diabetes, *Diabetes Metab. Rev.*, 5, 665, 1989.

11. Felber, J.-P., Ferrannini, E., Golay, A., Meyer, H. U., Theibaud, D., Curchod, B., Maeder, E., Jequier, E., DeFronzo, R. A., Role of lipid oxidation in pathogenesis of insulin resistance of obesity and Type II diabetes, *Diabetes*, 36, 1341, 1987.

12. Garvey, W. T., Insulin resistance and noninsulin-dependent diabetes mellitus: which horse is pulling the cart? *Diabetes Metabolism Rev.*, 5, 727, 1989.

13. Laakso, M., Malkki, M., Kekalainen, P., Kuusisto, J., Deeb, S. S., Insulin receptor substrate-1 variants in noninsulin-dependent diabetes, *J. Clin. Invest.*, 94, 1141, 1994.

14. Taylor, S. I., Accili, D., Imai, Y., Insulin resistance or deficiency: which is the primary cause of NIDDM? *Diabetes*, 43, 735, 1994.

15. Shepherd, P. R., Nave, B. T., O'Rahilly, S., The role of phosphoinositide 3-kinase in insulin signaling, *J. Mol. Endocrinol.*, 17, 175, 1996.

16. Vestergaard, H., Bjorbaek, C., Hansen, T., Larsen, F. S., Granner, D. K., Pedersen, O., Impaired activity and gene expression of hexokinase II in muscle from noninsulin-dependent diabetes mellitus patients, *J. Clin. Invest.*, 96, 2639, 1995.

17. Vogt, B., Muhlbacher, C., Carrascosa, J., Obermaier-Kusser, B., Seffer, E., Mushack, J., Pongratz, D., Haring, H. U., Subcellular distribution of GLUT 4 in the skeletal muscle of lean Type II (noninsulin-dependent) diabetic patients in the basal state, *Diabetologia*, 35, 456, 1992.

18. Zierath, J. R., Houseknecht, K. L., Kahn, B. B., Glucose transporters and diabetes, *Cell Dev. Biol.*, 7, 295, 1996.

19. Garvey, W. T., Maianu, L., Huecksteadt, T. P., Birnbaum, M. J., Molina, J. M., Ciaraldi, T. P., Pretranslational suppression of glucose transporter protein causes insulin resistance in adipocytes from patients with noninsulin-dependent diabetes mellitus and obesity, *J. Clin. Invest.*, 87, 1072, 1991.

20. Saad, M. F., Knowler, W. C., Pettitt, D. J., Nelson, R. G., Charles, M. A., Bennett, P. H., A two-step model for development of noninsulin-dependent diabetes, *Am. J. Med.*, 90, 229, 1991.

21. Porte, D., Jr., Kahn, S. E., The key role of islet dysfunction in Type II diabetes mellitus, *Clin. Invest. Med.*, 18, 247, 1995.

22. Weir, G. C., Bonner-Weir, S., Leahy, J. L., Islet mass and function in diabetes and transplantation, *Diabetes*, 39, 401, 1990.

23. Blondel, O., Bailbe, D., Portha, B., Relation of insulin deficiency to impaired insulin action in NIDDM adult rats given streptozotocin as neonates, *Diabetes*, 38, 610, 1989.

24. Weir, G. C., Clore, E. T., Zmachinsky, C. J., Bonner-Weir, S., Islet secretion in a new experimental model for noninsulin-dependent diabetes, *Diabetes*, 30, 590, 1981.

25. Wang, R. N., Bouwens, L., Kloppel, G., Beta-cell growth in adolescent and adult rats treated with streptozotocin during the neonatal period, *Diabetologia*, 39, 548, 1996.

26. Bonner-Weir, S., Trent, D. F., Honey, R. N., Weir, G. C., Responses of neonatal islets to streptozotocin: limited β-cell regeneration and hyperglycemia, *Diabetes*, 30, 64, 1981.

27. Iwase, M., Nunoi, K., Himeno, H., Yoshinari, M., Kikuchi, M., Maki, Y., Fujishima, M., Susceptibility to neonatal streptozotocin-induced diabetes in spontaneously hypertensive rats, *Pancreas*, 9, 344, 1994.

28. Schaffer, S. W., Wilson, G. L., Insulin resistance and mechanical dysfunction in hearts of Wistar rats with streptozotocin-induced noninsulin-dependent diabetes mellitus, *Diabetologia*, 36, 195, 1993.

29. Ashcroft, F. M., Proks, P., Smith, P. A., Ammala, C., Bokvist, K., Rorsman, P., Stimulus-secretion coupling in pancreatic β-cells, *J. Cell. Biochem.*, 55S, 54, 1994.

30. Giroix, M.-H., Portha, B., Kergoat, M., Bailbe, D., Picon, L., Glucose insensitivity and amino-acid hypersensitivity of insulin release in rats with noninsulin-dependent diabetes: a study with the perfused pancreas, *Diabetes*, 32, 445, 1983.

31. Grill, V., Sako, Y., Ostenson, C.-G., Jalkanen, P., Multiple abnormalities in insulin responses to nonglucose nutrients in neonatally streptozotocin diabetic rats, *Endocrinology*, 128, 2195, 1991.

32. Portha, B., Giroix, M.-H., Serradas, P., Welsh, N., Hellerstrom, C., Sener, A., Malaisse, W. J., Insulin production and glucose metabolism in isolated pancreatic islets of rats with NIDDM, *Diabetes*, 37, 1226, 1988.

33. Tsuji, K., Taminato, T., Ishida, H., Okamoto, Y., Tsuura, Y., Kato, S., Kurose, T., Okada, Y., Imura, H., Seino, Y., Selective impairment of the cytoplasmic Ca^{2+} response to glucose in pancreatic β-cells of streptozotocin-induced noninsulin-dependent diabetic rats, *Metabolism*, 42, 1424, 1993.

34. Kergoat, M., Giroix, M. H., Portha, B., Evidence for normal *in vitro* Ca^{2+}-stimulated insulin release in rats with noninsulin-dependent diabetes, *Diabete Metab.* (Paris), 12, 9, 1986.

35. Leahy, J. L., Bonner-Weir, S., Weir, G. C., Abnormal insulin secretion in a streptozotocin model of diabetes: effects of insulin treatment, *Diabetes*, 34, 660, 1985.

36. Serradas, P., Bailbe, D., Portha, B., Long-term gliclazide treatment improves the *in vitro* glucose-induced insulin release in rats with Type II (noninsulin-dependent) diabetes induced by neonatal streptozotocin, *Diabetologia*, 32, 577, 1989.

37. Schaffer, S. W., Warner, B. A., Wilson, G. L., Effects of chronic glipizide treatment on the NIDD heart, *Horm. Metab. Res.*, 25, 348, 1993.

38. Kergoat, M., Guerre-Millo, M., Lavau, M., Portha, B., Increased insulin action in rats with mild insulin deficiency induced by neonatal streptozotocin, *Am. J. Physiol.*, 260, E561, 1991.

39. Melin, B., Caron, M. Cherqui, G., Blivet, M.-J., Bailbe, D., Picard, J., Capeau, J., Portha, B., Increased insulin action in cultured hepatocytes from rats with diabetes induced by neonatal streptozotocin, *Endocrinology*, 128, 1693, 1991.

40. Fantus, I. G., Chayoth, R., O'Dea L., Marliss, E. B., Yale, J.-F., Grose, M., Insulin binding and glucose transport in adipocytes in neonatal streptozotocin-injected rat model of diabetes mellitus, *Diabetes*, 36, 54, 1987.

41. Trent, D. F., Fletcher, D. J., May, J. M., Bonner-Weir, S., Weir, G. C., Abnormal islet and adipocyte function in young β-cell-deficient rats with near-normoglycemia, *Diabetes*, 33, 170, 1984.

42. Grunberger, G., Nagy, K., Rempinski, D., Levy, J., Abnormal insulin receptor tyrosine kinase activity in kidney basolateral membranes from noninsulin-dependent diabetic rats. *J. Lab. Clin. Med.*, 115, 704, 1990.

43. Levy, J., Rempinski, D., Kuo, T. H., Hormone-specific defect in insulin regulation of (Ca^{++} + Mg^{++})-adenosine triphosphatase activity in kidney membranes from streptozocin noninsulin-dependent diabetic rats, *Metabolism*, 43, 604, 1994.

44. Karl, I. E., Gavin, J. R., III, Levy, J., Effect of insulin on glucose utilization in epitrochlearis muscle of rats with streptozocin-induced NIDDM, *Diabetes*, 39, 1106, 1990.

45. Schaffer, S. W., Tan, B. H., Wilson, G. L., Development of a cardiomyopathy in a model of noninsulin-dependent diabetes, *Am. J. Physiol.*, 248, H179, 1985.

46. Consoli, A., Nurjhan, N., Capani, F., Gerich, J., Predominant role of gluconeogenesis in increased hepatic glucose production in NIDDM, *Diabetes*, 38, 550, 1989.

47. Schaffer, S. W., Seyed-Mozaffari, M., Cutcliff, C. R., Wilson, G. L., Postreceptor myocardial metabolic defect in a rat model of noninsulin-dependent diabetes mellitus, *Diabetes*, 35, 593, 1986.

48. Schaffer, S. W., Cardiomyopathy associated with noninsulin-dependent diabetes, *Mol. Cell. Biochem.*, 107, 1, 1991.

49. Schaffer, S. W., Mozaffari, M. S., Artman, M., Wilson, G. L., Basis for myocardial mechanical defects associated with noninsulin-dependent diabetes, *Am. J. Physiol.*, 256, E25, 1989.

50. Takamatsu, T., Wier, W. G., Calcium waves in mammalian heart: quantification of origin, magnitude, waveform and velocity, *FASEB J.*, 4, 1519, 1990.

51. Lakatta, E. G., Functional implications of spontaneous sarcoplasmic reticulum Ca^{2+} release in the heart, *Cardiovasc. Res.*, 26, 193, 1992.

52. Alpert, N. R., Mulieri, L. A., Functional consequences of altered cardiac myosin isoenzymes, *Med. Sci. Sports Exerc.*, 18, 309, 1986.

53. Afzal, N., Pierce, G. N., Elimban, V. Beamish, R. E., Dhalla, N. S., Influence of verapamil on some subcellular defects in diabetic cardiomyopathy, *Am. J. Physiol.*, 256, E453, 1989.

54. Kitakaze, M., Weisman, H. F., Marban, E., Contractile dysfunction and ATP depletion after transient calcium overload in perfused ferret hearts, *Circulation*, 77, 685, 1988.

55. Jideama, N. M., Noland, T. A., Jr., Raynor, R. L., Blobe, G. C., Fabbro, D., Kazanietz, M. G., Blumberg, P. M., Hannun, Y. A., Kuo, J. F., Phosphorylation specificities of protein kinase C isozymes for bovine cardiac troponin I and troponin T and sites within these proteins and regulation of myofilament properties, *J. Biol. Chem.*, 271, 23277, 1996.

56. Venema, R. C., Kuo, J. F., Protein kinase C-mediated phosphorylation of troponin I and C-protein in isolated myocardial cells is associated with inhibition of myofibrillar actomyosin MgATPase, *J. Biol. Chem.*, 268, 2705, 1993.

57. Shattock, M. J., Bers, D. M., Rat vs. rabbit ventricle: Ca flux and intracellular Na assessed by ion-selective microelectrodes, *Am. J. Physiol.*, 256, C813, 1989.

58. Bridge, J. H. B., Smolley, J. R., Spitzer, K. W., The relationship between charge movements associated with I_{Ca} and I_{Na-Ca} in cardiac myocytes, *Science*, 248, 376, 1990.

59. Allo, S. N., Lincoln, T. M., Wilson, G. L., Green, F. J., Watanabe, A. M., Schaffer, S. W., Non-insulin-dependent diabetes-induced defects in cardiac cellular calcium regulation, *Am. J. Physiol.*, 260, C1165, 1991.

60. Schaffer, S. W., Mozaffari, M., Abnormal mechanical function in diabetes: relation to myocardial calcium handling, *Coronary Artery Dis.*, 7, 109, 1996.

61. Schaffer, S. W., Allo, S., Punna, S., White, T., Defective response to cAMP-dependent protein kinase in noninsulin-dependent diabetic heart, *Am. J. Physiol.*, 261, E369, 1991.

62. Ward, C. A., Moffat, M. P., Positive and negative inotropic effects of phorbol 12-myristate 13-acetate: relationship to PKC-dependence and changes in $[Ca^{2+}]_i$, *J. Mol. Cell. Cardiol.*, 24, 937, 1992.

63. Levy, J., Gavin, J. R., Hammerman, M. R., Avioli, L. V., $Ca^{++}-Mg^{++}$-ATPase activity in kidney basolateral membrane in noninsulin-dependent diabetic rats, *Diabetes*, 35, 899, 1986.

64. Levy, J., Teitelbaum, S. L., Gavin, J. R., Fausto, A., Kurose, H., Avioli, L. V., Bone calcification and calcium homeostasis in rats with noninsulin-dependent diabetes induced by streptozocin, *Diabetes*, 34, 365, 1985.

65. Iwase, M., Nunoi, K., Wakisaka, M., Wada, M., Kodama, T., Maki, Y., Fujishima, M., Effects of salt loading on glucose tolerance, blood pressure, and albuminuria in rats with noninsulin-dependent diabetes mellitus, *Metabolism*, 41, 969, 1992.

66. Levy, J., Avioli, L. V., Roberts, M. L., Gavin, J. R., $(Na^+ + K^+)$-ATPase activity in kidney basolateral membranes of noninsulin-dependent diabetic rats, *Biochem. Biophys. Res. Commun.*, 139, 1313, 1986.

67. Sato, T., Nara, Y., Note, S., Yamori, Y., New establishment of hypertensive diabetic animal models: neonatally streptozocin-treated spontaneously hypertensive rats, *Metabolism*, 36, 731, 1987.

68. Wakisaka, M., Nunoi, K., Iwase, M., Kikuchi, M., Maki, Y., Yamamato, K., Sadoshima, S., Fujishima, M., Early development of nephropathy in a new model of spontaneously hypertensive rat with noninsulin-dependent diabetes mellitus, *Diabetologia*, 31, 291, 1988.

69. Sripairojthikoon, W., Oparil, S., Wyss, J. M., Renal nerve contribution to NaCl-exacerabed hypertension in spontaneously hypertensive rats, *Hypertension*, 14, 184, 1989.

70. Sato, T., Nara, Y., Kato, Y., Yamori, Y., Hypertensive diabetic rats: different effects of streptozotocin treatment on blood pressure in adult SHR and in neonatal SHR, *Clin. Exp. Hyper. Theor. Pract.*, A13, 981, 1991.

71. Mozaffari, M. S., Warren, B. K., Russell, C. M., Schaffer, S. W., Renal function in the noninsulin-dependent diabetic rat: effects of unilateral nephrectomy, *J. Pharmacol. Toxicol. Methods*, 37, 197, 1997.

72. Haylor, J., Chowdry, J., Baillie, H., Cope, G., el Nahas, A. M., Renal function and nephrectomy in the dwarf rat following a reduction in renal mass, *Nephrol., Dialysis, Transplant.*, 11, 643, 1996.

73. Shohat, J., Erman, A., Boner, G., Rosenfield, J., Mechanisms of the early and late response to the kidney to contralateral nephrectomy, *Renal Physiol. Biochem.*, 14, 103, 1991.

74. Blantz, R. C., Paterson, O. W., Thomson, S. C., Tubuloglomerular feedback responses to acute contralateral nephrectomy, *Am. J. Physiol.*, 260, F749, 1991.

75. Roland, J. M., O'Hare, J. P., Valters, G., Corrall, R. J. M., Sodium retention in response to saline infusion in uncomplicated diabetes mellitus, *Diabetes Res.*, 3, 213, 1986.

76. Mbanya, J. C., Thomas, T. H., Taylor, R., Alberti, K. G. M. M., Wilkinson, R., Increased proximal tubular sodium reabsorption in hypertensive patients with Type II diabetes, *Diabetic Med.*, 6, 614, 1989.

77. Marchione, C.S., Tuman, R.W., Linogliride fumarate, an oral hypoglycemic agent, improves oral glucose tolerance in a rat model of noninsulin-dependent diabetes (NIDDM), *Drug Dev. Res.*, 17, 161, 1989.

78. Ohnota, H., Kitamura, T., Kinukawa, M., Hamano, S., Shibata, N. Miyata, H., Ujiie, A., A rapid-and short-acting hypoglycemic agent KAD-1229 improves post-prandial hyperglycemia and diabetic complications in streptozotocin-induced noninsulin-dependent diabetes mellitus rats, *Jpn. J. Pharmacol.*, 71, 315, 1996.

79. Shafrir, E., Development and consequences of insulin resistance: lessons from animals with hyperinsulinemia, *Diabetes & Metab.* (Paris), 22, 122, 1996.

80. Leiter, E. H., Coleman, D. L., Ingram, D. K., Reynolds, M. A., Influence of dietary carbohydrates on the induction of diabetes in C57BL/KsJ-db/db diabetes mice, *J. Nutr.*, 113, 184, 1983.

81. Marquie, G., Duhault, J., Jacotot, B., Diabetes mellitus in sand rats (*Psammomys obesus*): metabolic pattern during development of the diabetic syndrome, *Diabetes*, 33, 438, 1984.

82. Zhu, M., Noma, Y., Mizuno, A., Sano, T., Shima, K., Poor capacity for proliferation of pancreatic β-cells in Otsuka-Long-Evans-Tokushima Fatty rat: a model of spontaneous NIDDM, *Diabetes*, 45, 941, 1996.

83. Bisbis, S., Bailbe, D., Tormo, M-A, Picarel-Blanchot, F., Derouet, M., Simon, J., Portha, B., Insulin resistance in the GK rat: decreased receptor number but normal kinase activity in liver, *Am. J. Physiol.*, 65, E807, 1993.

84. Picarel-Blanchot, F., Berthelier, C., Bailbe, D., Portha, B., Impaired insulin secretion and excessive hepatic glucose production are both early events in the diabetic GK rat, *Am. J. Physiol.*, 271, E755, 1996.

85. Berdanier, C. D., The BHE rat: an animal model for the study of noninsulin-dependent diabetes mellitus, *FASEB J.*, 5, 2139, 1991.

12

Spontaneous Insulin-Dependent Diabetes Mellitus (IDDM) in Nonobese Diabetic (NOD) Mice: Comparisons with Experimentally Induced IDDM

Edward H. Leiter, Ivan C. Gerling, and Jeffrey C. Flynn

CONTENTS

12.1 Introduction

The inbred mouse has remained the premiere organism for analyzing the genetic basis for susceptibility/resistance to spontaneous or induced diseases of biomedical significance. However, until the appearance of spontaneous, T cell–mediated insulin-dependent diabetes mellitus (IDDM) in the Nonobese Diabetic (NOD) mouse strain, diabetes investigators seeking to utilize mouse models of IDDM were limited to the analysis of experimentally induced hyperglycemia. As described in this and other chapters of this volume, the pancreatic β-cell toxins, streptozotocin (STZ) and alloxan (AL), as well as certain human pathogenic viruses adapted for growth in mouse cells, have provided a mechanism for inducing hyperglycemia in otherwise normal mice. Indeed, some investigators have claimed that male mice rendered diabetic by multiple, low doses of STZ develop an autoimmune, T cell–mediated IDDM. The purpose of this chapter will first be to describe the strain–specific characteristics of NOD mice and then to review briefly the immunogenetic and pathophysiological features of spontaneous autoimmune IDDM development that sets this strain apart from other inbred strains of mice. Then, the basis for susceptibility in the NOD strain will be contrasted with what is known about differential susceptibility of mice to STZ, AL, and certain diabetogenic viruses.

12.2 The NOD Mouse

The descriptor "NOD" designates an inbred strain of albino mice developed by Makino et al.[1] in Japan. Descended from outbred Jcl:ICR (Swiss mice) progenitors, today's NOD mice represent the product of over 80 generations of sib matings. The origins of this strain in Japan are described in detail elsewhere.[1-3] It is notable that over the first 20 generations of sib matings, the strain was being maintained as a normoglycemic control line to match with another line being selected for impaired glucose tolerance (the NON strain). Once spontaneous development of IDDM was observed in a female of the "control" NOD strain at F20, development of frank hyperglycemia and glycosuria rather than normoglycemia became the selected phenotypes. Because not all NOD mice develop diabetes, it is recommended that the strain be referred to by its three letter abbreviation (NOD) instead of as Nonobese Diabetic. String abbreviations are standardly used to identify inbred strains (e.g., one refers to BALB mice instead of "Bagg Albino" mice, etc.).

12.2.1 Strain Description

Spontaneous development of autoimmune T cell–mediated IDDM in NOD mice of both sexes is the salient strain characteristic. The pathogenic role of autoreactive T cells in NOD mice has been well established.[4-8] The prediabetic period is characterized by a heavy leukocytic infiltration of the pancreas (insulitis). Insulitis initiates as early as 2 to 3 week postpartum in females, and slightly later in males. The intraislet leukocytes, primarily CD4+ and CD8+ T cells, with variable numbers of B lymphocytes and macrophages/dendritic cells, elicit destruction of only the β-cells in the pancreatic islets.[9,10] Onset of hyperglycemia and glycosuria is earlier in females than in males. Females also show an earlier age of onset and higher cumulative incidence of IDDM. Breeding females are particularly susceptible to early onset of hyperglycemia. Prophylactic measures, commonly giving young breeders a single injection of complete Freund's adjuvant (CFA, see below) are employed in some colonies to retard IDDM onset in breeding stock. The IDDM frequencies observed in virgin NOD mice vary widely between colonies, with male incidences being the most variable, ranging between 0 and 70% depending upon the colony.[11] This variability has been shown to be the consequence of environmental factors, both in the microbial and dietary environments.[12-14] This topic has been discussed extensively elsewhere.[3,15-18] Although investigators working with experimentally induced IDDM in mice and rats generally have not paid full heed to the physical and microbiological environment in which their mice or rats were housed, experience with the NOD mouse and the spontaneously diabetic BB rat model[19,20] has made it abundantly clear that these considerations are not trivial, and should be major concerns of any investigator using any rodent model of IDDM.

Detailed protocols describing the requirements for maintaining a specific pathogen-free (SPF) environment required to maintain a high frequency of IDDM in NOD mice of both sexes may be found in a contribution by one of the authors (EHL) in a recent supplement of *Current Protocols in Immunology.*[16] In the research colony of NOD/Lt mice maintained by one of the authors (EHL) at the Jackson Laboratory, approximately 80% of females maintained on chow diet are diabetic by 20 weeks of age, and 90% by 30 weeks. NOD/Lt male incidence is more variable, with approximately 20% diabetic by 20 weeks of age, and 40 to 70% diabetic by 40 weeks. Interestingly, even though penetrance of diabetes is suppressed in low-incidence colonies, such as the NOD/Wehi substrain, insulitis of variable severity is prevalent in most NOD mice.[21] In such colonies in which IDDM incidence is repressed because of undefined environmental or genetic influences, cyclophosphamide treatment has been effectively used to trigger IDDM onset.[22]

12.2.2 Other NOD Strain Characteristics

NOD mice exhibit a variety of interesting strain characteristics. They develop a progressively more severe hearing loss[23] that is apparently under polygenic control (Dr. Ken Johnson, the Jackson Laboratory, personal communication). Some of the unusual genetic features of the strain will be discussed in a following section. Nondiabetic NOD mice are exceptionally good breeders; females produce litters of 11 to 14 pups and successfully nurse the entire litter to weaning. Aging NOD mice spared an early death due to IDDM development are highly prone to tumor development. Lymphomas are the most common tumor, but a variety of other tumors, some relatively rare in mice, such as osteosarcomas, have been commonly recorded.[24] The high tumor susceptibility of the strain is reflected by the development of thymic lymphomas in 100% of T and B lymphocyte–deficient NOD/LtSz-*scid/scid* mice.[25] Leukocytic infiltrations are not limited to the pancreas and pancreatic islets of NOD mice. Lymphocytic infiltrates in thyroid (subclinical thyroiditis), submandibular salivary gland (sialoadenitis), lacrymal and Harderian glands (dacryoadenitis), kidney (focal glomerulonephritis), muscle (focal myositis), nerve (focal neuritis), and colon (focal colitis) have all been observed in aging NOD/Lt mice that have remained IDDM-free.[3] Hemolytic anemia accompanied by development of Coombs' positive autoantibodies, reticulocytosis, splenomegaly, and jaundice has been observed in aging (>200 days) mice of both the NOD/Wehi and NOD/Lt substrains.[26]

12.2.3   Immunodeficiencies Underlying Autoimmunity in NOD Mice

Although T cells have been shown to be essential mediators of β-cell destruction in both the BB-DP (diabetes prone) rat (described in Chapter 13 by Field and Butler) and in NOD mice, the two models superficially appear to be very different. BB-DP rats (a Wistar-like strain) are extremely immunodeficient, due to homozygosity for a single recessive gene (*Lyp*) producing T-lymphopenia. T-lymphopenia in these rats compromises their ability to reject allografts. In contrast, NOD mice rapidly reject allo- or xenografts, and appear to be "mirror images" of BB-DP rats in exhibiting a very high percentages of T cells (T-lymphoaccumulation) in peripheral lymphoid organs.[14] Yet the NOD-characteristic T-lymphoaccumulation results from polygenically controlled immunodeficiencies as profound as those produced solely by the *Lyp* gene in BB-DP rats.

   NOD mice exhibit a collection of immunodeficiencies in both innate and adaptive immunity.[25,27] A combination of these deficiencies allows release of increased numbers of potentially islet-autoreactive T cells into the periphery. The immunobiology of T cells and potential abnormalities in repertoire development in NOD mice have been reviewed recently.[28] Defects in the ability of NOD bone marrow-derived antigen-presenting cells (APC) to activate immunotolerogenic functions both intrathymically and in the periphery have been implicated.[14] These APC tolerogenic defects in NOD mice are controlled by both the unique MHC haplotype ($H2^{g7}$), and non-MHC genes that limit the ability of these cells to become functionally mature. Acquisition of T cell tolerance to low-abundance endocrine cell antigens may normally entail the spontaneous, transient expression of genes encoding these self-proteins within the thymus during the first week postpartum.[29] In NOD mice, defects have been identified in apoptotic death of thymocytes and in peripheral T cells.[30,31] This would lead to negative selection mechanisms being overwhelmed, and in part account for the NOD strain-characteristic delayed thymic involution[32] and concomitant colonization of the periphery with excessive numbers of long-lived T cells. Genetic ablation of a number of T cell receptor Vβ genes preferentially utilized by the NOD genome to generate the peripheral T cell repertoire of this strain fails to prevent IDDM development.[33] Moreover, when T cell receptor (TCR) gene utilization is examined in multiple islets obtained from a single NOD mouse, a spectrum of TCR clonotypes is represented.[28,34] These considerations would suggest that a wide spectrum of β-cell antigens, both soluble and membrane bound, rather than a single candidate autoantigen, constitute the targets of the islet-infiltrating T cells. It should not be overlooked that, although the NOD mouse serves as an excellent model for IDDM development in humans in many respects, certain strain–specific peculiarities, such as T-lymphoaccumulation, exist. Hence, it cannot be excluded that a more-limited repertoire of TCR and the β-cell autoantigens they recognize may serve as the focus of the autoimmune attack on human β-cells.

   While the "spillage" of autoreactive T cells into the periphery may reflect incomplete negative selection as a consequence of impaired apoptotic mechanisms, NOD mice are characterized by an inability to maintain adequate suppression of self-reactive T effectors in the periphery.[35] Treatments that accelerate diabetogenesis in young prediabetic NOD mice (neonatal administration of cyclosporine, adolescent thymectomy, and cyclophosphamide administration) are thought to impair peripheral suppressor function.[36] The potential pathogenic significance of this is well illustrated by NOR/Lt, a recombinant congenic strain produced by outcross of NOD/Lt with C57BLKS/J.[37] NOR/Lt mice share approximately 88% of their genome with NOD/Lt, including NOD alleles at numerous *Idd* susceptibility loci, including *H2^{g7}*.[38] Although T-lymphoaccumulation is present in NOR/Lt as it is in NOD/Lt, leukocytic infiltrates in the pancreas rarely transit from a peri-insular, perivascular to an intraislet localization. Yet autoimmune T effectors can be generated in NOR/Lt mice, since a low percentage of older mice can be rendered diabetic by cyclophosphamide treatment (unpublished results, EHL laboratory). Consistent with the possibility that NOR/Lt mice maintain better peripheral inhibition of autoreactive T cells was the demonstration of normalized activation of immunoregulatory T cells in a syngeneic mixed lymphocyte reaction (SMLR) in NOR/Lt compared with NOD/Lt.[37] Restoration of SMLR function by treatment of NOD mice *in vivo* with IL-2 correlated with protection from IDDM development.[39]

12.2.4 Other NOD Strain-Characteristic Immunodeficiencies

12.2.4.1 Antigen-Presenting Cells

Immunodeficiencies associated with NOD antigen-presenting functions have recently been reviewed.[40] These defects presumably account, in part, for why NOD mice do not tolerize well to self-antigens,[41] do not negatively select autoreactive T cells in the thymus, and/or do not suppress their function in the periphery.[42] Abnormal responses of NOD myelopoietic precursors to myelopoietic growth factors (CSF-1, GM-CSF, IL-3) and differentiation factors (interferon γ) contribute to their failure to mature completely into fully differentiated macrophages.[43-45] This immaturity is reflected by subnormal LPS-stimulated IL-1 secretion,[43,44] with the biological potency of the IL-1 secreted attenuated by a higher than normal production of IL-1 receptor antagonist (Serreze and Leiter, unpublished observations). This defect appears to be post-transcriptional, since IL-1 mRNA levels appear normal.[35,39] Several lines of evidence argue that this decreased IL-1 secretory capacity may be of pathogenic significance. IL-1 supplementation *in vitro* restores the ability of NOD APC to activate immunoregulatory T cells in an SMLR.[35] Further, IDDM is blocked in NOD mice treated with recombinant IL-1 *in vivo*.[46] Another aberrant function observed in NOD macrophages is that they lack normal regulation of the inducible prostaglandin E2 synthase gene (*Ptgs2* on Chromosome 1) and, hence, secrete higher than normal levels of prostaglandin E2.[47,48]

Defects in both the high-affinity Fcγ1 receptor on Chromosome 3[49] and the Fcγ2 receptor on Chromosome 1[50] have been reported. In human monocytes, signaling through the Fcγ receptors modulates the balance of IL-1/IL-1 receptor antagonist secreted,[51] such that these genetic defects may be associated with aberrant secretory responses exhibited by NOD/Lt macrophages in response to LPS stimulation. Both defects would also be expected to affect the ability of macrophages to phagocytose monomeric IgG2a and IgG2b antibodies, respectively. The mutation in the *Fcgr1* gene, eliminating 300 amino acids of the cytoplasmic tail of the molecule, was originally proposed as a candidate gene for *Idd10*, but recombination analysis has eliminated this possibility.[52] Interestingly, the frequency of IDDM was increased rather than decreased in an NOD congenic stock in which the defective *Fcγr2* locus on distal Chromosome 1 was replaced by a wild-type allele from C57BL6/J mice.[50]

12.2.4.2 T Cells

NOD CD4+ T-helper cell responses to antigenic stimulation are strongly skewed toward a T-helper 1–predominant cytokine profile. This may account, in part, for why NOD mice are strongly resistant to a variety of murine pathogenic agents, including most murine viruses tested. NOD T cells are robust producers of interferon gamma,[53,54] whereas NOD

CD4[+] T cells are especially low producers of IL-4,[55] and tend toward low production of IL-10.[56] Whereas NOD bone marrow stem cells do not respond normally to IL-3,[45] NOD/Lt T cells are high producers of IL-3. A strong non-MHC diabetes susceptibility genetic locus on Chromosome 3, designated *Idd3*, appears to be the IL-2 structural gene,[57] although splenocytes from NOD/Lt mice and SWR/Bm, an NOD-related control strain, secrete comparable levels of IL-2 *in vitro* when activated by Concanavalin A.[35] However, NOD spleens are enriched for T cells compared with SWR, such that, on a per cell basis, NOD T cells secrete less IL-2 after mitogenic or allogeneic stimulation. Hence, while the functional activity of the IL-2 produced by NOD T cells appears to be normal on a per molecule basis,[58] they produce less of this cytokine on a per T cell basis than do control strains. Combined with very low IL-4 production by NOD thymocytes, low IL-2 production in response to self-antigen presentation in the thymus may underlie some of the apoptotic defects that in turn produce peripheral T-lymphoaccumulation. Nevertheless, even after activation *in vitro* by IL-2, NOD T cells are still more resistant to apoptosis induction than are lymphocytes from other strains.[59]

12.2.4.3 *Natural Killer (NK) and NK1[+] T (NKT) Cells*

NK cells in NOD mice express the NK1.2 allotype and are detectable using a pan-NK monoclonal antibody (DX5, PharMingen, San Diego, CA). Although DX5 staining shows that NK cells are present in spleens of NOD mice, these cells are functionally deficient as measured by a greatly reduced ability to kill YAC-1 cell targets.[39,60,61] This deficiency was not corrected by treatment *in vivo* with IL-2 or poly I:C.[39] This functional deficiency undoubtedly represents one of the factors rendering NOD/LtSz-*scid/scid* mice exceptionally suitable for the growth of human tissues and cells.[62,63]

NKT cells are NK1[+] thymocytes as well as NK1[+] T cells in the periphery that are CD3[+], but negative for CD4 and/or CD8. These double-negative T cells are thought to represent an important IL-4-secreting population that primes development of CD4[+] T-helper 2 regulatory cells. NKT cells are also functionally deficient in NOD/Lt mice, as evidenced by the low secretion of IL-4 by NOD/Lt thymocytes[55] and by the finding that treatment of NOD/Lt mice with thymocyte preparations enriched for this double-negative population prevented IDDM development.[64] The deficiency in NOD thymocyte IL-4 production could be corrected *in vitro* by incubation with IL-7.[65]

12.2.4.4 *B Lymphocytes*

Autoantibodies appear to play a secondary role in IDDM pathogenesis in NOD mice.[66] However, B lymphocytes serving as APC to amplify T cell responses to β-cell autoantigens are essential diabetogenic catalysts in NOD mice. NOD mice rendered B lymphocyte–deficient by congenic transfer of a disrupted immunoglobulin heavy-chain gene (Igμ "knockout" mice) or anti-μ chain antibody treatment only rarely develop IDDM.[67-69] Some of the NOD strain–specific defects reflected by poor activation of regulatory T cells in a SMLR likely represent deficiencies in the B lymphocyte as well as the macrophage/dendritic cell population. These may include unstable MHC class II (I-A^{g7})/peptide complexes on NOD B cells.[70] NOD B lymphocytes, like T cells, exhibit extended survival *in vitro*.[71] In NOD/Lt mice, IgG2b represents the predominant subclass of autoantibodies to insulin[72] and another candidate β-cell autoantigen, glutamic acid decarboxylase (GAD).[73] Perhaps representing an example of substrain divergence, a predominance of IgG2a autoantibodies to GAD have been reported in another NOD substrain.[74]

12.2.5 Experimentally Induced Lesions

NOD mice are susceptible to a variety of experimentally induced disease syndromes, including chemically induced diabetes, lupus, colitis, encephalomyelitis, and thyroiditis.[26,75-78] Not surprisingly, young NOD/Lt males, like outbred CD-1 males, are susceptible to induction of IDDM by multidose streptozotocin (STZ).[75] This sensitivity is independent of autoimmune T cell involvement since NOD/LtSz-*scid/scid* males are even more sensitive to low doses of this diabetogen.[75] Injection of a single dose of 2.6×10^7 heat-killed *Mycobacterium tuberculosis* (bacillus Calmette-Guerin, or BCG) i.v. into 8-week-old NOD mice prevented diabetes but precipitated a syndrome similar to systemic lupus erythematosus.[79] Exposure of NOD/Lt mice to 3.5% dextran sodium sulfate in the drinking water for 5 days elicits a severe colitis.[80] Experimental allergic encephalomyelitis can be induced in NOD mice using a peptide fragment (residues 56-70) from proteolipid protein.[81]

12.2.6 Genetic Basis of IDDM Susceptibility

12.2.6.1 MHC

As is true for most other T cell–based autoimmune diseases, the MHC complex comprises the major component of this susceptibility. In the case of NOD mice, the MHC haplotype ($H2^{g7}$, Chromosome 17) is unique. Its diabetogenic contributions involve both a defective *H2-Ea* allele (homologous to *DR* in humans) as well as a rare *H2-Ab* allele encoding histidine at residue 56 and serine at 57 of the I-A β chain (homologous to "diabetogenic" HLA-*DQβ* nonaspartic acid[57] containing alleles). These contributions were demonstrated by construction of NOD transgenic mice in which site-specific mutagenesis was used to replace either the proline[56] with histidine or the serine[57] with aspartic acid.[82] Similarly, transgenic insertion of an expressible *H2-Ea^d* allele also protects.[73,83,84] Protection mediated by transgenic expression of I-E-molecules on NOD APC did not entail intrathymic clonal deletion of T-effector cells.[73] I-E mediated protection might be associated with differential level of autoantigen presentation in the periphery, since a Th1 → Th2 skewing was observed in T cell recall responses following priming with human recombinant GAD65, a model β-cell autoantigen.[73] However, the diabetogenic contributions are not limited to the MHC class II region. The entire haplotype is considered diabetogenic, since MHC class I genes, although not unique, are also essential for IDDM development. IDDM is absent in NOD mice congenic for a disrupted β2-microglobulin gene that prevents expression of cell-surface MHC class I molecules, and the production of CD8+ T cells.[85-87] Although splenic T cells from standard NOD/Lt mice rapidly transfer IDDM when adoptively transferred into T cell–deficient NOD/LtSz-*scid/scid* mice, these same cells fail to transfer IDDM adoptively when injected into a stock of MHC class I negative NOD/LtSz-*scid/scid* mice homozygous for a disrupted β2-microglobulin allele.[87] This latter study not only confirmed the requirement for CD8+ T cells in the initiation of β-cell lesions, but also used transplantation analysis to confirm the requirement for MHC class I on the β-cell targets.

NOD congenic stocks are made by outcrossing NOD to a strain carrying a chromosomal region of interest (the "donor" strain), followed by multiple backcross cycles to NOD, with selection at each backcross generation for heterozygosity for markers delineating the donor chromosomal region of interest. After a suitable number of backcross cycles (usually 12 unless a "speed congenic," see below, is made), heterozygotes are intercrossed to establish a congenic line. In NOD congenic stocks in which the diabetogenic $H2^{g7}$ haplotype is replaced by disparate MHC haplotypes ($H2^b$, $H2^{nb1}$, $H2^q$), insulitis and IDDM are prevented.[88] Additional evidence that MHC class II alleles do not represent the sole diabetogenic contributions within the H2^{g7} complex comes from the congenic transfer of the unique MHC haplotype of the related CTS/Shi strain onto the NOD/Shi genetic background. The CTS strain, selected for dominant cataract with microophthalmia, was produced in Japan from the same Clea:ICR progenitors that produced the NOD/Shi strain.[2] CTS mice have a rare MHC haplotype designated H2^{ct}. The MHC class II *H2-E* and *H2-A* alleles in this haplotype are identical to those of NOD, but the MHC class I genes at both *H2-K* and *H2-D* are distinct. The effect of congenic transfer of the H2^{ct} haplotype onto the NOD/Shi inbred background has been analyzed. After 13 backcross cycles to NOD, mice heterozygous for the H2^{g7} (NOD-type) and the H2^{ct} (CTS-type) were intercrossed to initiate a homozygous NOD.CTS-*H2^{ct}* congenic line. Both diabetes frequency and insulitis severity were reduced in the H2^{ct} homozygous mice when compared with segregants homozygous for H2^{g7}.[89] The reduced diabetogenic potency of the H2^{ct} thus provides strong support for the concept that, while the class II region is clearly important to disease development, other loci within the extended H2^{g7} haplotype also contribute. One of these has been dubbed *Idd16*, although the position of the locus in the complex was not established.[89] Even though the MHC class I alleles of NOD mice (*H2K^d*, *H2D^b*) are common in nonautoimmune-prone strains, they acquire in NOD mice a diabetogenic function — the selection and targeting of CD8$^+$ T cells essential for initiation of the diabetogenic process.[87] Thus, the class I alleles also contribute to the overall susceptibility represented by the extended H2^{g7} haplotype.

12.2.6.2 Non-MHC Loci

Whereas transfer of other MHC haplotypes onto the NOD strain background reduces or eliminates IDDM, transfer of the diabetogenic NOD H2^{g7} haplotype onto diabetes-resistant inbred strain backgrounds fails to trigger IDDM. Hence, contributions from non-MHC as well as MHC are required for diabetogenesis. Genetic segregation analysis following outcross of NOD with diabetes-resistant inbred strains demonstrates IDDM inheritance as a polygenic threshold liability.[27,90] Some of the non-MHC IDDM susceptibility (*Idd*) loci have been mapped to chromosomal regions associated with other spontaneous or experimentally induced autoimmune diseases in mice.[91] Outcrossing NOD to other inbred strains has demonstrated the numbers and locations of the non-MHC genes are predicated upon the degree of relatedness of the strain chosen for outcross with NOD. Individually, none is essential for conferring complete IDDM susceptibility or resistance. The strength and potential function of non-MHC loci are analyzed by construction of partially resistant congenic stocks of NOD mice carrying chromosomal segments from donor strains known to carry resistance loci.[38,92] The availability of highly polymorphic simple sequence repeat-based microsatellites makes it possible to create "speed congenics" based upon knowledge of what chromosome regions are essential for diabetogenesis.[93] A listing of the currently identified "*Idd*" regions may be found elsewhere.[27] Not all susceptibility genes derive from NOD, as illustrated by *Idd7* (Chromosome 7), where the autoimmune diabetes-resistant progenitor strain carries the more–diabetogenic allele.[90,94] Outcross of NOD/Jos mice with SPRET/Ei, an inbred strain recently derived from wild *M. spretus*, results in a complex comingling of genes predisposing to both Type I and Type II diabetes.[95]

12.2.6.3 Subcongenic Analysis to Identify Idd Genes and Their Functions

By definition, any locus that affects susceptibility/resistance to IDDM development in NOD mice is an *Idd* locus. Once segregation analysis identifies linkage of a discrete chromosomal region to IDDM or to a subdiabetogenic phenotype (insulitis), subcongenic analysis is required to refine the map position of the putative gene. Initially, only one *Idd* (*Idd3*) was reported on Chromosome 3,[96] but subsequent studies, including subcongenic analysis, showed at least four *Idd* loci on this chromosome.[52] Subcongenic analysis indicates that the IL-2 structural gene itself may be *Idd3*.[97] The NOD allele at the β2-microglobulin locus (*B2m^a*) is an excellent illustration of the complexity of diabetes genetics in this mouse. The diabetes-protective effect of a functionally disrupted β2-microglobulin gene has been discussed above. The NOD β2-microglobulin allele (*B2m^a*) is neither uncommon nor defective. Yet it may be one of several genes within the *Idd13* region on Chromosome 2 that promotes diabetogenesis by affecting the conformation of MHC class I molecules on APCs.[98] It illustrates the likelihood that common alleles can acquire diabetogenic functions when paired with certain other genes that themselves may not be inherently diabetogenic (e.g., the "common" MHC class I loci in the *H2^g7* haplotype).

12.2.6.4 Environmental Effects on Idd Gene Penetrance

The NOD mouse has provided researchers with the most-compelling evidence to date that environmental factors are important modulators of *Idd* gene functions. Insulitic damage can be restricted to subclinical levels if NOD mice are exposed to environmental pathogens or immunomodulatory substances (including a surprising variety of cytokines). There are now well over 100 different therapeutic interventions reported in the literature.[99] The ease with which autoimmune T-effector functions of NOD mice can be downregulated by environmental stimuli indicate that, in a natural environment, IDDM development would be a relatively rare event. Indeed, the wide variation in IDDM frequencies in NOD colonies worldwide, and, especially in males, is most likely the consequence of environmental factors.[100,101] Transfer of NOD males from a conventional mouseroom in Japan into germ-free conditions raised the male diabetes incidence from 6 to 70%.[61] Exposure of NOD mice to a variety of murine viruses (encephalomyocarditis virus, lymphocytic choriomeningitis virus, and murine hepatitis virus) prevents diabetes development.[17,102,103] These infectious agents apparently protect by providing general immunostimulation since treatment of prediabetic NOD mice with various types of exogenous immunomodulators, including bacterial antigens (CFA, BCG, OK432), cytokines (including IL-1, TNFα, IL-2, IL-4, IL-10, TGFβ, and interferon γ), and poly I:C all circumvent diabetes development (reviewed in References 12 and 99). Diabetogenic catalysts are also present in natural-ingredient diets which contain lipoidal moieties that are absent or present in low concentration in semipurified diets.[104] The parenteral administration of bacterial preparations activating acute-phase responses (CFA, BCG, OK432) represents the most potent immunomodulatory treatments. In contrast to a demonstrated role for viral triggers in BB rats,[20,105] NOD mice seem unsuitable as models for investigating whether or not viruses are diabetogenic triggers in human populations because viral exposures protect against, rather than precipitate IDDM.[101]

Certain peripheral immunoregulatory functions observed to be defective in NOD mice maintained in SPF environments can be ameliorated when mice are maintained in pathogen-compromised environments. Defects in the degree of cytokine-elicited differentiation of APC from bone marrow have been associated with inefficient presentation of self-antigens.[43,44] Inefficient presentation of self-antigens by NOD APC may explain not only the defective immunoregulatory functions of these cells as exemplified by defective T-suppressor cell functions measured *in vitro*, but also the subnormal secretion of monokines by peripheral macrophages in response to LPS stimulation.[42] Presumably, immunomodulatory effects mediated via environmental components serve to upregulate certain of these defective APC functions, resulting either in more-normal thymic elimination of autoreactive T cells or more-potent activation of immunoregulatory T cells in the periphery, or both.

12.3 Experimentally Induced IDDM Models in Mice

12.3.1 Multiple Low-Dose Streptozotocin

12.3.1.1 Model Overview

The fungal antibiotic, STZ, comprises a nitrosamide methylnitrosourea group linked to the C-2 position of D-glucose. As reviewed by Wilson and Leiter,[106] STZ rapidly and spontaneously breaks down inside β-cells to produce highly reactive carbamoylating and alkylating species. These ions alkylate intracellular macromolecules, including DNA. Resultant DNA strand breaks in turn induce poly ADP-ribose polymerase (PARP) activity.[107,108] PARP degrades limiting intracellular pools of reduced nicotine adenine dinucleotides necessary to maintain the redox state in β-cells. The multiple low-dose STZ (MDSTZ) diabetic male mouse, originally described by Like and Rossini,[109] represents one of the most useful tools available to researchers interested in analyzing the pathogenic effects of chronic hyperglycemia in an insulin-dependent diabetic syndrome. Mice are considerably more resistant than rats to STZ, such that considerably higher single doses are necessary to elicit hyperglycemia rapidly in 100% of injected mice of either sex. For inbred strains, single doses of at least 150 mg/kg or higher are required to elicit chronic hyperglycemia. These single high STZ doses are associated with serious collateral damage to other organs, rapid weight loss, and high mortality. Because of a mouse's small size and high basal metabolic rate, the resultant severe hyperglycemia is very difficult to manage by insulin administration. In contrast to the high mortality induced by single high doses of STZ in mice of both sexes, males of selected inbred strains can be rendered chronically diabetic (mean nonfasting plasma glucose between 300 and 600 mg/dl) by daily administration over 3 to 5 days of smaller STZ doses. The MDSTZ regimen is highly strain and age dependent, but typically ranges between 30 to 40 mg/kg × 5 days for highly sensitive adolescent males (such as CD-1 and NOD/LtSz-*scid/scid* males) and 60 mg/kg body weight × 5 days for resistant CBA/J males. Hyperglycemic mice do not show the precipitous rapid weight loss observed after single high-dose STZ administration, and will survive for months with chronic hyperglycemia without insulin therapy. Indeed, males of strains with intermediate susceptibility (e.g., C57BL/6J, BALB/cByJ) may eventually exhibit a spontaneous remission, indicating that not all β-cell function is destroyed. Because a level of stable hyperglycemia can be achieved that is not associated with rapid weight loss and requirement for insulin therapy, MDSTZ diabetic males are ideal for evaluation of islet transplantation protocols. They are robust enough to survive the transplantation surgery and can easily be cured by syngeneic islets provided in sufficient numbers.[110,111] Unlike spontaneously diabetic NOD mice, which rapidly reject islet syngrafts, there is no comparable autoimmune memory in mice rendered hyperglycemic by MDSTZ.[112] Thus, immunomodulative therapies designed to maintain allografted or xenografted islets can also be evaluated in the absence of a preexisting β-cell autoimmunity.

12.3.1.2 Etiopathogenesis

The high affinity for STZ uptake into rodent pancreatic β-cells, mediated via GLUT-2 transporters,[113] is discussed in detail elsewhere in this volume (see Chapter 1). In mice, massive necrosis of the pancreatic β-cell mass follows within hours after administration of a single high dose of STZ, with nonfasting hyperglycemia presenting within 24 to 48 h

TABLE 12.1

Mouse Strain (Male) Susceptibilities to MDSTZ Induced IDDM

High Susceptibility	Intermediate Susceptibility	Resistant
CD-1[a 109]	C57BL/6J[132]	FVB/N[140]
NOD/Lt[a 75]	C57BL/10J[159]	SWR/J (EHL, unpublished)
NON/Lt[a] (EHL, unpublished)	C3H/HeJ[162]	BALB/cJ[15]
ALS/Lt (EHL, unpublished)	C3H/OuJ[162]	A/J[235]
C57BLKS/J[a 132]	BALB/cByJ[15]	
C3H.SW/SnJ[162]	DBA/2J[235]	
CBA/J[161]	ALR/Lt[a] (EHL, unpublished)	

Note: Once daily injections of 40 mg/kg × 5 days; diabetogenic response assessed by plasma glucose measurement 16 days after last injection (experiment day 21). High susceptibility = plasma glucose >500 mg/dl; intermediate susceptibility = 300–400 mg/dl; resistant = < 250 mg/dl.

[a] Insulitis development within days post-STZ treatment.

postadministration. As reviewed in Wilson and Leiter,[106] MDSTZ diabetes elicited by doses ≥ 40 mg/kg body weight represents a diabetic condition in which the primary etiopathological effect is clearly produced by cumulative β-cytotoxic effects of STZ. Longitudinal analyses of the 40 mg/kg × 5 day MDSTZ model in which β-cell loss is quantified demonstrates that massive β-cell destruction occurs cumulatively over the 5-day STZ exposure period.[114,115] In inbred C57BLKS/J males, each daily 40 mg/kg "subdiabetogenic" dose of STZ destroyed or functionally impaired a percentage of the β-cells, such that on experiment day 6 (1 day after the last injection), a 64% reduction in islet volume and an 84% reduction in insulin secretory capacity by perfused pancreas was shown.[114]

Insulitis, prevalent 5 to 6 days after the last STZ injection in CD-1 and C57BLKS/J males,[116-118] is transient and is not a consistent feature of this model in all inbred strains of mice (Table 12.1). Several days before heavy insulitis develops in MDSTZ-treated CD-1 males, aberrant type C retroviral particles were observed budding intracellularly into the cisternae of the rough endoplasmic reticulum of pre-necrotic β-cells.[109,117] A recent report suggests apoptotic cell death is responsible for IDDM in MDSTZ-treated C57BL6/J males,[115] but the percentage of nuclei deemed apoptotic by light microscopic examination was low. Ultrastructural analysis of MDSTZ damaged CD-1 and C57BLKS/J male β-cells *in situ* show that necrotic cell death predominates.[116,118] Arteriolar blood enters the mouse islet via capillaries directed toward the islet center, and then perfuses from the center outward toward venular capillary beds at the periphery.[119] Whether MDSTZ induced β-cell death is by apoptosis or necrosis probably depends upon the ambient level of STZ surrounding each β-cell.[120]

One of the most contentious issues associated with the MDSTZ model has been the pathogenic contribution made by T cells in those strains where insulitis is a feature. That this reactive insulitis might be an essential component of the model was indicated by the finding that hyperglycemia, usually developing a week or so after the last STZ injection, could be blocked by antilymphocyte serum or a variety of antibodies to cell surface markers on either APCs or on T cells (reviewed by Kolb and Kroncke[121]). It was hypothesized that STZ induced necrosis (or apoptosis) of a few β-cells led to presentation of sequestered self-antigens such as heat shock (stress) proteins,[122] retroviral antigens,[123] or neoantigens generated by direct alkylation of proteins by STZ.[111] This presentation of sequestered or novel antigens, in turn, was hypothesized to elicit a T cell–mediated destruction of the mass of the β-cells, already structurally weakened and perhaps antigenically altered by MDSTZ exposure.[121]

Literature dealing with the requirement for T cells in this model prior to 1993 has been critically reviewed in several places.[106,121] Much of the earlier debate centered around the issue of whether or not athymic nude (*nu/nu*) males are susceptible to MDSTZ induced diabetes. The focus of the debate continues to be whether insulitis represents a secondary response to inflammation induced by the direct β-cell cytotoxic effects of STZ or whether it represented an autoimmune, T cell–initiated and T cell–mediated insulitic destruction as observed in NOD mice. The use of STZ doses lower than 40 mg/kg × 5 days in highly sensitive CD-1 males has delineated a T cell contribution. CD-1 males treated with MDSTZ (30 mg/kg × 5 days or less)[124,125] develop a marked insulitis and progressively more severe hyperglycemia. In contrast, T cell–deficient CD-1-*nu/nu* males, although susceptible to the 40 mg/kg × 5 day regimen, showed attenuated susceptibility to the lower MDSTZ regimen.[124] An immunocytochemical analysis of the CD-1 *nu/+* pancreas showed that CD4[+] T cells predominated, with CD8[+] T cells scattered throughout, and B lymphocytes accumulating over time around foci of CD4[+] T cells.[126] A similar immunocytochemical picture, with the additional documentation of Mac-1[+] positive islet-infiltrating macrophages, was reported for "Swiss" males (essentially the same as CD-1) treated with the 40 mg/kg × 5 day dose regimen.[127]

Since some authors refer to MDSTZ elicited insulitis as "autoimmune" insulitis, a comparison to the NOD model of spontaneous IDDM recognized to be autoimmune in etiology is warranted. The comparison of the two models in Table 12.2 illustrates how strikingly different they are. The most salient difference is that T cells from prediabetic or diabetic NOD mice will adoptively transfer IDDM into NOD/LtSz-*scid/scid* recipients, whereas T cells from young NOD/Lt males made diabetic by MDSTZ will not.[75] The finding that T and B lymphocyte–deficient NOD and C.B-17-*scid/scid* mice are highly sensitive to MDSTZ[75,128] is evidence for direct β-cytotoxicity as the main pathogenic mediator. STZ mediates DNA alkylation and double-strand breaks, and the *scid* mutation imparts an inability to rejoin coding ends of DNA. Accordingly, the high sensitivity of *scid* mice may represent a deleterious synergism between the STZ-mediated DNA strand breaks coupled with the *scid* mutation-induced defect in repair. This is perhaps evidenced by the report that CB.17-*scid* females are also susceptible to MDSTZ induced IDDM.[128] Nevertheless, the striking differences between the spontaneous vs. the induced IDDM models enumerated in Table 12.2 suggest that β-cell autoreactive T cells play a secondary role in the chemically induced model. Indeed, the 40 mg/kg × 5 day MDSTZ regimen has been shown to suppress T cell responsiveness to mitogens.[129] Although this immunosuppression arguably could be limited to a regulatory, and not an effector population, this argument seems unlikely since cyclophosphamide, like MDSTZ, exerts a strong, but transient immunosuppressive effect, yet cyclophosphamide prevents MDSTZ induced hyperglycemia.[130] Hence, MDSTZ administration does not release indigenous autoimmune T-effector cells in the same way that cyclophosphamide treatment of prediabetic NOD mice accelerates T cell–mediated autoimmunity.[131]

Although T cells certainly may contribute to inflammatory damage in the heavy MDSTZ induced insulitis observed in outbred CD-1 males,[124] their presence is clearly not obligatory in inbred strains.[75,124,128,132-134] Studies designed to elucidate pathogenic contributions of T cells in inbred strains, particularly efforts to induce CD8[+] T cell tolerance to STZ altered islets in C57BLKS/J, have been reported.[135-137] However, interpretation of such studies is difficult because complex paradigms requiring additional single or multiple injections of STZ to demonstrate abrogation of tolerance were employed subsequent to an initial treatment of five injections. Following priming of popliteal leukocytes with STZ *in vivo*, T cells from popliteal nodes showed a blastogenic response *in vitro* to syngeneic islets previously exposed to STZ *in vitro*.[138] This indicates that β-cell surface proteins altered by the glucopyranose ring

TABLE 12.2

Comparison of Spontaneous Diabetes in NOD Mice vs. MDSTZ Induced IDDM

Phenotype/Treatment	NOD Mouse*	MDSTZ
Etiopathogenesis	Autoimmune, presence of both CD4+ and CD8+ T cell effectors are mandatory	Direct β-cell cytotoxicity; inflammation, but T cells not mandatory
Insulitis present	Yes	Strain dependent, transient[155]
MHC restricted	Yes	No[163]
Adoptively transferred	Yes	No[75]
Cured by islet transplants	No	Yes[236]
Gender bias	Female	Male[156]
Prevented by immunomodulation	Yes	Yes[121]
Cyclosporine treatment	Prevents IDDM	Exacerbates IDDM[237]
Androgen treatment	Prevents IDDM	Exacerbates IDDM[157]
CFA treatment	Prevents IDDM	Exacerbates IDDM[144]
Poly I:C treatment	Prevents IDDM	Exacerbates IDDM[238]
Viral exposure	Prevents IDDM	Exacerbates IDDM[212]
Cytochrome P450 induction	Associated with prevention	Associated with acceleration[158]

* The reader is referred to the review articles on NOD mice cited for references. A recently published textbook describing NOD mice is also available.[239]

of STZ may indeed be immunogenic *in vivo*.[138] However, use of STZ to generate altered forms of native proteins is distinctly different from development of spontaneous IDDM in NOD mice, wherein autoimmunity entails a presumed loss of tolerance to native self-antigens.

The advent of transgenic technology has provided researchers with an MDSTZ model in which T cell activation in response to STZ induced beta cell alterations is clearly a major pathogenic event. Mouse β-cells do not constitutively express the B7-1 (CD80) T cell costimulatory molecule expressed by "professional" APC. Following T cell receptor cross-linking to an antigen on the surface of β-cells (presumably presented by MHC class I molecules to CD8+ T cells), B7-1 provides a second activation signal by binding to the CD28 T cell receptor. When NOD mice transgenically express the B7-1 gene ligated to an insulin promoter, diabetogenesis is markedly accelerated due to activation of the CD28 receptor on CD8+ T cells in the insulitic infiltrate.[139] In contrast, when an insulin promoter-B7-1 transgene was microinjected into zygotes of FVB/N strain mice,[140] the transgenic mice produced exhibited only a low incidence of spontaneous IDDM (currently 3%, personal communication, Dr. David Harlan, Naval Medical Research Institute, Bethesda, MD). However, after treatment with a very low MDSTZ regimen (dose of 20 mg/kg × 5 days), *female* mice, after a 26 to 100 day latency period, developed glycosuria.[140] This pathogenesis could be blocked by treatment with anti-CD8 monoclonal antibody. Immunocytochemical staining showed heavy intraislet infiltration of both CD4+ and CD8+ T cell subsets. However, RIP-B7-1 activated T cells from diabetic FVB donors have thus far failed to transfer adoptively IDDM into naive recipients whose β-cells have not been exposed to STZ (Dr. David Harlan, personal communication). Thus, this immune-mediated model clearly is the model of choice if the investigator is interested in analyzing T cell responses to STZ altered self-antigens, or STZ induced neoantigens. Another interesting transgenic model producing accelerated activation of immune effectors entails transgenic expression of interferon α (IFNα) in β-cells driven by an insulin promoter. This constitutive expression at high levels renders males susceptible to hyperglycemia induction by 25 mg/kg × 5 days, and was associated with upregulated expression of other proinflammatory cytokines within the islets.[125]

12.3.1.3 Immunopathology: The Role of Acute Inflammatory Reactants

If NOD mice are treated with a relatively high dose of STZ at a point where the insulitic lesions are extensive and destructive, β-cell damage mediated by STZ synergizes with indigenous autoimmunity to accelerate IDDM onset.[141] However, MDSTZ administered to young prediabetic NOD/Lt females reduces frequency of spontaneous IDDM development.[75] Whereas CFA, a nonspecific immune activator, prevents IDDM development in NOD mice,[142] it augments STZ induced hyperglycemia in other strains.[143,144] Data provided below establish that the timing of exposure to an acute inflammatory shock can either prevent or precipitate IDDM in the MDSTZ model.

One of the simplest compounds capable of blocking IDDM development in NOD/Lt mice is gallium nitrate. Gallium nitrate has been used in the treatment of certain malignancies as well as Paget's disease in humans,[145] and has been used to suppress experimental allergic encephalomyelitis induction in rats.[146] Data in Figure 12.1 show the diabetes-protective effect of chronic treatment of young prediabetic NOD/Lt females with gallium nitrate, beginning at 6 weeks and continuing to 20 weeks of age. Treatment entailed an initial injection i.p. of 45 mg/kg, followed by once weekly injections i.p. of 15 mg/kg. Interestingly, although heavy insulitis developed in the gallium-treated group, protection was unequivocal, and extended to a 5-week period after cessation of gallium injections (see Figure 12.1). Gallium interferes with the cellular uptake of iron by competitively displacing iron from transferrin.[147] Transferrin–gallium complexes are also able to target transferrin receptor–bearing T and B lymphocytes and interfere with their proliferation and function.[148] Detailed investigations of gallium effects on the immune system indicated that the initial dose of 45 mg/kg was associated with acute (but transient) systemic toxicity, manifested peritoneal hemorrhage including large numbers of mast cells, as well as histological evidence of hepatotoxicity and nephrotoxicity. Further, this systemic response to heavy metal–induced tissue damage led to upregulated activity of the innate immune system. This was evidenced by higher levels of LPS-stimulated IL-1 secretion from peritoneal macrophages (EHL laboratory, unpublished). Treatment of NOD mice with another metal salt, lithium chloride, also retards IDDM.[149]

If the nonspecific toxic effects of the 45 mg/kg initiating dose of gallium nitrate produced transiently high levels of acute-phase reactants, administration of gallium nitrate prior to MDSTZ in 6-week-old prediabetic NOD/Lt males might exert an effect different from that when the tissue-damaging high dose of gallium was coadministered with the first of the five MDSTZ injections. As shown in Figure 12.2, this differential effect, dependent upon time of gallium administration, was indeed observed. By using a MDSTZ regimen of 25 mg/kg × 5, coadministration of gallium markedly exacerbated the diabetogenic action of MDSTZ (Figure 12.2A). In contrast, administration of gallium prior to MDSTZ administration significantly ($P < 0.01$) attenuated the diabetogenic damage mediated by this low MDSTZ regimen (Figure 12.2B). The effect of gallium predosing would be consistent with the protective effect of gallium in circumventing overt IDDM in NOD/Lt females. Presumably, the upregulation of immune function elicited by the release of acute-phase reactants leads to a more-regulated peripheral T cell repertoire. This is consistent with the finding that treatment of young NOD mice with CFA, BCG, poly I:C, IL-2, IL-1, TNFα, IFNγ, TGFβ, IL-4, and IL-10 all repress spontaneous diabetogenesis (reviewed by Atkinson[99]).

The point of these model experiments with gallium nitrate is to illustrate the important contributions of the innate immune system in mediating β-cell damage during and immediately after the exposure to each cumulative STZ dose in the MDSTZ paradigm. The proinflammatory effects of STZ on macrophages has been reviewed.[121] In NOD/LtSz-*scid/scid* mice treated with a very low MDSTZ regimen (30 mg/kg × 5), there is rapid

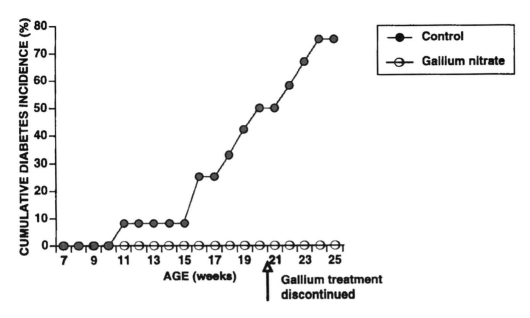

FIGURE 12.1
Chronic treatment with gallium nitrate circumvents development of spontaneous IDDM in NOD/Lt females compared with vehicle control (n = 12/group).

influx into the damaged islets of BM8+ (a scavenger macrophage marker) macrophages (Dr. Hemmo Drexhage, Erasmus University, Rotterdam, personal communication). Pre-treatment of males with colloidal silica, a macrophage toxin, can block MDSTZ hyperglycemia.[150] However, interpretation of the protective mechanism is complicated by the finding that administration of colloidal silica increases rather than decreases pancreatic macrophage content.[7] Insulin has been shown to be a Macrophage chemoattractant,[151] and Macrophage will develop spontaneous nonspecific cytotoxicity against islet cells *in vitro*.[152] Macrophage-mediated cytotoxicity entails nitric oxide release.[153] Two monokines, IL-1 and TNFα, especially in combination with IFNγ, are extremely cytotoxic to cultured islet cells via mechanisms entailing free radical generation and lipid peroxidation.[154] Figure 12.3 presents a schematic diagram suggesting the complex interactions potentially underlying β-cell destruction in inbred strains in which insulitis is a feature of MDSTZ induced diabetes.

12.3.1.4 Genetics
Strain differences in responsiveness to once daily STZ injections of 40 mg/kg body weight × 5 days were first shown by Rossini and Like.[155] A listing of various strain sensitivities to MDSTZ-induced IDDM (40 mg/kg × 5 regimen) is given in Table 12.1. As mentioned above, MDSTZ responsiveness was male sex limited. Castration of highly sensitive, outbred CD-1 males blocked hyperglycemia, while testosterone administration enhanced hyperglycemic responses in females and castrated males.[156] Estrogen administration to males was suppressive.[157] Hence, genes whose expression is sex limited or androgen controlled are likely to be important regulators of susceptibility and resistance. Some of these genes may encode gender-specific P450-linked enzymes, since induction of P450 activity in CD-1 females with phenobarbital attenuated their resistance.[158] Interestingly, the reverse holds for the NOD model of autoimmune IDDM. NOD/Lt females are at higher risk than males. High penetrance of underlying *Idd* genes is observed when

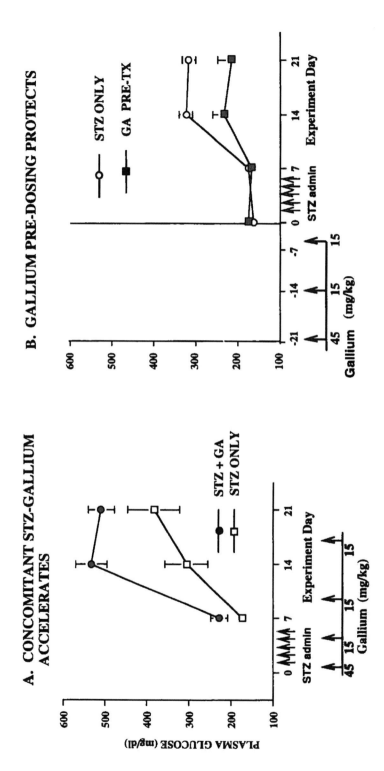

FIGURE 12.2
Gallium nitrate accelerates IDDM (A) when injected concomitantly with MDSTZ, but prevents IDDM (B) when predosed prior to MDSTZ administration. Data are for 6-week-old NOD/Lt males, n = 8/group treated with 25 mg STZ/kg body weight × 5 days).

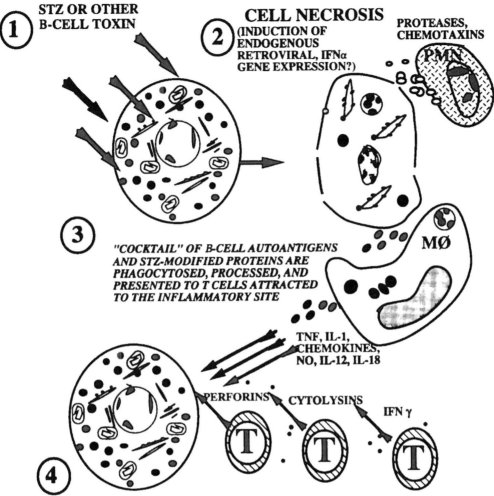

FIGURE 12.3

Schematic representation of potential pathogenic interactions between the innate and acquired immune system in synergizing with STZ to mediate β-cell destruction in inbred mouse strains in which insulitis is a feature of the model.

NOD/Lt mice of both sexes are fed complex chow diets.[104] These chow diets suppress hepatic P450 activities in contrast to diabetes-retardant semipurified diets that maintain higher rates of catabolism of the progesterone ring via P450-linked pathways.[88] Although not as yet proved, genes controlling defenses against free radical–mediated damage may distinguish certain MDSTZ diabetes susceptible from resistant backgrounds (see Section 12.4).

In humans, BB rats, and NOD mice, genes within the MHC comprise a major contribution toward IDDM susceptibility. As discussed above, the *H2g7* complex on Chromosome

17 contains multiple immunoregulatory loci controlling diabetogenesis in NOD mice. Young prediabetic NOD males are also strongly susceptible to MDSTZ induced IDDM.[75] Initially, studies employing *H2*-congenic stocks of mice on the C57B10/J (B10) inbred background indicated no association of the *H2^b* haplotype with MDSTZ sensitivity,[159] but subsequent analyses using various congenic stocks did suggest a gene controlling sensitivity mapped proximal to the *H2-D* locus.[160,161] However, the MHC associations were not consistent when different inbred strain backgrounds were analyzed, indicating that non-MHC background differences, probably associated with differential androgen sensitivity,[162] were equally likely to explain the response differences. A critical evaluation of the potential protective role of the *H2^b* haplotype was performed by congenic transfer from the relatively MDSTZ- and insulitis-resistant C57BL/6J (B6) background onto the highly susceptible C57BLKS/J (BKS) background. No loss of sensitivity to insulitis and hyperglycemia induction was observed in BKS.B6-*H2 ^b* congenic males at the seventh backcross generation.[163] Currently at the 20th backcross generation, males of this stock continue to manifest the full MDSTZ sensitivity of standard BKS males. Absence of a strong MHC association in the MDSTZ model is in contrast to IDDM in humans, BB rats, and NOD mice, but is consistent with male sex-limited susceptibility to virally induced diabetes.[164] In both the viral and MDSTZ models, increased sensitivity to, or availability of, endogenous androgens appears to be a common feature of male mice from those inbred strains showing high sensitivity to hyperglycemia induction.[106]

Most efforts to map genes controlling susceptibility to MDSTZ were performed prior to the "genetic revolution" that has provided the molecular resources for genome-wide scanning associated with the polymerase chain reaction (PCR). An early study analyzing the genetic basis for MDSTZ susceptibility in BALB/cByJ males vs. resistance in the BALB/cJ substrain suggested that a single gene difference might account for the phenotypes.[15] Although genetic polymorphisms detected by classical isoenzyme or immunophenotypic analysis on Chromosomes 5, 12, and 17 were recognized, susceptibility was not mapped to any of the known polymorphisms. In the course of this analysis, an effect of environment was elucidated. BALB/cByJ males responded to MDSTZ when obtained from a colony exposed to Minute Virus of Mice (MVM) showed attenuated responsiveness when rederived free of this virus.[15] Again, this represents another major difference between pathogenesis elicited in the MDSTZ model vs. the spontaneous diabetes developing in NOD mice. In the latter, exposure to pathogens reduces rather than enhances penetrance of diabetes susceptibility genes.[12]

As mentioned above, MDSTZ administration to CD-1 males is associated with activation of an endogenous C-type retroviral genome.[109,117] In prenecrotic NOD/Lt β-cells, a similar defective intracellular C-type retrovirus has been observed to bud into the cisternae of the rough endoplasmic reticulum, instead of being shed from the cell surface.[165] Of the non-Swiss-derived strains, C57BLKS/J represents a recombinant congenic stock between C57BL6/J and another inbred strain, probably DBA/2J.[166] A distinct retrovirus, an intracellular intracisternal type A particle is induced by hyperglycemia in C57BLKS/J and DBA/2J β-cells, but not C57BL/6J.[167] There is an apparent conformational molecular mimicry between the group-specific antigen (p73) of this particle and the insulin molecule.[72] Hence, a proviral gene or genes encoding for endogenous retroviruses whose expression is activated either by STZ mediated DNA strand breaks or by elevated ambient blood glucose levels, or both, could represent the source of immunogenic neoantigens (see Figure 12.3). The possibility that expression of endogenous type C retroviral genomes in humans with IDDM may represent a triggering neoantigen has been suggested by recent data.[168] Obviously, knowledge of the genetic control of MDSTZ responsiveness is scant. However, as noted in the section below describing alloxan-induced diabetes (Section 12.4), genetic tools are now available to allow identification of major genes. This is particularly true since two strains being currently analyzed for the genetic basis of alloxan susceptibility/resistance also show an identical pattern of susceptibility/resistance to MDSTZ.

12.4 Alloxan Diabetes

12.4.1 Inbred Strain Sensitivity

Alloxan (AL) has been employed for over five decades as a selective β-cell toxin for the induction of IDDM.[169] Like STZ, AL is a potent β-cell-selective toxin in mice as well as in rats when administered intravenously in single high dose. Its selective toxicity to β-cells has been attributed both to rapid cellular uptake by β-cells coupled with an exquisite sensitivity of β-cells to peroxide formation.[170] Detailed mechanisms of AL toxicity are detailed in Chapter 10. Like STZ, AL is extremely unstable in aqueous solutions at neutral pH. A half-life of 2.8 min was reported after intravenous administration of 50 or 100 mg/kg of AL into ICR mice; by 10 min, it is virtually undetectable in serum.[171] Because of its structural resemblance to glucose, AL is rapidly taken up by GLUT-2 transporters into mouse β-cells, and there spontaneously decomposes to dialuric acid (see Washburn and Wolf[172] for recent review). Dialuric acid undergoes redox cycling in the presence of physiological reducing agents, especially glutathione, generating potent superoxide/hydroxyl free radicals and inhibiting thiol-dependent enzymes including glucokinase and hexokinase.[173] The diabetogenic effect of AL is rapid, as evidenced by an acute hypoglycemia within an hour postadministration, followed by frank hyperglycemia within 48 h.[174] Electron microscopic analysis shows β-cells are undergoing a necrotic cell death.[175] Both AL and STZ toxicity was reported to entail induction of poly(ADP-ribose) synthetase (PARPP) for unscheduled DNA repair synthesis in rat islets exposed to AL.[176] However, only STZ, and not AL, was observed to induce PARPP, leading to the conclusion that STZ and AL exerted their major cytotoxic effects via different mechanisms.[177] High concentrations of 3-*O*-methyl-glucose, an inhibitor of glucose and of AL uptake into β-cells,[178] inhibit AL-mediated β-cell necrosis *in vivo*, but not *in vitro*.[175] Hence, it is unclear whether or not uptake of AL is required to mediate its necrotic effects on β-cell membranes *in vitro*.

Although high AL doses (100 to 150 mg/kg) have been used to produce diabetes in mice, these doses are probably higher than necessary, producing unwanted collateral damage and rapid mortality. Dependent upon inbred strain and sex, AL doses between 50 and 80 mg/kg body weight are usually effective in producing chronic hyperglycemia.[179-182] The dose should be empirically established by the investigator since there may be multiple variables affecting how mice will respond. For example, two inbred strains, ALS and ALR, were selected in Japan for susceptibility and resistance, respectively, to a lower dose of alloxan (47 mg/kg for females; 45 mg/kg for males).[183] One of the authors of the chapter (EHL) has imported both of these strains to the Jackson Laboratory. In this new vivarium (with different diet, etc.), a slightly higher dose (52 mg/kg) is required to observe the differential susceptibility distinguishing these two strains. Table 12.3 lists various strains reported to be susceptible or resistant to single AL injections when tested at a lower threshold level between 25 to 50 mg/kg. It is noteworthy that strains susceptible to lower AL doses are generally the same strains susceptible to MDSTZ (C57BLKS/J, DBA/2J, ALS/Lt) while those resistant to lower AL doses are also resistant to MDSTZ (e.g., C3H, ALR/Lt). However, there are exceptions — e.g., it is observed that young

TABLE 12.3

Differential Sensitivity of Various Inbred Mouse Strains to
Hyperglycemia Induction within 7 days after Tail Vein Injections
of Diabetogenic Threshold Doses (40–50 mg/kg) of Alloxan

Resistant	Susceptible
C3H[182]	C57BLKS/J[180]
ALR[183]	ALS[183]
DDK[179]	DBA/2[182]
	NOD/Lt*(EHL, unpublished)
C57BL/6J[180]	NON/Lt (EHL, unpublished)
NC[179]	RR[179]

* Partially responsive (1/5 males; 2/5 females hyperglycemic at day 7).

NOD/Lt mice are highly susceptible to MDSTZ (40 mg/kg × 5 administered i.p.), but less susceptible to administration i.v. of 52 mg/kg AL.

12.4.2   Physiological Basis for Variation in Alloxan Sensitivity in Mice

Because AL is a potent generator of ·OH radicals, it represents a useful probe to elucidate the genetic mechanisms controlling the β-cell defenses against oxygen free radical–mediated damage. The high β-cell toxicity of AL is not only due to its selective uptake by GLUT-2 glucose transporters in β-cells, but also due to the low β-cell content of glutathione and of antioxidant enzymes (superoxide dismutase, or SOD, catalase, glutathione peroxidase, and reductase) capable of scavenging oxygen free radicals.[184-186] Lower than normal concentrations of SOD have been reported in islets of NOD mice[187] and BB rats, although this finding was not produced in another NOD study using essentially the same methods.[188] Indeed, mouse β-cells appear to maintain the lowest concentrations of antioxidant enzymes and glutathione compared with either rat or human islets.[189] Antioxidant defenses in human islets are further enhanced over those in rodent islets by the presence of higher levels of heat shock proteins, especially Hsp70.[186] The current controversies regarding whether or not suppression of human β-cell function by cytokine exposure *in vitro* requires nitric oxide (NO)[190-192] may in part be a reflection of genetically determined differences in the level of antioxidant defenses extant in the cadaveric islets employed in the various studies. The new mouse models described below, with drastically different systemic abilities to handle free radical toxicity, could provide important insights into this controversy. Perhaps because of the rapid rate of spontaneous AL decomposition in serum, strain-dependent differences in clearance rates have not been shown to be a contributor to differential diabetogenic susceptibilities among strains.

12.4.3   Genetic Control of Susceptibility to Alloxan: ALS and ALR Mice

Inbreeding of outbred ICR (Swiss Hauschka) mice in Japan has been an ongoing process since the end of World War II. The NOD, NON, ILI, and CTS strains are the most notable examples of how valuable this effort has been to understanding of the immunogenetic and pathophysiological bases of IDDM development.[2] Adding to this effort, Ino et al.[183] inbred CD-1 (essentially ICR) mice with selection for AL susceptibility vs. resistance to the potent diabetogenic agent alloxan. Selection was based upon diabetogenic responsiveness to an AL dose representing the ED_{50} for the starting population (47 mg/kg for females; 45 mg/kg for males). After a litter was born and weaned, the parents and some of the progeny were treated with AL to select for high vs. low incidence lines based on blood glucose levels at 7 days post-treatment. It should be noted that the selection doses used were at the lower threshold for diabetogenic responses for most inbred strains, in which ED_{50} is attained only at a dose of 60 mg/kg or higher.[181] This technique of high–low selection was successful, as demonstrated by the high sensitivity of ALS mice vs. the relative resistance of ALR mice.[183] These two strains have been imported by one of the authors (EHL) to the Jackson Laboratory. The Jackson Laboratory substrains are designated ALS/Lt and ALR/Lt. At a dose of 52 mg/kg of AL monohydrate, 6- to 7-week-ALS/Lt mice of both sexes are consistently diabetic at experiment day 7 (mean plasma glucose >400 mg/dl), whereas ALR/Lt mice are not. The resistance of ALR/Lt mice is relative and not absolute, since a dose of 60 mg/kg renders most of them diabetic by experiment day 7. A preliminary genetic comparison of ALS and ALR strains in Japan has been reported using "classical" screening methods (isozymes, immunophenotypic typing, etc.).[193] Preliminary analysis of the genomes of the ALS/Lt and ALR/Lt strains using simple sequence repeat length polymorphisms indicates the two strains differ at approximately 25% of the polymorphic loci tested. Genetic segregation analysis will establish whether the differential sensitivity of the two strains is under monogenic, oligogenic, or polygenic control.

Only a single study exists in which an AL-resistant strain (C3H) was mated to an AL-sensitive strain (DBA/2J), and the F1 progeny examined.[182] F1 hybrids were as resistant as C3H parentals, indicating resistance was dominant. This resistance correlated with higher levels of glutathione in blood of resistant C3H and F1 mice as compared with susceptible DBA/2J mice.[182] Preliminary evidence from analysis of the mice at the Jackson Laboratory indicate that a similar elevation in blood and tissue levels of glutathione levels may distinguish untreated ALR from ALS mice. If confirmed, this would indicate that genetically controlled differences in ability to dissipate free radicals may well distinguish individuals systemically, and perhaps at the β-cell level. Recent model studies in transgenic mice support this possibility. Transgenic mice have been produced in which multiple copies of the *Sod1* gene (Cu-Zn SOD) have been introduced either on the endogenous genomic promoter,[194] or ligated to the rat insulin promoter to limit expression to β-cells.[195] This change in expression of Cu-Zn SOD systemically reduced the sensitivity of transgene-positive mice to both AL- and STZ-mediated β-cell damage. Alternatively, or in addition, genetic differences in AL susceptibility could entail differences in uptake mechanisms. Human β-cells have a tenfold lower uptake of AL than do mouse islets, perhaps because GLUT-1 rather than GLUT-2 predominates in the former. Accordingly, differences in ability to transport these toxins, as well as greater ability to dissipate oxygen free radicals, may distinguish human from rodent islets.[189]

12.5 Virus-Induced Glucose Intolerance in Mice

Epidemiological studies associate serologic reactivity to human pathogenic viruses with IDDM onset in children, raising the possibility that certain viruses represent diabetogenic catalysts in genetically susceptible individuals.[167,196-199] β-cell cytolytic viruses could directly produce IDDM by infecting and destroying the majority of β-cells in the pancreas. A less infective or cytolytic variant might produce a comparable level of damage by eliciting immune autoreactivity if lysis of a few acutely infected β-cells led to exposure of sequestered autoantigens analogous to STZ altered "self" molecules. Alternatively, persistently infected β-cells might incorporate viral antigens into their cell membranes, triggering anti-β cell immunity or impairing β-cell function, or both. Finally, the viral infection may trigger IDDM not by a direct attack on the β-cells, but rather by a systemic effect whereby certain cytokines, perhaps immune interferons, impair immunosuppression of autoimmune effector cells that are present in the periphery of rodents (both rats and mice) that nominally do not develop IDDM. The existence of the latter pathway has been clearly demonstrated by the diabetogenic triggering action of the Kilham rat virus (KRV) in BB-DR (diabetes-resistant) rats (see Chapter 13). The unexpected finding that exposure of NOD mice and BB-DP (diabetes-prone) rats to most viruses upregulates cytokine communication in such a way to prevent IDDM only serves to emphasize the potential of viruses to modulate IDDM susceptibility in these two models. Obviously, children identified as having genetic susceptibility to IDDM (e.g., high-risk HLA haplotypes coupled with familial history of IDDM) cannot be experimentally infected with human viruses to test their capacity to serve as diabetogenic triggers. However, susceptible strains of inbred mice can be used as surrogate hosts to assess diabetogenic potential of human viruses. This was illustrated by the use of mice to confirm "Koch's postulates" in a case of a 10-year-old male Caucasian who developed diabetic ketoacidosis 3 days after experiencing an influenza-like illness. The child died 7 days after hospital admission. Pieces of his pancreas were homogenized, and following incubation with a variety of cell lines, a Coxsackie B4 virus was isolated.[200] This pancreatic viral isolate, but not one from the heart of the same patient, produced overt hyperglycemia in 9 of 13 SJL/J males that persisted for 2 weeks postinoculation, thereby confirming Koch's postulate regarding the pathogenicity of the infectious agent. In addition to variable insulitis, histopathological analysis of these mice showed acute myopericarditis and menigoencephalitis. The purpose of the following sections will not be to recapitulate evidence that viruses are diabetogenic triggers, but rather to illustrate briefly how mice present research tools to address the question.

12.5.1   Adaptation of Human Viruses for Growth in Mice

Among the various human viruses adapted for growth in mouse cells are the RNA-containing picornaviruses Coxsackie B4 (CB4), encephalomyocarditis (EMC-D and M variants), and Mengo-2T, as well as two other double-stranded RNA viruses, reovirus and lymphocytic choriomeningitis virus (LMCV, Armstrong variant). Primary isolates of these human pathogenic agents are generally not pancreatotrophic or lytic to mouse β-cells and must be adapted for growth either by inoculation into suckling mice, or by passage in cultured mouse β-cells. The picornaviruses adapted for growth in mice are primarily tropic for pancreatic exocrine and myocardial tissues, but tropism of picornavirus and reovirus for β-cells can be increased by serial passage in primary cultures of mouse embryonic fibroblasts or islet cells.[201]

12.5.2   Differential Inbred Strain Susceptibility to Human Viruses Adapted for Growth in Use

Table 12.4 contains a survey from the literature of strains deemed to be susceptible or resistant to the diabetogenic action of various human viruses adapted for growth in mouse cells. Unless neonates are inoculated, either male mice or testosterone-treated females must be used since androgens act synergistically with pancreatropic viruses to impair glucose tolerance.[202] In most cases, transient, impaired glucose tolerance (IGT) is reported rather than development of a chronic IDDM syndrome. Indeed, as mentioned above, inflammation of the heart and the nervous system is often a consequence of infection with EMC-M or D variants or CB4, such that mice die of causes other than diabetes. This is illustrated by the finding that C57BL/6J mice, resistant to the diabetogenic action of CB4 virus, exhibited early lethality higher than in strains susceptible to IGT. Strains such as

TABLE 12.4

Differential Sensitivity of Various Inbred Mouse Strains
to Impaired Glucose Tolerance Elicited by Viral Infection

Virus	Resistant	Susceptible
EMC-D or M variant	C57BL/6J[240]	SJL/J[241]
	CBA/J[241]	SWR/J[241]
	C3H/HeJ[240]	DBA/1J[241]
	AKR/J[241]	DBA/2J[240]
	BALBc/J[240]	BALB/cCum[208]
Mengo 2T	—	SJL[241]
		C57BL/6J[241]
		CBA/J[241]
		C3H/HeJ[241]
		AKR/J[241]
		CE/J[241]
CB4	C57BL/6J[a 242]	SJL/J[242]
	CBA/J[200]	SWR/J[242]
	AKR/J[242]	
	BALBc/J	
	DBA/1J[164]	
	DBA/2J[242]	
	C3H/HeJ[203]	
Reo	—	SJL/J[201]

ᵃ High mortality without pancreatic lesions.

C3H/HeJ, resistant to development of IGT in response to EMC and CB4, nonetheless develop severe pancreatitis affecting the exocrine parenchyma, but not the islets.[203] Among inbred strains, the SJL/J male stands out as being susceptible to IGT or overt diabetes induction by the human viruses described in Table 12.4. Although omitted from Table 12.4 because they are not inbred, CD-1 males (essentially the same as ICR Swiss) are generally quite susceptible to IGT development.

12.5.3 Mechanism of Differential Strain Sensitivity to Virus-Induced IGT

VCAM-1 has been identified as an EMC viral receptor on mouse vascular endothelial cells.[204] Although differences in viral receptors on endothelium could potentially limit exposure of β-cells to virus, possible strain differences in viral receptor numbers on β-cells cannot explain differential susceptibility to induction of IGT. When β-cells from C57BL/6J mice are infected *in vitro* with EMC-M virus, cytopathic changes are as severe as observed in cultured β-cells from noninbred CD-1 mice, whereas *in vivo* only CD-1 males develop IGT.[205] The IFN system has been implicated as a major determinant of strain sensitivity, with diabetes-resistant C57BL/6J males generating a high IFN response against this variant.[203] A single nucleotide substitution at codon 776 of the VP1 capsid protein (causing replacement of a threonine with an alanine residue in the EMC-D variant) is thought to be responsible for its diabetogenicity.[196] A nondiabetogenic EMC-B variant has been associated with higher IFN production,[206] and coadministration of B and D variants prevents IGT induced by the D variant (reviewed by Ramsingh et al.[197]). However, the protective effects of IFN were strain dependent, with diabetogenicity of the EMC-D variant blocked by IFNβ or IFN inducers in SWR/J, but not in outbred ICR Swiss males.[207]

As in the MDSTZ model, the issue of whether T cells are required for EMC-mediated pathogenesis has been controversial. Requirement for T cells has definitively been ruled out in the Mengo viral infection model (reviewed by Yoon[196]). A T cell dependency to EMC-M has been shown in one substrain of BALB/c males (BALB/cBy), but not in another substrain (BALB/cCum) or in DBA/2J males.[208,209] The fact that outbred CD-1 males (with highly polymorphic MHC haplotypes represented) are generally susceptible argues against a specific MHC requirement for presentation of diabetogenic viral epitopes. The timing of IFN exposure may critically effect β-cell function, since treatment of ICR Swiss mice with either IFNβ or IFNγ 4 days after EMC-D inoculation exacerbated rather than diminished frequency and severity of IGT.[210] Acceleration of IDDM onset by poly I:C in prediabetic BB-DP rats has been associated with induced expression of IFNα mRNA in islets, and high levels of this cytokine were induced both in pancreata of MDSTZ-treated CD-1 male mice[125] and in selected human IDDM cases.[211] The "innocent bystander" concept posits that viral expression within islets or in endothelium/ductal cells adjacent to islets elicits induction of combinations of β-cytotoxic lymphokines (interferons) and monokines. Hence, viruses may trigger IDDM by inducing synthesis of a deleterious cascade of cytopathic cytokines in the islet environment that kill β-cells via generation of cytotoxic free radicals (reviewed by Rewers and Atkinson[198]). This could be the mechanism whereby a subdiabetogenic dose of STZ followed by CB4 virus infection synergized to produce greater than additive diabetogenic damage to β-cells in both mice and in Patas mon-keys.[196,212] Experimental infection of BB-DP rats with LCMV protects against IDDM devel-opment, as it does in the NOD mouse.[102,213] Further, diabetes induced in BB-DR/Wor rats exposed to KRV and then further challenged by systemic poly I:C treatment indicate that the effects of virally induced IFNs are likely to be on immunoregulatory cells rather than directly on the β-cells.[20,214] Macrophages and macrophage-derived monokines have been shown to be important for virus catalyzed diabetogenesis in this model.[215] Similarly, depletion of macrophages also protects DBA/2J mice from EMC-induced myocarditis and diabetes.[216] Thus, the diabetogenic consequences of viral infection in these models is not limited to direct lytic effects on β-cells, but also may entail systemic effects on immuno-regulatory cells as well. It should be noted, however, that interpretation of results from immunomodulation of virus-infected animals can be difficult, since both antiviral and autoimmune responses can be influenced by the manipulations.

12.5.4 Coxsackie Virus: A Molecular Mimic of Glutamic Acid Decarboxylase, a Candidate β-Cell Autoantigen?

CB4 virus has been reported to alter lymphocyte repertoire preceding onset of IGT in CD-1 male mice.[217] An ongoing debate in the immunology of diabetes concerns the potential immunomodulatory properties of P2-C, a nonstructural Coxsackie protein involved in viral RNA replication. P2-C shows a modest level of structural homology to both isoforms of GAD (GAD65 and GAD67), leading to the speculation that this viral protein, localizing within host target cells, has sufficient cross-reactivity to a GAD epitope that it can break T cell tolerance to GAD in β-cells. Years before onset of clinical IDDM in children, high titers of GAD autoantibodies, when present in combination with antibodies to other islet autoantigens, are reasonably predictive of the presence of an underlying, destructive insulitic process in the islets.[218] GAD65 and GAD67 are cytosolic enzymes producing γ-aminobutyric acid (GABA), an inhibitory neurotransmitter. GABA is found in both human and rodent islets, and GAD protein is detectable by Western blot in human and rat islets.[219] Although relatively high concentrations of GABA have been reported in NOD islets,[220] neither GAD67 nor GAD65 protein has been detectable by Western blot in islets of young prediabetic NOD/Lt mice.[221] Nonetheless, early spontaneous T cell responses to synthetic 20-mer GAD65 peptides have been observed in spleens of NOD mice by some workers,[222] but not others.[73] A 20-mer peptide containing an identical six amino acid sequence (PEVKEK) contained in P2-C and GAD65/67, administered intranasally to prediabetic NOD mice in a mixture with two additional peptides, was protective.[223] In contrast, administration of a 20-mer GAD65 peptide containing the PEVKEK sequence intrathymically into young NOD mice was marginally protective, whereas injected syngeneic islet cells were clearly protective.[224] The MHC class II I-A^{g7} molecule of NOD mice is particularly efficient in presenting to CD4$^+$ T cells both the 20-mer GAD65 and P2-C sequence similarity peptides spanning the PEVKEK sequence.[225] However, when overlapping 15-mer GAD peptides were analyzed, different immunodominant epitopes presented by I-A^{g7}, not including the Coxsackie sequence similarity region, were reported.[226] It is clear that induction of hyperglycemia by CB4 (E2 strain) is not MHC restricted, since both outbred CD-1 (multiple MHC haplotypes represented) and SJL/J (H2^s) males develop hyperglycemia in association with upregulated islet expression of a 64-kDa protein presumed to be GAD.[227] The MHC class II genes of SJL/J were found to be poor presenters (to CD4$^+$ T cells) of the sequence similarity peptide from Coxsackie or GAD65, yet SJL/J represents one of the most susceptible inbred strains to CB4-induced hyperglycemia. It is unlikely that CB4 infection would trigger diabetes in NOD mice (by molecular mimicry or any other mechanism), since diabetogenesis in this strain is promoted in an SPF environment, whereas exposure to viruses upregulates protective immunoregulatory networks and reduces diabetes frequency. The influence of cross-reactive CB4 viral epitopes on induction of hyperglycemia in NOD-congenic stocks that do not develop IDDM spontaneously, or in the strains that traditionally are used to study CB4-induced hyperglycemia, remains to be established. If it is possible to alter the PEVKEK region of the virus by targeted mutagenesis without changing its biological and infectious characteristics, it should be possible at least to address the significance of this homology to GAD molecules.

It is unlikely that a single pathogenic mechanism is involved in CB4 virus-induced hyperglycemia. The E2 strain has been shown initially to establish a productive lytic infection, induce production of antibodies to a 64-kDa mouse islet protein, and later establish a persistent infection.[228] This persistent infection was associated with a reduced ability of the remaining β-cells to produce insulin mRNA and with both a reduction in insulin production and in content per islet.[229] This indicates that three different mechanisms (lysis, autoimmunity, and functional impairment) all may be involved in reducing the insulin output from the pancreas of CB4-infected mice below a level that can sustain normoglycemia.

12.5.5   Retroviruses as Diabetogenic Catalysts

Susceptibility of mice to diabetes induced by either MDSTZ or by single gene obesity mutations has been correlated with β-cell ability to express endogenous retroviral particles.[123] A higher-order molecular conformational mimicry exists between insulin and the group-specific antigen of the murine intracisternal type A particle (IAP) retrovirus.[72] Acceleration of IDDM in NOD mice by cyclophosphamide was associated with upregulation of expression of endogenous retroviral genomes.[230] These latter particles included xenotropic C-type retroviral particles as well as IAP.[165] The potential diabetogenic significance of upregulated retroviral gene expression in stressed β-cells has remained enigmatic; for example, derepression of IAP gene expression is a frequent finding in mouse neoplasms. Indeed, an NOD β-cell line (NIT-1) produced from neoplastic islets sheds a type C retrovirus not normally expressed in untransformed NOD/Lt β-cells.[231] Recently, the question of the pathogenic significance of retroviral gene expression in β-cells has been examined with renewed interest following the report that an endogenous retrovirus had been isolated from the pancreas of a child with IDDM[232] (see note added in proof). What was particularly intriguing about this finding was that an N-terminal peptide made from one of the retroviral proteins functioned as a "superantigen," activating CD4[+] T cells with a Vβ7 T cell receptor. This was the prevalent clonotype originally isolated as islet reactive from the pancreas of the diabetic child, leading to the speculation that a "superantigen-like" trigger had precipitated IDDM.[233] The unusual aspect of the superantigen peptide is that it derived from the envelope portion of the retroviral genome, and not the 5' long terminal repeat (LTR), the source of the mouse mammary tumor virus (MMTV) superantigen. Evidence for retroviral expression was found in the pancreas of another child who had died following acute IDDM development, but not in control pancreata. Whether human endogenous retroviral (HERV) sequences embedded in the human genome can be activated (perhaps by cytokines induced by infection with other viruses?) remains to be established. Notice has recently been taken that a close homology exists between the C-terminal of IL-2 and the transmembrane envelope glycoprotein (gp41) of the human immunodeficiency virus (HIV).[234] A 6-mer peptide (LEHLLL) in the sequence similarity region reportedly binds to the IL-2 receptor, raising the possibility that β-cell expression of this segment of an HERV genome could activate T cells infiltrating into the pancreas.[234] Undoubtedly, this question will be addressed using transgenic mouse models expressing the HIV gp41 sequence ligated to an insulin promoter to target expression to β-cells.

Note Added in Proof:

Unfortunately, this observation has not been replicated by other laboratories or by the original authors, and apparently represents a technical artifact. See:

Murphy, V. J., Harrison, L. C., Rudort, W. A., Luppi, P., Trucco, M., Fierabracci, A., Biro, P. A., and Bottazzo, G.-F., Retroviral superantigens and type 1 diabetes mellitus, *Cell*, 95, 9, 1998.

Löwer, R., Tonjes, R. R., Boller, K., Denner, J., Kaiser, B., Phelps, R. C., Löwer, J., Kurth, R., Badenhoop, K., Donner, H., Usadel, K. H., Miethke, T., Lapatschek, M., and Wagner, H., Development of insulin-dependent diabetes mellitus does not depend on specific expression of the human endogenous retrovirus HERV-K [In Process Citation], *Cell*, 95, 11, 1998.

Lan, M. S., Mason, A., Coutant, R., Chen, Q. Y., Vargas, A., Rao, J., Gomez, R., Chalow, S., Garry, R., and Maclaren, N. K., HERV K10s and immune mediated (type 1) diabetes, *Cell*, 95, 14, 1998.

Conrad, B., In response to Murphy et al., Lower et al., and Lan et al., *Cell*, 95, 16, 1998.

Acknowledgments

The writing of this chapter was supported by NIH grants DK36175 and DK27722 and a grant from the Juvenile Diabetes Foundation, International (E.H.L), as well as fellowship grants from the American Diabetes Association (I.G.) and NIH DK07449 (J.F.). Dr. Dave Serreze and Ms. Emmie Chen (the Jackson Laboratory) are thanked for their participation in analysis of gallium effects on NOD mice. Dr. Nicholas Gerber (Ohio State University) is thanked for providing gallium nitrate. Drs. Dave Serreze and Clayton Mathews of the Jackson Laboratory are thanked for their critical reviews. Dr. Mathews kindly provided unpublished information on the alloxan sensitivity of NOD/Lt and NON/Lt mice.

References

1. Makino, S., Kunimoto, K., Muraoka, Y., Mizushima, Y., Katagiri, K., and Tochino, Y., Breeding of a non-obese, diabetic strain of mice. *Exp. Anim.* 29, 1, 1980.
2. Kikutani, H. and Makino, S., The murine autoimmune diabetes model: NOD and related strains. In *Advances in Immunology*, Vol. 51, Dixon, F.J., Ed., Academic Press, New York, 1992, 285.
3. Leiter, E.H., NOD mice and related strains: origins, husbandry, and biology. In *NOD Mice and Related Strains: Research Applications in Diabetes, AIDS, Cancer, and Other Diseases*, Leiter, E.H., and Atkinson, M.A., Eds., R.G. Landes, Austin, 1998, 1.
4. Harada, M. and Makino, S., Suppression of overt diabetes in NOD mice by antithymocyte serum or anti-Thy 1.2 antibody, *Exp. Anim.* 35, 501, 1986.
5. Miller, B.J., Appel, M.C., O'Neil, J.J., and Wicker, L.S., Both the Lyt-2+ and L3T4+ T cell subsets are required for the transfer of diabetes in nonobese diabetic mice. *J. Immunol.* 140, 52, 1988.
6. Bendelac, A., Carnaud, C., Boitard, C., and Bach, J.F., Syngeneic transfer of autoimmune diabetes from diabetic NOD mice to healthy neonates: requirement for both L3T4+ and Lyt-2+ T cells. *J. Exp. Med.* 166, 823, 1987.
7. Christianson, S.W., Shultz, L.D., and Leiter, E.H., Adoptive transfer of diabetes into immuno-deficient NOD-*scid/scid* mice: relative contributions of CD4+ and CD8+ T lymphocytes from diabetic vs. prediabetic NOD.NON-Thy-1ª donors. *Diabetes* 42, 44, 1993.
8. Bach, J., Autoimmunity and type-1 diabetes. (review), *Trends Endocrinol.* 8, 71, 1997.
9. Fujino-Kurihara, H., Fujita, H., Hakura, A., Nonaka, K., and Tarui, S., Morphological aspects on pancreatic islets of non-obese diabetic (NOD) mice. *Virchows Arch. Cell Pathol.* 49, 107, 1985.
10. Jarpe, A.J., Hickman, M.R., Anderson, J.T., Winter, W.E., and Peck, A.B., Flow cytometric enumeration of mononuclear cell populations infiltrating the islets of Langerhans in prediabetic NOD mice: development of a model of autoimmune insulitis for type 1 diabetes. *Reg. Immunol.* 3, 305, 1991.
11. Pozzilli, P., Signore, A., Williams, A., and Beales, P., NOD mouse colonies around the world — recent facts and figures. *Immunol. Today* 14, 193, 1993.
12. Bowman, M.A., Leiter, E.H., and Atkinson, M.A., Autoimmune diabetes in NOD mice: a genetic programme interruptible by environmental manipulation. *Immunol. Today* 15, 115, 1994.
13. Hoorfar, J., Buschard, K., and Dagnaes-Hansen, F., Prophylactic nutritional modification of the incidence of diabetes in autoimmune non-obese diabetic (NOD) mice. *Br. J. Nutr.* 69, 597, 1993.
14. Serreze, D.V. and Leiter, E.H., Insulin dependent diabetes mellitus (IDDM) in NOD mice and BB rats: origins in hematopoietic stem cell defects and implications for therapy. In *Lessons from Animal Diabetes. V*, Shafrir, E., Ed, Smith-Gordon, London, 1995, 59.
15. Leiter, E.H., Le, P.H., Prochazka, M., Worthen, S.M., and Huppi, K., Genetic and environmental control of diabetes induction by multi-dose streptozotocin in two BALB/c substrains. *Diabetes Res.* 9, 5, 1988.
16. Leiter, E., The NOD mouse: a model for insulin dependent diabetes mellitus. In *Current Protocols in Immunology*, Vol. 3, Coligan, J.E., Kruisbeek, A.M., Margulies, D.M., Shevach, E.M., and Strober, W., Eds, John Wiley & Sons, New York, 1997, 15.
17. Wilberz, S., Partke, H.J., Dagnaes-Hansen, F., and Herberg, L., Persistent MHV (mouse hepatitis virus) infection reduces the incidence of diabetes mellitus in non-obese diabetic mice. *Diabetologia* 34, 2, 1991.
18. Ohsugi, T. and Kurosawa, T., Increased incidence of diabetes mellitus in specific pathogen-eliminated offspring produced by embryo transfer in NOD mice with low incidence of the disease. *Lab. Anim. Sci.* 44, 386, 1994.
19. Like, A., Guberski, D., and Butler, L., Influence of environmental viral agents on frequency and tempo of diabetes mellitus in BB/Wor rats. *Diabetes* 40, 259, 1991.
20. Ellerman, K.E., Richards, C.A., Guberski, D.L., Shek, W.R., and Like, A.A., Kilham rat virus triggers T-cell-dependent autoimmune diabetes in multiple strains of rats. *Diabetes* 45, 557, 1996.
21. Baxter, A.G., Adams, M.A., and Mandel, T.E., Comparison of high and low diabetes incidence NOD mouse strains. *Diabetes* 38, 1296, 1989.

22. Baxter, A.G. and Mandel, T.E., Accelerated diabetes in non-obese diabetic (NOD) mice differing in incidence of spontaneous disease. *Clin. Exp. Immunol.* 85, 464, 1991.
23. Atkinson, M., Gendreau, P., Ellis, T., and Pettitto, J., NOD mice as a model for inherited deafness. *Diabetologia* 40, 868, 1997.
24. Leiter, E.H., The NOD mouse meets the "Nerup Hypothesis." Is diabetogenesis the result of a collection of common alleles present in unfavorable combinations? In *Frontiers in Diabetes Research: Lessons from Animal Diabetes III.*, Vardi, P. and Shafrir, E., Eds., Smith-Gordon., London, 1990, 54.
25. Shultz, L.D., Schweitzer, P.A., Christianson, S.W., Gott, B., Birdsall-Maller, I., Tennent, B., McKenna, S., Mobraaten, L., Rajan, T.V., Greiner, D.L., and Leiter, E.H., Multiple defects in innate and adaptive immunological function in NOD/LtSz-*scid* mice. *J. Immunol.* 154, 180, 1995.
26. Baxter, A.G. and Mandel, T.E., Hemolytic anemia in non-obese diabetic mice. *Eur. J. Immunol.* 21, 2051, 1991.
27. Leiter, E.H., Genetics and immunogenetics of NOD mice and related strains. In *NOD Mice and Related Strains: Research Applications in Diabetes, AIDS, Cancer, and Other Diseases*, Leiter, E.H. and Atkinson, M.A., Eds, R.G. Landes, Austin, 1998, 37.
28. Serreze, D.V., The identity and ontogenic origins of autoreactive T lymphocytes in NOD mice. In *NOD Mice and Related Strains: Research Applications in Diabetes, AIDS, Cancer, and Other Diseases*, Leiter, E.H., and Atkinson, M.A., Eds, R.G. Landes, Austin, 1998, 71.
29. Smith, K., Olson, D., Hirose, R., and Hanahan, D., Pancreatic gene expression in rare cells of thymic medulla: evidence for functional contribution to T cell tolerance. *Int. Immunol.* 9, 1355, 1997.
30. Colucci, F., Cilio, C.M., Lejon, K., Goncalves, C.P., Bergman, M.L., and Holmberg, D., Programmed cell death in the pathogenesis of murine IDDM: resistance to apoptosis induced in lymphocytes by cyclophosphamide. *J. Autoimmunity* 9, 271, 1996.
31. Colucci, F., Bergman, M.-L., Penha-Gonclaves, C., Cilio, C., and Holmberg, D., Apoptosis resistance of nonobese diabetic peripheral lymphocytes linked to the Idd5 diabetes susceptibility region. *Proc. Natl. Acad. Sci. U.S.A.*, 94, 8670, 1997.
32. Cetkovic-Cvrlje, M. and Leiter, E., Mono-ADP ribosyltransferase genes and diabetes in NOD mice: is there a relationship? In *ADP-Ribosylation in Animal Tissues: Structure, Function and Biology of Mono(ADP-Ribosyl)Transferase and Related Enzymes*, Haag, F. and Koch-Nolte, F., Eds, Plenum Press, New York, 1997, 217.
33. Livingstone, A., Edwards, C.T., Shizuru, J.A., and Fathman, C.G., Genetic analysis of diabetes in the nonobese diabetic mouse. I. MHC and T cell receptor β gene expression. *J. Immunol.* 146, 529, 1991.
34. Sarukhan, A., Bedossa, P., Garchon, H.J., Bach, J.F., and Carnaud, C., Molecular analysis of TCR junctional variability in individual infiltrated islets of non-obese diabetic mice: evidence for the constitution of largely autonomous T cell foci within the same pancreas. *Int Immunol*, 7, 139, 1995.
35. Serreze, D.V. and Leiter, E.H., Defective activation of T suppressor cell function in nonobese diabetic mice. Potential relation to cytokine deficiencies. *J. Immunol.* 140, 3801, 1988.
36. Bach, J.-F., Insulin-dependent diabetes mellitus as an autoimmune disease. *Endocrine Rev.* 15, 516, 1994.
37. Prochazka, M., Serreze, D.V., Frankel, W.N., and Leiter, E.H., NOR/Lt; MHC-matched diabetes-resistant control strain for NOD mice. *Diabetes* 41, 98, 1992.
38. Serreze, D.V., Prochazka, M., Reifsnyder, P.C., Bridgett, M.M., and Leiter, E.H., Use of recombinant congenic and congenic strains of NOD mice to identify a new insulin dependent diabetes resistance gene. *J. Exp. Med.* 80, 1553, 1994.
39. Serreze, D.V., Hamaguchi, K., and Leiter, E.H., Immunostimulation circumvents diabetes in NOD/Lt mice. *J. Autoimmunity* 2, 759, 1990.
40. Clare-Salzler, M., The immunopathogenic roles of antigen presenting cells in the NOD mouse. In *NOD Mice and Related Strains: Research Applications in Diabetes, AIDS, Cancer, and Other Diseases*, Leiter, E.H., and Atkinson, M.A., Eds, R.G. Landes, Austin, 1998, 101.
41. Shimada, A., Charlton, B., Rohane, P., Taylor-Edwards, C., and Fathman, C.G., Immune regulation in type 1 diabetes. *J. Autoimmunity* 9, 263, 1996.

42. Serreze, D.V., Autoimmune diabetes results from genetic defects manifest by antigen presenting cells. *FASEB J.*, 7, 1092, 1993.
43. Serreze, D.V., Gaskins, H.R., and Leiter, E.H., Defects in the differentiation and function of antigen presenting cells in NOD/Lt mice. *J. Immunol.* 150, 2534, 1993.
44. Serreze, D.V., Gaedeke, J.W., and Leiter, E.H., Hematopoietic stem cell defects underlying abnormal macrophage development and maturation in NOD/Lt mice: defective regulation of cytokine receptors and protein kinase C. *Proc. Natl. Acad. Sci. U.S.A.*, 90, 9625, 1993.
45. Langmuir, P.B., Bridgett, M.M., Bothwell, A.L.M., and Crispe, I.N., Bone marrow abnormalities in the non-obese diabetic mouse. *Int. Immunol.* 5, 169, 1993.
46. Jacob, C.O., Aiso, S., Michie, S.A., McDevitt, H.O., and Acha-Orbea, H., Prevention of diabetes in nonobese diabetic mice by tumor necrosis factor (TNF); similarities between TNF-a and interleukin 1. *Proc. Natl. Acad. Sci. U.S.A.*, 87, 968, 1990.
47. Xie, T., Hofig, A., Yui, M., Wakeland, E., Reddy, S., Hershman, H., Wicker, L., Peterson, L., and Clare-Salzler, M., Spontaneous prostaglandin synthase-2 (Ptgs2) gene expression in macrophages of NOD and congenic mice. *Autoimmunity* 21, 17, 1995.
48. Xie, T., Reddy, S., Hofig, A., Litherland, S., Herschman, H., Myrick, C., Wakeland, E., Wicker, L., and Clare-Salzler, M., Regulation of prostaglandin synthase-2 (Pgs-2) in NOD macrophages. *Autoimmunity* 24 (Suppl. 1), 23, 1996.
49. Prins, J.-B., Todd, J., Rodriques, N., Ghosh, S., Hogarth, P., Wicker, L., Gaffney, E., Podolin, P., Fischer, P., Sirotina, A., and Peterson, L., Linkage on chromosome 3 of autoimmune diabetes and defective Fc receptor for IgG in NOD mice. *Science* 260, 695, 1993.
50. Luan, J., Monteiro, R., Sautes, C., Fluteau, G., Eloy, L., Fridman, W., Bach, J., and Garchon, H., Defective Fc gamma RII gene expression in macrophages of NOD mice — genetic linkage with upregulation of IgG1 and IgG2b in serum. *J Immunol.* 157, 4707, 1996.
51. Marsh, C.B., Pope, H.A., and Wewers, M.D., FCγ receptor cross-linking downregulates IL-1 receptor antagonist and induces IL-1β in mononuclear phagocytes stimulated with endotoxin or *Staphylococcus aureus*. *J. Immunol.* 152, 4604, 1994.
52. Podolin, P.L., Denny, P., Todd, J.A., Lyons, P.A., Lord, C.J., Peterson, L.B., Hill, N.J., and Wicker, L.S., Congenic mapping of the insulin-dependent diabetes (*Idd*) gene, *Idd10*, localizes 2 genes mediating the *Idd10* effect and eliminates the candidate *Fcgr1*. *J. Immunol.* 159, 1835, 1997.
53. Tsumura, H., Komada, H., Ito, Y., and Shimura, K., *In vitro* and *in vivo* interferon production in NOD mice. *Lab. Anim. Sci.* 39, 575, 1989.
54. Liblau, R.S., Singer, S.M., and McDevitt, H.O., Th1 and Th2 CD4(+) T cells in the pathogenesis of organ-specific autoimmune diseases. *Immunol Today* 16, 34, 1995.
55. Rapoport, M.J., Jaramillo, A., Zipris, D., Lazarus, A.H., Serreze, D.V., Leiter, E.H., Cyopick, P., Danska, J.S., and Delovitch, T.L., IL-4 reverses thymic T cell anergy and prevents the onset of diabetes in NOD mice. *J. Exp. Med.* 178, 87, 1993.
56. Rabinovitch, A., Immunoregulatory and cytokine imbalances in the pathogenesis of IDDM. *Diabetes* 43, 613, 1994.
57. Lord, C.J., Bohlander, S.K., Hopes, E.A., Montague, C.T., Hill, N.J., Prins, J.B., Renjilian, R.J., Peterson, L.B., Wicker, L.S., Todd, J.A., and Denny, P., Mapping the diabetes polygene Idd3 on mouse chromosome 3 by use of novel congenic strains. *Mamm Genome* 6, 563, 1995.
58. Chesnut, K., Shie, J.-X., Cheng, I., Muralidharan, K., and Wakeland, E.K., Characterization of candidate genes for IDD susceptibility from the diabetes-prone NOD mouse strain. *Mamm. Genome.* 4, 549, 1993.
59. Garchon, H.-J., Luan, J.-J., Eloy, L., Bédossa, P., and Bach, J.-F., Genetic analysis of immune dysfunction in non-obese diabetic (NOD) mice: mapping of a susceptibility locus close to the *Bcl-2* gene correlates with increased resistance of NOD T cells to apoptosis induction *Eur. J. Immunol.* 24, 380, 1994.
60. Kataoka, S., Satoh, J., Fujiya, H., Toyota, T., Suzuki, R., Itoh, K., and Kumagai, K., Immunologic aspects of the nonobese diabetic (NOD) mouse. Abnormalities of cellular immunity. *Diabetes* 32, 247, 1983.

61. Suzuki, T., Yamada, T., Takao, T., Fujimura, T., Kawamura, E., Shimizu, Z. M., Yamashita, R., and Nomoto, K., Diabetogenic effects of lymphocyte transfusion on the NOD or NOD nude mouse. In *Immune-Deficient Animals in Biomedical Research*, J. Rygaard, N.B., N. Graem, M. Sprang-Thomsen, Eds, Karger, Basel, 1987, 112.

62. Christianson, S.W., Greiner, D.L., Hesselton, R.A., Leif, J.H., Wagar, E.J., Schweitzer, P.B., Rajan, T.V., Gott, B., Roopenian, D.C., and Shultz, L.D., Enhanced human CD4⁺ T cell engraftment in β₂-microglobulin-deficient NOD-*scid* mice. *J. Immunol.* 158, 3578, 1997.

63. Greiner, D.L. and Shultz, L.D., The use of NOD/LtSz-*scid/scid* mice in biomedical research. In *NOD Mice and Related Strains: Research Applications in Diabetes, AIDS, Cancer, and Other Diseases*, Leiter, E.H., and Atkinson, M.A., Eds, R.G. Landes, Austin, 1998, 173.

64. Baxter, A.G., Kinder, S.J., Hammond, K.J.L., Scollary, R., and Godfrey, D.I., Association between alpha-beta-TCR⁺CD4⁻CD8⁻T-cell deficiency and IDDM in NOD/Lt mice. *Diabetes* 46, 572, 1997.

65. Gombert, J.M., Tancredebohin, E., Hameg, A., Leitedemoraes, M.D., Vicari, A., Bach, J.-F., and Herbelin, A., IL-7 reverses NK1(+) T cell-defective IL-4 production in the non-obese diabetic mouse. *Int. Immunol.* 8, 1751, 1996.

66. Bendelac, A., Boitard, C., Bedossa, P., Bazin, H., Bach, J.-F., and Carnaud, C., Adoptive T cell transfer of autoimmune nonobese diabetic mouse diabetes does not require recruitment of host B lymphocytes. *J. Immunol.* 141, 2625, 1988.

67. Serreze, D.V., Chapman, H.D., Varnum, D.S., Hanson, M.S., Reifsnyder, P.C., Richard, S.D., Fleming, S.A., Leiter, E.H., and Shultz, L.D., B lymphocytes are essential for the initiation of T cell-mediated autoimmune diabetes: analysis of a new "speed congenic" stock of NOD*Igμ^null* mice. *J. Exp. Med.* 184, 2049, 1996.

68. Akashi, T., Nagafuchi, S., Anzai, K., Kondo, S., Kitamura, D., Wakana, S., Ono, J., Kiruchi, M., Niho, Y., and Watanabe, T., Direct evidence for the contribution of B cells to the progression of insulitis and the development of diabetes in non-obese diabetic mice. *Int. Immunol.* 9, 1159, 1997.

69. Noorchashm, H., Noorchashm, N., Kern, J., Rostami, S.Y., Barker, C.F., and Naji, A., B-cells are required for the initiation of insulitis and sialitis in nonobese diabetic mice. *Diabetes* 46, 941, 1997.

70. Carrasco-Marins, E., Shimizu, J., Kanagawa, O., and Unanue, E., The class II MHC I-A^{g7} molecules from nonobese diabetic mice are poor peptide binders. *J. Immunol.* 156, 450, 1996.

71. Leijon, K., Hammarström, B., and Holmberg, D., Non-obese diabetic (NOD) mice display enhanced immune responses and prolonged survival of lymphoid cells. *Int. Immunol.* 6, 339, 1994.

72. Serreze, D.V., Leiter, E.H., Kuff, E.L., Jardieu, P., and Ishizaka, K., Molecular mimicry between insulin and retroviral antigen p73. Development of cross-reactive autoantibodies in sera of NOD and C57BL/KsJ-*db/db* mice, *Diabetes*, 37, 351, 1988.

73. Hanson, M.S., Cetkovic-Cvrlje, M., Ramiya, V., Atkinson, M., Maclaren, N., Singh, B., Elliott, J., Serreze, D., and Leiter, E., Quantitative thresholds of MHC class II I-E expression on hematopoietically derived APC in transgenic NOD/Lt mice determine level of diabetes resistance and indicate mechanism of protection. *J. Immunol.* 157, 1279, 1996.

74. Lenschow, D., Herold, K., Rhee, L., Patel, B., Koons, A., Qin, H., Fuchs, E., Singh, B., Thompson, C., and Bluestone, J., CD28/B7 regulation of Th1 and Th2 subsets in the development of autoimmune diabetes. *Immunity* 5, 285, 1996.

75. Gerling, I.C., Freidman, H., Greiner, D.L., Shultz, L.D., and Leiter, E.H., Multiple low dose streptozotocin-induced diabetes in NOD-*scid/scid* mice in the absence of functional lymphocytes. *Diabetes* 43, 433, 1994.

76. Shimada, A., Rohane, P., Fathman, C.G., and Charlton, B., Pathogenic and protective roles of CD45RB(low) CD4(+) cells correlate with cytokine profiles in the spontaneously autoimmune diabetic mouse. *Diabetes* 45, 71, 1996.

77. Amor, S., Oneill, J.K., Morris, M.M., Smith, R.M., Wraith, D.C., Groome, N., Travers, P.J., and Baker, D., Encephalitogenic epitopes of myelin basic protein, proteolipid protein, and myelin oligodendrocyte glycoprotein for experimental allergic encephalomyelitis induction in biozzi ABH (h-2A(g7)) mice share an amino acid motif. *J Immunol.* 156, 3000, 1996.

78. Many, M.C., Maniratu, S., and Denef, J.F., The nonobese diabetic (NOD) mose — an animal model for autoimmune thyroiditis. *Exp. Clin. Endocrinol. Diabetes* 104, 17, 1996.

79. Baxter, A.G., Horsfall, A.C., Healey, D., Ozegbe, P., Day, S., Williams, D.G., and Cooke, A., Mycobacteria precipitate an SLE-like syndrome in diabetes-prone NOD mice. *Immunology* 83, 227, 1994.

80. Mahler, M., Leiter, E.H., Birkenmeier, E.H., Bristol, I.J., Elson, C.O., and Sundberg, J.P., Differential susceptibility of inbred mouse strains to dextran sulfate sodium-induced colitis. *Am. J. Physiol.* 274, G544, 1998.

81. Amor, S., Baker, D., Groome, N., and Turk, J.L., Identification of major encephalitogenic epitope of proteolipid protein (residues 56-70) for the induction of experimental allergic encephalomyelitis in Biozzi AB/H and nonobese diabetic mice. *J. Immunol.* 150, 5666, 1993.

82. Slattery, R., Transgenic approaches to understanding the role of MHC genes in insulin dependent diabetes mellitus. II. The non-obese diabetic (NOD) mouse. *Baillieres Clin. Endocrinol. Metab.* 5, 449, 1991.

83. Uehira, M., Uno, M., Kurner, T., Kikutani, H., Mori, K., Inomoto, K., Uede, T., Miyazaki, J., Nishimoto, H., Kishimoto, T., and Yamamura, K., Development of autoimmune insulitis is prevented in Eα^d but not in Aβ^k NOD transgenic mice. *Int. Immunol.* 1, 209, 1989.

84. Lund, T., O'Reilly, L., Hutchings, P., Kanagawa, O., Simpson, E.R.G., Chandler, P., Dyson, J., Picard, J.K., Edwards, A., Kioussis, D., and Cooke, A., Prevention of insulin-dependent diabetes mellitus in non-obese diabetic mice by transgenes encoding modified I-A β-chain or normal I-E α-chain. *Nature* 345, 727, 1990.

85. Serreze, D.V., Leiter, E.H., Christianson, G.J., Greiner, D., and Roopenian, D.C., MHC class I deficient NOD-*B2m^null* mice are diabetes and insulitis resistant. *Diabetes* 43, 505, 1994.

86. Wicker, L.S., Leiter, E.H., Todd, J.A., Renjilian, R.J., Peterson, E., Fischer, P.A., Podolin, P.L., Zijlstra, M., Jaenisch, R., and Peterson, L.B., β2 microglobulin-deficient NOD mice do not develop insulitis or diabetes. *Diabetes* 43, 500, 1994.

87. Serreze, D.V., Chapman, H.C., Gerling, I.C., Leiter, E.H., and Shultz, L.D., Initiation of autoimmune diabetes in NOD/Lt mice is MHC class I-dependent. *J. Immunol.* 158, 3978, 1997.

88. Serreze, D.V. and Leiter, E.H., Genetic and pathogenic basis for autoimmune diabetes in NOD mice. *Curr. Opin. Immunol.* 6, 900, 1994.

89. Ikegami, H., Makino, S., Yamato, Y., Ueda, H., Sakamoto, T., Takekawa, K., and Ogihara, T., Identification of a new susceptibility locus for insulin dependent diabetes mellitus by ancestral haplotype congenic mapping. *J. Clin. Invest.* 96, 1936, 1995.

90. McAleer, M.A., Reifsnyder, P., Palmer, S.M., Prochazka, M., Love, J.M., Copeman, J.B., Powell, E.E., Rodrigues, N.R., Prins, J.-B., Serreze, D.V., DeLarto, N.H., Wicker, L.S., Peterson, L.B., Shork, N., Todd, J.A., and Leiter, E.H., Crosses of NOD mice with the related NON strain: a polygenic model for Type I diabetes. *Diabetes* 44, 1186, 1995.

91. Vyse, T.J. and Todd, J.A., Genetic analysis of autoimmune disease. *Cell* 85, 311, 1996.

92. Wicker, L.S., Todd, J.A., and Peterson, L.B., Genetic control of autoimmune diabetes in the NOD mouse. *Annu. Rev. Immunol.* 13, 179, 1995.

93. Wakeland, E., Morel, L., Achey, K., Yui, M., and Longmate, J., Speed congenics: a classic technique in the fast lane (relatively speaking). *Immunol. Today* 18, 472, 1997.

94. Ghosh, S., Palmer, S.M., Rodrigues, N.R., Cordell, H.J., Hearne, C.M., Cornall, R.J., Prins, J.-B., McShane, P., Lathrop, G.M., Peterson, L.B., Wicker, L.S., and Todd, J.A., Polygenic control of autoimmune diabetes in nonobese diabetic mice. *Nature Genet.* 4, 404, 1993.

95. Hattori, M., Yamato, E., Matsumoto, E., Itoh, N., Toyonaga, T., Petruzzelli, M., Fukuda, M., Kobayashi, M., and Chapman, V., Occurrence of preType I diabetes (pre-IDDM) and Type II diabetes (NIDDM) in BC1 [(NOD × *Mus spretus*)F1 × NOD] mice. In *Lessons from Animal Diabetes*, VI, Shafrir, E., Ed, Birkhaüser, Boston, 1996, 83.

96. Todd, J.A., Aitman, T.J., Cornall, R.J., Ghosh, S., Hall, J.R.S., Hearne, C.M., Knight, A.M., Love, J.M., McAleer, M.A., Prins, J.-B., Rodrigues, N., Lathrop, M., Pressey, A., DeLarato, N.H., Peterson, L.B., and Wicker, L.S., Genetic analysis of autoimmune type 1 diabetes mellitus in mice. *Nature* 351, 542, 1991.

97. Denny, P., Lord, C.J., Levy, E.R., Wicker, L.S., Hill, N.J., Podolin, P.L., Todd, J.A., Goy, J.V., Peterson, L.B., and Lyons, P.A., Mapping of the IDDM locus *Idd3* to a 0.35 cM interval containing the Interleukin-2 gene. *Diabetes* 46, 695, 1997.

98. Serreze, D.V., Bridgett, M.B., Chapman, H.D., Chen, E., Richard, S.B., and Leiter, E.H., Sub-congenic analysis of the *Idd13* locus in NOD/Lt mice: evidence for several susceptibility genes including a possible diabetogenic role for β2-microglobulin. *J. Immunol.* 160, 1472, 1998.

99. Atkinson, M.A., NOD mice as a model for therapeutic interventions in human insulin dependent diabetes mellitus. In *NOD Mice and Related Strains: Research Applications in Diabetes, AIDS, Cancer, and Other Diseases*, Leiter, E.H., and Atkinson, M.A., Eds., R.G. Landes, Austin, 1998, 145.

100. Leiter, E.H., The role of environmental factors in modulating insulin dependent diabetes. In *Current Topics in Immunology and Microbiology. The Role of Microorganisms in Non-infectious Disease*. de Vries, R., Cohen, I., and van Rood, J., Eds., Springer Verlag, Berlin, 1990, 39.

101. Leiter, E.H., The nonobese diabetic mouse: a model for analyzing the interplay between heredity and environment in development of autoimmune disease. *ILAR News* 35, 4, 1993.

102. Oldstone, M.B.A., Prevention of type 1 diabetes in nonobese diabetic mice by virus infection. *Science* 23, 500, 1988.

103. Hermite, L., Vialettes, B., Naquet, P., Atlan, C., Payan, M.-J., and Vague, P., Paradoxical lessening of autoimmune processes in non-obese diabetic mice after infection with the diabetogenic variant of encephalomyocarditis virus. *Eur. J. Immunol.* 20, 1297, 1990.

104. Coleman, D.L., Kuzava, J.E., and Leiter, E.H., Effect of diet on the incidence of diabetes in non-obese diabetic (NOD) mice. *Diabetes* 39, 432, 1990.

105. Guberski, D., Thomas, V., Shek, W., Like, A., Handler, E., Rossini, A., Wallace, J., and Welsh, R., Induction of Type I diabetes by Kilham's rat virus in diabetes-resistant BB/Wor rats. *Science* 254, 1010, 1991.

106. Wilson, G.L. and Leiter, E.H., Streptozotocin interactions with pancreatic β cells and the induction of insulin dependent diabetes. In *Current Topics in Microbiology and Immunobiology* Dyrberg, T., Ed, Springer Verlag, Berlin, 1990, 27.

107. Okamoto, H., Takasawa, S., and Tohgo, A., New aspects of the physiological significance of NAD, poly ADP-ribose and cyclic ADP-ribose. *Biochimie* 77, 356, 1995.

108. Heller, B., Wang, Z.Q., Wagner, E.F., Radons, J., Burkle, A., Fehsel, K., Burkart, V., and Kolb, H., Inactivation of the poly(ADP-ribose) polymerase gene affects oxygen radical and nitric oxide toxicity in islet cells. *J Biol Chem* 270, 11176, 1995.

109. Like, A.A. and Rossini, A.A., Streptozotocin-induced pancreatic insulitis: new model of diabetes mellitus. *Science* 193, 415, 1976.

110. Leiter, E.H., Analysis of differential survival of syngeneic islets transplanted into hyperglycemic C57BL/KsJ vs. C57BL/6J mice. *Transplantation* 44, 401, 1987.

111. Weide, L.G. and Lacy, P.E., Low-dose streptozotocin-induced autoimmune diabetes in islet transplantation model. *Diabetes* 40, 1157, 1991.

112. Prowse, S.J., Steele, E.J., and Lafferty, K.J., Islet allografting without immunosuppression: reversal of insulitis-associated diabetes and a case of spontaneous juvenile onset diabetes in mice. *Aust.J. Exp. Biol. Med. Sci.* 60, 619, 1982.

113. Wang, Z. and Gleichmann, H., GLUT2 in pancreatic islets: crucial target molecule in diabetes induced with multiple low doses of streptozotocin in mice. *Diabetes* 47, 50, 1998.

114. Bonnevie-Nielsen, V., Steffes, M.W., and Lernmark, Å., A major loss in islet mass and B-cell function precedes hyperglycemia in mice given multiple low doses of streptozotocin. *Diabetes* 30, 424, 1981.

115. O'Brien, B.A., Harmon, B.V., Cameron, D.P., and Allan, D.J., Beta-cell apoptosis is responsible for the development of IDDM in the multiple low-dose streptozotocin model. *J. Pathol.* 178, 176, 1996.

116. Like, A.A., Appel, M.C., Williams, R.M., and Rossini, A.A., Streptozotocin-induced pancreatic insulitis in mice. *Lab. Invest.* 38, 470, 1978.

117. Appel, M.C., Rossini, A.A., Williams, R.M., and Like, A.A., Viral studies in streptozotocin-induced pancreatic insulitis. *Diabetologia* 15, 327, 1978.

118. Cossel, L., Schneider, E., Kuttler, B., Schmidt, S., Wohlrab, F., Schade, J., and Bochmann, C., Low dose streptozotocin induced diabetes in mice. *Exp Clin Endocrinol.* 85, 7, 1985.

119. Bonner-Weir, S., The microvasculature of the pancreas, with emphasis on that of the islets of Langerhans. In *The Pancreas: Biology, Pathobiology, and Disease*, Go, V.L.W., Ed., Raven Press, New York, 1993, 759.

120. Saini, K.S., Thompson, C., Winterford, C.M., Walker, N.I., and Cameron, D.P., Streptozotocin at low doses induces apoptosis and at high doses causes necrosis in a murine pancreatic beta cell line, INS-1. *Biochem. Mol. Biol. Int.* 39, 1229, 1996.

121. Kolb, H. and Kroncke, K.-D., IDDM. Lessons from the low-dose streptozotocin model in mice. *Diabetes Rev.* 1, 116, 1993.

122. Elias, D., Meilin, A., Ablamuni, V., Birk, O.S., Carmi, P., Konenwai, S., and Cohen, I.R., HSP60 peptide therapy of NOD mouse diabetes induces a TH2 cytokine burst and downregulates autoimmunity to various beta-cell antigens. *Diabetes* 46, 758, 1997.

123. Leiter, E.H. and Hamaguchi, K., Viruses and diabetes: diabetogenic role for endogenous retroviruses in NOD mice? *J. Autoimmunity* 3 (Suppl), 31, 1990.

124. Nakamura, M., Nagafuchi, S., Yamaguchi, K., and Takaki, R., The role of thymic immunity and insulitis in the development of streptozocin-induced diabetes in mice. *Diabetes* 33, 894, 1984.

125. Huang, X.J., Hultgren, B., Dybdal, N., and Stewart, T.A., Islet expression of interferon-alpha precedes diabetes in both the BB rat and streptozotocin-treated mice. *Immunity* 1, 469, 1994.

126. Iwakiri, R., Nagafuchi, S., Kounoue, E., Nakamura, M., Kikuchi, M., Nakano, S., and Niho, Y., Immunohistochemical study of insulitis induced by multiple low does of streptozocin in CD-1 mice. *Diabetes Res. Clin. Pract.* 9, 75, 1990.

127. Reddy, S., Wu, D., and Poole, C.A., Glutamic acid decarboxylase 65 and 67 isoforms in fetal, neonatal and adult porcine islets: predominant beta cell co-localization by light and confocal microscopy. *J. Autoimmunity* 9, 21, 1996.

128. Reddy, S., Wu, D., and Elliott, R.B., Low dose streptozotocin causes diabetes in severe combined immunodeficient (scid) mice without immune cell infiltration of the pancreatic islets. *Autoimmunity* 20, 83, 1995.

129. Itoh, M., Funauchi, M., Sato, K., Fukuma, N., Hirooka, Y., and Nihei, N., Abnormal lymphocyte function precedes hyperglyceemia in mice treated with multiple low doses of streptozotocin. *Diabetologia* 27, 109, 1984.

130. Yanagawa, T., Maruyama, T., Takei, I., Asaba, Y., Takahashi, T., Ishi, T., Kataoka, K., Saruta, T., Minoshima, S., and Shimizu, N., The suppressive effect of cyclophosphamide on low-dose streptozotocin-induced diabetes in mice. *Diabetes Res.* 12, 79, 1989.

131. Harada, M. and Makino, S., Promotion of spontaneous diabetes in non-obese diabetes-prone mice with cyclophosphamide. *Diabetologia* 27, 604, 1984.

132. Leiter, E., Multiple low dose streptozotocin-induced hyperglycemia and insulitis in C57BL mice: influence of inbred background, sex, and thymus. *Proc. Natl. Acad. Sci. U.S.A.*, 79, 630, 1982.

133. Leiter, E.H., Beamer, W.G., and Shultz, L.D., The effect of immunosuppression on streptozotocin-induced diabetes in C57BL/KsJ mice. *Diabetes* 32, 148, 1983.

134. Dayer-Metroz, M.-D., Kimoto, M., Izui, S., Vassalli, P., and Renold, A.E., Effect of helper and/or cytotoxic T-lymphocyte depletion on low-dose streptozotocin-induced diabetes in C57BL/6J mice. *Diabetes* 37, 1082, 1988.

135. Herold, K.C., Montag, A.G., and Buckingham, F., Induction of tolerance to autoimmune diabetes with islet antigens. *J. Exp. Med.* 176, 1107, 1992.

136. Baumann, E.E., Buckingham, F., and Herold, K.C., Development of tolerance to autoimmune diabetes following intrathymic islet transplantation involves CD8+ diabertogenic T-cells. *Pediat. Res.* 37, 85, 1995.

137. Baumann, E.E., Buckingham, F., and Herold, K.C., Intrathymic transplantation of islet antigen affects CD8+ diabetogenic T-cells resulting in tolerance to autoimmune IDDM. *Diabetes* 44, 871, 1995.

138. Klinkhammer, C., Popowa, P., and Gleichmann, H., Specific immunity to streptozocin: cellular requirements for induction of lymphoproliferation. *Diabetes* 37, 74, 1988.

139. Wong, S., Guerder, S., Visintin, I., Reich, E.P., Swenson, K.E., Flavell, R.A., and Janeway, C.A., Expression of the co-stimulator molecule B7-1 in pancreatic beta-cells accelerates diabetes in the NOD mouse. *Diabetes* 44, 326, 1995.

140. Harlan, D.M., Barnett, M.A., Abe, R., Pechhold, K., Patterson, N.B., Gray, G.S., and June, C.H., Very-low-dose streptozotocin induces diabetes in insulin promoter-mB7-1 transgenic mice. *Diabetes* 44, 816, 1995.

141. Ihm, S.H., Lee, K.U., McArthur, R.G., and Yoon, J.-W., Predisposing effect of anti-beta cell autoimmune process in NOD mice on the induction of diabetes by environmental insults. *Diabetologia* 33, 709, 1990.

142. McInerney, M.F., Pek, S.B., and Thomas, D.W., Prevention of insulitis and diabetes onset by treatment with complete Freund's adjuvant in NOD mice. *Diabetes* 40, 715, 1991.

143. Richens, E.R. and Behbehani, K., The effect of adjuvants on immune function in the multi-low dose streptozotocin model of murine diabetes. *Int. J. Tissue Reac.* 4, 207, 1988.

144. Kohnert, K.-D., Ziegler, B., Fält, K., and Ziegler, M., Augmentation of steptozotocin-induced hyperglycemia in mice by prior treatment with complete Freund's adjuvant. *Int. J. Pancreatol.* 4, 321, 1989.

145. Matkovic, V., Apseloff, G., Shepard, D.R., and Gerber, N., Use of gallium to treat Paget's disease of bone: a pilot study. *Lancet* 335, 72, 1990.

146. Whitacre, C., Apseloff, G., Cox, K., Matkovic, V., Jewell, S., and Gerber, N., Suppression of experimental autoimmune encephalomyelitis by gallium nitrate. *J. Neuroimmunol.* 39, 175, 1992.

147. Chitambar, R.C., Seigneuret, M.C., Matthaeus, W.G., and Lum, L.G., Modulation of lymphocyte proliferation and immunoglobulin production by transferrin-gallium. *Cancer Res.* 49, 1125, 1989.

148. Chitamber, C.R., Craig, A., and Ash, R.C., Transferrin receptor-mediated suppression of *in vitro* hematopoiesis by transferrin-gallium. *Exp. Hematol.* 17, 418, 1989.

149. Lenz, S.P., Pak, C., and Hart, D.A., Low-dose LICL treatment enhances survival and inhibits pancreatic beta-cell destruction in the NOD model and type-I diabetes. *Lithium* 5, 139, 1994.

150. Oschilewski, M., Schwab, E., Kiesel, U., Opitz, U., Stunkel, K., Kolb-Bachofen, V., and Kolb, H., Administration of silica or monoclonal antibody to Thy-1 prevents low-dose streptozotocin-induced diabetes in mice. *Immunol. Lett.* 12, 289, 1986.

151. Leiter, E.H., Murine macrophages and pancreatic β cells. Chemotactic properties of insulin and β-cytostatic action of interleukin 1. *J. Exp. Med.* 166, 1174, 1987.

152. Kroncke, K.D., Funda, J., Berschick, B., Kolb, H., and Kolb Bachofen, V., Macrophage cytotoxicity towards isolated rat islet cells: neither lysis nor its protection by nicotinamide are beta-cell specific. *Diabetologia* 34, 232, 1991.

153. Kröncke, K.-D., Kolb-Bachofen, V., Berschick, B., Burkart, V., and Kolb, H., Activated macrophages kill pancreatic syngeneic islet cells via arginine-dependent nitric oxide generation. *Biochem. Biophys. Res. Commun.* 175, 752, 1991.

154. Rabinovitch, A., Suarez, W.L., Thomas, P.D., Strynadka, K., and Simpson, I., Cytotoxic effects of cytokines on rat islets: evidence for involvement of free radicals and lipid peroxidation. *Diabetologia* 35, 409, 1992.

155. Rossini, A.A., Appel, M.C., Williams, R.M., and Like, A.A., Genetic influence of the streptozotocin-induced insulitis and hyperglycemia. *Diabetes* 26, 916, 1977.

156. Rossini, A.A., Williams, R.M., Appel, M.C., and Like, A.A., Sex differences in the multiple-dose streptozotocin model of diabetes. *Endocrinology* 103, 1518, 1978.

157. Paik, S.-G., Michelis, M.A., Kim, Y.T., and Shin, S., Induction of insulin dependent diabetes by streptozotocin: inhibition by estrogens and potentiation by androgens. *Diabetes* 31, 724, 1982.

158. Maclaren, N.K., Neufeld, M., McLaughlin, J.V., and Taylor, G., Androgen sensitization of streptozotocin-induced diabetes in mice. *Diabetes* 29, 710, 1980.

159. Kromann, H., Christy, M., Egeberg, J., Lernmark, A., and Nerup, J., Absence of H-2 genetic influence on streptozotocin-induced diabetes in mice. *Diabetologia* 23, 114, 1982.

160. Kiesel, U., Falkenberg, F.W., and Kolb, H., Genetic control of low-dose streptozotocin-induced autoimmune diabetes in mice. *J. Immunol.* 130, 1719, 1983.

161. Wolf, J., Lilly, F., and Shin, S., The influence of genetic background on the susceptibility of inbred mice to streptozotocin-induced diabetes. *Diabetes* 33, 567, 1984.

162. Le, P.H., Leiter, E.H., and Leydendecker, J.R., Genetic control of susceptibility to streptozotocin diabetes in inbred mice: effect of testosterone and H-2 haplotype. *Endocrinology* 116, 2450, 1985.

163. Leiter, E.H., Le, P.H., and Coleman, D.L., Susceptibility to *db* gene and streptozotocin-induced diabetes in C57BL mice: control by gender-associated, MHC-unlinked traits. *Immunogenetics* 26, 6, 1987.

164. Yoon, J.-W. and Ray, U.R., Perspectives on the role of viruses in insulin-dependent diabetes. *Diabetes Care* 8, 39, 1986.

165. Gaskins, H.R., Prochazka, M., Hamaguchi, K., Serreze, D.V., and Leiter, E.H., Beta cell expression of endogenous xenotropic retrovirus distinguishes diabetes susceptible NOD/Lt from resistant NON/Lt mice. *J. Clin. Invest.* 90, 2220, 1992.
166. Naggert, J.K., Mu, M.-L., Frankel, W.F., and Paigen, B., Genomic analysis of the C57BL/Ks mouse strain. *Mamm. Genome.* 6, 131, 1995.
167. Leiter, E.H. and Wilson, G.L., Viral interactions with pancreatic β cells. In *The Pathology of the Endocrine Pancreas in Diabetes*. Lefebvre, P.J. and Pipeleers, D., Eds, Springer Verlag, Berlin, 1988, 85.
168. Conrad, B., Weidmann, E., Trucco, G., Rudert, W.A., Behboo, R., Ricordi, C., Rodriquezrilo, H., Finegold, D., and Trucco, M., Evidence for superantigen involvement in insulin-dependent diabetes mellitus aetiology. *Nature* 371, 351, 1994.
169. Rerup, C.C., Drugs producing diabetes through damage of the insulin secreting cells. *Pharmacol. Rev.* 22, 485, 1970.
170. Malaisse, W.J., Malaisse Lagae, F., Sener, A., and Pipeleers, D.G., Determinants of the selective toxicity of alloxan to the pancreatic B cell. *Proc. Natl. Acad. Sci. U.S.A.*, 79, 927, 1982.
171. Waguri, M., Yamamoto, K., Yamamori, K., Watada, H., Miyagawa, J.I., Kajimoto, Y., Yoshiuchi, I., Tochino, Y., Nakajima, H., and Itoh, N., Demonstration of two different processes of beta-cell regeneration in a new diabetic mouse model induced by selective perfusion of alloxan. *Diabetes* 46, 1281, 1997.
172. Washburn, M.P. and Wells, W.W., Glutathione-dependent reduction of alloxan to dialuric acid-catalyzed by thioltransferase (Glutaredoxin) — a possible role for thioltransferase in alloxan toxicity. *Free Radical Biol.* 23, 563, 1997.
173. Lenzen, S. and Panten, U., Alloxan: history and mechanism of action. *Diabetologia* 31, 337, 1988.
174. Jansson, L. and Sandler, S., Alloxan-induced diabetes in the mouse: time course of pancreatic B-cell destruction as reflected in an increased islet vascular permeability. *Virchows Arch. A Pathol. Anat. Histopathol.* 410, 17, 1986.
175. Jörns, A., Munday, R., Tiedge, M., and Lenzen, S., Comparative toxicity of alloxan, N-alkyla-lloxans and ninhydrin to isolated pancreatic islets *in vitro. J. Endocrinol.* 155, 283, 1997.
176. Yamamoto, H., Uchigata, Y., and Okamoto, H., Streptozotocin and alloxan induce DNA strand breaks and poly(ADP-ribose) synthetase in pancreatic islets. *Nature* 294, 284, 1981.
177. Sandler, S. and Swenne, I., Streptozotocin, but not alloxan, induces DNA repair synthesis in mouse pancreatic islets *in vitro. Diabetologia* 25, 444, 1983.
178. Weaver, D.C., McDaniel, M.L., and Lacy, P.E., Alloxan uptake by isolated rat islets of Langerhans. *Endocrinology* 102, 1847, 1978.
179. Ino, T. and Yoshikawa, S., Alloxan diabetes in different strains of mice. *Exp. Anim.* 15, 97, 1966.
180. Cohn, J.A. and Cerami, A., The influence of genetic background on the susceptibility of mice to diabetes induced by alloxan and on recovery from alloxan diabetes. *Diabetologia* 17, 187, 1979.
181. Martinez, C., Grande, F., and Bittner, J.J., Alloxan diabetes in different strains of mice. *Proc. Soc. Exp. Biol. Med.* 87, 236, 1954.
182. Swenson, F.J., Martinez, C., and Lazarow, A., Blood glutathione and alloxan susceptibility in inbred mice. *Proc. Soc. Exp. Biol. Med.* 100, 6, 1959.
183. Ino, T., Kawamoto, Y., Sato, K., Nishikawa, K., Yamada, A., Ishibashi, K., and Sekiguchi, F., Selection of mouse strains showing high and low incidences of alloxan-induced diabetes. *Exp. Anim.* 40, 61, 1991.
184. Grankvist, K., Marklund, S.L., and Täljedal, I.-B., CuZn-superoxide dismutase, Mn-superoxide dismutase, catalase, and gluthathione peroxidase in pancreatic islets and other tissues in the mouse. *Biochem. J.* 199, 393, 1981.
185. Lenzen, S., Drinkgern, J., and Tiedge, M., Low antioxidant enzyme gene expression in pancreatic islets compared with various other mouse tissues *Free Radical Biol. Med.* 20, 463, 1996.
186. Welsh, N., Margulis, B., Borg, L.A., Wiklund, H.J., Saldeen, J., Flodstrom, M., Mello, M.A., Andersson, A., Pipeleers, D.G., and Hellerstrom, C., Differences in the expression of heat-shock proteins and antioxidant enzymes between human and rodent pancreatic islets: implications for the pathogenesis of insulin-dependent diabetes mellitus. *Mol. Med.* 1, 806, 1995.
187. Papaccio, G., Franscatore, S., Pisanti, F., Latronico, M., and Linn, T., Superoxide dismutase in the nonobese diabetic (NOD) mouse: a dynamic time-course study. *Life Sci.* 56, 2223, 1995.

188. Cornelius, I.G., Luttge, B.G., and Peck, A.B., Anti-oxidant enzyme activities in IDD prone and IDD resistant mice: a comparative study. *Free Radical Biol. Med.* 14, 409, 1993.

189. Eizirik, D.L., Beta-cell defence and repair mechanisms in human pancreatic islets. *Horm. Metab. Res.* 28, 302, 1996.

190. Rabinovitch, A., Suarez-Pinzon, W.L., Strynadka, K., Schulz, R., Lakey, J.R.T., Warnock, G.L., and Rajotte, R.V., Human pancreatic islet beta-cell destruction by cytokines is independent of nitric oxide production. *J. Clin. Endocrinol. Metab.* 79, 1058, 1994.

191. Eizirik, D.L., Pipeleers, D.G., Ling, Z., Welsh, N., Hellerstrom, C., and Andersson, A., Major species differences between humans and rodents in the susceptibility to pancreatic beta-cell injury. *Proc. Natl. Acad. Sci. U.S.A.*, 91, 9253, 1994.

192 Corbett, J.A., Sweetland, M.A., Wang, J.L., Lancaster, J.R., Jr., and McDaniel, M.L., Nitric oxide mediates cytokine-induced inhibition of insulin secretion by human islets of Langerhans. *Proc. Natl. Acad. Sci. U.S.A.* 90, 1731, 1993.

193. Sekiguchi, F., Ishibashi, K., Katoh, H., Kawamoto, Y., and Ino, T., Genetic profile of alloxan-induced diabetes-susceptible mice (ALS) and resistant mice (ALR). *Exp. Anim.* 39, 269, 1990.

194. Kubisch, H.M., Wang, J.Q., Luche, R., Carlson, E., Bray, T.M., Epstein, C.J., and Phillips, J.P., Transgenic copper/zinc superoxide dismutase modulates susceptibility to Type I diabetes. *Proc. Natl. Acad. Sci. U.S.A.*, 91, 9956, 1994.

195. Kubisch, H., Wang, J., Bray, T., and Phillips, J., Targeted overexpression of Cu/Zn superoxide dismutase protects pancreatic β-cells against oxidative stress. *Diabetes* 46, 1563, 1997.

196. Yoon, J.-W., Role of viruses in the pathogenesis of IDDM. *Ann. Med.* 23, 437, 1991.

197. Ramsingh, A.I., Chapman, N., and Tracy, S., Coxsackieviruses and Diabetes (Review) *Bioessays* 19, 793, 1997.

198. Rewers, M. and Atkinson, M., The possible role of enteroviruses in diabetes mellitus. In *Human Enterovirus Infections*, Rotbart, H.A., Ed, *Amer. Soc. Microbiol.*, Washington, D.C., 1995, 353.

199. Graves, P.M., Norris, J.M., Pallansch, M.A., Gerling, I.C., and Rewers, M., The role of enteroviral infections in the development of IDDM — limitations of current approaches. *Diabetes* 46, 161, 1997.

200. Yoon, J.-W., Austin, M., Onodera, T., and Notkins, A.L., Virus-induced diabetes mellitus: isolation of a virus from the pancreas of a child with diabetic ketoacidosis. *N. Engl. J. Med.* 300, 1173, 1979.

201. Onodera, T., Jenson, A.B., Yoon, J.-W., and Notkins, A.L., Virus-induced diabetes mellitus: reovirus infection of pancreatic β-cells in mice. *Science* 201, 529, 1978.

202. Giron, D.J. and Patterson, R.R., Effects of steroid hormones on virus-induced diabetes mellitus. *Infect. Immun.* 37, 820, 1982.

203. Gaines, K.L., Kayes, S.G., and Wilson, G.L., Altered pathogenesis in encephalomyocarditis virus (D variant)-infected diabetes-susceptible and resistant strains of mice. *Diabetologia* 29, 313, 1986.

204. Huber, S.A., VCAM-1 is a receptor for encephalomyocarditis virus on murine vascular endothelial cells. *J. Virol.* 68, 3453, 1994.

205. Wilson, G.L., D'Andrea, B.J., Bellomo, S.C., and Craighead, J.E., Encephalomyocarditis virus infection of cultured murine pancreatic β-cells. *Nature* 285, 112, 1980.

206. Jordan, G.W. and Cohen, S.W., Encephalomyocarditis virus-induced diabetes mellitus in mice: model of viral pathogenesis. *Rev. Infect. Dis.* 9, 917, 1987.

207. Giron, D.J., Cohen, S.J., Lyons, S.P., Wahrton, C.H., and Cerutis, D.R., Inhibition of virus-induced diabetes mellitus by interferon is influenced by the host strain. *Proc. Soc. Exp. Biol. Med.* 173, 328, 1983.

208. Huber, S.A., Babu, P.G., and Craighead, J.E., Genetic influences on the immunologic pathogenesis of encephalomyocarditis (EMC) virus-induced diabetes mellitus. *Diabetes* 34, 1186, 1985.

209. Babu, P.G., Huber, S.A., and Craighead, J.E., Contrasting features of T-lymphocyte-mediated diabetes in encephalomyocarditis virus-infected Balb/cBy and Balb/cCum mice. *Am. J. Pathol.* 124, 193, 1986.

210. Gould, C.L., McMannama, K.G., Bigley, N.J., and Giron, D.J., Exacerbation of the pathogenesis of the diabetogenic variant of encephalomyocarditis virus in mice by interferon. *J. Interferon Res.* 5, 33, 1985.
211. Foulis, A.K., The pathology of the endocrine pancreas in type 1 (insulin-dependent) diabetes mellitus. *APMIS* 104, 161, 1996.
212. Toniolo, A., Onodera, T., Yoon, J.-W., and Notkins, A.L., Induction of diabetes by cumulative environmental insults from viruses and chemicals. *Nature* 288, 383, 1980.
213. Schwimmbeck, P.L., Dyrberg, T., and Oldstone, M.B.A., Abrogation of diabetes in BB rats by acute virus infection. *J. Immunol.* 140, 3394, 1988.
214. Brown, D.W., Welsh, R.M., and Like, A.A., Infection of peripancreatic lymph nodes but not islets precedes Kilham rat virus-induced diabetes in BB/Wor rats. *J. Virol.* 67, 5873, 1993.
215. Chung, Y.H., Jun, H.S., Kang, Y., Hirasawa, K., Lee, B.R., Vanrooij, N., and Yoon, J.-W., Role of macrophages and macrophage-derived cytokines in the pathogenesis of Kilham rat virus-induced autoimmune diabetes in diabetes-resistant biobreeding rats. *J. Immunol.* 159, 466, 1997.
216. Hirasawa, K., Tsutsui, S., Takeda, M., Mizutani, M., Itagaki, S., and Doi, K., Depletion of Mac1-positive macrophages protects DBA/2 mice from encephalomyocarditis virus-induced myocarditis and diabetes. *J. Gen. Virol.* 77, 737, 1996.
217. Chatterjee, N.K., Hou, J., Dockstader, P., and Charbonneau, T., Coxsackievirus B4 infection alters thymic, splenic, and peripheral lymphocyte repertoire preceding onset of hyperglycemia in mice. *J. Med. Virol.* 38, 124, 1992.
218. Palmer, J.P., Ed., Prediction, Prevention and Genetic Counseling in IDDM. John Wiley, New York, 1995.
219. Kim, J., Richter, W., Aanstoot, H.-J., Shi, Y., Fu, Q., Rajotte, R., Warnock, G., and Baekkeskov, S., Differential expression of GAD65 and GAD67 in human, rat, and mouse pancreatic islets. *Diabetes* 42, 1799, 1993.
220. Saravia-Fernandez, R., Faveeuw, C., Blasquez-Bulant, C., Tappaz, M., Throsby, M., Pelletier, G., Vaudry, H., Dardenne, M., and Homo-Delarche, F., Localization of γ-aminobutyric acid and glutamic acid decarboxylase in the pancrease of the nonobese diabetic mouse. *Endocrinology* 137, 3497, 1996.
221. Bridgett, M.M., Cetkovic-Cvrlje, M., Narayanswami, S., Lambert, J., O'Rourke, R., Shi, Y., Baekkeskov, S., Ramiya, V., and Leiter, E.H., Differential protection in two transgenic lines of NOD/Lt mice hyperexpressing the autoantigen GAD65 in pancreatic beta cells. *Diabetes*, 47, 1848, 1998.
222. Kaufman, D.L., Erlander, M.G., Clare-Salzler, M., Atkinson, M.A., Maclaren, N.K., and Tobin, A.J., Autoimmunity to two forms of glutamate decarboxylase in insulin-dependent diabetes mellitus. *J. Clin. Invest.* 89, 283, 1992.
223. Tian, J., Atkinson, M.A., Clare-Salzler, M., Herschenfeld, A., Forsthuber, T., Lehmann, P.V., and Kaufman, D.L., Nasal administration of glutamate decarboxylase (GAD65) peptides induces Th2 responses and prevents murine insulin-dependent diabetes. *J. Exp. Med.* 183, 1561, 1996.
224. Gerling, I.C., Atkinson, M.A., and Leiter, E.H., The thymus as a site for evaluating the potency of candidate β cell autoantigens in NOD mice. *J. Autoimmunity* 7, 851, 1994.
225. Tian, J., Lehmann, P.V., and Kaufman, D.L., T cell cross-reactivity between Coxsackie and glutamate decarboxylase is associated with a murine diabetes susceptibility allele. *J. Exp. Med.* 180, 1979, 1994.
226. Chao, C.C. and McDevitt, H.O., Identification of immunogenic epitopes of GAD-65 presented by A^{g7} in nonobese diabetic mice. *Immunogeneties* 46, 29, 1997.
227. Gerling, I. and Chatterjee, N.K., Autoanigen (64000-M$_r$) expression in Coxsackievirus B4-induced experimental diabetes. In *Current Topics in Microbiology and Immunology: The Role of Viruses and the Immune System in Diabetes Mellitus,* Vol. 156, Dyrberg, T., Ed., Springer-Verlag, Berlin, 1990, 55.
228. Gerling, I.C., Chatterjee, N.K., and Nejman, C., Coxsackie B4-induced development of autoantibodies to 64,000 Mr autoantigen and hyprglycemia in mice. *Autoimmunity* 10, 49, 1991.
229. Chatterjee, N.K., and Nejman, C., Insulin mRNA content in pancreatic beta cells of Coxsackie B4-induced diabetic mice. *Mol. Cell. Endocrinol.* 55, 193, 1988.

230. Suenaga, K. and Yoon, J.-W., Association of β-cell-specific expression of endogenous retrovirus with development of insulitis and diabetes in NOD mouse. *Diabetes* 37, 1722, 1988.
231. Hamaguchi, K., Gaskins, H.R., and Leiter, E.H., NIT-1, a pancreatic β cell line established from a transgenic NOD/Lt mouse. *Diabetes* 40, 842, 1991.
232. Conrad, B., Weissmah, R.N., Schuppac, J., Boni, J., Mach, B., and Arcari, R., A human endogenous retroviral superantigen as candidate autoimmune gene in type 1 diabetes. *Cell* 90, 303, 1997.
233. Conrad, B. and Trucco, M., Superantigens as etiopathogenetic factors in the development of insulin-dependent diabetes mellitus. *Diabetes Metab. Rev.* 10, 309, 1994.
234. Signore, A., Procaccini, E., Chianelli, M., and Pozzilli, P., Retroviruses and diabetes in animal models: hypotheses for the induction of the disease. *Diabete Metab.* 21, 147, 1995.
235. Zunino, S.J., Interleukin-1 promotes hyperglycemia and insulitis in mice normally resistant to streptozotocin-induced diabetes. *Am. J. Pathol.* 145, 661, 1994.
236. Andersson, A., Islet implantation normalizes hyperglycemia caused by streptozotocin-induced insulitis. *Lancet* 1, 581, 1979.
237. Sai, P., Maugendre, D., Loreal, O., Maurel, C., and Pogu, S., Effects of cyclosporin on autoimmune diabetes induced in mice by streptozotocin. *Diabete Metab.* 14, 455, 1988.
238. Stewart, T.A., Hultgren, B., Huang, X., Pitts-Meek, S., Hully, J., and MacLachlan, N.J., Induction of type 1 diabetes by interferon-α in transgenic mice. *Science* 260, 1942, 1993.
239. Leiter, E.H. and Atkinson, M.A., Eds., *NOD Mice and Related Strains: Research Applications in Diabetes, AIDS, Cancer, and Other Diseases*, Molecular Biology Intelligence Unit, R.G. Landes, Austin, 1998.
240. Craighead, J.E., Animal model of human disease. Mice infected with the M variant of encephalomyocarditis virus. *Am. J. Pathol.* 76, 537, 1975.
241. Yoon, J.-W., The role of viruses and environmental factors in the induction of diabetes. In *Current Topics in Microbiology and Immunology* Vol. 164, Dyrberg, T., Ed., Springer-Verlag, Berlin, 1991, 95.
242. Webb, S.R. and Madge, G.E., The role of host genetics in the pathogenesis of Coxsackievirus infection in the pancrease of mice. *J. Infect. Dis.* 141, 47, 1980.

13

The BB Rat: A Unique Model of Human Type I Diabetes

Catherine J. Field and Shannon C. Butler

CONTENTS

The importance of animal models in the study of diabetes is beyond dispute; they have provided an opportunity for detailed study of the multitude of factors contributing to the syndrome of diabetes that is not feasible in the afflicted human. The BB rat is one of two unique rodent models that spontaneously develops insulin-dependent (Type I) diabetes similar to humans. BB rats have been used extensively as a metabolic model of diabetes for clinical study, basic research, and by those interested in the multifactorial etiology and treatment of Type I diabetes. The many homologies with the human disease and some of the unique features of the BB rat will be highlighted in this chapter.

13.1 History

Spontaneous diabetes in the BB Wistar rat was initially diagnosed in 1974 by the Chappel brothers at the BioBreeding Laboratories commercial breeding facility in Ottawa, Ontario, Canada in a noninbred but closed outbred colony of Wistar rats.[1] It was decided to name this syndrome BB after the initials of the breeding laboratory in which they were discovered.[1] The original diabetic progeny were carefully maintained with daily injections of insulin, and a breeding colony of diabetic rats established in 1977 under the management of Pierre Thibert, Director of the Animal Resources Division, Health Protection Branch, Health Canada. BB rats (diabetic prone and control line) from the original Ottawa colony are still available to researchers. All BB rat colonies in existence today are descendants of the original Ottawa colony. BB sublines have been subsequently derived by several laboratories from the original outbred BioBreeding stock, and these lines vary in the frequency and severity of diabetes, likely a reflection of genetic diversity.[2-4] In parallel to the Ottawa colony, a major inbreeding program though the National Institutes of Health was established in 1977 by Dr. A. A. Like and his associates at the University of Massachusetts.[5] The animals in the Worchester colony have now been inbred for many generations in viral/antigen-free conditions becoming a central source of BB rats for many researchers.[5] A nomenclature system exists that identifies the specific pedigree of BB rats available to researchers,[4] and a detailed description of the different strains of BB rats is published.[5,6] The nomenclature indicates the source of BB rats (e.g., BB/Wor to identify rats that originate from the Worchester colony, BB/E from the Edinburgh colony, BB/Ottawa from the Ottawa colony, BB/OK from the Ottawa-Kalsburg colony, etc.). Although there is considerable confusion regarding the nomenclature of BB rats, for the sake of this chapter DR-BB rats will be used to designate diabetes-resistant rats and DP-BB rats to represent diabetes-prone BB rats. If further information on the colony origin is desired, the reader is encouraged to consult the original papers.

13.2 Clinical and Metabolic Presentation

The clinical presentation of diabetes in the BB rat is similar to that of its human counterpart. Marked hyperglycemia, glycosuria, and weight loss occur within a day of onset and are associated with decreased plasma insulin that, untreated, will result in ketoacidosis within several days.[1,7,8] Like the NOD mouse, the BB rat is one of the few rodent models in which significant ketosis occurs in the absence of obesity. Unlike most NOD mouse colonies, both sexes of BB rats are equally affected.[1] BB diabetes appears (first detection of sustained glycosuria) during adolescence/early adulthood which corresponds to 60 to 120 days in the rat.[1,5,7-9] BB diabetic rats experience selective and complete destruction of pancreatic β-cells (islets of Langerhans).[1,10] The pancreas of the afflicted animal has less than 0.1% of normal insulin content, and light microscope examination of the pancreas at the end stage of the disease shows small islets containing virtually no β-cells.[1] The reported diabetes incidence rates (30 to 90%) vary between colonies.[5,11,12] Provision of exogenous insulin will control most of the metabolic derangement that reoccurs if insulin is stopped.[1]

The progression from normal to severely decompensated glucose homeostasis occurs very rapidly, over intervals of hours to a few days.[13] BB diabetic rats will die from severe hyperglycemia (>500 mg/dl) and ketoacidosis within 1 to 2 weeks of onset unless exogenous insulin is provided. There are no clear clinical indexes, such as changes in body weight and food intake,[13] of impending diabetes in DP-BB rats. A short period of glucose intolerance has been reported to occur 2 to 3 days prior to the onset of diabetes, but rats are usually mildly hyperglycemic by the time this is documented.[13,14] The sudden onset of diabetes is followed by rapid "clinical" deterioration with many metabolic abnormalities analogous to those in human diabetes. Despite hyperphagia and polydipsia, weight loss is rapid, continuous, and associated with total depletion of visible fat stores.[8] The lack of insulin results in net total body protein loss,[7] and urea nitrogen excretion doubles with onset of diabetes.[7,8] Decreased physical activity and tachypnea occur in untreated animals. The impact of hypoinsulinemia upon fat metabolism is evident by a rise in plasma free fatty acids, and this augments ketogenesis.[8] If exogenous insulin is not provided, this generalized catabolic state results in death. Spontaneous remission of diabetes after insulin is required is very rare.

The BB rat has been used to elucidate the pathophysiology of the metabolic changes in the diabetic state and has resulted in major insights into the control of insulin synthesis, secretion, and action. Insulin responses to other metabolic perturbants such as arginine remain normal or increased in both prediabetic and newly diabetic rats.[1] By using clamp techniques, insulin sensitivity is reported to be normal during the impaired glucose tolerance period preceding diabetes, but hepatic and peripheral insulin resistance appear at the onset of diabetes.[12] On the first day of diabetes, there is an increased basal hepatic glucose production, which is the consequence of both hypoglycemia and hepatic insulin resistance.[12] However, during hyperinsulinemic clamps, a decreased insulin sensitivity was observed in diabetic rats at both submaximal and maximal insulin concentrations, suggesting that decreased basal insulin concentration may be responsible for the insulin resistance at the onset of diabetes in the BB rat.[12] Hyperglucagonemia[1,13,15] and other endocrine abnormalities characteristic of insulin-dependent diabetes mellitus (IDDM, i.e., decreased growth hormone secretion in response to standard perturbants[16] and elevated plasma concentrations of somatostatin[16,17]) have been described after diabetes develops in BB rats.

13.3 Autoimmune Etiology

Parallels are often drawn between many facets of the etiology of human Type I diabetes and the BB rat model. A number of endogenous and external contributing factors have been identified. Similar endogenous pathological mechanisms have been described for both human and BB rat diabetes. Both forms have been screened for the presence of autoimmune factors or triggers of the disease, by examining humoral and cellular immune constituents. The criteria necessary to establish that a disease is autoimmune in origin include (1) direct proof, such as the transfer of the disease by either pathogenic autoantibodies or autoreactive T cells; (2) indirect evidence based on the development of the autoimmune disease in experimental animals; and (3) circumstantial evidence arising from distinctive clinical clues, such as lymphocytic infiltration of the affected organ, association with other autoimmune diseases, correlation with particular human leukocyte antigen (HLA) haplotypes, or benefit from immunosuppressive therapy.[18] Understanding of the autoimmune process involved in the pathogenesis of Type I diabetes has considerably improved through studies of this unique animal model, which spontaneously develops autoimmune diabetes.

The presence of autoreactive cell populations in the BB rat[19-22] clearly implicates the immune system in the process of β-cell destruction. However, it does not indicate whether the immune system is in any way abnormal or it is just responding to a signal (antigen) that is inappropriately expressed. Below is a brief synopsis of the current understanding of the autoimmune nature of this disease as acquired from studies using the BB rat. Most evidence supports T cells as playing a central role in the pathogenesis of diabetes in the BB rat. A number of molecules — cytokines, nitric oxide — and other immune cells — macrophages, natural killer (NK) cells — that normally interact within T cells are also activated during the attack on the β-cell. Although not yet definitively identified, current evidence suggests that the autoantigen expressed on the pancreas is that of a normal pancreatic protein.

13.3.1 Insulitis

The development of diabetes in the BB rat is associated with an inflammatory lymphocytic infiltration in the islets of Langerhans,[1,14,20,23-27] termed insulitis, similar to that observed in the islets of humans with Type I diabetes.[1,28,29] Because the pancreas is not easily accessible to clinical investigation in humans and most pathological events are not detected until overt diabetes is manifested, most of the current knowledge on the pathogenesis of Type I diabetes has come from animal studies, particularly those in the BB rat. Pronounced insulitis is seen in the BB rat both at the time of and immediately prior to the onset of hyperglycemia.[13,30-32] It has been reported that early in the disease process the islets are enlarged, poorly delineated, and infiltrated with lymphocytes and debris-laden macrophages, progressing to multicellular insulitis at or around the time of clinical onset.[30,33] Histopathological examination of serial pancreatic biopsies suggests that the lesions may actually start as early as 2 to 3 weeks before the clinical onset of overt diabetes.[31,32,34] After the onset of hyperglycemia, the infiltrating cells disappear, leaving end-stage islets devoid of β-cells.[1] Immune destruction is limited to the β-cell, despite infiltrating lymphoid cells throughout the pancreas. The α- and δ-cells and exocrine pancreatic functions are preserved.[1] Additionally, early periductular and infiltrative insulitis, consisting mainly of mononuclear cells, has been reported in DP-BB rats that do not develop diabetes.[5,13,31,32,35]

T cells (both CD4[+] and CD8[+]), β-cells, macrophages, dendritic cells, and NK cells have all been found in human[28,29] and BB rat[1,13,14,20,23-27,31,32] islets at the time of diabetes onset. In the BB rat, macrophages and T cells appear to be present in the initial pancreatic infiltrate, which is then followed by a more-generalized multicellular insulitis.[36] Eosinophils, although frequently the mediators of tissue damage in allergic disease and in parasitic infestations, have not been consistently seen in BB rat islets.[14,37] Participatory roles in the autoimmune etiology have been proposed for each of the immune cell types that infiltrate the pancreas during the immune attack. Like the human disease[26], many of the infiltrating immune cells in the BB rat[38] expressed major histocompatabilty complex (MHC) class II antigens, indicative of an activated state. Immune cells isolated from the pancreas of BB rats have been shown *in vitro* to be much stronger mediators of islet cell destruction *in vitro* than immune cells derived from other sites in the body.[39]

13.3.2 Role of the β-Cell

It is still not definitely decided whether the β-cell is intrinsically abnormal or is an innocent bystander that is destroyed by an abnormal immune system.[40] Most available data suggest that DP-BB rat β-cells are intrinsically normal.[41] The exceptions are discussed below. In humans, aberrant (inappropriate or untimely) expression of class II and hyperexpression of class I antigens are seen on the β-cells in patients with newly diagnosed with diabetes.[26,42,43] This is postulated to result in immunogenic presentation of autoantigens by the β-cell to helper T cells. With the exception of one report of the expression of class II antigens on the surface of BB rat β-cells that were in the process of being destroyed,[44] most studies indicate that BB rat β-cells do not express Ia[+] antigens.[40] However, the hyperexpression of class I antigens has been reported on islets and exocrine cells in diabetic BB rats.[45-47] A venular defect, specific to the pancreas of both DP and DR-BB rats has been described.[48] It has been suggested that the BB rat contains a population of adherent intravascular monocytes that can be induced to cause venular leakage.[5] This defect is observed in other, nondiabetic rat strains and at present its relationship to diabetes pathogenesis is not clear.[5] Despite these observations, the best support for a limited role of abnormal islets comes from transplantation studies. These studies clearly demonstrate that the disease will recur when islets from DR-BB rats are transplanted into BB diabetic rats.[37] This rapid recurrence of diabetes is consistent with what has been observed in humans when a diabetic monozygotic twin receives a pancreas transplant from a nonconcordant nondiabetic sibling.[49]

13.3.2.1 Autoantigens

The presence of autoantibodies directed at a number of self-components has been identified in humans around and after the clinical diagnosis of diabetes.[50] These may be either the instigator of the pancreatic β-cell attack or a secondary symptom of β-cell destruction. In human research, cow's milk[51] and insulin[52] autoantibodies have been found in children with recently diagnosed diabetes at higher levels than in children without diabetes. Commonly speculated autoantigens in the BB rat have included a number of endocrine and pancreatic factors that could be targets or triggers of the autoimmune process (Table 13.1). Islet cell surface antibodies (ICSA) have been reported in the BB rat.[53] These autoantibodies develop in some but perhaps not all DP-BB rats 4 to 8 weeks prior to the onset of overt diabetes.[19] The presence of autoantibodies may vary between genetic strains, and they are not generally found to be an accurate predictor of disease onset.[54] Islet cell cytoplasmic autoantibodies have not been found.[20,21] The presence of autoantibodies to

TABLE 13.1

Characteristics of Autoimmune Diabetes in the DP-BB Rat

β-Cell autoantibodies	Carboxypeptidase H, GAD subunits, ICSA, proinsulin, sulfatide, a 38-kDa β-cell antigen, insulin (controversial)
Autoantibodies to other organs/tissues	Antiendothelial cell, antilymphocyte, antiparietal cell, antismooth muscle, antithymocyte, antithyroglobulin
Cells involved in the etiology	*Primary:* T cells (CD2⁺, CD4⁺, CD8⁺ and RT6⁻), or absence of RT6⁺ T cells *Secondary:* Macrophages, NK cells
Molecules involved in the etiology (from *in vitro* studies)	Destructive (*in vitro*): Th1 cytokines (IL-1, IL-2, TNF-α IFN-γ, IL-12) and nitric oxide Protective (*in vitro*): Th2 cytokines (IL-4, IL-5, IL-10)
Disease accelerators	Poly I:C, cyclophosphamide, diet (nonpurified chow diet, cow's milk protein), viral infection (encephalomycarditis or Coxsackie B virus), cytokines (controversial): IL-1, IL-2
Disease inhibitors	Acivicin, azasparine, CFA, cyclosporine, cyclosporine plus deoxyspergulain, 2' deoxycoformycin, glipizide, insulin, nicotinamide, silica TNF-α Cytotoxic antibodies against: CD2⁺ cells, IFN-γ Early introduction of purified and hydrolyzed casein-based diets Infection with encephalomycarditis virus

Abbreviations used: CFA, complete Freund's adjuvant; GAD, glutamic acid decarboxylase; ICSA, islet cell surface antigens; IL, interleukin; INF, interferon; NK, natural killer cells; Poly I:C polyinosinic polycytidylic acid; TNF, tumor necrosis factor. See text of chapter for appropriate references.

Table adapted from that by Rossini et al. 1995.[22]

insulin in the BB rat remains controversial.[22] Autoantibodies have been detected in BB rats with specificity for a 38-kDa β-cell antigen,[55] glutamic acid decarboxylase (GAD) subunits,[22] carboxypeptidase H,[22] and sulfatide.[56] Furthermore, injecting young DP-BB rats with GAD65 did not alter the incidence of diabetes, suggesting the role of these autoantigens in diabetes may be limited.[57] Other autoreactive T cells have been reported in BB rats, directed to proinsulin.[58] T cells reactive to the cow's milk constituent bovine serum albumin (BSA) have been found in the children with recently diagnosed diabetes.[59] However, injecting BSA into young DP-BB rats did not alter the expression of diabetes.[57] A potentially predictive discovery of autoantibodies directed at T lymphocytes in BB rats was reported,[60] with detectable antibody titers prior to the onset of diabetes.[61] Several nonpancreatic BB autoantibodies have been reported in DP-BB rats, including those reactive to thyroid colloid antigens, smooth muscle, gastric parietal cells, and thymocytes (see Table 13.1).[21] Antiendothelial cell antibodies have been identified early in the disease process in DP-BB rats and in RT6-depleted DR-BB rats.[62] The presence of these autoantibodies early in the disease process and their ability to induce pancreatic vascular leakage suggest that they may participate in diabetes pathogenesis.[62] In conclusion, although there is considerable evidence that autoantigens exist in the BB rat, a clear identification of these and their role in the pathogenesis of diabetes remains to be determined.

13.3.2.2 β-Cell Turnover

Lack of information on the nature of the β-cell target antigen lends support for an interesting hypothesis that suggests that expression of a potential "autoantigen" on DP-BB rat pancreas occur early in life when tolerance to self is being established. The trigger for the immune attack may occur as a result of altered β-cells mass dynamics. The β-cells of the islets of Langerhans, like most other tissues, are dynamic and adaptable to changes in demand for their secretory product, insulin.[63-66] The replication rate of β-cells in the adult rodent pancreas is reported to be about 3% per day,[63,67] however, it has been demonstrated that rodent β-cell mass increases more than tenfold between 10 days and 7 months of age.[68] β-cell mass is regulated by rates of proliferation and differentiation of embryonic ductal precursors (neogenesis) and the process of cell death via apoptosis (programmed cell death) and/or necrosis. Available data suggest that β-cell replicative capacity remains normal even during the immune attack.[69-71] Programmed death or apoptosis is a characteristic of a number of cell populations. The contribution of apoptosis to the dynamics of β-cell mass has only recently been investigated in other models of β-cell metabolism in the rat.[72] Although apoptosis is part of normal pancreatic development, altered cell death could expose the immune system to potential autoantigens present on the dying cells. In support of this theory there is evidence that reductions in β-cell mass may occur before the appearance of insulitis in the BB rat.[73,74] Alternatively, a wave of neogenesis follows a period of increased cell death.[75] The process of increased cell growth/differentiation would increase β-cell metabolism and could potentially alter the expression of antigens on the β-cell surface. There is indirect evidence for altered neogenesis in the BB rat. Chronic prophylactic insulin administration to young DP rats reduces the metabolic demands on the pancreas (therefore neogenesis[63]) and decreases the incidence of diabetes and insulitis in DR-BB rats.[76-80] Additionally, an increased body weight (therefore, increased metabolic demand on the pancreas) in the juvenile period was found to increase the risk of diabetes in the DP-BB rat.[11]

13.3.3   Immune Mediators of β-Cell Destruction

Despite extensive studies in the DP-BB rat, the precise immune mechanisms that initiate, amplify, and mediate β-cell destruction remain unknown. Although strong evidence in the BB rat supports diabetes as a T cell–dependent autoimmune disease, one cannot rule out the involvement of other mononuclear cells in the destruction of pancreatic β-cells. There are considerable data to support many different cell types participating to varying degrees in the attack on the β-cell (see Table 13.1). The definitive manner in which each cell population is involved in pancreatic destruction remains to be determined.

13.3.3.1   T Cells

One of the most important criteria for establishing the existence of an autoimmune disease is the ability to transfer the disease with immune cells into naive recipients. The existence of passive transfer methodology has made a variety of investigations in the BB rat possible that could not be performed in humans. The autoimmune etiology of diabetes in the BB rat has been confirmed by several protocols of adoptive transfer. Diabetes can be transferred to young DP-BB rats by injection of Concanavalin A (Con A)–stimulated splenocytes from newly diagnosed diabetic BB rats.[81-83] With this method, diabetes is induced in 50% of young DP recipient rats at an age (<60 days) when less than 0.5% of the rats would spontaneously develop diabetes. Diabetes can also be adoptively transferred using the same method to histocompatible (RT1ᵘ) non-BB rats if the recipients are first immunosuppressed.[82,84] In a third model of adoptive transfer, insulitis, but not overt diabetes, can be transferred to nude mice using Con A-stimulated diabetic rat splenocytes.[85,86]

  T cells are a major cell population in spleen, and strong evidence points to autoreactive T cells (both CD4⁺ and CD8⁺) being major players in the pathogenesis of diabetes. *In vivo* administration of a cytotoxic T cell antibody (anti-CD2) prevents young DP-BB rats from developing diabetes.[87,88] Although most CD8+ cells in BB rats are largely immature, short-lived, and very few in number,[24,89-92] their role with respect to the autoimmune disease in BB rats cannot be ignored. The removal of CD8+ cells *in vivo* with specific monoclonal antibodies was demonstrated to prevent or significantly reduce the incidence of spontaneous BB diabetes.[87,93,94] CD8+ cells are necessary for the successful transfer of diabetes to DP-BB rats.[95] Both these pieces of evidence suggest that CD8+ cells contain autoreactive properties that are essential for the development of diabetes. BB rats possess functional CD8+ peripheral T cells[96] that fail to express the RT6.1 surface alloantigen.[97,98] This has led to the suggestion that BB rat lacks a suppressor population that prevents autoimmune diabetes from occurring. Likewise, there is considerable evidence to support a role of CD4+ cells in the pathogenesis of BB rat diabetes. Activated CD4+ T lymphocytes from BB rats are particularly effective at transferring diabetes to young DP recipient animals,[99] and depletion of CD4+ T cells prevents diabetes in DP-BB rats.[93] CD4+ cells from DP rats are reported to have a defective expression of the CD45R marker, suggesting that they are immature and possibly autoreactive.[100] Infusing "normal mature" CD4+ (w3/25+) cells from DR rats to young DP-BB rats prevents diabetes.[101] In conclusion, it has been demonstrated that both CD4+ and CD8+ T cells are required for efficient transfer of autoimmunity in the BB rat.[102] It appears that in the BB rat, similar to the NOD mouse,[103,104] the initiation of the immune attack appears to be a T cell–mediated process.

13.3.3.2 *RT6+ T cells*

Decreased levels of peripheral T cells in the DP-BB rat can be accounted for almost exclusively by the absence of T cells that express the surface antigen RT6.[97,98] The RT6 rat alloantigen system was first described in the 1970s[105] and has been used for cell tracing in adoptive transfer experiments and for investigations of T cell development and differentiation.[106] RT6 is a nonglycosylated 21-kDa surface molecule, linked to the cell surface by a glycosylphosphatidlyinositol-linked anchor, that is expressed on mature CD4+ and CD8+ cells in the periphery of the rat.[107-112] The RT6 alloantigen of the rat is expressed on most peripheral T cells but not on thymocytes and thus represents, in this species, a marker for postthymic T lymphocyte maturation.[113,114] Two forms of the molecule are known, RT6.1 and RT6.2, with molecular weights of 25 to 35 and 24 to 26 kDa, respectively.[115] BB rats express the RT6.1 form.[116] In the DR-BB rat and other nondiabetic rat strains, the RT6 differential alloantigen is expressed on approximately 70% of CD8+, approximately 50% of CD4+ peripheral T cells,[108,109,117,118] and is also found on most CD45+ T cells.[112,119] DP rats express about 10% of the RT6 protein present on lymphocytes of DR rats.[107] The expression of RT6 on intraepithelial cells does not differ between DR and DP rats.[112,114] Recently, it was suggested that an RT6 expression defect may also be present in some DR-BB rats by the observation of the expression of a low RT6^{low} phenotype.[120]

There is considerable evidence to demonstrate that a deficiency in peripheral RT6+ T cells is critically important in the susceptibility to diabetes in the BB rat.[121-128] A single transfusion of 50 to 200 × 10^6 normal histocompatible RT6+ T cells from DR-BB rats or other strains to young (<30 days old) DP-BB rats prevents diabetes, provided the graft is accepted.[116,125] These grafted RT6+ DP rats are not only resistant to spontaneous diabetes but also to the adoptive transfer of diabetes with Con A–activated spleen cells from diabetic animals.[125] The most convincing evidence for the importance of RT6+ cells comes from studies depleting DR-BB rats with an antibody against RT6. Immune elimination of RT6+ T lymphocytes from DR-BB/Wor rats by administration of anti-RT6 lymphotoxic antibody at 30 days of age precipitates diabetes within 2 to 4 weeks in 50% of these rats.[126] If the depleting monoclonal antibody is combined with polyinosinic polycytidylic acid (Poly I:C, an inducer of interferons), the proportion of DR-BB rats that develop diabetes can be increased to 90%.[128] In other DR-BB rat colonies and other non-BB MHC congenic rat strains (YOS and LEW rats) depletion of RT6[+] cells results in variable rates of insulitis but fails to induce diabetes.[36,62,106,126,129-131] This suggests that for most DR-BB rats a deficiency of RT6[+] cells alone is not enough to lead to diabetes.

The precise mechanism by which RT6[+] cells suppress autoimmune destruction of β-cells is not known, but evidence suggests that the RT6 antigen exerts a regulatory influence on the rat immune system. The structure and function of the RT6 gene in the DR-BB rat appears to be normal,[107,114] supporting the occurrence of a maturation defect that results in the failure of the DR-BB rat to express RT6.[97,132] RT6[+] cells are expressed on mature T cells,[113,133] and, although RT6 is not expressed in the thymus, all peripheral RT6[+] T cells are believed to be thymus derived.[112] It has been suggested that there is an abnormal maturation of CD4-CD8[+] thymocytes[134] and a failure of these cells to be exported from the thymus and/or to survive and differentiate into RT6[+] T cells in the peripheral lymphoid tissues of the DP-BB rat.[98] There is also evidence supporting abnormal precursor development and differentiation of early T cell progenitor cells in bone marrow.[132]

RT6 may be part of a signaling complex and functions as an accessory molecule, suppressing the autoimmune process via altered T cell function.[113,133,135,136] In DR rats RT6[+] cells have been found to respond to mitogenic and allogenic stimulation and to secrete interleukin 2 (IL-2) *in vitro* and participate *in vivo* in graft vs. host and delayed-type hypersensitivity reactions.[137,138] The functional importance of RT6 is supported by the observation that grafting RT6[+] cells in the DP-BB rat not only prevents diabetes but also restores immune T cell responses.[112] RT6-mediated signaling events may prime T cells to respond to exogenous cytokines, suggesting a possible mechanism by which surface RT6 may influence T cell function.[133] Based on *in vitro* data, RT6[+] cells regulate other effectors, such as NK cells, cytotoxic T cells, and autoreactive antibodies.[116,137] The cytokine profile found in the insulitis in β-cells during disease onset suggests that Th1 lymphocytes predominate over Th2 lymphocytes, and it is proposed that RT6[+] cells regulate autoimmunity by modulating the balance between Th1- and Th2-type cells.[113] The connection between the failure to express RT6 in the BB rat to human diabetes has not yet been made. A human RT6 gene has been described but appears not to be functional.[139]

13.3.3.3 Abnormal T Cell Development

There is considerable evidence that the breakdown in self-tolerance occurs as a result of a defect in T cell development. Autoimmunity can be viewed as unchecked destructive activity of self-reactive clones that escaped elimination or regulation in the thymus. Positive selection of immunocompetent T cells and negative selection (clonal deletion) of autoreactive T cells both occur in the thymus.[140] The escape of T cells from negative selection has been proposed by several groups as a contributor to BB rat autoimmunity.[96,141] A defect in either negative or positive selection in the thymus could potentially result in both the loss of T cells and the release of autoreactive T cells. The thymus of the DP-BB rat appears to be of normal size and histology.[142] The absolute number of thymocytes, their expression of CD4, TCR-αβ, and *in vitro* response to mitogens do not differ between DR and DP rats.[89,134,142,143] However, neonatal thymectomy prevents BB rat diabetes,[76,144] and there are data to suggest that double-negative (possibly autoreactive) T cells may escape from the T cell depletion process in the thymus.[145]

The fact that neonatal thymectomy in the DP-BB rat prevents diabetes is not inconsistent with a prethymic defect, as maturation within a normal thymus may be required for abnormal prothymocytes to be produced. Indeed, there are thymic maturation abnormalities in the DP-BB rat that may contribute to the release of potential autoreactive immature T cells into the general circulation. Support for altered thymic development in the DP rat comes from experiments that implant a small amount of MHC-compatible islet tissue into the thymus of neonatal DP-BB rats. This prevents diabetes and insulitis from developing.[146] It has been suggested that intrathymic transplantation of islets into neonatal BB rats alters T cell development by promoting the deletion or functional inactivation of antigen-specific clones (against the β-cells) before their migration to the periphery.[146] The observation of a lower proportion of mature CD4-CD8+ thymocytes and an increased proportion of a less mature phenotype[134,141,147-149] supports the hypothesis of inadequate negative selection of maturing T cells. This abnormality along the maturation route would contribute to both the peripheral T lymphopenia and autoreactivity in the DP rat. T cells from DP-BB rats released from the thymus have an unusually short life span compared with peripheral T cells of DR or other non-diabetes-prone lines.[106] The molecular defect in this cell is not known. However, a CD4-dependent signaling abnormality in DP-BB peripheral T cells appears during maturation.[150] Additionally, an abnormality in the activity of the enzyme nucleoside phosphorylase has been reported in BB rat thymocytes.[151]

In conclusion, combination of thymic antigen-presenting abnormalities and/or thymic epithelial defects in the DP-BB rat would impair the ability of the thymus to select negatively or positively developing T cells. Thymocyte selection, clonal deletion, or elimination of self-reactive T cell clones (negative selection) is hypothesized to result from interaction of precursor cells with MHC class II antigens expressed on the thymic epithelium and bone marrow–derived thymic antigen-presenting cells.[152,153] Both bone marrow and the thymic microenvironment have been shown to contribute to the generation of peripheral T cell abnormalities in the BB rat.[121,122,132,141,154-159]

13.3.3.4 Altered Energy Metabolism of Immune Cells

An early event of mitogen stimulation in lymphocytes results in a dramatic enhancement in the rates of glucose transport[160-164] and metabolism.[160-164] Increased anaerobic glycolysis, the conversion of glucose to lactate, may be important for both the initiation and continuation of the highly active metabolic state induced by immune stimuli. Blocking glucose transport or utilization completely obliterates the mitogenic responses of lymphocytes.[165-167] Glutamine is both an oxidative substrate and an important source of nitrogen for *de novo* synthesis of pyrimidine and purine nucleotides, and amino sugars in lymphocytes.[168] Blocking glutamine metabolism, with a glutamine analog, prevented diabetes in young DP-BB rats,[169] suggesting that glutamine metabolism by cells is important for the diabetes process. Thus, substrate utilization is critically important to immune cells and can be used as a marker of activation. Freshly isolated splenocytes from diabetic BB rats have increased glucose and glutamine metabolism and higher rates of ATP production than DR-BB rats, consistent with immune cells being immunologically activated *in vivo*.[151,170,171] Enriched CD4+ T cell preparations from diabetic BB rats demonstrated a 1.6- and 5.4-fold increase in the production of metabolites from glucose and glutamine, respectively.[172] Consistent with a state of immune activation, an increased adenosine deaminase activity has also been reported in diabetic BB rat splenocytes and mesenteric lymph nodes.[151] Intervention demonstrated to prevent diabetes, such as feeding a semipurified casein diet, has been demonstrated to reduce energy metabolism in young DP-BB rats.[173] Interestingly, a subnormal production of reducing equivalents from pyruvate was also found, suggesting the possibility of an innate redox anomaly in immune cells from the BB rat.[170,171]

13.3.3.5 Role of Macrophages

Macrophages are present in the islets early in the autoimmune process.[174-176] Activated macrophages *in vitro* demonstrate direct cytotoxicity against isolated rat islet cells but not similarly isolated hepatocytes and thyroid cells, suggesting a pathogenic role for macrophages in the destruction of islets.[9,177] In support of this, *in vivo* alteration of macrophage infiltration into the islets suppresses the development of diabetes.[175] For example, intraperitoneal administration of silica to young DP-BB rats, which is selectively toxic to macrophages, prevents insulitis and diabetes in the BB rat[174,178-180] and reduces class I MHC expression on macrophages in islets.[38] These studies support that immigration of macrophages into the islet is an essential prerequisite for the disease process.

Several mechanisms have been proposed for macrophage-induced β-cell destruction. There is evidence that prevention of both insulitis and diabetes in silica-treated young BB rats appears to be due to a decrease in macrophage-dependent T and NK cell cytotoxicity rather than silica treatment altering the susceptibility of islets to insulitis.[180] Alternatively, macrophage-mediated injury may be the result of cytokine release. *In vitro* IL-1 and tumor necrosis factor (TNF)-α have direct cytotoxic effects on pancreatic islets.[181-187] These two cytokines are produced by activated macrophages,[185] and macrophages are metabolically activated in BB rats around the time of diabetes onset.[151] Consistent with this hypothesis, the expression of IL-1[188] and TNF-α[189] in DP-BB rat macrophages has been reported to be upregulated.

Although the role of macrophages is not completely identified, there are data to support that free oxygen radical damage to islet cells may be involved. Macrophages produce toxic amounts of nitric oxide. This is formed by the inducible nitric oxide synthase enzyme during the conversion of L-arginine to L-citrulline.[190,191] Nitric is produced through the actions of two enzymes, inducible and constitutive nitric oxide synthase (iNOS and cNOS, respectively). Of particular interest is iNOS, the enzyme form that exists in macrophages and pancreatic β-cells.[192] Coculturing macrophages and islets with the iNOS inhibitor L-NMA (*N*-methyl-L-arginine) reduces macrophage destruction of islets *in vitro*.[9] It has been proposed that nitric oxide kills islet cells by inhibiting the actions of the mitochondrial enzyme aconitase[193] and inducing rapid induction of DHA damage via excessive activation of poly(ADP-ribose) polymerase, a nuclear enzyme involved in DNA repair.[194] This nuclear enzyme uses NAD as a substrate, and depletion of cellular NAD stores results in cell death.[9] Providing nicotinamide at high doses, which scavenges hydroxyl free radicals[195,196] but is not toxic to islet cells or macrophages,[177] prevents or slows the manifestation of diabetes in NOD mice.[197,198] Inhibition of nitric oxide production reduces macrophage killing of islets *in vitro*.[199] However, *in vivo* injection or oral application of iNOS inhibitors (such as aminoguanidine) to BB rats results in only a weak, if any, inhibitory effect on the development of diabetes.[9,200,201]

13.3.3.6 Role of Natural Killer Cells

NK cells are large granular CD3-CD8+ (OX19-/OX8+ in the rat) lymphocytes, found predominantly in the spleen and peripheral blood, that exhibit spontaneous cytotoxicity against various targets.[202-204] NK cells are a major cell population present in the inflamed islets during the prediabetes process[39] and compared with DR-BB rats or other rat strains, DP-BB rats have a relative increase in the number[171,205] and activity[173,205] of NK cells in blood and spleen. In fact, large granular lymphocytes with NK activity account for the majority of BB rat peripheral blood lymphocytes expressing CD8.[25,94,205] These observations, together with *in vitro* data demonstrating that NK cells isolated from diabetic and prediabetic DP-BB are spontaneously cytotoxic to islet cells,[25,94,186,206] implicate NK cells in the pathogenesis of diabetes in the BB rat. Consistent with the BB rat, an increased number[207] and activity[208] of NK cells have been reported in human IDDM. However, although NK cells may be involved in the insult on the β-cell, the autoimmune destruction of BB rat pancreatic β-cells can occur in the absence of NK cells. *In vivo* depletion of NK cells with a monoclonal antibody (3.2.3) failed to prevent adoptive transfer of diabetes by diabetogenic T cells.[95]

13.3.3.7 Cytokines

Once the appropriate stimulus is provided, T cells become activated and divide into various subgroups. The CD4+ helper T cells are differentiated into Th1 and Th2 subsets based on the types of molecules they produce. The interactions between immune and inflammatory cells are mediated in a large part by these molecules (proteins), termed *cytokines*, that are able to promote cell growth, differentiation, and functional activation.[209] Cytokines represent the cell-to-cell communication network necessary to mediate a T cell response to an antigen and induce an inflammatory response. It is believed that damage to the insulin-producing β-cells by the infiltrating mononuclear cells is caused by cytokines (see Table 13.1). The balance of cytokines produced appears to be critical to the generation of the autoimmune reaction.[210,211] In the pancreas of diabetic BB rats, inflammatory mediators including IL-1, IL-6, and TNF-α have been found.[148] Consistent with the presence of these proinflammatory cytokines the expression of mRNA for interferon-γ (IFN-γ), IL-12, and IL-2 have been reported in pancreatic islets of DP-BB rats[212,213] and RT6-depleted DR-BB rats[213] prior to and after diabetes onset. The profile of cytokines in islets has led to the hypothesis that a strong Th1 (inflammatory) response predominates over a protective Th2 (humoral or suppressive) response.[213,214] *In vitro* IL-1 and TNF-α are cytotoxic to human pancreatic islet monolayer culture.[215] High β-cell activity increases the susceptibility of β-cells to these two cytokines.[216] Culturing of BB lymphocytes with allogenic islets results in an increased release of IFN-γ and IL-2.[217] Th2 cells secrete IL-4, IL-5, and IL-10, cytokines which mediate a humoral or antibody response and inhibit the Th1 cells inflammatory response.

13.3.3.8 Altered Balance between Effector and Regulatory Cells

One of the most comprehensive models developed to describe the immune etiology in the BB rat is that by Rossini and co-workers.[5,218] They hypothesized that on a susceptible genetic background, expression of diabetes depends on a "balance" between the β-cell cytotoxic effector (diabetogenic) cells and the functioning regulatory cells that should normally prevent β-cell destruction. An imbalance between diabetogenic and regulatory T cell populations would result in the expression of diabetes in the BB rat. This is consistent with the data suggesting that the β-cell itself is intrinsically normal,[41] but there are a number of immune cell populations in the BB rat that are cytotoxic against the β-cell. Although activated T cells of BB rats do not kill islet cells *in vitro*,[219] T cells, particularly those that do not express the RT6 alloantigen, are central in the pathogenesis of diabetes in the BB rat. A number of molecules (e.g., cytokines, nitric oxide) and other immune cells that normally interact with T cells are activated/produced and participate in the direct killing of islet cells. Effector cells are clearly not the only prerequisite for the development of diabetes. A large number of DR rats do not develop the disease despite the fact that they have β-cell cytotoxic effector cells. These DR rats can become diabetic if their immune system is altered with cyclophosphamide,[83] low dose irradiation,[220] or elimination of RT6+ T cells,[221] supporting the importance of a regulatory population of cells in the etiology. In conclusion, this hypothesis suggests that the expression of diabetes in the BB rat appears to be a function of the relative balance between RT6- autoreactive cells and a population of regulatory cells that express the RT6 alloantigen.

13.4 Abnormal Immunity

13.4.1 Cellular Immunity

Although there are cellular and humoral immune changes reported in humans prior to the onset of diabetes[222,223] and as a consequence of poor glycemic control,[224,225] the immunological defects of the BB rat are more severe than those in humans, particularly those at the cellular level. Despite these differences, studies aimed at identifying the abnormalities in cellular immunity in the BB rat may provide clues to the still unknown immunopathogenetic mechanisms in the human disease.

From birth, DR-BB rats have a profound lymphopenia that involves primary and secondary lymphoid tissues and is most evident for T-suppressor cells, particularly those expressing the RT6 differential alloantigen.[14,86,92,170,226] Lymphopenia is a unique feature of the BB rat, as human IDDM has not been associated with lymphopenia or defects in proportion of T and B lymphocytes.[227,228] In contrast to DP rats, DR-BB rats have normal numbers of all lymphocyte phenotypes.[97] Lymphopenia in the DP rat is characterized by a severe reduction in the number of CD4+ T cells (fourfold reduction) and a virtual absence of CD8+ cells (15-fold reduction) in peripheral circulation and most lymphoid tissues.[24,89-92,171] Lymphopenia in the DP-BB rat is present from birth and does not differ between DP rats who do and do not develop diabetes.[92] Thus, T-lymphopenia appears necessary for the disease to develop but is not alone sufficient for the development of insulitis and hyperglycemia in BB rat.[229,230] As already discussed, possible causes for lymphopenia include impaired maturation and differentiation and/or an excessive rate of destruction of lymphocytes.[98]

Despite lymphopenia, the remaining immune cells in the periphery of DP-BB rats, both prior to and during the disease onset, demonstrate a marked decrease in their response to T cell mitogens[23,89,96,142,149,170,171,188,231-233] and alloantigenic cells in a mixed lymphocyte culture.[23,89,91,118,143] Production of cytokines such as IL-2 after Con A stimulation is also reported to be reduced.[188,231] To what extent the defects in cellular immune responses represent an intrinsic abnormality and to what degree they reflect the altered distribution of lymphocyte populations are still not known. However, defective cytotoxic activity of isolated DP CD8+ cells against allogeneic cells and virally infected target cells has been reported.[233-235] This functional immunodeficiency may account for the relative inability of DP-BB rats, to reject skin allografts across both major and minor histocompatibility barriers[89] and the enhanced susceptibility of DP rats to infection and virus-induced immunosuppression.[31,40,60,236,237] The inability to reject skin grafts does not appear to be a general defect in mounting immune memory by BB-DP rats, as a second graft is rejected in an accelerated manner.[238] Delayed-type hypersensitivity does not appear to be as severely affected as other T cell functions in the BB rat.[239]

Surprisingly, purified DP T cells are reported to exhibit normal proliferative response to mitogen.[231] It has been suggested that reduced T cell function of BB DP cells, at least in part, may be due to suppression by macrophages. Depletion of adherent cells bearing the Fc receptor (primarily macrophages) was reported to improve, although not completely restore, the mitogenic and alloantigenic response of BB spleen cells.[89,188] Another suggestion for poor mitogen response is the possibility of a reduced number of IL-2 receptors and/or binding of IL-2 to its receptor.[240] A membrane defect is supported by the observation that stimulating DP cells with phorbol esters and Ionomycin (agents that bypass membrane-binding steps in activation) improve DP lymphocyte proliferation[170] and IL-2 receptor expression.[241] In conclusion, BB rats are essentially immunodeficient. The principal characteristic of the immunodeficiency is severe T-lymphopenia and T cell dysfunction. The role of these abnormalities in the development of diabetes is not clear as they are present in all DP rats, whether or not they develop diabetes.

13.4.2   Humoral Immunity

Because of the severe T cell lymphopenia in the DR rat, the proportion of β-cells is higher in both primary and secondary lymphoid.[171,173] The actual number of β-cells and immunoglobulin levels in most DP-BB rat lymphoid organs are not different from DR rats.[89] Whereas a subnormal response to T-dependent antigens is observed in the DP-BB rat, direct testing of the ability of BB rats to mount an antibody response to various injected immunogens has suggested that response to T-independent antigens is normal.[242] Therefore, except for the indirect evidence for the humoral arm of the immune system contributing to the pathogenesis of autoimmune disease, humoral immunity in the DP rat does not appear to differ from that of DR rats.

13.5   Genetic Predisposition and Triggering Signals in the BB Rat

Type I diabetes was one of the first autoimmune diseases in humans to be shown to be associated with HLA.[243] In the human disease, particular HLA molecules are associated with susceptibility, others with protection, whereas still others appear neutral. Many genes (perhaps more than 18 in the human) may modify the risk of developing diabetes.[244-246] For example, the class II HLA-DR3 and DR4 loci appear to have a highly specific linkage to the development of diabetes, and the DQ and DR4 molecules may jointly determine susceptibility or protection.[246] Extensive studies done to date have demonstrated that, similar to the human disease[244] and NOD mouse,[247] diabetes in the BB-DP rat is a heritable disorder with strong immunogenetic associations. Classical breeding studies, involving multiple crossing studies, have been done to define the inheritance of autoimmune diabetes in this animal model. Several modes of diabetes inheritance have been proposed[5] and at least three independent recessive unlinked genes may be necessary for susceptibility to diabetes in the BB rat.[248,249] Differences between studies in the identification genes are most likely due to the use of different (genetic and phenotypic) BB rat sublines[5] and to the use of genetically different inbred and outbred diabetes-resistant rat strains (BN, BUF, DA, LEW, Fischer, WF, etc.) in the crossing studies.[123,127,249-254]

One of the independent genes necessary for susceptibility to diabetes involves a gene associated with the rat MHC. The MHC in the rat, similar to the human HLA, is a group of genetically linked loci coding for cell surface glycoproteins, which play a major role in self vs. nonself immunological discrimination. The rat MHC (RT1) comprises a number of class I loci (RT1A, RT1E, and RT1C) flanking a pair of class II loci (RT1B and RT1D).[255] Two types of class II molecules specified by the RT1B and RT1D loci are analogous with the murine loci H-2-1A and -IE, respectively, and with the human loci HLA-DQ and HLA-DR, respectively.[255,256] Expression of the disease is independent of class I haplotype, but requires the presence of at least one class II RT1u allele.[14,248,251,257] This is similar to the human disease, where only one copy of the permissive class II allele is necessary.[246] Class II gene products are surface molecules that bind peptide fragments of foreign or self-antigens and present them to T cells in the thymus. They are thought to be involved in positive and negative selection.[256] The class II gene of the RT1^u complex in BB rat linked to diabetes susceptibility has been named *Iddm 2*.[248,251,258,259] There is no evidence that these class II molecules of the DP-BB rat are abnormal, as unaltered class II molecules of the u haplotype support the autoimmune response in the BB rat.[260] Despite the evidence in human Type I genetic studies,[246] the region around position 57 of the class II β chains of nondiabetes-prone Lewis rats and Buffalo rats appears to be identical to that found in the BB rat.[260] The RT1A locus is not involved in diabetes expression.[261] Additional genes are necessary for expression of diabetes, as depletion of the RT6.1 alloantigen in the YO and Lewis strains will not result in diabetes despite also having an RT1^u MHC haplotype phenotype.[62,106,131]

Lymphopenia is inherited independently of the MHC gene. Lymphopenia is caused by homozygosity for a second recessive allele of a single gene (*lyp* or *Iddm-l*), which has been mapped to the proximity of the neuropeptide Y gene on rat Chromosome 4.[123,262,263] This gene or gene cluster is considered by many as essential for the development of diabetes in BB rats.[123,262,263] It is believed that abnormalities in postthymic T cell development in the BB rat results in part from the *IDDM-1* gene defect in hemopoietic stem cells.[123,132] Recently, it was reported that inheritance of the *lyp* gene is associated with a unique cytokine profile consistent with those involved in β-cell destruction.[264,265] A subline of DP-BB rats has been developed that is nonlymphopenic and has normal T lymphocytes subsets,[266] suggesting that expression of the gene for lymphopenia may not be an obligate immunogenetic feature in BB rat diabetes. This suggests the disease is more similar to the human disease, where severe lymphopenia does not occur.

Since class I molecules are important restrictive elements for T cell selection of targets and play a key role in antigen presentation, alterations of these molecules have been sought in the BB rat. Although the hyperexpression of some class I molecules has been reported in the BB rat, the appearance of the disease appears to be independent of class I haplotype.[46] More recently, a third non-MHC gene (*Iddm 3*) linked to the expression of diabetes has been recently found in the BB rat.[123,267]

13.6 Environmental Triggers of Diabetes

While genetic susceptibility is important, in humans the concordance rates for diabetes between identical twins is less than 33%, indicating that the etiology of Type I diabetes is complex and dependent on environmental factors.[268-270] Similarly, despite many generations of selective inbreeding, not all DP-BB rats develop diabetes, suggesting that environmental factors also interact with genetic susceptibility in the BB rat. One of the greatest challenges now being addressed through the use of the BB rat model is that of unraveling the environmental trigger(s) of the autoimmune process. Similar to the human disease, there is considerable evidence in the BB rat to suggest a role of environmental factors in the pathogenesis of diabetes (seeTable 13.1).

13.6.1 Diet

There is considerable epidemiological data to suggest that diet is an important environmental factor in the etiology of human Type I diabetes.[271-278] These studies suggest that a shorter duration of breast-feeding (replacing human milk with cow's milk–based formula) increases the risk of diabetes in genetically susceptible individuals.[271-278] To date, the strongest evidence for diet in the etiology of diabetes comes from the BB rat and the NOD mouse models of diabetes. The onset of diabetes in these rodents can be substantially delayed or prevented by early dietary intervention[279-287] by a yet-to-be established mechanism.

In the rodent studies, diet and diet ingredients are categorized as protective (those that delay or reduce the incidence of diabetes) or as permissive (those that reduce the age of onset and increase the incidence of diabetes). The categorization of diets is based on changing the high incidence of diabetes in DP-BB rats fed nonpurified (standard rat chow) diets. It is now well documented that replacing cereal-based rodent weanling diets (chow) with a number of defined semipurified, purified, and elemental diets decreases the incidence of diabetes by at least 50% in BB rats[38,280,282-285] and NOD mice.[279,286] The question emerges: Are these protective diets simply decreasing the exposure of the animal to a diabetogen (protein or other compound) present in chow or are they modulating the development of the autoimmune process?

Although designed to meet the macro- and micronutrient requirements of rodents, chow is a cereal-based open formula, which includes wheat, corn, and soy proteins with some milk ingredients.[288] Not surprisingly, the composition of the "protective" and "permissive" diets used in the rodent studies differs dramatically in both the raw ingredients and resulting nutrient content and composition. The most-striking macronutrient differences between these diets are the concentrations and sources of proteins, carbohydrates, and fats. Several research groups have attempted to add back ingredients/nutrients to the protective (low-incidence) diets to measure their effect on diabetes incidences. Elliott and Martin[282] in 1984 were the first to suggest skim milk protein (possibly BSA) as a possible trigger of diabetes in the BB rat. It has been suggested that the immune response to pancreatic autoantigens might involve the potential sequence similarity of cow's milk proteins to a pancreatic antigen (molecular mimicry).[289] In support of this hypothesis, immunoglobulins against BSA have been found in BB animals near the peak onset period for diabetes[38] and feeding specific animal chows that do not contain milk protein (including BSA) reduces the incidence of BB rat diabetes in some studies.[271] However, further research indicates that milk protein is not the sole "diabetogenic" component in chow, since its removal from chow does not completely prevent BB rat diabetes.[290,291]

It has been demonstrated that replacing casein in these protective diets with soy protein results in an incidence of diabetes lower than chow but higher than casein-based diets.[281] These observations are interesting, as soy and cow's milk are the proteins used in commercially available infant formula. Epidemiological and serological data in humans suggest a relationship between decreased exposure to breast milk (by the feeding of infant formula[115,272,292] or the early introduction of foods[272]) and the incidence of Type I diabetes. One of the earliest foods introduced to infants is cereal. In the BB rat and NOD mouse, the wheat proteins, present in chow but absent in the protective diets, have been suggested to be diabetogenic.[282,285] Although reported diabetes incidence was higher when wheat proteins where added to the diet, the resulting diabetes incidence was still lower than in animals fed chow or milk-based diets.[285] Replacement of casein in purified diets with alternative protein sources, such as rapeseed flour, peanut meal, kidney beans, fish meal, hydrolyzed lactoalbumin, wheat germ, alfalfa seeds, brewer's yeast, red lentils, and plant mixtures, increased the onset and incidence of diabetes and insulitis relative to casein-based diets in some studies[280,281,287] but not in others.[285] However, it is difficult to attribute, in the BB rat, changes in the onset and incidence of diabetes to plant proteins per se since the plant protein sources added to the semipurified protective diets were impure, with up to 75% of their composition as complex carbohydrates.[280,287] Thus, the relative importance of plant proteins vs. complex carbohydrate in the pathogenesis of diabetes in the BB rat is not known. Although few studies have been done, the content and composition of dietary fat do not appear to affect the onset and expression of diabetes in the BB rat significantly.[284] Similar to other autoimmune diseases,[293] feeding an essential fatty acid diet suppresses the immune system and reduces the incidence of BB rat diabetes.[294] To date, definite diabetogenic ingredient(s) in chow have not been identified, although the search continues.

The protective effect of diets is influenced by both the timing of initial exposure and the duration of the exposure. It is reported that initial exposure to a protective diet must occur at least from weaning.[38,280,284,291,295] However, by weaning (20 to 24 days) rats will have consumed some maternal diet, which in most studies was the permissive chow diet. This may help account for incomplete disease protection when feeding a protective diet. The duration of dietary exposure is also important because feeding semipurified diets from weaning and delaying exposure to chow diets until 50 days of age shifted the onset of the disease to a later age but did not ultimately change the incidence of diabetes.[295] Moreover, BB rats,[38] like the NOD mice,[287] appear protected from diabetes if fed the protective diet until 100 days of age, then fed chow. These observations are consistent with human studies that suggest extending the length of breast-feeding may reduce the risk for Type I diabetes.[272] Thus, an alternative hypothesis to the mechanism of diet protection is that diet modulates the development of the autoimmune process.

The gut represents the largest immune organ in the body, and migration of immune cells to the rat gut begins during the first postnatal week and is not complete until approximately 4 weeks of age.[296] This corresponds to the period when diet modulates the expression of autoimmune diabetes in the BB rat. Maturation of the gut-associated lymphoid tissue relies on the presence of antigens,[296] and there is evidence that gut-associated lymphoid tissue function is affected by nutritional status.[297] The gut of the young animal is permeable to macromolecules (undigested and partially digested food antigens) that can enter the circulation and induce antibody production.[298] There are phenotypic and functional differences in immune cells in the neonatal as compared with the mature adult gut.[299] Consistent with this hypothesis, DP-BB rats exposed to cow's milk protein later in life are not as susceptible to its diabetogenic effects.[291] In addition, early diet (less than 5 weeks postweaning) has been shown to have irreversible effects on gut size and possibly nutrient transport, providing the basis for the concept of "critical period programming."[300] Differences in the development of the intestine have been reported between DP and DR-BB rats.[301]

The effect of protective diets may involve their immunostimulatory/immunosuppressive effect on the developing immune system in the BB rat. There is evidence that some plant (soy, wheat, and alfalfa) and milk proteins may alter pancreatic expression of an antigen or modulate immune autoreactivity.[38] Feeding a protective diet was demonstrated to affect pancreatic MHC class I expression,[284,302] reduce energy metabolism and cytotoxicity of immune cells,[173] modulate cytokine profiles in the pancreas,[295] and alter T cell function.[173] These diet alterations in immune parameters demonstrate the immunomodulatory impact of diet in the BB rat. In conclusion, similar to the human disease, early diet plays a critical role in the expression of BB rat diabetes. Identification of the mechanism by which early diet alters the expression of diabetes in the DP-BB rat will ultimately lead to dietary recommendations aimed at reducing the risk of diabetes in genetically susceptible individuals.

13.6.2 Viruses

Viral infection has long been suspected to play a role in the pathogenesis of human IDDM.[303] Associations of diabetes with mumps, Coxsackie B4, and CMV virus have been reported.[303,304] Similarly, there is considerable evidence in the NOD mouse of the involvement of viruses in the expression of diabetes.[305,306] However, the possibility of viral involvement in BB rat diabetes is less clear and appears to be linked to genetic susceptibility. Infection of DP-BB rats infected with encephalomycarditis virus or Coxsackie B virus[307] induces diabetes.[307] Interestingly, if DP rats were transfused with DR spleen cells prior to viral infection, they did not develop diabetes.[5] However, lymphocytic choriomeningitis virus infection results in a lower incidence of diabetes in DP-BB rats.[60] Infecting DR-BB rats with Kilham rat virus induces these rats to develop autoimmune diabetes similar to the DP-BB rat.[147,308-310] The Kilham rat virus has also been shown to trigger autoimmune diabetes in other RT1^u rat strains that are normally resistant to diabetes.[309] A spontaneous infection of a Worchester colony with a viral pathogens (most likely Kilham rat virus) was reported to increase the incidence of diabetes and reduce the age of onset of diabetes in DP-BB rats.[5,147]

There is limited evidence that viruses are directly cytotoxic to the β-cell. One hypothesis for the role of viruses suggests that IFN-γ production following local viral infection could result in induction of MHC class II antigen expression on endocrine epithelial cells enabling these cells to present self-antigens to autoreactive T cells.[26,311] Others have suggested that viruses may act by amplifying the immune response of preexisting autoreactive cell populations or by affecting the function of regulatory cell populations or the susceptibility of the β-cell to immune damage.[5] The evidence from work with Coxsackie B and encephalomycarditis virus would suggest that raising BB rats under gnotobiotic conditions would reduce the incidence of diabetes. This, however, does not occur as DP-BB rats raised under gnotobiotic conditions are reported to have the same[312] or even a higher[5] incidence of spontaneous diabetes than DP-BB rats raised in standard conditions. On the other hand, raising DR-BB rats under gnotobiotic conditions reduces their susceptibility to various methods of inducing diabetes.[5] In the NOD mouse, there is considerable evidence to suggest vertical transmission of an infectious agent such as retrovirus.[313] In the BB rat the possible contribution of retroviral infection remains controversial.[22]

13.6.3   Other

There have been very few additional reports on other possible environmental triggers of diabetes in the BB rat. In a preliminary study, psychological stress such as restraint, rotation, crowding, and resocialization, independent of weight gain or food intake, significantly reduced the average age of onset and increased the incidence of diabetes in BB rats.[314]

13.7   Prevention of Diabetes in the BB Rat

The BB rat has been invaluable in the progress of work aimed at developing prevention strategies for Type I diabetes. Prevention strategies can be classified into primary, secondary, and tertiary interventions.[315] Primary prevention refers to an early intervention, prior to any abnormality in serological markers of autoimmunity or in β-cell secretory response. Secondary prevention involves an intervention initiated in response to the presence of one or both of these abnormalities, and tertiary prevention is an intervention initiated soon after diagnosis designed to preserve residual β-cell function. Diabetes can be prevented or delayed in the BB rat using a number of different treatments (see Table 13.1). The following sections will examine the current understanding of prevention of diabetes in the BB rat.

13.7.1 Immunosuppression

13.7.1.1 Pharmacological Agents

The evidence in favor of a causative role of immune cells, particularly T cells in the pathogenesis of Type I diabetes, has led to the use of immunosuppressive agents early in the disease process to prevent or halt the immune attack on the islets. Systemic immunosuppression with cyclosporine, azathioprine, and azathiaporine plus prednisone can slow and sometime arrest the progress of Type I diabetes in humans.[232] Similarly, in the BB rat, immunosuppressive agents have been shown to delay or prevent the development of diabetes mellitus. Cyclosporine A (CsA) prevents the development of diabetes and insulitis in DP-BB rats when administered continually from an early age (prior to 40 days of age).[316-319] CsA induces a selective inhibition of cell-mediated immunity (depression of IL-2 production and abrogation of suppression of insulin syntheses) without clear-cut effects on autoantibody formation.[320] Unfortunately, CsA has many toxic side effects to both the BB rat and humans that would limit its use clinically in the prediabetes state.[232] More recently, CsA in combination with another immunosuppressive agent, deoxyspergulain (DSP), was shown to provide, at a lower CsA dose, protective effects in the DP rat with fewer side effects.[321] The early success with CsA has led to subsequent studies demonstrating the efficacy of other immunosuppressive agents at successfully reducing diabetes in the BB rat. These include administration of 2' deoxycoformycin,[322] oral azasparine (SK & F 106610),[323] the sulfonylurea glipizide,[324] and the glutamine antimetabolite acivicin.[169] As discussed earlier, depleting young DP rat of macrophages with intraperitoneal administration of silica, an agent known to destroy macrophages, reduces the incidence of autoimmune diabetes.[178] The use of pharmacological agents in the BB rat has provided both evidence for the immune system in the etiology of diabetes and potential agents for the remission of disease processes and symptoms in the human disease.

13.7.1.2 Cytokines

Cytokines are found in the islets prior to and during the clinical expression of the disease in both the BB rat[148,212-214,325] and humans.[185] The types of cytokines present and their effect on β-cells *in vitro*[185,216,217] suggest that diabetes results from an imbalance of a Th1 response dominating over a protective Th2 response.[213] This would suggest that the provision of Th1 cytokines (TNF, IFN-γ, IL-1, IL-12, and IL-2) would accelerate the onset of BB diabetes while the provision of Th2 cytokines (IL-4, IL-10) would prevent or delay the onset of BB diabetes. Indeed, some of the immunomodulatory treatments that prevent BB diabetes result in a Th2 cytokine pattern in the islet.[185,212,295,326] Increasing serum IFN-α through the administration of Poly I:C accelerates diabetes onset in DP-BB rats[327,328] and induces diabetes in DR-BB rats,[329] but not Wistar rats.[330] The IFN-α-inducing activity of Poly I:C in the DR-BB rat has been shown to act in a dose-dependent manner[330] and may alter the number and activity of NK cells.[329,330] However, many of the studies that provide either Th1 or Th2 cytokines *in vivo* to DP-BB rats have produced less-convincing results. Contrary to the hypothesis of a dominant Th1 response, injecting rats with TNF-α reduced diabetes incidence and insulitis severity in DP rats.[331,332] Injecting young DP rats with IL-2 is reported to both induce and protect DP-BB rats from diabetes.[333] Studies investigating the impact of IL-1 on diabetes in the BB rat have also been inconsistent. Providing IL-1 to DP animals is reported to accelerate[334] or to have no effect on diabetes onset in DP-BB rats.[301] *In vivo* treatments with cytokines can be complicated by changes in food intake and body weight in the rats, which will independently affect the incidence of diabetes. Additionally, the dose, frequency of injections, age of treatment, and strain of BB rat studied are all likely to impact on the results of these type of studies.

13.7.1.3 Antibodies

The use of specific cytotoxic antibodies directed against the autoimmune cell(s) has been used as a method of altering the course of BB rat diabetes. Cytotoxic antibodies to T cells,[93] CD2[+] T cells,[87] the inflammatory cytokine IFN-γ[335] have all been reported to exert protective influences in the course of diabetes of the DP-BB rat.

13.7.2 Immunomodulation

13.7.2.1 Complete Freund's Adjuvant (CFA)

Although normally considered an immunostimulatory adjuvant, CFA, a mixture of mycobacterial cell wall and mineral oil, has demonstrated protective influences in DP-BB rats, preventing them from developing diabetes.[336] Timed injections of CFA between 9 and 28 days of age reduces diabetes incidence and the degree of insulitis in DP-BB rats.[336] Further work has found that the transfer of splenic cells from CFA-treated DP rats prevents young DP rats from developing diabetes.[337] The protective influences of CFA have been attributed to a number of possible immunoenhancing mechanisms, such as increasing natural suppressor lymphocytes and/or altering immunoregulatory cytokine production.[338] Administration of CFA was found to change the production of suppressive cytokines such as TNF-β.[219] Leukocytes isolated from DP pancreas had high levels of IFN-γ and IL-2 mRNA, but both DR and DP rats treated with CFA had lower levels of mRNA for these inflammatory cytokines.[212]

13.7.2.2 Free Radical Scavengers

There is considerable evidence that the production of free radicals by immune cells is involved in β-cell destruction.[339] Providing compounds that scavenge hydoxyl free radicals (e.g., nicotinamide) delays the onset of BB rat diabetes.[196] BB rats treated with nitric oxide inhibitors have been reported to have a lower incidence[201] or delayed the onset[200] of diabetes in some studies. The clinical value of therapeutic interventions aimed at reducing free radical damage has been dampened by the observation by others that *in vivo* inhibition of nitric oxide had little influence on diabetes incidence in BB rats.[9,200,201]

13.7.2.3 Oral Tolerance

Oral tolerance is defined as hyporesponsiveness to a previously encountered protein antigen after earlier oral administration of the antigen.[340] Potential antigens are introduced orally at doses that will initiate, in the gut-associated lymphoid tissue, a suppressive immune response. This ability to induce "tolerance" to autoantigens has considerable therapeutic potential for the treatment of autoimmune disorders,[341,342] including Type I diabetes.[343] For example, tolerance has been induced in animal models of rheumatoid arthritis using collagen as the target autoantigen.[344] In the case of Type I diabetes mellitus, delivering pancreatic candidate autoantigens, such as GAD65, insulin and proinsulin, has been proposed.[345] The administration of oral human insulin to prevent the immune attack on β-cells is now being tested on its effect of modulating the expression of HLA antigens associated with diabetes susceptibility in a Phase II clinical trial.[345]

The mucosal surface (at the gut, respiratory tract, genitourinary tracts) provides a unique interface for antigen and suppressive factors, which may further prevent a systemic immune response. At the mucosa, T-helper cells influence tolerance induction via a Th2 cytokine profile while suppressing inflammatory Th1 lymphocyte actions. These gut-derived cells that have been exposed to diet can migrate to the systemic circulation and ultimately reach other organs, such as the pancreas. Upon reaching areas of autodestruction (i.e., the pancreas), the tolerized lymphocytes could exert nonspecific "bystander suppression" via the Th2 cytokine profile, and reduce autoinflammation and cytolysis (or the Th1 response).[346]

Inducing therapeutic oral tolerance to rodent diabetes has been attempted with mixed success. Providing oral doses of insulin and GAD65 has been demonstrated to reduce the incidence of diabetes in the NOD mice.[347] However, gavaging young DP-BB rats with insulin did not alter the onset or incidence of diabetes, implying the absence of tolerance.[348] Several factors remain to be established before oral tolerance can be ruled out as a possible treatment in BB rats. These include identification of the potential antigens for use in this procedure, the optimum age at which to initiate antigen exposure,[349,350] the appropriate dose to induce suppression and initiate a Th2 response,[345,351] the impact of BB rat lymphopenia on the process[348] and the possible role of other dietary constituents in facilitating tolerance.

13.7.2.4 Insulin Treatment

Early administration of insulin (prior to the development of overt diabetes) has been indicated as a method of reducing diabetes onset and incidence. Prophylactic insulin treatment is postulated to reduce β-cell activity, and decrease the expression of the putative β-cell antigen that initiates the disease process. Prophylactic insulin administration to young DP-BB rats reduced the incidence of diabetes.[77] Daily injections of exogenous insulin also protected RT6-depleted DR-BB rats from developing diabetes.[352] Similarly, administration of glipizide, a sulfonylurea that reduced insulin secretion, reduces diabetes incidence and delays disease onset in DP-BB rats.[324]

13.8 Multiorgan Pathophysiology

13.8.1 Multiple Organ Complications of Diabetes

BB rats are prone to organ system changes similar to human diabetes complications. A comprehensive autopsy study has been reported on BB rats.[353] In insulin-treated BB rats that have survived for months to years, pathological changes in the retina,[354-357] myocardium,[358-361] kidney,[353,362-367] liver,[353,368,369] stomach,[353] colon,[370] gonads,[371-373] thyroid,[353] bone,[374] and peripheral nerves[375-383] have been reported. The most common cause of morbidity and mortality in humans with Type I diabetes is vascular disease, but atherosclerosis and severe microangiopathy do not occur in the BB diabetic rat.[353]

In contrast to the human disease, both DR and DP rats have an increased susceptibility to pulmonary infections.[31,353] Many colonies of BB rats have been maintained in pathogen-free environments to prevent epidemics, particularly of *Mycoplasma pneumoniae* which is often fatal.[6] However, most significant strain-related lesions in the BB rat involve the lymph nodes. Mesenteric lymph nodes of DP rats are often enlarged, lymphocyte depleted, and show absence of germinal centers,[31] and frequently lymphomas/granulomas are found in the mesenteric lymph nodes and colon.[353,384] It is hypothesized that the high incidence of lymphomas in the DP-BB rat is due to the expansion of β-cells in lymphoid organs.[385,386]

13.8.2   The Thyroid

During recent years, an increasing number of cases of concurrent Type I diabetes and other organ-specific autoimmune diseases have been reported.[387] After the pancreas, the thyroid gland is by far the most common endocrine organ affected in human Type I diabetes.[387] As with human Type I diabetes, thyroiditis is common in DP-BB rats and occurs in some DR-BB rats.[372,388,389] Thyroiditis is characterized by the infiltration of dendritic cells throughout the thyroid gland[27] and the presence of antithyroid colloid autoantibodies and antithyroglobulin antibodies[20] are found in both DR and DP sublines. Thyrocytoxic autoantibodies have also been reported in both strains of BB rat.[21] However, the thyroid lesion in the BB rat does not progress to overt hypothyroidism.[388,390,391] The incidence of thyroiditis in BB rats varies in the different genetic sublines.[390,391] Recently, it was proposed that the BB rat could be a useful model to study thyroiditis.[392]

Generally, the interventions employed to protect against the onset of autoimmune diabetes in the BB rat are not effective at preventing autoimmune thyroid complications.[352,393] Similarly, administering L-thyroxin or methimazole is protective against thyroiditis in the BB rat, but does not alter the incidence of diabetes.[393] Thyroiditis may be induced with high dietary intake of iodine.[393,394] As with the diabetic syndrome of the BB rat, etiological associations have included genetics, MHC haplotype, and environmental factors. Lymphopenia is involved in the development of the thyroiditis in the DP-BB rat.[395] Thyroiditis can also be induced in DR-BB rats by *in vivo* depletion of RT6 lymphocytes.[213] It has been hypothesized that cytokine production in the thyroid may account for altered susceptibility to thyroiditis between BB rat strains.[213]

13.9   The Use of the BB Rat as a Model for Transplantation Studies

In humans, pancreatic allografts are quickly rejected because of their high immunogenicity in contrast to those of liver, heart, or kidney.[396] Transplantation of both allogeneic and syngeneic islets into nonprivileged sites in the BB rat leads rapidly to graft destruction.[37,116,397] The BB rat has been used as a model to study tolerance to transplanted tissues.[398] Successful tissue transplantation in humans currently requires general immunosuppression.[49] Improved graft survival has been shown to occur in transplanted BB rats when combined with anti-ICAM-1 and LFA-1 monoclonal antibody therapy.[116] Immune-privileged sites for transplantation have also been explored. For example, intrathymic transplantation of MHC-compatible islets into DP-BB rats has been shown to prolong normoglycemia.[399] Ultimately, the use of the BB rat to study transplantation may translate into new molecular and cellular understanding of tolerance and interventions that will cure and prevent insulin-dependent diabetes.

13.10 Care and Breeding of BB Rats

Specific instructions on the care and maintenance of BB rats can be obtained from the animal suppliers. Below are some general guidelines that the authors have developed during their 10-years experience with BB rats. From the age of 60 days, BB rats should be monitored for the appearance of diabetes. Daily weight monitoring is sufficient initially. As hyperglycemia appears at the onset of diabetes, any change in body weight should be followed up by monitoring urinary glucose. Diabetes is usually confirmed by a 3+ urinary glucose followed by a nonfasting measure of blood glucose (via a tail vein) of >200 mg/dl (11 mM). Blood glucose can be measured using a portable glucosmeter. Once diabetes is confirmed, exogenous insulin should be provided.

For standard maintenance of diabetic BB rats, one subcutaneous injection of a long-acting insulin is given. This is usually administered prior to beginning of the housing dark cycle in the neck region with a pediatric insulin syringe. The authors use a long-acting human insulin; others use U-40 protamine zinc insulin.[6] Insulin doses range from 1 to 8 units/day/rat, and the dosage is adjusted according to the degree of glycosuria present at the time insulin is given. Failure to administer insulin results in ketoacidosis within 48 h and death (within days) unless treatment is resumed. Weight losses of greater than 2 g should be compensated with increasing the exogenous insulin dose by approximately 1 unit. Once adjusted, the insulin dose is rarely reduced. If animals are to be maintained for a significant period of time (> 14 days), insulin implants should be considered.

After about 7 days of exogenous subcutaneous insulin injections, the authors implant a commercially available sustained-release insulin implant in the neck scruff of the rat (Linplant®, Linshin Canada Ltd., Ontario, Canada). Implantation in this region, rather than the rat's flank, reduces the incidence of infections and prevents the rat from accessing it. Following the dosage recommended by the supplier, insulin implants last about 60 days in BB rats. The body weight of the implanted rat is monitored two times per week and weight losses of greater than 5 g are followed up by urinary and/or blood glucose determinations. Once hyperglycemia is confirmed, exogenous insulin is begun again following the above procedure. When the necessary insulin dose is greater than 5 units, the rats are reimplanted with new insulin implants. For breeder diabetic males, due to the appearance of diabetic complications, the rats are generally implanted three times before retiring them.

Male and female diabetic BB rats are capable of breeding, but litters from diabetic dams, particularly those with uncontrolled hyperglycemia, tend to be small and result in high perinatal mortality.[6] The breeding of diabetic males to nondiabetic females has proved to be the most successful breeding strategy. To maintain a high incidence of diabetes in the authors' colony (a small BB/Ottawa colony), outbreeding of a diabetic male to a nondiabetic DP female from a litter with a high incidence of diabetes is maintained. Other colonies, such as that in Worchester, are maintained as inbred with a diabetic male bred to a nondiabetic sibling.[6] Generally, outbreeding results in larger litter sizes (8 to 14 pups/dam). If the female rat becomes diabetic during the pregnancy, this presents difficulties in management with a poor pregnancy outcome;[6] therefore, females are monitored for glycosuria and glycemia during pregnancy.

There are reports that DP rats do not survive well for extended periods of time (50 ± 32 days) after the onset of diabetes.[400] It was speculated that this poor prognosis was due to their profound immunodeficient state.[400] Many colonies are maintained in a pathogen-free environment.[6] The authors have not had to maintain their colony in a pathogen-free environment; however, special care must be taken to maintain a clean environment that minimizes exposure to antigens and common rat viruses. For this reason, it is prudent to segregate BB rats from other rat colonies. Standard laboratory chow, due to its high fiber content and slower carbohydrate absorption, allows one to maintain adequate glycemic control. If semipurified diets are being fed, care should be taken to ensure a carbohydrate source that promotes a low glycemic response.

13.11 Conclusions

Although the exact etiology for the development of Type I diabetes mellitus in the BB rat remains unclear, its many similarities to the human disease suggest it is influenced by both genetic and environmental factors. Although it is well established that β-cells are destroyed through an inflammatory process, the pathological events that initiate the process are not well understood. The spontaneously diabetic BB rat has and will continue to contribute to a more complete understanding of the etiology, pathogenesis, prevention, and treatment of autoimmune-mediated diabetes.

Acknowledgments

The authors would like to acknowledge the editorial assistance of S. Massimino in the preparation of this chapter. C. J. Field is a recipient of a Canadian Diabetes Association scholarship.

References

1. Nakhooda AF, Like AA, Chappel CI, Murray, FT, Marliss EB, The spontaneously diabetic Wistar rat. Metabolic and morphologic studies, *Diabetes*, 26(2), 100, 1977.
2. Marliss EB, Nakhooda AF, Poussier P, Clinical forms and natural history of the diabetic syndrome and insulin and glucagon secretion in the BB rat, *Metab. Clin. Exp.*, 32(7 Suppl. 1), 11, 1983.
3. Nakhooda AF, Poussier P, Marliss EB, Insulin and glucagon secretion in BB wistar rats with impaired glucose tolerance, *Diabetologia*, 24(1), 58, 1983.
4. Prins JB, Herberg L, Den Bieman M, Van Zutphen B, Genetic characterization and interrelationship of inbred lines of diabetes-prone and not diabetes-prone BB rats, in *Frontiers in Diabetes Research. Lessons from Animal Diabetes III*, Shafrir E., Ed., Smith-Gordon, London, 1991, 19.
5. Crisa L, Mordes JP, Rossini AA, Autoimmune diabetes mellitus in the BB rat, *Diabetes Metabolism Reviews*, 8(1), 4, 1992.
6. Mordes JP, Desemone J, Rossini AA, The BB rat, *Diabetes Metabolism Reviews*, 3(3), 725, 1987.
7. Nakhooda AF, Wei CN, Marliss EB, Muscle protein catabolism in diabetes: 3-methylhistidine excretion in the spontaneously diabetic "BB" rat, *Metabolism: Clinical & Experimental*, 29(12), 1272, 1980.
8. Marliss EB, Recommended nomenclature for the spontaneously diabetic syndrome of the BB rat, *Metabolism: Clinical & Experimental*, 32(7 Suppl. 1), 6, 1983.

9. Burkart V, Kolb H, Macrophages in islet destruction in autoimmune diabetes mellitus, *Immunobiology*, 195(4-5), 601, 1996.
10. Chappel CI, Chappel WR, The discovery and development of the BB rat colony: an animal model of spontaneous diabetes mellitus, *Metabolism: Clinical & Experimental*, 32(7 Suppl. 1), 8, 1983.
11. Pedersen CR, Bock T, Hansen SV, Hansen MW, Buschard K, High juvenile body weight and low insulin levels as markers preceding early diabetes in the BB rat, *Autoimmunity*, 17(4), 261, 1994.
12. Baudon MA, Ferre P, Penicaud L, Maulard P, Ktorza A, Castano L, Girard J, Normal insulin sensitivity during the phase of glucose intolerance but insulin resistance at the onset of diabetes in the spontaneously diabetic BB rat, *Diabetologia*, 32(12), 839, 1989.
13. Nakhooda AF, Like AA, Chappel CI, Wei CN, Marliss EB, The spontaneously diabetic Wistar rat (the "BB" rat). Studies prior to and during development of the overt syndrome, *Diabetologia*, 14(3), 199, 1978.
14. Parfrey NA, Prud'homme GJ, Colle E, Fuks A, Seemayer TA, Guttmann RD, Ono SJ, Immunologic and genetic studies of diabetes in the BB rat, *Critical Reviews in Immunology*, 9(1), 45, 1989.
15. Nakhooda AF, Sima AA, Poussier P, Marliss EB, Passive transfer of insulitis from the "BB" rat to the nude mouse, *Endocrinology*, 109(6), 2264, 1981.
16. Tannenbaum GS, Colle E, Wanamaker L, Gurd W, Goldman H, Seemayer TA, Dynamic time-course studies of the spontaneously diabetic BB Wistar rat. II. Insulin-, glucagon-, and somatostatin-reactive cells in the pancreas, *Endocrinology*, 109(6), 1880, 1981.
17. Patel YC, Wheatley T, Malaisse-Lagae F, Orci L, Elevated portal and peripheral blood concentration of immunoreactive somatostatin in spontaneously diabetic (BBL) Wistar rats: suppression with insulin, *Diabetes*, 29(9), 757, 1980.
18. Guillausseau PJ, Tielmans D, Virally-Monod M, Assayag M, Diabetes: from phenotypes to genotypes, *Diabetes & Metabolism*, 23 (Suppl. 2), 14, 1997.
19. Dyrberg T, Poussier P, Nakhooda F, Marliss EB, Lernmark, A, Islet cell surface and lymphocyte antibodies often precede the spontaneous diabetes in the BB rat, *Diabetologia*, 26(2), 159, 1984.
20. Like AA, Butler L, Williams RM, Appel, MC, Weringer EJ, Rossini AA, Spontaneous autoimmune diabetes mellitus in the BB rat, *Diabetes*, 31 (Suppl. 1, Pt. 2), 7, 1982.
21. Maclaren NK, Elder ME, Robbins VW, Riley WJ, Autoimmune diatheses and T lymphocyte immunoincompetences in BB rats, *Metabolism: Clinical & Experimental*, 32 (7 Suppl. 1), 92, 1983.
22. Rossini AA, Handler ES, Mordes JP, Greiner DL, Human autoimmune diabetes mellitus: lessons from BB rats and NOD mice — caveat emptor, *Clinical Immunology & Immunopathology*, 74(1), 2, 1995.
23. Bellgrau D, Naji A, Silvers WK, Markmann JF, Barker CF, Spontaneous diabetes in BB rats: evidence for a T cell dependent immune response defect, *Diabetologia*, 23(4), 359, 1982.
24. Jackson R, Rassi N, Crump T, Haynes B, Eisenbarth GS, The BB diabetic rat. Profound T-cell lymphocytopenia, *Diabetes*, 30(10), 887, 1981.
25. MacKay P, Jacobson J, Rabinovitch A, Spontaneous diabetes mellitus in the Bio-Breeding/Worcester rat. Evidence *in vitro* for natural killer cell lysis of islet cells, *Journal of Clinical Investigation*, 77(3), 916, 1986.
26. Bottazzo GF, Dean BM, McNally JM, MacKay EH, Swift PG, Gamble DR, *In situ* characterization of autoimmune phenomena and expression of HLA molecules in the pancreas in diabetic insulitis, *New England Journal of Medicine*, 313(6), 353, 1985.
27. Voorbij HA, Jeucken PH, Kabel PJ, De Haan M, Drexhage, HA, Dendritic cells and scavenger macrophages in pancreatic islets of prediabetic BB rats, *Diabetes*, 38(12), 1623, 1989.
28. Shehadeh NN, Lafferty KJ, The role of T cells in the development of autoimmune diabetes, *Diabetes Review*, 1 141, 1993.
29. Karounos DG, Thomas JW, Recognition of common islet antigen by autoantibodies from NOD mice and humans with IDDM, *Diabetes*, 39(9), 1085, 1990.
30. Seemayer TA, Tannenbaum GS, Goldman H, Colle E, Dynamic time course studies of the spontaneously diabetic BB Wistar rat. III. Light-microscopic and ultrastructural observations of pancreatic islets of Langerhans, *American Journal of Pathology*, 106(2), 237, 1982.

31. Seemayer TA, Colle E, Tannenbaum GS, Oligny LL, Guttmann, RD, Goldman H, Spontaneous diabetes mellitus syndrome in the rat. III. Pancreatic alterations in aglycosuric and untreated diabetic BB Wistar-derived rats, *Metabolism: Clinical & Experimental*, 32(7 Suppl. 1), 26, 1983.
32. Logothetopoulos J, Valiquette N, Madura E, Cvet D, The onset and progression of pancreatic insulitis in the overt, spontaneously diabetic, young adult BB rat studied by pancreatic biopsy, *Diabetes*, 33(1), 33, 1984.
33. Kolb H, Kantwerk G, Treichel U, Kurner T, Kiessel U, Hoppe T, Kolb-Bachofen V, Prospective analysis of islet lesions in BB rats. *Diabetologia*, 29, 559A, 1986.
34. Gomez Dumm CL, Semino MC, Gagliardino JJ, Quantitative morphological changes in endocrine pancreas of rats with spontaneous diabetes mellitus, *Vichows Archiv. B. Cell Pathology* 57, 375, 1989.
35. Seemayer TA, Schurch W, Kalant N, B cell lymphoproliferation in spontaneously diabetic BB Wistar rats, *Diabetologia*, 23(3), 261, 1982.
36. Jiang Z, Handler ES, Rossini AA, Woda, BA, Immunopathology of diabetes in the RT6-depleted diabetes-resistant BB/Wor rat, *American Journal of Pathology*, 137(4), 767, 1990.
37. Prowse SJ, Bellgrau D, Lafferty KJ, Islet allografts are destroyed by disease occurrence in the spontaneously diabetic BB rat, *Diabetes*, 35(1), 110, 1986.
38. Scott FW, Marliss EB, Conference summary: diet as an environmental factor in development of insulin-dependent diabetes mellitus, *Canadian Journal of Physiology & Pharmacology*, 69(3), 311, 1991.
39. Hosszufalusi N, Chan E, Teruya M, Takei S, Granger G, Charles MA, Quantitative phenotypic and functional analyses of islet immune cells before and after diabetes onset in the BB rat, *Diabetologia*, 36(11), 1146, 1993.
40. Mordes JP, Rossini AA, Keys to understanding autoimmune diabetes mellitus: the animal models of insulin-dependent diabetes mellitus, *Clin Immunol Allergy*, 1 29, 1987.
41. Yale JF, Grose M, Videtic GM, Marliss EB, Sensitivity of BB rat beta cells as determined by dose–responses to the cytotoxic effects of streptozotocin and alloxan, *Diabetes Research*, 3(3), 161, 1986.
42. Foulis AK, Farquharson MA, Aberrant expression of HLA-DR antigens by insulin-containing beta-cells in recent-onset Type I diabetes mellitus, *Diabetes*, 35(11), 1215, 1986.
43. Foulis AK, Farquharson MA, Hardman R, Aberrant expression of class II major histocompatibility complex molecules by B cells and hyperexpression of class I major histocompatibility complex molecules by insulin containing islets in Type I (insulin-dependent) diabetes mellitus, *Diabetologia*, 30(5), 333, 1987.
44. Dean BM, Walker R, Bone AJ, Baird JD, Cooke A, Pre-diabetes in the spontaneously diabetic BB/E rat: lymphocyte subpopulations in the pancreatic infiltrate and expression of rat MHC class II molecules in endocrine cells, *Diabetologia*, 28(7), 464, 1985.
45. Weringer EJ, Like AA, Identification of T cell subsets and class I and class II antigen expression in islet grafts and pancreatic islets of diabetic BioBreeding/Worcester rats, *American Journal of Pathology*, 132(2), 292, 1988.
46. Bone AJ, Walker R, Varey AM, Cooke A, Baird JD, Effect of cyclosporin on pancreatic events and development of diabetes in BB/Edinburgh rats, *Diabetes*, 39(4), 508, 1990.
47. Ono SJ, Issa-Chergui B, Colle E, Guttmann RD, Seemayer, TA, Fuks A, IDDM in BB rats. Enhanced MHC class I heavy-chain gene expression in pancreatic islets, *Diabetes*, 37(10), 1411, 1988.
48. Majno G, Joris I, Handler ES, Desemone J, Mordes JP, Rossini AA, A pancreatic venular defect in the BB/Wor rat, *American Journal of Pathology*, 128(2), 210, 1987.
49. Sutherland D, Sibley R, Chinn P, Michael A, Srikanta S et al., Twin to twin pancreas transplantation (Tx): reversal and reenactment of the pathogenesis of Type I diabetes, *Clinical Research*, 32, 561A, 1984.
50. Harrison LC, Islet cell antigens in insulin-dependent diabetes: Pandora's box revisited, *Immunology Today*, 13(9), 348, 1992.
51. Dahlquist G, Savilahti E, Landin-Olsson M, An increased level of antibodies to beta-lactoglobulin is a risk determinant for early-onset Type I (insulin-dependent) diabetes mellitus independent of islet cell antibodies and early introduction of cow's milk, *Diabetologia*, 35(10), 980, 1992.

52. Casali P, Nakamura M, Ginsberg-Fellner F, Notkins AL, Frequency of B cells committed to the production of antibodies to insulin in newly diagnosed patients with insulin-dependent diabetes mellitus and generation of high affinity human monoclonal IgG to insulin, *Journal of Immunology*, 144(10), 3741, 1990.

53. Dyrberg T, Nakhooda AF, Baekkeskov S, Lernmark A, Poussier P, Marliss EB, Islet cell surface antibodies and lymphocyte antibodies in the spontaneously diabetic BB Wistar rat, *Diabetes*, 31(3), 278, 1982.

54. Schlosser M, Ziegler B, Augstein P, Kloting I, Ziegler M, Occurrence of islet cell reactive autoantibodies in diabetes-prone BB/OK rats is not associated with the onset of diabetes: a cross-sectional study of BB rats and their diabetes-resistant congenic strains, *Diabetes Research*, 26(2), 67, 1994.

55. Ko IY, Ihm SH, Yoon JW, Studies on autoimmunity for initiation of beta-cell destruction. VIII. Pancreatic beta-cell dependent autoantibody to a 38 kilodalton protein precedes the clinical onset of diabetes in BB rats, *Diabetologia*, 34(8), 548, 1991.

56. Buschard K, Josefsen K, Horn T, Fredman P, Sulphatide and sulfatide antibodies in insulin-dependent diabetes mellitus, *Lancet*, 342(8875), 840, 1993.

57. Petersen JS, MacKay P, Plesner A, Karlsen A, Gotfredsen C, Verland S, Michelsen B, Dyrberg T, Treatment with gad65 or bsa does not protect against diabetes in bb rats, *Autoimmunity*, 25(3), 129, 1997.

58. Griffin AC, Zhao WG, Wegmann KW, Hickey WF, Experimental autoimmune insulitis induction by T lymphocytes specific for a peptide of proinsulin, *American Journal of Pathology*, 147(3), 845, 1995.

59. Cheung R, Karjalainen J, Vandermeulen J, Singal DP, Dosch HM, T cells from children with IDDM are sensitized to bovine serum albumin, *Scandinavian Journal of Immunology*, 40(6), 623, 1994.

60. Dyrberg T, Schwimmbeck PL, Oldstone MB, Inhibition of diabetes in BB rats by virus infection, *Journal of Clinical Investigation*, 81(3), 928, 1988.

61. Bertrand S, Vigeant C, Yale JF, Predictive value of lymphocyte antibodies for the appearance of diabetes in BB rats, *Diabetes*, 43(1), 137, 1994.

62. Doukas J, Majno G, Mordes JP, Anti-endothelial cell autoantibodies in BB rats with spontaneous and induced IDDM, *Diabetes*, 45(9), 1209, 1996.

63. Bonner-Weir S, Deery D, Leahy JL, Weir GC, Compensatory growth of pancreatic beta-cells in adult rats after short-term glucose infusion, *Diabetes*, 38(1), 49, 1989.

64. Ogawa A, Johnson JH, Ohneda M, McAllister CT, Inman L, Alam T, Unger RH, Roles of insulin resistance and beta-cell dysfunction in dexamethasone-induced diabetes, *Journal of Clinical Investigation*, 90(2), 497, 1992.

65. Marynissen G, Malaisse WJ, Van Assche FA, Influence of lactation on morphometric and secretory variables in pancreatic beta-cell of mildly diabetic rats, *Diabetes*, 36(8), 883, 1987.

66. Chen L, Appel MC, Alam T, Miyaura C, Sestak A, O'Neil J, Unger RH, Newgard CB, Factors regulating islet regeneration in the post-insulinoma NEDH rat, *Advances in Experimental Medicine & Biology*, 321 71, 1992.

67. Swenne I, Effects of aging on the regenerative capacity of the pancreatic B-cell of the rat, *Diabetes*, 32(1), 14, 1983.

68. McEvoy RC, Changes in the volumes of the A-, B-, and D-cell populations in the pancreatic islets during the postnatal development of the rat, *Diabetes*, 30(10), 813, 1981.

69. Bone AJ, Walker R, Dean BM, Baird JD, Cooke A, Pre-diabetes in the spontaneously diabetic BB/E rat: pancreatic infiltration and islet cell proliferation, *Acta Endocrinologica*, 115(4), 447, 1987.

70. Dunger A, Lucke S, Kloting I, Hahn HJ, 3H-Thymidine incorporation into islets obtained from prediabetic BB rats, *Experimental & Clinical Endocrinology*, 93(2–3), 267, 1989.

71. Komiya I, Baetens D, Kuwajima M, Orci L, Unger RH, Compensatory capabilities of islets of BB/Wor rats exposed to sustained hyperglycemia, *Metabolism: Clinical & Experimental*, 39(6), 614, 1990.

72. Scaglia L, Smith FE, Bonner-Weir S, Programmed cell death in post-partum involuting islets. *Diabetes*, 42 (Suppl. 1), 11A, 1993.

73. Lucke S, Besch W, Kauert C, Hahn HJ, The endocrine pancreas of BB/OK-rats before and at diagnosis of hyperglycemia, *Experimental & Clinical Endocrinology*, 91(2), 161, 1988.

74. Lohr M, Markholst H, Dyrberg T, Kloppel G, Oberholzer M, Lernmark A, Insulitis and diabetes are preceded by a decrease in beta cell volume in diabetes-prone BB rats, *Pancreas*, 4(1), 95, 1989.

75. Finegood DT, Scaglia L, Bonner-Weir S, Dynamics of beta-cell mass in the growing rat pancreas. Estimation with a simple mathematical model, *Diabetes*, 44(3), 249, 1995.

76. Like AA, Insulin injections prevent diabetes (DB) in Biobreeding/Worcester (BB/Wor) rats. *Diabetes*, 35(Suppl. 1), 74A, 1986.

77. Gotfredsen CF, Buschard K, Frandsen EK, Reduction of diabetes incidence of BB Wistar rats by early prophylactic insulin treatment of diabetes-prone animals, *Diabetologia*, 28(12), 933, 1985.

78. Appel MC, O'Neil JJ, Prevention of spontaneous diabetes in the BB/W rat by insulin treatment. *Pancreas*, 1, 356, 1986.

79. Vlahos WD, Seemayer TA, Yale JF, Diabetes prevention in BB rats by inhibition of endogenous insulin secretion, *Metabolism: Clinical & Experimental*, 40(8), 825, 1991.

80. Buschard K, The functional state of the beta cells in the pathogenesis of insulin-dependent diabetes mellitus, *Autoimmunity*, 10(1), 65, 1991.

81. Koevary S, Rossini A, Stoller W, Chick W, Williams RM, Passive transfer of diabetes in the BB/W rat, *Science*, 220(4598), 727, 1983.

82. Koevary SB, Williams DE, Williams RM, Chick WL, Passive transfer of diabetes from BB/W to Wistar-Furth rats, *Journal of Clinical Investigation*, 75(6), 1904, 1985.

83. Like AA, Weringer EJ, Holdash A, McGill P, Atkinson D, Rossini AA, Adoptive transfer of autoimmune diabetes mellitus in biobreeding/Worcester (BB/W) inbred and hybrid rats, *Journal of Immunology*, 134(3), 1583, 1985.

84. Handler ES, Mordes JP, McKeever U, Nakamura N, Bernhard, J, Greiner DL, Rossini AA, Effects of irradiation on diabetes in the BB/Wor rat, *Autoimmunity*, 4(1–2), 21, 1989.

85. Nakhooda AF, Sole MJ, Marliss EB, Adrenergic regulation of glucagon and insulin secretion during immobilization stress in normal and spontaneously diabetic BB rats, *American Journal of Physiology*, 240(4), E373, 1981.

86. Poussier P, Nakhooda AF, Sima AA, Marliss EB, Passive transfer of insulitis and lymphopenia in the BB rat, *Metabolism: Clinical & Experimental*, 32 (7 Suppl. 1), 73, 1983.

87. Barlow AK, Like AA, Anti-CD2 monoclonal antibodies prevent spontaneous and adoptive transfer of diabetes in the BB/Wor rat, *American Journal of Pathology*, 141(5), 1043, 1992.

88. Ellerman K, Wrobleski M, Rabinovitch A, Like A, Natural killer cell depletion and diabetes mellitus in the BB/Wor rat, *Diabetologia*, 36(7), 596, 1993.

89. Elder ME, Maclaren NK, Identification of profound peripheral T lymphocyte immunodeficiencies in the spontaneously diabetic BB rat, *Journal of Immunology*, 130(4), 1723, 1983.

90. Woda BA, Padden C, Mitogen responsiveness of lymphocytes from the BB/W rat, *Diabetes*, 35(5), 513, 1986.

91. Naji A, Silvers WK, Kimura H, Bellgrau D, Markmann JF, Barker CF, Analytical and functional studies on the T cells of untreated and immunologically tolerant diabetes-prone BB rats, *Journal of Immunology*, 130(5), 2168, 1983.

92. Yale JF, Grose M, Marliss EB, Time course of the lymphopenia in BB rats. Relation to the onset of diabetes, *Diabetes*, 34(10), 955, 1985.

93. Like AA, Guberski DL, Butler L, Diabetic BioBreeding/Worcester (BB/Wor) rats need not be lymphopenic, *Journal of Immunology*, 136(9), 3254, 1986.

94. Jacobson JD, Markmann JF, Brayman KL, Barker CF, Naji A, Prevention of recurrent autoimmune diabetes in BB rats by anti-asialo-GM1 antibody, *Diabetes*, 37(6), 838, 1988.

95. Edouard P, Hiserodt JC, Plamondon C, Poussier P, CD8+ T-cells are required for adoptive transfer of the BB rat diabetic syndrome, *Diabetes*, 42(3), 390, 1993.

96. Bellgrau D, Lagarde AC, Cytotoxic T-cell precursors with low-level CD8 in the diabetes-prone Biobreeding rat: implications for generation of an autoimmune T-cell repertoire, *Proceedings of the National Academy of Sciences of the United States of America*, 87(1), 313, 1990.

97. Crisa L, Greiner DL, Mordes JP, MacDonald RG, Handler ES, Czech MP, Rossini AA, Biochemical studies of RT6 alloantigens in BB/Wor and normal rats. Evidence for intact unexpressed RT6a structural gene in diabetes-prone BB rats, *Diabetes*, 39(10), 1279, 1990.

98. Zadeh HH, Greiner DL, Wu DY, Tausche F, Goldschneider I, Abnormalities in the export and fate of recent thymic emigrants in diabetes-prone BB/W rats, *Autoimmunity*, 24(1), 35, 1996.

99. Metroz-Dayer MD, Mouland A, Brideau C, Duhamel D, Poussier P, Adoptive transfer of diabetes in BB rats induced by CD4 T lymphocytes, *Diabetes*, 39(8), 928, 1990.

100. Groen H, van der Berk JM, Nieuwenhuis P, Kampinga J, Peripheral T cells in diabetes prone (DP) BB rats are CD45R-negative, *Thymus*, 14(1–3), 145, 1989.

101. Mordes JP, Gallina DL, Handler ES, Greiner DL, Nakamura, N, Pelletier A, Rossini AA, Transfusions enriched for W3/25+ helper/inducer T lymphocytes prevent spontaneous diabetes in the BB/W rat, *Diabetologia*, 30(1), 22, 1987.

102. Whalen BJ, Greiner DL, Mordes JP, Rossini AA, Adoptive transfer of autoimmune diabetes mellitus to athymic rats: synergy of CD4$^+$ and CD8$^+$ T cells and prevention by RT6$^+$ T cells, *Journal of Autoimmunity*, 7(6), 819, 1994.

103. Miller BJ, Appel MC, O'Neil JJ, Wicker, LS, Both the Lyt-2+ and L3T4+ T cell subsets are required for the transfer of diabetes in nonobese diabetic mice, *Journal of Immunology*, 140(1), 52, 1988.

104. Kurasawa K, Sakamoto A, Maeda T, Sumida T, Ito I, Tomioka H, Yoshida S, Koike T, Short-term administration of anti-L3T4 MoAb prevents diabetes in NOD mice, *Clinical & Experimental Immunology*, 91(3), 376, 1993.

105. Lubaroff DM, Butcher GW, DeWitt C, Gill TJ, III, Gunther E, Howard JC, Wonigeit K, Fourth international workshop on alloantigenic systems in the rat, *Transplantation Proceedings*, 15 1683, 1983.

106. McKeever U, Mordes JP, Greiner DL, Appel MC, Rozing J, Handler ES, Rossini AA, Adoptive transfer of autoimmune diabetes and thyroiditis to athymic rats, *Proceedings of the National Academy of Sciences of the United States of America*, 87(19), 7618, 1990.

107. Crisa L, Sarkar P, Waite DJ, Friedrich FH, Koch-Nolte, Rajan TV, Mordes JP, Handler ES, Thiele HG, Rossini AA et al., An RT6a gene is transcribed and translated in lymphopenic diabetes-prone BB rats, *Diabetes*, 42(5), 688, 1993.

108. Mojcik CF, Greiner DL, Medlock ES, Komschlies KL, Goldschneider I, Characterization of RT6 bearing rat lymphocytes. I. Ontogeny of the RT6$^+$ subset, *Cellular Immunology*, 114(2), 336, 1988.

109. Mojcik CF, Greiner DL, Goldschneider I, Characterization of RT6-bearing rat lymphocytes. II. Developmental relationships of RT6- and RT6$^+$ T cells, *Developmental Immunology*, 1(3), 191, 1991.

110. Thiele HG, Koch F, Hamann A, Arndt R, Biochemical characterization of the T-cell alloantigen RT-6.2, *Immunology*, 59(2), 195, 1986.

111. Koch F, Thiele HG, Low MG, Release of the rat T cell alloantigen RT-6.2 from cell membranes by phosphatidylinositol-specific phospholipase C, *Journal of Experimental Medicine*, 164(4), 1338, 1986.

112. Waite DJ, Appel MC, Handler ES, Mordes JP, Rossini AA, Greiner DL, Ontogeny and immunohistochemical localization of thymus-dependent and thymus-independent RT6 cells in the rat, *American Journal of Pathology*, 148(6), 2043, 1996.

113. Greiner DL, Malkani S, Kanaitsuka T, Bortell R, Doukas, J, Rigby M, Whalen B, Stevens LA, Moss J, Mordes JP, Rossini AA, The T cell marker RT6 in a rat model of autoimmune diabetes, *Advances in Experimental Medicine & Biology*, 419 209, 1997.

114. Fangmann J, Schwinzer R, Hedrich HJ, Kloting I, Wonigeit, K, Diabetes-prone BB rats express the RT6 alloantigen on intestinal intraepithelial lymphocytes, *European Journal of Immunology*, 21(9), 2011, 1991.

115. Scott J, The spontaneously diabetic BB rat: sites of the defects leading to autoimmunity and diabetes mellitus. A review, *Current Topics in Microbiology & Immunology* 156 1, 1990.

116. Uchikoshi F, Ito T, Kamiike W, Nakao H, Makino S, Miyasaka M, Nozawa M, Matsuda H, Restoration of immune abnormalities in diabetic BB rats after pancreas transplantation. I. Macrochimerism of donor-graft-derived RT6$^+$ T cells responsible for restoration of immune responsiveness and suppression of autoimmune reaction, *Transplantation*, 61(11), 1629, 1996.

117. Thiele HG, Koch F, Kashan A, Postnatal distribution profiles of Thy-1+ and RT6 cells in peripheral lymph nodes of DA rats, *Transplantation Proceedings*, 19, 3157, 1987.

118. Greiner DL, Handler ES, Nakano K, Mordes, JP, Rossini AA, Absence of the RT-6 T cell subset in diabetes-prone BB/W rats, *Journal of Immunology*, 136(1), 148, 1986.

119. Groen H, Klatter FA, Brons NH, Wubbena AS, Nieuwenhuis, P, Kampinga J, High-frequency, but reduced absolute numbers of recent thymic migrants among peripheral blood T lymphocytes in diabetes-prone BB rats, *Cellular Immunology*, 163(1), 113, 1995.

120. Haag F, Nolte F, Lernmark A, Simrell C, Thiele HG, Analysis of T-cell surface marker profiles during the postnatal ontogeny of normal and diabetes-prone rats, *Transplantation Proceedings*, 25(5), 2831, 1993.

121. Georgiou HM, Bellgrau D, Thymus transplantation and disease prevention in the diabetes-prone Bio-Breeding rat, *Journal of Immunology*, 142(10), 3400, 1989.

122. Georgiou HM, Lagarde AC, Bellgrau D, T cell dysfunction in the diabetes-prone BB rat. A role for thymic migrants that are not T cell precursors, *Journal of Experimental Medicine*, 167(1), 132, 1988.

123. Jacob HJ, Pettersson A, Wilson D, Mao Y, Lernmark A, Lander ES, Genetic dissection of autoimmune Type I diabetes in the BB rat, *Nature Genetics*, 2(1), 56, 1992.

124. Rossini AA, Mordes JP, Greiner DL, Nakano K, Appel MC, Handler ES, Spleen cell transfusion in the Bio-Breeding/Worcester rat. Prevention of diabetes, major histocompatibility complex restriction, and long-term persistence of transfused cells, *Journal of Clinical Investigation*, 77(4), 1399, 1986.

125. Burstein D, Mordes JP, Greiner DL, Stein D, Nakamura N, Handler ES, Rossini AA, Prevention of diabetes in BB/Wor rat by single transfusion of spleen cells. Parameters that affect degree of protection, *Diabetes*, 38(1), 24, 1989.

126. Greiner DL, Mordes JP, Handler ES, Angelillo M, Nakamura N, Rossini AA, Depletion of RT6.1+ T lymphocytes induces diabetes in resistant biobreeding/Worcester (BB/W) rats, *Journal of Experimental Medicine*, 166(2), 461, 1987.

127. Markholst H, Eastman S, Wilson D, Andreasen BE, Lernmark A, Diabetes segregates as a single locus in crosses between inbred BB rats prone or resistant to diabetes, *Journal of Experimental Medicine*, 174(1), 297, 1991.

128. Thomas VA, Woda BA, Handler ES, Greiner, DL, Mordes JP, Rossini AA, Altered expression of diabetes in BB/Wor rats by exposure to viral pathogens, *Diabetes*, 40(2), 255, 1991.

129. Like AA, Depletion of RT6.1+ T lymphocytes alone is insufficient to induce diabetes in diabetes-resistant BB/Wor rats, *American Journal of Pathology*, 136(3), 565, 1990.

130. Ellerman K, Like AA, Regulatory T cells in rat autoimmune diabetes are strain dependent. *Diabetes*, 44(Suppl. 1), 138A, 1995.

131. Whalen BJ, Doukas J, Mordes JP, Rossini AA, Greiner DL, Induction of insulin-dependent diabetes mellitus in PVG.RT1(u) rats, *Transplantation Proceedings*, 29(3), 1684, 1997.

132. Angelillo M, Greiner DL, Mordes JP, Handler ES, Nakamura N, McKeever U, Rossini A, Absence of RT6+ T cells in diabetes-prone BioBreeding/Worcester rats is due to genetic and cell developmental defects, *Journal of Immunology*, 141(12), 4146, 1988.

133. Rigby MR, Bortell R, Greiner DL, Czech MP, Klarlund JK, Mordes JP, Rossini AA, The rat T-cell surface protein RT6 is associated with src family tyrosine kinases and generates an activation signal, *Diabetes*, 45(10), 1419, 1996.

134. Plamondon C, Kottis V, Brideau C, Metroz-Dayer MD, Poussier P, Abnormal thymocyte maturation in spontaneously diabetic BB rats involves the deletion of CD4-8+ cells, *Journal of Immunology*, 144(3), 923, 1990.

135. Krensky AM, Sanchez-Madrid F, Robbins E, Nagy JA, Springer TA, Burakoff SJ, The functional significance, distribution, and structure of LFA-1, LFA-2, and LFA-3: cell surface antigens associated with CTL-target interactions, *Journal of Immunology*, 131(2), 611, 1983.

136. Williams AF, Barclay AN, Clark SJ, Paterson DJ, Willis AC, Similarities in sequences and cellular expression between rat CD2 and CD4 antigens, *Journal of Experimental Medicine*, 165(2), 368, 1987.

137. Hunt HD, Lubaroff DM, Identification of functional T cell subsets and surface antigen changes during activation as they relate to RT6, *Cellular Immunology*, 143(1), 194, 1992.

138. Ernst DN, Lubaroff DM, Membrane antigen phenotype of sensitized T lymphocytes mediating tuberculin-delayed hypersensitivity in rats, *Cellular Immunology*, 88(2), 436, 1984.

139. Haag F, Koch-Nolte F, Kuhl M, Lorenzen S, Thiele HG, Premature stop codons inactivate the RT6 genes of the human and chimpanzee species, *Journal of Molecular Biology*, 243(3), 537, 1994.

140. Ramsdell F, Fowlkes BJ, Clonal deletion vs. clonal anergy: the role of the thymus in inducing self tolerance, *Science*, 248(4961), 1342, 1990.

141. Groen H, Klatter FA, Brons NH, Mesander G, Nieuwenhuis P, Kampinga J, Abnormal thymocyte subset distribution and differential reduction of CD4+ and CD8+ T cell subsets during peripheral maturation in diabetes-prone BioBreeding rats, *Journal of Immunology*, 156(3), 1269, 1996.

142. Jackson R, Kadison P, Buse J, Rassi N, Jegasothy B, Eisenbarth GS, Lymphocyte abnormalities in the BB rat, *Metabolism: Clinical & Experimental*, 32 (7 Suppl. 1), 83, 1983.

143. Naji A, Kimura H, Silvers WK, Barker CF, Numerical and functional abnormality of T suppressor cells in diabetic rats, *Surgery*, 94(2), 235, 1983.

144. Like AA, Kislauskis E, Williams RR, Rossini AA, Neonatal thymectomy prevents spontaneous diabetes mellitus in the BB/W rat, *Science*, 216(4546), 644, 1982.

145. Hosszufalusi N, Chan E, Granger G, Charles MA, Quantitative analyses comparing all major spleen cell phenotypes in BB and normal rats: autoimmune imbalance and double negative T cells associated with resistant, prone and diabetic animals, *Journal of Autoimmunity*, 5(3), 305, 1992.

146. Posselt AM, Barker CF, Friedman AL, Naji, A, Prevention of autoimmune diabetes in the BB rat by intrathymic islet transplantation at birth, *Science*, 256(5061), 1321, 1992.

147. Like AA, Guberski DL, Butler L, Influence of environmental viral agents on frequency and tempo of diabetes mellitus in BB/Wor rats, *Diabetes*, 40(2), 259, 1991.

148. Jiang Z, Woda BA, Cytokine gene expression in the islets of the diabetic Biobreeding/Worcester rat, *Journal of Immunology*, 146(9), 2990, 1991.

149. Tullin S, Farris P, Petersen JS, Hornum L, Jackerott M, Markholst H, A pronounced thymic B cell deficiency in the spontaneously diabetic BB rat, *Journal of Immunology*, 158(11), 5554, 1997.

150. Bellgrau D, Redd JM, Sellins KS, Peculiar T-cell signaling does not preclude positive selection in the diabetes-prone BB rat, *Diabetes*, 43(1), 47, 1994.

151. Wu G, Marliss EB, Deficiency of purine nucleoside phosphorylase activity in thymocytes from the immunodeficient diabetic BB rat, *Clinical & Experimental Immunology*, 86(2), 260, 1991.

152. Hodes RJ, Sharrow SO, Solomon A, Failure of T cell receptor V beta negative selection in an athymic environment, *Science*, 246(4933), 1041, 1989.

153. Fry AM, Jones LA, Kruisbeek AM, Matis LA, Thymic requirement for clonal deletion during T cell development, *Science*, 246(4933), 1044, 1989.

154. Doukas J, Mordes JP, Swymer C, Niedzwiecki D, Mason R, Rozing J, Rossini AA, Greiner DL, Thymic epithelial defects and predisposition to autoimmune disease in BB rats, *American Journal of Pathology*, 145(6), 1517, 1994.

155. Francfort JW, Barker CF, Kimura H, Silvers WK, Frohman, M, Naji A, Increased incidence of Ia antigen-bearing T lymphocytes in the spontaneously diabetic BB rat, *Journal of Immunology*, 134(3), 1577, 1985.

156. Scott J, Engelhard VH, Benjamin DC, Bone marrow irradiation chimeras in the BB rat: evidence suggesting two defects leading to diabetes and lymphopenia, *Diabetologia*, 30(10), 774, 1987.

157. Rozing J, Coolen C, Tielen FJ, Weegenaar J, Schuurman, HJ, Greiner DL, Rossini AA, Defects in the thymic epithelial stroma of diabetes prone BB rats, *Thymus*, 14(1-3), 125, 1989.

158. Naji A, Silvers WK, Bellgrau D, Anderson AO, Plotkin S, Barker CF, Prevention of diabetes in rats by bone marrow transplantation, *Annals of Surgery*, 194 328, 1981.

159. Greiner DL, Mordes JP, Handler ES, Nakamura N, Angelillo, M, Rossini AA, Prothymocyte development in diabetes-prone BB rats: description of a defect that predisposes to immune abnormalities, *Transplantation Proceedings*, 19(1 Pt 2), 976, 1987.

160. Helderman JH, Role of insulin in the intermediary metabolism of the activated thymic-derived lymphocyte, *Journal of Clinical Investigation*, 67(6), 1636, 1981.

161. Brand K, Williams JF, Weidemann MJ, Glucose and glutamine metabolism in rat thymocytes, *Biochemical Journal*, 221(2), 471, 1984.

162. Roos D, Loos JA, Changes in the carbohydrate metabolism of mitogenically stimulated human peripheral lymphocytes. II. Relative importance of glycolysis and oxidative phosphorylation on phytohaemagglutinin stimulation, *Experimental Cell Research*, 77(1), 127, 1973.

163. Hume DA, Radik JL, Ferber E, Weidemann MJ, Aerobic glycolysis and lymphocyte transformation, *Biochemical Journal*, 174(3), 703, 1978.
164. Brand K, Leibold W, Luppa P, Schoerner C, Schulz A, Metabolic alterations associated with proliferation of mitogen-activated lymphocytes and of lymphoblastoid cell lines: evaluation of glucose and glutamine metabolism, *Immunobiology*, 173(1), 23, 1986.
165. Jacobs DB, Lee TP, Jung CY, Mookerjee BK, Mechanism of mitogen-induced stimulation of glucose transport in human peripheral blood mononuclear cells. Evidence of an intracellular reserve pool of glucose carriers and their recruitment, *Journal of Clinical Investigation*, 83(2), 437, 1989.
166. Resch K, Prester M, Ferber E, Gelfand EW, The inhibition of initial steps of lymphocyte transformation by cytochalasin B1, *Journal of Immunology*, 117(5 Pt. 1), 1705, 1976.
167. Mookerjee BK, Jung CY, The effects of cytochalasins on lymphocytes: mechanism of action of Cytochalasin A on responses to phytomitogens, *Journal of Immunology*, 128(5), 2153, 1982.
168. Szondy Z, Newsholme EA, The effect of glutamine concentration on the activity of carbamoyl-phosphate synthase II and on the incorporation of [3H]thymidine into DNA in rat mesenteric lymphocytes stimulated by phytohaemagglutinin, *Biochemical Journal*, 261(3), 979, 1989.
169. Misra M, Duguid WP, Marliss EB, Prevention of diabetes in the spontaneously diabetic BB rat by the glutamine antimetabolite acivicin, *Canadian Journal of Physiology & Pharmacology* 74(2), 163, 1996.
170. Field CJ, Chayoth R, Montambault M, Marliss EB, Enhanced 2-deoxy-D-glucose uptake and metabolism in splenocytes from diabetic and diabetes-prone BB rats. Further evidence to support prior *in vivo* activation, *Journal of Biological Chemistry*, 266(6), 3675, 1991.
171. Field CJ, Wu G, Metroz-Dayer MD, Montambault M, Marliss, EB, Lactate production is the major metabolic fate of glucose in splenocytes and is altered in spontaneously diabetic BB rats, *Biochemical Journal*, 272(2), 445, 1990.
172. Field CJ, Wu G, Marliss EB, Enhanced metabolism of glucose and glutamine in mesenteric lymph node lymphocytes from spontaneously diabetic BB rats, *Canadian Journal of Physiology & Pharmacology*, 72(7), 827, 1994.
173. Field CJ, A diet producing a low diabetes incidence modifies immune abnormalities in diabetes-prone BB rats, *Journal of Nutrition*, 125(10), 2595, 1995.
174. Lee KU, Kim MK, Amano K, Pak CY, Jaworski MA, Mehta JG, Yoon JW, Preferential infiltration of macrophages during early stages of insulitis in diabetes-prone BB rats, *Diabetes*, 37(8), 1053, 1988.
175. Hanenberg H, Kolb-Bachofen V, Kantwerk-Funke G, Kolb H, Macrophage infiltration precedes and is a prerequisite for lymphocytic insulitis in pancreatic islets of pre-diabetic BB rats, *Diabetologia*, 32(2), 126, 1989.
176. Kolb-Bachofen V, Kolb H, "Single cell infiltration" of pancreatic islets: an alternative concept of B-islet cell destruction, *Diabetologia*, 27, 297, 1984.
177. Kroncke KD, Funda J, Berschick B, Kolb H, Kolb-Bachofen V, Macrophage cytotoxicity towards isolated rat islet cells: neither lysis nor its protection by nicotinamide are beta-cell specific, *Diabetologia*, 34(4), 232, 1991.
178. Oschilewski U, Kiesel U, Kolb H, Administration of silica prevents diabetes in BB-rats, *Diabetes*, 34(2), 197, 1985.
179. Kiesel U, Oschilewski M, Kantwerk G, Maruta M, Hanenber H, Treichel U, Kolb-Bachofen V, Hartung HP, Kolb H, Essential role of macrophages in the development of Type I diabetes in BB rats, *Transplantaton Proceedings*, 6 1525, 1986.
180. Amano K, Yoon JW, Studies on autoimmunity for initiation of beta-cell destruction. V. Decrease of macrophage-dependent T lymphocytes and natural killer cytotoxicity in silica-treated BB rats, *Diabetes*, 39(5), 590, 1990.
181. Mandrup-Poulsen T, Bendtzen K, Nerup J, Dinarello CA, Svenson M, Nielsen JH, Affinity-purified human interleukin I is cytotoxic to isolated islets of Langerhans, *Diabetologia*, 29(1), 63, 1986.
182. Sandler S, Andersson A, Hellerstrom C, Inhibitory effects of interleukin 1 on insulin secretion, insulin biosynthesis, and oxidative metabolism of isolated rat pancreatic islets, *Endocrinology*, 121(4), 1424, 1987.

183. Rabinovitch A, Pukel C, Baquerizo H, Mackay P, Immunological mechanisms of islet B cell destruction; cytotoxic cells and cytokines, in *Frontiers in Diabetes Research. Lessons from Animal Diabetes II*, Shafrir E and Renold AE, Eds., John Libbey, London, 1988, 52.

184. Wogensen LD, Kolb-Bachofen V, Christensen P, Dinarello, CA, Mandrup-Poulsen T, Martin S, Nerup J, Functional and morphological effects of interleukin-1 beta on the perfused rat pancreas, *Diabetologia*, 33(1), 15, 1990.

185. Rabinovitch A, Immunoregulatory and cytokine imbalances in the pathogenesis of IDDM. Therapeutic intervention by immunostimulation? *Diabetes*, 43(5), 613, 1994.

186. Pukel C, Baquerizo H, Rabinovitch A, Interleukin 2 activates BB/W diabetic rat lymphoid cells cytotoxic to islet cells, *Diabetes*, 36(11), 1217, 1987.

187. Mandrup-Poulsen T, Bendtzen K, Dinarello CA, Nerup J, Human tumor necrosis factor potentiates human interleukin 1-mediated rat pancreatic beta-cell cytotoxicity, *Journal of Immunology*, 139(12), 4077, 1987.

188. Prud'homme GJ, Fuks A, Colle E, Guttmann RD, Isolation of T-lymphocyte lines with specificity for islet cell antigens from spontaneously diabetic (insulin-dependent) rats, *Diabetes*, 33(8), 801, 1984.

189. Rothe H, Fehsel K, Kolb H, Tumour necrosis factor alpha production is upregulated in diabetes prone BB rats, *Diabetologia*, 33(9), 573, 1990.

190. Andrade J, Conde M, Sobrino F, Bedoya FJ, Activation of peritoneal macrophages during the prediabetic phase in low-dose streptozotocin-treated mice, *FEBS Letters*, 327(1), 32, 1993.

191. Moncada S, Palmer RM, Higgs EA, Nitric oxide: physiology, pathophysiology, and pharmacology, *Pharmacological Reviews*, 43(2), 109, 1991.

192. Kolb H, Kolb-Bachofen V, Nitric oxide: a pathogenetic factor in autoimmunity, *Immunology Today*, 13(5), 157, 1992.

193. Welsh N, Eizirik DL, Bendtzen K, Sandler S, Interleukin-1 beta-induced nitric oxide production in isolated rat pancreatic islets requires gene transcription and may lead to inhibition of the Krebs cycle enzyme aconitase, *Endocrinology*, 129(6), 3167, 1991.

194. Fehsel K, Jalowy A, Qi S, Burkart V, Hartmann B, Kolb H, Islet cell DNA is a target of inflammatory attack by nitric oxide, *Diabetes*, 42(3), 496, 1993.

195. Wilson GL, Patton NJ, McCord JM, Mullins DW, Mossman BT, Mechanisms of streptozotocin- and alloxan-induced damage in rat B cells, *Diabetologia*, 27(6), 587, 1984.

196. LeDoux SP, Hall CR, Forbes PM, Patton NJ, Wilson GL, Mechanisms of nicotinamide and thymidine protection from alloxan and streptozocin toxicity, *Diabetes*, 37(8), 1015, 1988.

197. Yamada K, Nonaka K, Hanafusa T, Miyazaki A, Toyoshima H, Tarui S, Preventive and therapeutic effects of large-dose nicotinamide injections on diabetes associated with insulitis. An observation in nonobese diabetic (NOD) mice, *Diabetes*, 31(9), 749, 1982.

198. Nakajima H, Fujino-Kurihara H, Hanafusa T et al., Nicotinamide prevents the development of cyclophosphamide-induced diabetes mellitus in male non-obese diabetic (NOD) mice, *Biomedical Research*, 6 185, 1985.

199. Corbett JA, McDaniel ML, Does nitric oxide mediate autoimmune destruction of beta-cells? Possible therapeutic interventions in IDDM, *Diabetes*, 41(8), 897, 1992.

200. Wu G, Nitric oxide synthesis and the effect of aminoguanidine and NG-monomethyl-L-arginine on the onset of diabetes in the spontaneously diabetic BB rat, *Diabetes*, 44(3), 360, 1995.

201. Lindsay RM, Smith W, Rossiter SP, McIntyre MA, Williams BC, Baird JD, N-omega-nitro-L-arginine methyl ester reduces the incidence of IDDM in BB/E rats, *Diabetes*, 44(3), 365, 1995.

202. Ortaldo JR, Herberman RB, Heterogeneity of natural killer cells, *Annual Review of Immunology* 2 359, 1984.

203. Herberman RB, Reynolds CW, Ortaldo JR, Mechanism of cytotoxicity by natural killer (NK) cells, *Annual Review of Immunology* 4 651, 1986.

204. Ortaldo JR, Reynolds CW, Natural killer activity: definition of a function rather than a cell type, *Journal of Immunology* 138(12), 4545, 1987.

205. Woda BA, Biron CA, Natural killer cell number and function in the spontaneously diabetic BB/W rat, *Journal of Immunology* 137(6), 1860, 1986.

206. Nakamura N, Woda BA, Tafuri A, Greiner DL, Reynolds CW, Ortaldo J, Chick W, Handler ES, Mordes JP, Rossini AA, Intrinsic cytotoxicity of natural killer cells to pancreatic islets *in vitro*, *Diabetes*, 39(7), 836, 1990.

207. Pozzilli P, Sensi M, Gorsuch A, Bottazzo, GF, Cudworth AG, Evidence for raised K-cell levels in type-I diabetes, *Lancet*, 2(8135), 173, 1979.

208. Sensi M, Pozzilli P, Gorsuch AN, Bottazzo GF, Cudworth AG, Increased killer cell activity in insulin dependent (Type 1) diabetes mellitus, *Diabetologia*, 20(2), 106, 1981.

209. Mizel SB, The interleukins, *FASEB Journal*, 3(12), 2379, 1989.

210. Healey D, Ozegbe P, Arden S, Chandler P, Hutton J, Cooke A, *In vivo* activity and *in vitro* specificity of CD4⁺ Th1 and Th2 cells derived from the spleens of diabetic NOD mice, *Journal of Clinical Investigation*, 95(6), 2979, 1995.

211. Katz JD, Benoist C, Mathis D, T helper cell subsets in insulin-dependent diabetes, *Science*, 268(5214), 1185, 1995.

212. Rabinovitch A, Suarez-Pinzon W, El-Sheikh A, Sorensen O, Power RF, Cytokine gene expression in pancreatic islet-infiltrating leukocytes of BB rats: expression of Th1 cytokines correlates with beta-cell destructive insulitis and IDDM, *Diabetes*, 45(6), 749, 1996.

213. Zipris D, Evidence that Th1 lymphocytes predominate in islet inflammation and thyroiditis in the BioBreeding (BB) rat, *Journal of Autoimmunity* 9(3), 315, 1996.

214. Bellgrau D, Stenger D, Richards C, Bao F, The diabetic BB rat. Neither Th1 nor Th2? *Hormone & Metabolic Research*, 28(6), 299, 1996.

215. Rabinovitch A, Sumoski W, Rajotte RV, Warnock GL, Cytotoxic effects of cytokines on human pancreatic islet cells in monolayer culture, *Journal of Clinical Endocrinology & Metabolism*, 71(1), 152, 1990.

216. Dunger A, Schroder D, Augstein P, Witstruck T, Wachlin G, Vogt L, Ziegler B, Schmidt S, Impact of metabolic activity of beta cells on cytokine-induced damage and recovery of rat pancreatic islets, *Acta Diabetologica*, 32(4), 217, 1995.

217. Kuttler B, Rosing K, Hahn HJ, Anti-CD4/CyA therapy causes prevention of autoimmune but not allogeneic destruction of grafted islets in BB rats, *Transplantation Proceedings*, 29(4), 2163, 1997.

218. Rossini AA, Greiner DL, Friedman HP, Mordes JP, Immunopathogenesis of diabetes mellitus, *Diabetes Reviews*, 1(1), 43, 1993.

219. Lapchak PH, Guilbert LJ, Rabinovitch A, Tumor necrosis factor production is deficient in diabetes-prone BB rats and can be corrected by complete Freund's adjuvant: a possible immunoregulatory role of tumor necrosis factor in the prevention of diabetes, *Clinical Immunology & Immunopathology*, 65(2), 129, 1992.

220. Handler ES, Mordes JP, Geisberg M, Nakano K, Rossini AA, Effect of ultraviolet (UVB) and X-irradiation on diabetes prone and resistant BB/W rats. *Diabetes*, 34 (Suppl. 1), 69A, 1985.

221. Mordes JP, Greiner DL, Handler ES, Nakamura N, Rossini AA, Possible role of RT-6+ lymphocytes in the pathogenesis of BB/W rat diabetes. *Diabetologia*, 29, 574A, 1986.

222. Tun RY, Peakman M, Alviggi L, Hussain MJ, Lo SS, Shattock M, Pyke DA, Bottazzo GF, Vergani D, Leslie RD, Importance of persistent cellular and humoral immune changes before diabetes develops: prospective study of identical twins, *British Medical Journal*, 308(6936), 1063, 1994.

223. Faustman D, Eisenbarth G, Daley J, Breitmeyer J, Abnormal T-lymphocyte subsets in Type I diabetes, *Diabetes*, 38(11), 1462, 1989.

224. Rayfield EJ, Ault MJ, Keusch GT, Brothers MJ, Nechemias C, Smith H, Infection and diabetes: the case for glucose control, *American Journal of Medicine*, 72(3), 439, 1982.

225. Selam JL, Clot J, Andary M, Mirouze J, Circulating lymphocyte subpopulations in juvenile insulin-dependent diabetes. Correction of abnormalities by adequate blood glucose control, *Diabetologia*, 16(1), 35, 1979.

226. Poussier P, Nakhooda AF, Falk JA, Lee C, Marliss EB, Lymphopenia and abnormal lymphocyte subsets in the "BB" rat: relationship to the diabetic syndrome, *Endocrinology* 110(5), 1825, 1982.

227. MacCuish AC, Urbaniak SJ, Campbell CJ, Duncan LJ, Irvine WJ, Phytohemagglutinin transformation and circulating lymphocyte subpopulations in insulin-dependent diabetic patients, *Diabetes*, 23(8), 708, 1974.

228. Hann S, Kaye R, Falkner B, Subpopulations of peripheral lymphocytes in juvenile diabetes, *Diabetes*, 25(2), 101, 1976.
229. Guttmann RD, Colle E, Michel F, Seemayer T, Spontaneous diabetes mellitus syndrome in the rat. II. T lymphopenia and its association with clinical disease and pancreatic lymphocytic infiltration, *Journal of Immunology*, 130(4), 1732, 1983.
230. Colle E, Fuks A, Poussier P, Edouard P, Guttmann RD, Polygenic nature of spontaneous diabetes in the rat. Permissive MHC haplotype and presence of the lymphopenic trait of the BB rat are not sufficient to produce susceptibility, *Diabetes*, 41(12), 1617, 1992.
231. Woda BA, Like AA, Padden C, McFadden ML, Deficiency of phenotypic cytotoxic-suppressor T lymphocytes in the BB/W rat, *Journal of Immunology*, 136(3), 856, 1986.
232. Rossini AA, Mordes JP, Pelletier AM, Like AA, Transfusions of whole blood prevent spontaneous diabetes mellitus in the BB/W rat, *Science*, 219(4587), 975, 1983.
233. Woda BA, Padden C, BioBreeding/Worcester (BB/Wor) rats are deficient in the generation of functional cytotoxic T cells, *Journal of Immunology*, 139(5), 1514, 1987.
234. Prud'homme GJ, Lapchak PH, Parfrey NA, Colle E, Guttmann, RD, Autoimmunity-prone BB rats lack functional cytotoxic T cells, *Cellular Immunology*, 114(1), 198, 1988.
235. Oldstone MB, Tishon A, Schwimmbeck PL, Shyp S, Lewicki H, Dyrberg T, Cytotoxic T lymphocytes do not control lymphocytic choriomeningitis virus infection of BB diabetes-prone rats, *Journal of General Virology*, 71(4), 785, 1990.
236. Yale JF, Marliss EB, Altered immunity and diabetes in the BB rat, *Clinical & Experimental Immunology*, 57(1), 1, 1984.
237. Prud'homme GJ, Colle E, Fuks A, Goldner-Sauve A, Guttmann RD, Cellular immune abnormalities and autoreactive T lymphocytes in insulin dependent diabetes mellitus in rats, *Immunology Today*, 6 160, 1985.
238. Mathieu C, Kuttler B, Waer M, Bouillon, R, Hahn HJ, Spontaneous reestablishment of self-tolerance in BB/Pfd rats, *Transplantation*, 58(3), 349, 1994.
239. Guttmann RD, Christou N, Fuks A, Colle E, Genetic studies of delayed-type hypersensitivity and concanavalin A responses in inbred rats, *Transplantation Proceedings*, 17 1849, 1985.
240. Weringer EJ, Woodland R, Defective interleukin-2 autocrine regulation of T-lymphocytes in the BB/Wor diabetes-prone rat, in *Frontiers in Diabetes Research. Lessons from Animal Diabetes III*, Shafrir E. Ed., Smith-Gordon, London, 1991, 99.
241. Metroz-Dayer MD, Marliss EB, Poussier P, Evidence that macrophage mediated T cell dysfunction in the diabetic BB rat occurs at the level of calcium mobilization, *Diabetes Research Clinical Practice*, 5 (Suppl. 1), S531, 1988.
242. Gosselin E, Woodland R, Mordes JP, Pelletier A, Rossini AA, Antibody responses to T-dependent antigens are defective in the BB/W rat and the diabetes resistant W-line, *Diabetes*, 34 (Suppl. 1), 66A, 1985.
243. Singal DP, Blajchman MA, Histocompatibility (HL-A) antigens, lymphocytotoxic antibodies and tissue antibodies in patients with diabetes mellitus, *Diabetes*, 22(6), 429, 1973.
244. Davies JL, Kawaguchi Y, Bennett ST, Copeman JB, Cordell HJ, Pritchard LE, Reed PW, Gough SC, Jenkins SC, Palmer SM et al., A genome-wide search for human Type I diabetes susceptibility genes, *Nature*, 371(6493), 130, 1994.
245. Rich SS, Positional cloning works: identification of genes that cause IDDM, *Diabetes*, 44(2), 139, 1995.
246. Thorsby E, Invited anniversary review: HLA associated diseases, *Human Immunology*, 53(1), 1, 1997.
247. Kolb H, Mouse models of insulin dependent diabetes: low-dose streptozocin-induced diabetes and nonobese diabetic (NOD) mice, *Diabetes-Metabolism Reviews*, 3(3), 751, 1987.
248. Colle E, Guttmann RD, Seemayer T, Spontaneous diabetes mellitus syndrome in the rat. I. Association with the major histocompatibility complex, *Journal of Experimental Medicine*, 154(4), 1237, 1981.
249. Jackson RA, Buse JB, Rifai R, Pelletier D, Milford EL, Carpenter CB, Eisenbarth GS, Williams RM, Two genes required for diabetes in BB rats. Evidence from cyclical intercrosses and backcrosses, *Journal of Experimental Medicine*, 159(6), 1629, 1984.

250. Colle E, Guttmann RD, Seemayer TA, Association of spontaneous thyroiditis with the major histocompatibility complex of the rat, *Endocrinology*, 116(4), 1243, 1985.
251. Colle E, Guttmann RD, Fuks A, Seemayer TA, Prud'homme GJ, Genetics of the spontaneous diabetic syndrome. Interaction of MHC and non-MHC-associated factors, *Molecular Biology & Medicine*, 3(1), 13, 1986.
252. Kloting I, Stark O, Genetic studies of IDDM in BB rats: the incidence of diabetes in F2 and first backcross hybrids allows rejection of the recessive hypothesis, *Experimental & Clinical Endocrinology*, 89(3), 312, 1987.
253. Kloting I, Vogt L, Coat colour phenotype, leucopenia, and insulin-dependent diabetes mellitus (IDDM) in BB rats, *Diabetes Research and Clinical Ex*, 15, 37, 1990.
254. Markholst H, Jackerott M, Andreasen BE, Segregation analysis of diabetogenic alleles in a cross between BB rats and Brown Norway rats, *Diabetologia*, 36 (Suppl. 1), A91, 1993.
255. Gill TJ III, Kunz HW, Misra DN, Hassett AL, The major histocompatibility complex of the rat, *Transplantation*, 43(6), 773, 1987.
256. Howard JC, The major histocompatibility complex of the rat: a partial review, *Metabolism: Clinical & Experimental*, 32 (7 Suppl. 1), 41, 1983.
257. Colle E, Guttmann RD, Seemayer TA, Michel F, Spontaneous diabetes mellitus syndrome in the rat. IV. Immunogenetic interactions of MHC and non-MHC components of the syndrome, *Metabolism: Clinical & Experimental*, 32 (7 Suppl. 1), 54, 1983.
258. Colle E, Guttmann RD, Fuks A, Insulin-dependent diabetes mellitus is associated with genes that map to the right of the class I RT1.A locus of the major histocompatibility complex of the rat, *Diabetes*, 35(4), 454, 1986.
259. Colle E, Ono SJ, Fuks A, Guttmann RD, Seemayer TA, Association of susceptibility to spontaneous diabetes in rat with genes of major histocompatibility complex, *Diabetes*, 37(10), 1438, 1988.
260. Holowachuk EW, Greer MK, Unaltered class II histocompatibility antigens and pathogenesis of IDDM in BB rats, *Diabetes*, 38(2), 267, 1989.
261. Ono SJ, Fuks A, Guttmann RD, Colle E, Susceptibility and resistance genes to insulin-dependent diabetes mellitus in the BB rat, *Experimental & Clinical Immunogenetics*, 6(2), 169, 1989.
262. Hornum L, Jackerott M, Markholst H, The rat T-cell lymphopenia resistance gene (Lyp) maps between D4Mit6 and Npy on RN04, *Mammalian Genome*, 6(5), 371, 1995.
263. Jacob HJ, Pettersson A, Wilson D, Mao Y, Lernmark A, Lander ES, Genetic dissection of autoimmune Type-1 diabetes in the BB rat, *Nature Genetics*, 7, 215, 1994.
264. Gold DP, Shaikewitz ST, Mueller D, Redd JR, Sellins KS, Pettersson A, Lernmark A, Bellgrau D, T cells from BB-DP rats show a unique cytokine mRNA profile associated with the IDDM1 susceptibility gene, Lyp, *Autoimmunity*, 22(3), 149, 1995.
265. Bieg S, Moller C, Olsson T, Lernmark A, The lymphopenia (lyp) gene controls the intrathymic cytokine ratio in congenic biobreeding rats, *Diabetologia*, 40(7), 786, 1997.
266. Like AA, McGill PD, Sroczynski E, Adult thymectomy prevents diabetes mellitus in BB/W rats, *Diabetologia*, 29, 565a, 1986.
267. Kloting I, Vogt L, Serikawa T, Locus on chromosome 18 cosegregates with diabetes in the BB/OK rat subline, *Diabete et Metabolisme*, 21(5), 338, 1995.
268. Tosi G, Facchin A, Pinelli L, Accolla RS, Assessment of the DQB1-DQA1 complete genotype allows best prediction for IDDM, *Diabetes Care*, 17(9), 1045, 1994.
269. Dahlquist G, Environmental risk factors in human Type I diabetes — an epidemiological perspective, *Diabetes-Metabolism Reviews*, 11(1), 37, 1995.
270. Olmos P, A'Hern R, Heaton DA, Millward BA, Risley D, Pyke DA, Leslie RD, The significance of the concordance rate for Type I (insulin-dependent) diabetes in identical twins, *Diabetologia*, 31(10), 747, 1988.
271. Dosch HM, Karjalainen J, Morkowski J, Martin JM, Robinson BH, Nutritional triggers of IDDM, *Pediatric and Adolescent Endocrinology*, 21 202, 1992.
272. Kostraba JN, Cruickshanks KJ, Lawler-Heavner J, Jobim LF, Rewers MJ, Gay EC, Chase HP, Klingensmith G, Hamman RF, Early exposure to cow's milk and solid foods in infancy, genetic predisposition, and risk of IDDM, *Diabetes*, 42(2), 288, 1993.
273. Scott FW, Norris JM, Kolb H, Milk and Type I diabetes, *Diabetes Care*, 19(4), 379, 1996.

274. Virtanen SM, Aro A, Dietary factors in the aetiology of diabetes, *Annals of Medicine*, 26(6), 469, 1994.

275. Gerstein HC, Cow's milk exposure and Type I diabetes mellitus. A critical overview of the clinical literature, *Diabetes Care*, 17(1), 13, 1994.

276. Mayer EJ, Hamman RF, Gay EC, Lezotte DC, Savitz DA, Klingensmith GJ, Reduced risk of IDDM among breast-fed children. The Colorado IDDM Registry, *Diabetes*, 37(12), 1625, 1988.

277. Borch-Johnsen K, Joner G, Mandrup-Poulsen T, Christy M, Zachau-Christiansen B, Kastrup K, Nerup J, Relation between breast-feeding and incidence rates of insulin-dependent diabetes mellitus. A hypothesis, *Lancet*, 2(8411), 1083, 1984.

278. Nigro G, Campea L, De Novellis A, Orsini M, Breast-feeding and insulin-dependent diabetes mellitus, *Lancet*, 1(8426), 467, 1985.

279. Elliott RB, Reddy SN, Bibby NJ, Kida K, Dietary prevention of diabetes in the non-obese diabetic mouse, *Diabetologia*, 31(1), 62, 1988.

280. Hoorfar J, Scott FW, Cloutier HE, Dietary plant materials and development of diabetes in the BB rat, *Journal of Nutrition*, 121(6), 908, 1991.

281. Hoorfar J, Buschard K, Brogren CH, Impact of dietary protein and fat source on the development of insulin-dependent diabetes in the BB rat, *Diabetes Research*, 20(1), 33, 1992.

282. Elliott RB, Martin JM, Dietary protein: a trigger of insulin-dependent diabetes in the BB rat? *Diabetologia*, 26(4), 297, 1984.

283. Scott FW, Mongeau R, Kardish M, Hatina G, Trick KD, Wojcinski Z, Diet can prevent diabetes in the BB rat, *Diabetes*, 34(10), 1059, 1985.

284. Issa-Chergui B, Guttmann RD, Seemayer TA, Kelley VE, Colle E, The effect of diet on the spontaneous insulin dependent diabetic syndrome in the rat, *Diabetes Research*, 9(2), 81, 1988.

285. Scott FW, Daneman D, Martin JM, Evidence for a critical role of diet in the development of insulin-dependent diabetes mellitus, *Diabetes Research*, 7(4), 153, 1988.

286. Coleman DL, Kuzava JE, Leiter EH, Effect of diet on incidence of diabetes in nonobese diabetic mice, *Diabetes*, 39(4), 432, 1990.

287. Hoorfar J, Buschard K, Dagnaes-Hansen F, Prophylactic nutritional modification of the incidence of diabetes in autoimmune non-obese diabetic (NOD) mice, *British Journal of Nutrition*, 69(2), 597, 1993.

288. Report of the American Institute of Nutrition Ad Hoc Committee on Standards for Nutritional Studies, 1994.

289. Glerum M, Robinson BH, Martin JM, Could bovine serum albumin be the initiating antigen ultimately responsible for the development of insulin dependent diabetes mellitus? *Diabetes Research*, 10(3), 103, 1989.

290. Malkani S, Nompleggi D, Hansen JW, Greiner DL, Mordes JP, Rossini AA, Dietary cow's milk protein does not alter the frequency of diabetes in the BB rat, *Diabetes*, 46(7), 1133, 1997.

291. Daneman D, Fishman L, Clarson C, Martin JM, Dietary triggers of insulin-dependent diabetes in the BB rat, *Diabetes Research*, 5(2), 93, 1987.

292. Karjalainen J, Martin JM, Knip M, Ilonen J, Robinson BH, Savilahti E, Akerblom HK, Dosch HM, A bovine albumin peptide as a possible trigger of insulin- dependent diabetes mellitus, *New England Journal of Medicine*, 327(5), 302, 1992.

293. Fernandes G, Dietary lipids and risk of autoimmune disease, *Clinical Immunology & Immunopathology*, 72(2), 193, 1994.

294. Lefkowith J, Schreiner G, Cormier J, Handler ES, Driscoll HK, Greiner D, Mordes JP, Rossini AA, Prevention of diabetes in the BB rat by essential fatty acid deficiency. Relationship between physiological and biochemical changes, *Journal of Experimental Medicine*, 171(3), 729, 1990.

295. Scott FW, Cloutier HE, Kleemann R, Woerz-Pagenstert U, Rowsell P, Modler HW, Kolb H, Potential mechanisms by which certain foods promote or inhibit the development of spontaneous diabetes in BB rats; dose, timing, early effect on islet area, and switch in infiltrate from TH1 to TH2 cells, *Diabetes*, 46(4), 589, 1997.

296. Biewenga J, van Rees EP, Sminia T, Induction and regulation of IgA responses in the microenvironment of the gut, *Clinical Immunology & Immunopathology*, 67(1), 1, 1993.

297. Cerf-Bensussan N, Guy-Grand D, Intestinal intraepithelial lymphocytes, *Gastroenterology Clinics of North America*, 20(3), 549, 1991.

298. Cunningham-Rundles C, Brandeis WE, Good RA, Day NK, Milk precipitins, circulating immune complexes, and IgA deficiency, *Proceedings of the National Academy of Sciences of the United States of America*, 75(7), 3387, 1978.

299. Wilson CB, Penix L, Weaver WM, Melvin A, Lewis DB, Ontogeny of T lymphocyte function in the neonate, *American Journal of Reproductive Immunology*, 28(3–4), 132, 1992.

300. Karasov WH, Solberg DH, Chang SD, Hughes M, Stein ED, Diamond JM, Is intestinal transport of sugars and amino acids subject to critical-period programming? *American Journal of Physiology*, 249(6 Pt. 1), G770, 1985.

301. Reimer RA, Field CJ, McBurney MI, Ontogenic changes in proglucagon mRNA in bb diabetes prone and normal rats weaned onto a chow diet, *Diabetologia*, 40(8), 871, 1997.

302. Li XB, Scott FW, Park YH, Yoon JW, Low incidence of autoimmune Type I diabetes in BB rats fed a hydrolysed casein-based diet associated with early inhibition of non-macrophage-dependent hyperexpression of MHC class I molecules on beta cells, *Diabetologia*, 38(10), 1138, 1995.

303. Yoon JW, The role of viruses and environmental factors in the induction of diabetes, *Current Topics in Microbiology & Immunology*, 164, 95, 1990.

304. Craighead JE, Workshop on viral infection and diabetes mellitus in man, *Journal of Infectious Diseases*, 125(5), 568, 1972.

305. Ramsingh AI, Chapman N, Tracy S, Coxsackie viruses and diabetes, *Bioessays*, 19(9), 793, 1997.

306. Leiter EH, Hamaguchi K, Viruses and diabetes: diabetogenic role for endogenous retroviruses in NOD mice? *Journal of Autoimmunity*, 3 (Suppl. 1), 31, 1990.

307. Berdanier CD, Diet, autoimmunity, and insulin-dependent diabetes mellitus: a controversy, *Proceedings of the Society for Experimental Biology & Medicine*, 209(3), 223, 1995.

308. Brown DW, Welsh RM, Like AA, Infection of peripancreatic lymph nodes but not islets precedes Kilham rat virus-induced diabetes in BB/Wor rats, *Journal of Virology*, 67(10), 5873, 1993.

309. Ellerman KE, Richards CA, Guberski DL, Shek WR, Like AA, Kilham rat triggers T-cell-dependent autoimmune diabetes in multiple strains of rat, *Diabetes*, 45(5), 557, 1996.

310. Guberski DL, Thomas VA, Shek WR, Like AA, Handler ES, Rossini AA, Wallace JE, Welsh RM, Induction of Type I diabetes by Kilham's rat virus in diabetes-resistant BB/Wor rats *Science*, 254(5034), 1010, 1991. [Published erratum appears in *Science*, 255(5043), 383, 1992].

311. Hanafusa T, Pujol-Borrell R, Chiovato L, Russell RC, Doniach D, Bottazzo GF, Aberrant expression of HLA-DR antigen on thyrocytes in Graves' disease: relevance for autoimmunity, *Lancet*, 2(8359), 1111, 1983.

312. Rossini AA, Williams RM, Mordes JP, Appel MC, Like AA, Spontaneous diabetes in the gnotobiotic BB/W rat, *Diabetes*, 28(11), 1031, 1979.

313. Szopa TM, Titchener PA, Portwood ND, Taylor KW, Diabetes mellitus due to viruses — some recent developments, *Diabetologia*, 36(8), 687, 1993.

314. Carter WR, Herrman J, Stokes K, Cox DJ, Promotion of diabetes onset by stress in the BB rat, *Diabetologia*, 30(8), 674, 1987.

315. Muir A, Schatz DA, Maclaren NK, The pathogenesis, prediction, and prevention of insulin-dependent diabetes mellitus, *Endocrinology & Metabolism Clinics of North America*, 21(2), 199, 1992.

316. Jaworski MA, Honore L, Jewell LD, Mehta JG, McGuire-Clark P, Schouls JJ, Yap WY, Cyclosporin prophylaxis induces long-term prevention of diabetes, and inhibits lymphocytic infiltration in multiple target tissues in the high-risk BB rat, *Diabetes Research*, 3(1), 1, 1986.

317. Yale JF, Grose M, Seemayer TA, Marliss EB, Immunological and metabolic concomitants of cyclosporin prevention of diabetes in BB rats, *Diabetes*, 36(6), 749, 1987.

318. Laupacis A, Stiller CR, Gardell C, Keown P, Dupre J, Wallace AC, Thibert P, Cyclosporin prevents diabetes in BB Wistar rats, *Lancet*, 1(8314–5), 10, 1983.

319. Like AA, Dirodi V, Thomas S, Guberski DL, Rossini AA, Prevention of diabetes mellitus in the BB/W rat with cyclosporin-A, *American Journal of Pathology*, 117(1), 92, 1984.

320. Bach JF, Mechanisms of autoimmunity in insulin-dependent diabetes mellitus, *Clinical & Experimental Immunology*, 72(1), 1, 1988.

321. Di Marco R, Zaccone P, Magro G, Grasso S, Lunetta M, Barcellini W, Nicolosi VM, Meroni PL, Nicoletti F, Synergistic effect of deoxyspergualin (DSP) and cyclosporin A (CsA) in the prevention of spontaneous autoimmune diabetes in BB rats, *Clinical & Experimental Immunology*, 105(2), 338, 1996.

322. Thliveris JA, Begleiter A, Manchur D, Johnston JB, Immunotherapy for insulin-dependent diabetes mellitus in the "BB" rat, *Life Sciences*, 61(3), 283, 1997.

323. Rabinovitch A, Roles of cytokines in IDDM pathogenesis and islet B-cell destruction, *Diabetes Reviews*, 1(2), 215, 1993.

324. Hosszufalusi N, Reinherz L, Takei S, Chan E, Charles MA, Glipizide-induced prevention of diabetes and autoimmune events in the BB rat, *Journal of Autoimmunity*, 7(6), 753, 1994.

325. Rabinovitch A, Suarez WL, Qin HY, Power RF, Badger AM, Prevention of diabetes and induction of non-specific suppressor cell activity in the BB rat by an immunomodulatory azaspirane, SK&F 106610, *Journal of Autoimmunity*, 6(1), 39, 1993.

326. Kolb H, Worz-Pagenstert U, Kleemann R, Rothe H, Rowsell P, Scott FW, Cytokine gene expression in the BB rat pancreas: natural course and impact of bacterial vaccines, *Diabetologia*, 39(12), 1448, 1996.

327. Ewel C, Sobel DO, Zeligs B, Abbassi V, Bellanti JA, The role of alpha interferon in the pathogenesis of diabetes mellitus, *Diabetes*, 38 (Suppl. 2), 73a, 1989.

328. Ewel CH, Sobel DO, Zeligs BJ, Bellanti JA, Poly I:C accelerates development of diabetes mellitus in diabetes-prone BB rat, *Diabetes*, 41(8), 1016, 1992.

329. Sobel DO, Newsome J, Ewel CH, Bellanti JA, Abbassi V, Creswell K, Blair O, Poly I:C induces development of diabetes mellitus in BB rat, *Diabetes*, 41(4), 515, 1992.

330. Sobel DO, Azumi N, Creswell K, Holterman D, Blair OC, Bellanti JA, Abbassi V, Hiserodt JC, The role of NK cell activity in the pathogenesis of poly I:C accelerated and spontaneous diabetes in the diabetes prone BB rat, *Journal of Autoimmunity*, 8(6), 843, 1995.

331. Satoh J, Seino H, Shintani S, Tanaka S, Ohteki T, Masuda T, Nobunaga T, Toyota T, Inhibition of Type I diabetes in BB rats with recombinant human tumor necrosis factor-alpha, *Journal of Immunology*, 145(5), 1395, 1990.

332. Takahashi K, Satoh J, Seino H, Zhu XP, Sagara M, Masuda T, Toyota T, Prevention of Type I diabetes with lymphotoxin in BB rats, *Clinical Immunology & Immunopathology*, 69(3), 318, 1993.

333. Zielasek J, Burkart V, Naylor P, Goldstein A, Kiesel U, Kolb H, Interleukin-2-dependent control of disease development in spontaneously diabetic BB rats, *Immunology*, 69(2), 209, 1990.

334. Wilson CA, Jacobs C, Baker P, Baskin DG, Dower S, Lernmark A, Toivola B, Vertrees S, Wilson D, IL-1 beta modulation of spontaneous autoimmune diabetes and thyroiditis in the BB rat, *Journal of Immunology*, 144(10), 3784, 1990.

335. Nicoletti F, Zaccone P, Di Marco R, Lunetta M, Magro G, Grasso S, Meroni P, Garotta G, Prevention of spontaneous autoimmune diabetes in diabetes-prone BB rats by prophylactic treatment with anti-rat interferon-gamma antibody, *Endocrinology*, 138(1), 281, 1997.

336. Sadelain MW, Qin HY, Sumoski W, Parfrey N, Singh B, Rabinovitch A, Prevention of diabetes in the BB rat by early immunotherapy using Freund's adjuvant, *Journal of Autoimmunity*, 3(6), 671, 1990.

337. Qin HY, Suarez WL, Parfrey N, Power RF, Rabinovitch A, Mechanisms of complete Freund's adjuvant protection against diabetes in BB rats: induction of non-specific suppressor cells, *Autoimmunity*, 12(3), 193, 1992.

338. Singh B, Rabinovitch A, Influence of microbial agents on the development and prevention of autoimmune diabetes, *Autoimmunity*, 15(3), 209, 1993.

339. Mandrup-Poulsen T, Corbett JA, McDaniel ML, Nerup J, What are the types and cellular sources of free radicals in the pathogenesis of Type I (insulin-dependent) diabetes mellitus? *Diabetologia*, 36(5), 470, 1993.

340. Mowat AM, The regulation of immune responses to dietary protein antigens, *Immunology Today*, 8 93, 1987.

341. Weiner HL, Friedman A, Miller A, Khoury SJ, al-Sabbagh A, Santos L, Sayegh M, Nussenblatt RB, Trentham DE, Hafler DA, Oral tolerance: immunologic mechanisms and treatment of animal and human organ-specific autoimmune diseases by oral administration of autoantigens, *Annual Review of Immunology*, 12, 809, 1994.

342. Amital H, Swissa M, Bar-Dayan Y, Buskila D, Shoenfeld Y, New therapeutic avenues in autoimmunity, *Research in Immunology*, 147(6), 361, 1996.

343. Muir A, Schatz D, Maclaren N, Antigen-specific immunotherapy: oral tolerance and subcutaneous immunization in the treatment of insulin-dependent diabetes, *Diabetes-Metabolism Reviews*, 9(4), 279, 1993.

344. Thompson HS, Staines NA, Gastric administration of Type II collagen delays the onset and severity of collagen-induced arthritis in rats, *Clinical & Experimental Immunology*, 64(3), 581, 1986.

345. Weiner HL, Oral tolerance: immune mechanisms and treatment of autoimmune diseases, *Immunology Today*, 18(7), 335, 1997.

346. Miller A, Lider O, Weiner HL, Antigen-driven bystander suppression after oral administration of antigens, *Journal of Experimental Medicine*, 174(4), 791, 1991.

347. Maron R, Blogg NS, Polanski M, Hancock W, Weiner HL, Oral tolerance to insulin and the insulin B-chain: cell lines and cytokine patterns, *Annals of the New York Academy of Sciences*, 778, 346, 1996.

348. Mordes JP, Schirf B, Roipko D, Greiner DL, Weiner H, Nelson P, Rossini AA, Oral insulin does not prevent insulin-dependent diabetes mellitus in BB rats, *Annals of the New York Academy of Sciences*, 778, 418, 1996.

349. Strobel S, Dietary manipulation and induction of tolerance, *Journal of Pediatrics*, 121(5 Pt. 2), S74, 1992.

350. Strobel S, Neonatal oral tolerance, *Annals of the New York Academy of Sciences*, 778, 88, 1996.

351. Bergerot I, Fabien N, Mayer A, Thivolet, C, Active suppression of diabetes after oral administration of insulin is determined by antigen dosage, *Annals of the New York Academy of Sciences*, 778 362, 1996.

352. Gottlieb PA, Handler ES, Appel MC, Greiner DL, Mordes JP, Rossini AA, Insulin treatment prevents diabetes mellitus but not thyroiditis in RT6-depleted diabetes resistant BB/Wor rats, *Diabetologia*, 34(5), 296, 1991.

353. Wright JR, Jr., Yates AJ, Sharma HM, Thibert P, Pathological lesions in the spontaneously diabetic BB Wistar rat: a comprehensive autopsy study, *Metabolism: Clinical & Experimental*, 32(7 Suppl. 1), 101, 1983.

354. Sima AA, Yagihashi S, Central-peripheral distal axonopathy in the spontaneously diabetic BB-rat: ultrastructural and morphometric findings, *Diabetes Research & Clinical Practice*, 1(5), 289, 1985.

355. Fitzgerald ME, Caldwell RB, The retinal microvasculature of spontaneously diabetic BB rats: structure and luminal surface properties, *Microvascular Research*, 39(1), 15, 1990.

356. Chakrabarti S, Sima AA, Lee J, Brachet P, Dicou E, Nerve growth factor (NGF), proNGF and NGF receptor-like immunoreactivity in BB rat retina, *Brain Research*, 523(1), 11, 1990.

357. Caldwell RB, Fitzgerald ME, The choriocapillaris in spontaneously diabetic rats, *Microvascular Research*, 42(3), 229, 1991.

358. Miller TB, Jr., Altered regulation of cardiac glycogen metabolism in spontaneously diabetic rats, *American Journal of Physiology*, 245(4), E379, 1983.

359. Malhotra A, Mordes JP, McDermott L, Schaible TF, Abnormal cardiac biochemistry in spontaneously diabetic Bio-Breeding/Worcester rat, *American Journal of Physiology*, 249(5 Pt. 2), H1051, 1985.

360. Rodrigues B, McGrath GM, McNeill JH, Cardiac function in spontaneously diabetic BB rats treated with low and high dose insulin, *Canadian Journal of Physiology & Pharmacology*, 67(6), 629, 1989.

361. Krizsan-Agbas D, Bunag RD, Normotensive diabetic BB/W rats show enhanced reflex tachycardia, *Diabetes*, 40(11), 1504, 1991.

362. Cohen AJ, McCarthy DM, Rossetti RR, Renin secretion by the spontaneously diabetic rat, *Diabetes*, 35(3), 341, 1986.

363. Brown DM, Steffes MW, Thibert P, Azar S, Mauer SM, Glomerular manifestations of diabetes in the BB rat, *Metabolism: Clinical & Experimental*, 32 (7 Suppl. 1), 131, 1983.

364. Cohen AJ, Mcgill PD, Rossetti RG, Guberski DL, Like AA, Glomerulopathy in spontaneously diabetic rat. Impact of glycemic control, *Diabetes*, 36(8), 944, 1987.

365. Chakrabarti S, Ma N, Sima AA, Reduced number of anionic sites is associated with glomerular basement membrane thickening in the diabetic BB-rat, *Diabetologia*, 32(11), 826, 1989.

366. Chakrabarti S, Sima AA, Effect of aldose reductase inhibition and insulin treatment on retinal capillary basement membrane thickening in BB rats, *Diabetes*, 38(9), 1181, 1989.

367. Sharma K, Ziyadeh FN, Hyperglycemia and diabetic kidney disease. The case for transforming growth factor-β as a key mediator, *Diabetes*, 44(10), 1139, 1995.

368. Appel MC, Like AA, Rossini AA, Carp DB, Miller TB, Jr., Hepatic carbohydrate metabolism in the spontaneously diabetic Bio-Breeding Worcester rat, *American Journal of Physiology* 240(2), E83, 1981.

369. Ruggere MD, Patel YC, Impaired hepatic metabolism of somatostatin-14 and somatostatin-28 in spontaneously diabetic BB rats, *Endocrinology*, 115(1), 244, 1984.

370. Meehan CJ, Fleming S, Smith W, Baird JD, Idiopathic megacolon in the BB rat, *International Journal of Experimental Pathology*, 75(1), 37, 1994.

371. Cameron DF, Rountree J, Schultz RE, Repetta D, Murray, FT, Sustained hyperglycemia results in testicular dysfunction and reduced fertility potential in BBWOR diabetic rats, *American Journal of Physiology*, 259(6 Pt. 1), E881, 1990.

372. Wright JR, Jr., Yates AJ, Sharma HM, Shim C, Tigner RL, Thibert P, Testicular atrophy in the spontaneously diabetic BB Wistar rat, *American Journal of Pathology*, 108(1), 72, 1982.

373. Murray FT, Cameron DF, Orth JM, Katovich MJ, Gonadal dysfunction in the spontaneously diabetic BB rat: alterations of testes morphology, serum testosterone and LH, *Hormone & Metabolic Research*, 17(10), 495, 1985.

374. Verhaeghe J, van Herck E, Visser WJ, Suiker AM, Thomasset M, Einhorn TA, Faierman E, Bouillon R, Bone and mineral metabolism in BB rats with long-term diabetes. Decreased bone turnover and osteoporosis, *Diabetes*, 39(4), 477, 1990.

375. Sima AA, Thibert P, Proximal motor neuropathy in the BB-Wistar rat, *Diabetes*, 31(9), 784, 1982.

376. Longhurst PA, Urinary bladder function 6 months after the onset of diabetes in the spontaneously diabetic BB rat, *Journal of Urology*, 145(2), 417, 1991.

377. Zhang WX, Chakrabarti S, Greene DA, Sima AA, Diabetic autonomic neuropathy in BB rats and effect of ARI treatment on heart-rate variability and vagus nerve structure, *Diabetes*, 39(5), 613, 1990.

378. Sima AA, Prashar A, Zhang WX, Chakrabarti S, Greene DA, Preventive effect of long-term aldose reductase inhibition (ponalrestat) on nerve conduction and sural nerve structure in the spontaneously diabetic Bio-Breeding rat, *Journal of Clinical Investigation*, 85(5), 1410, 1990.

379. Burchiel KJ, Russell LC, Lee RP, Sima AA, Spontaneous activity of primary afferent neurons in diabetic BB/Wistar rats. A possible mechanism of chronic diabetic neuropathic pain, *Diabetes*, 34(11), 1210, 1985.

380. Yagihashi S, Sima AA, Diabetic autonomic neuropathy in the BB rat. Ultrastructural and morphometric changes in sympathetic nerves, *Diabetes*, 34(6), 558, 1985.

381. Sima AA, Can the BB-rat help to unravel diabetic neuropathy? *Neuropathology & Applied Neurobiology*, 11(4), 253, 1985.

382. Yagihashi S, Sima AA, Diabetic autonomic neuropathy. The distribution of structural changes in sympathetic nerves of the BB rat, *American Journal of Pathology*, 121(1), 138, 1985.

383. Yu O, Ouyang A, Distribution of beta-adrenoceptor subtypes in gastrointestinal tract of non-diabetic and diabetic BB rats. A longitudinal study, *Digestive Diseases & Sciences*, 42(6), 1146, 1997.

384. Kalant N, Seemayer T, Malignant lymphoma in spontaneously diabetic rats, *New England Journal of Medicine*, 300(13), 737, 1979.

385. Friedman DF, Cho EA, Goldman J, Carmack CE, Besa EC, Hardy RR, Silberstein LE, The role of clonal selection in the pathogenesis of an autoreactive human B cell lymphoma, *Journal of Experimental Medicine*, 174(3), 525, 1991.

386. Shirai T, Hirose S, Okada T, Nishimura H, CD5+ B cells in autoimmune disease and lymphoid malignancy, *Clinical Immunology & Immunopathology*, 59(2), 173, 1991.

387. Presotto F, Betterle C, Insulin-dependent diabetes mellitus: a constellation of autoimmune diseases, *Journal Pediatric Endocrinology and Metabolism*, 10(5), 455, 1997.

388. Sternthal E, Like AA, Sarantis K, Braverman LE, Lymphocytic thyroiditis and diabetes in the BB/W rat. A new model of autoimmune endocrinopathy, *Diabetes*, 30(12), 1058, 1981.

389. Voorby HA, Van der Gaag RD, Jeucken PH, Bloot AM, Drexhage HA, The goitre of the BB/O rat: an animal-model for studying the role of immunoglobulins stimulating growth of thyroid cells, *Clinical & Experimental Immunology* 76(2), 290, 1989.

390. Rajatanavin R, Appel MC, Alex S, Yang YN, Reinhardt W, Braverman LE, Variable incidence of spontaneous and iodine induced lymphocytic thyroiditis in different lines of the BB/W rat. *Endocrine Society, 71st Annual Meeting*, Seattle, WA, 1989, 477.

391. Rajatanavin R, Appel MC, Reinhardt W, Alex S, Yang YN, Braverman LE, Variable prevalence of lymphocytic thyroiditis among diabetes-prone sublines of BB/W or rats, *Endocrinology,* 128(1), 153, 1991.

392. Delemarre FG, Simons PJ, Drexhage HA, Histomorphological aspects of the development of thyroid autoimmune diseases: consequences for our understanding of endocrine ophthalmopathy, *Thyroid*, 6(4), 369, 1996.

393. Allen EM, Appel MC, Braverman LE, The effect of iodide ingestion on the development of spontaneous lymphocytic thyroiditis in the diabetes-prone BB/W rat, *Endocrinology,* 118(5), 1977, 1986.

394. Sundick RS, Bagchi N, Brown TR, The role of iodine in thyroid autoimmunity: from chickens to humans: a review, *Autoimmunity,* 13(1), 61, 1992.

395. Awata T, Guberski DL, Like AA, Genetics of the BB rat: association of autoimmune disorders (diabetes, insulitis, and thyroiditis) with lymphopenia and major histocompatibility complex class II, *Endocrinology,* 136(12), 5731, 1995.

396. Yamamoto S, Ito T, Nakata S, Nozaki S, Uchikoshi F, Shirakura R, Kamiike W, Miyata M, Matsuda H, The rejection mechanism of rat pancreaticoduodenal allografts with a class I MHC disparity, *Transplantation*, 57(8), 1217, 1994.

397. Gottlieb PA, Berrios JP, Mariani G, Handler ES, Greiner D, Mordes JP, Rossini AA, Autoimmune destruction of islets transplanted into RT6-depleted diabetes-resistant BB/Wor rats, *Diabetes*, 39(5), 643, 1990.

398. Markmann JF, Woehrle M, Roza A, Barker CF, Naji A, Islet transplantation to study autoimmune pathogenesis of diabetes in BB rat, *Hormone & Metabolic Research*, Suppl. 25, 116, 1990.

399. Posselt AM, Naji A, Roark JH, Markmann JF, Barker CF, Intrathymic islet transplantation in the spontaneously diabetic BB rat, *Annals of Surgery,* 214(4), 363, 1991.

400. Uchikoshi F, Ito T, Kamiike W, Yamamoto S, Nozaki S, Nakata S, Shirakura R, Miyata M, Matsuda H, Nakao H et al., Restoration of defective immune responses in diabetic BB rats after successful pancreas transplantation, *Transplantation Proceedings*, 26(2), 956, 1994.

14

Noninsulin-Dependent Animal Models of Diabetes Mellitus

Christopher H. S. McIntosh and Raymond A. Pederson

CONTENTS

14.1 General Introduction

Type II or noninsulin-dependent diabetes mellitus (NIDDM) is the most common form of diabetes, accounting for ~85% of cases.[1,2] It has been estimated that approximately 3% of the world population (~100 million people) suffer from the disease[2] and, since there is also an increasing prevalence, it is clearly imperative that a better understanding of its underlying causes is developed. The most important characteristic of NIDDM, inappropriate and chronic hyperglycemia and glucose intolerance, is associated with several metabolic derangements, but all patients exhibit two common features: pancreatic β-cell dysfunction and peripheral and hepatic insulin resistance, leading to decreased skeletal muscle and white adipose tissue glucose utilization, and increased hepatic glucose production. A combination of both insulin resistance and impaired insulin secretion is required for NIDDM to manifest itself. Apart from rare conditions of insulin receptor mutations, resistance alone does not normally result in NIDDM, providing that the β-cell has the ability to compensate for the degree of insulin resistance.[2] Therefore, at least two genetic defects are generally involved in NIDDM. Elucidation of the origins of these defects, and development of more satisfactory therapies than are currently available are objectives that can only be realized through experimentation with appropriate animal models. The objective of this chapter is to provide an update on some of the animal models currently available. At the onset of writing it soon became apparent that a fully comprehensive assessment of the massive literature on the subject was both impossible and undesirable in view of the excellence of previously published reviews. Those from Bray and York[3,4] and Herberg and Coleman[5] on the metabolic characteristics of the Mendelian mouse models should be consulted for the important literature up until 1979. A number of excellent general reviews have summarized more recent studies,[6-10] and more specific reviews will be referred to whenever possible.

14.2 Aspects of Human NIDDM Studied in Animal Models

It has been established through numerous epidemiological, adoption, and twin studies that dietary and environmental triggers and genetic susceptibility determinants are important etiological factors for human NIDDM.[1,2,11] However, the molecular basis underlying the inherited susceptibility is largely unknown, and several environmental factors, including a sedentary lifestyle, drugs, and diet, have all been implicated.[13] It is now recognized that most of the difficulty in determining factors involved in the development of most forms of human NIDDM is related to the polygenic nature of the disease.[1,14] Human studies have revealed mutations in a number of candidate NIDDM genes including those for insulin, the insulin receptor, glucokinase, and mitochondrial tRNA, and identified them as primary lesions in well-defined subtypes of diabetes.[1,11] However, although estimates vary and there are racial differences, these types of diabetes account for only 1 to 2% of the total, and the underlying causes of the majority of human obesity and NIDDM probably depend on the particular mixture of genes involved. Nevertheless, further understanding of the link between such mutations and the phenotype expressed could provide useful clues regarding associated metabolic alterations in polygenic types of NIDDM, and introduction of these mutations into animal models provides one way of facilitating their study. In humans, obesity is one of the strongest risk factors for NIDDM, and the search for obesity genes in animals is therefore intimately connected to the search for diabetogenic genes. As with NIDDM, evidence for human genes controlling body weight and composition has arisen from different sources, including adoption and twin studies. However, the identification of human genes by techniques such as positional cloning has proved extremely difficult, and studies on animal models are proving invaluable. Additionally, studies on specific forms of early-onset forms of obesity, such as the Prader–Willi and Bardet–Biedl syndromes, have resulted in their genetic mapping to specific chromosome sites.[14] The identification of mutations and imprinting defects responsible for these rare autosomal genetic syndromes may also lead to the generation of new animal models. At present, four major types of animals are being used to develop a better understanding of diabetes: (1) Mendelian monogenic obese and diabetic mice and rats; (2) polygenic obese and diabetic animals; (3) transgenic and knockout mice; (4) and obese animals produced by chemical treatment or surgical (hypothalamic) manipulation. This chapter will focus on small-animal genetic models which have provided the most important insights into the origins of NIDDM, with some consideration given to transgenic and knockout animals. The reader is directed to reviews on surgical[15] and chemical[6,13,16,17] induction of obesity and diabetes and an excellent comprehensive review of primate models,[18] for further information in these areas, since they will not be discussed due to space limitations.

14.3 Advantages of Animal Models for Studying NIDDM

The overriding reason for using animal models of diabetes is that experiments can be performed that are not possible in humans, particularly those involving tissue sampling for assessment of specific biochemical, metabolic, hormonal, and morphological parameters. More specific advantages include[8-10]

1. Programmed breeding allows the production of animal lines that are genetically homogeneous, and systematic identification of specific genes can be performed.
2. Several distinct autosomal and polygenic rodent genetic models are available.
3. Environmental factors, which impact on the development of diabetes, can be controlled.
4. Hypotheses regarding the roles of specific genes can be tested in identified genetic models, using techniques, such as positional cloning, and via the use of transgenic animals.
5. The synteny between rodent and human genes allows transfer of information to facilitate identification of homologous genes. The recent success in identifying specific gene defects in mouse models of obesity[8-10,19] has already led to the identification of similar gene defects in humans.[20,21]

Animals that exhibit hyperglycemia and glucose intolerance resulting from insulin resistance and/or pancreatic β-cell malfunction can be considered appropriate models for NIDDM. Expression of the phenotype is variable among different strains and is dependent upon both genetic background and environmental factors. The majority of animal obesity models are characterized by hyperglycemia and hyperinsulinemia at some stage of life and have, therefore, been used to study the development of NIDDM. This chapter will consider what has already been learned from the study of such animals and future prospects. With regard to the development of both inherited and acquired hyperglycemia, the following areas have been extensively studied:

1. The biochemical basis of insulin-resistant glucose metabolism in liver and skeletal muscle;
2. The causes of elevated hepatic glucose production, and reduced metabolic clearance rate of glucose in the basal state;
3. The underlying causes of abnormal insulin secretion;
4. The origins of elevated circulating proinsulin.

Further studies on these specific biochemical abnormalities will no doubt lead to an even clearer picture of the events involved.

Animals exhibiting spontaneous obesity/diabetes have been obtained in two ways.[8] First, there are those animals discovered or inbred after the fortuitous observation of compromised glycemic control and which maintained this deficiency through subsequent generations. This includes both monogenic and polygenic strains.[8] The second approach has been to select animals with NIDDM-like syndromes from nondiabetic outbred populations, and to produce a colony by repeated inbreeding using responsiveness to a glucose load as a selection procedure. These animals are normally polygenic. A major breakthrough in the use of animal models was the identification of leptin as a signaling molecule involved in the regulation of appetite and energy metabolism.[22] This discovery opened a new era in obesity research, which has proved crucial for understanding the link between obesity and NIDDM. All of the other genes responsible for the monogenic rodent obesity syndromes currently studied have now been identified, and these animals will be described first.

14.4 Monogenic Animal Models of Obesity and NIDDM

The defining phenotypes of the monogenic rodent models include obesity, hyperinsulinemia, transient or sustained hyperglycemia, and hyperlipidemia.[9,19,21] Autosomal recessive animals may also exhibit hyperphagia, defective thermoregulation, hypogonadism, and sterility. All of the monogenic syndromes have now been mapped to defined autosomal loci, and current studies are directed at understanding how the genetic defects result in increased energy intake, decreased energy expenditure, and/or preferential partitioning of ingested calories into fat depots,[19] ultimately leading to obesity and, in some cases, NIDDM. Table 14.1 summarizes the identified genes and chromosomal loci of the different strains of animals, as summarized by Chagnon and Bouchard.[21]

TABLE 14.1

Single Gene Mutation Models of Obesity

Strain	Gene	Inheritance	Mouse/Rat Chromosome	Human Chromosome
Mouse				
Yellow	A^y, A^{vy}, A^{iy}, A^{sy}, A^{iapy}	Autosomal dominant	2	20q13 (20q11.2)
Obese	*ob*, *ob²ʲ*	Autosomal recessive	6	7q31.3
Diabetes	*db*, *db²ʲ*, *db³ʲ*, *db^ad*, *db^pas*, *db⁵ʲ*	Autosomal recessive	4	1p31-p21
Fat	*fat*	Autosomal recessive	8	4q32
Tubby	*tub*	Autosomal recessive	7	11p15.4
Rat				
Fatty	*fa*	Autosomal recessive	5	1p31-p21
Corpulent	*fa^cp*	Autosomal recessive	5	1p31-p21

Note: Although the alternative nomenclature *ob* = *Lep^ob*, *db* = *Lep^db*, *fat* = *Cpe^fat* is now appearing in the literature, the more conventional form is used in this chapter.

14.4.1   Obese and Diabetic Mice

The early literature on the *ob* and *db* mouse has been reviewed extensively[3-5] and these overviews will be referred to whenever possible. The obese mutation was detected in noninbred mouse stock and was subsequently maintained in the C57BL/6J strain.[23] Two alleles have been described: *ob* and *ob²ʲ*. The diabetes (*db*) mutation occurred in the C57BL/KsJ inbred strain, and two further *db* strains, *db²ʲ* and *db³ʲ*, arose in the Jackson laboratories.[24] Both *ob* and *db* are autosomal recessive with full penetrance. The adipose (*ad*) mutant described by Falconer and Isaacson[25] was found later to be an allele of diabetes and has been renamed *db*ᵃᵈ. The phenotype appears to be almost identical to *db* when the alleles are bred on the same background.[23] Homozygous *ob* and *db* mutants of both sexes are generally infertile, although *ob/ob* males can occasionally reproduce if maintained on a restricted diet.[26] Obese and diabetes mutants are bred by heterozygote mating.[23] There is a defect in thermogenesis in both *ob* and *db* strains, which is detectable early in life as a lower core temperature.[19] There are also similar hormonal abnormalities. Although the expression of the syndromes diverges with age, at 8 to 12 weeks both *ob/ob* and *db/db* mice demonstrate hyperglycemia, hyperinsulinemia, and hypercorticosteronism.

The obese phenotype is characterized by extreme insulin resistance, glucose intolerance, and mild hyperglycemia,[3,4] and, therefore, exhibits many of the characteristics of NIDDM.[8] These traits are more marked when the *ob* gene is expressed on the C57BL/KsJ background.[8] Abnormalities in *ob/ob* mice can be detected early in life: impaired thermogenesis is detectable at 10 days. There is both marked hyperphagia and inappropriately decreased energy expenditure. Weight gain is rapid, resulting in increased carcass lipid by 3 weeks and visually obvious obesity by ~4 weeks.[9] Adiposity, which is a result of hypertrophy in several adipose tissue depots, peaks at maturity and is a result of both increased lipogenesis and decreased lipolysis. Animals continue to synthesize, and fail to mobilize, fat even following calorie restriction.[3,4] Enlargement of fat depots precedes the development of a progressive increase in circulating insulin. At 20 to 28 days, extremely high levels of hyperinsulinemia are observed in both fasting and fed states,[9] and both the number and size of pancreatic β-cells are increased.[4] Hyperinsulinemia is accompanied by decreased glucose tolerance. Serum insulin eventually reaches a peak and then falls, and this is followed by improvement and normalization of glucose tolerance, a stable serum insulin level, and decrease in body weight. Insulin resistance is accompanied by hepatic glucose overproduction, increased activity of gluconeogenic enzymes, and decreased activity of glycolytic and glycogen-synthesizing enzymes. Lipogenesis in both liver and adipose tissue is increased. Fasting triglycerides and cholesterol are increased two- to threefold and corticosterone three- to fourfold in adult mice. Despite the extreme insulin resistance, severe diabetes is not normally a characteristic of the *ob/ob* mouse, although colonies of mice in some centers exhibit a more severe diabetes-like syndrome.[5]

When expressed on the C57BL/KsJ background, *db* mice are obese, hyperphagic, exhibit low energy expenditure, and are severely hyperglycemic and diabetic.[23,24] Plasma insulin is increased as early as 10 days, and peaks at six to ten times normal by 2 to 3 months, when animals are severely hyperglycemic. Insulin levels drop rapidly to near normal values, at which time islets are hyperplastic and hypertrophic. This is followed by progressive degranulation and necrosis, and the islet insulin content becomes greatly reduced. Glucose-induced insulin secretion is severely decreased, and there is a rapid rise in blood glucose to over 22 mM until death at 5 to 8 months of age.[23,24] Hyperglycemia in the *db/db* mouse is more severe than in the *ob/ob* mouse, and animals show vascular abnormalities. Mice with a second allele, *db²ʲ*, exhibit mild diabetes but greatly elevated insulin levels throughout life. The phenotypic expression is very similar to the C57BL/6J *ob* mouse. However, when the *db²ʲ* allele is introduced onto the C57BL/KsJ background, offspring are indistinguishable from the *db* animals, emphasizing the importance of genetic back-ground on gene expression.[5] The *db³ʲ* mutation, arose in the 129/J mouse strain and has severe obesity, hypoglycemia rather than hyperglycemia, marked hyperinsulinemia, and greatly enlarged islets.[23,24]

14.4.1.1 Identification of the Obese Gene and Leptin

In a series of experiments, Coleman[23,24] established parabiotic unions between *ob/ob* or *db/db* mice with normal mice of the same genetic background. Parabiosis of normal animals with *db/db* mice resulted in death from starvation of the normal partner. When *db/db* mice were joined with *ob/ob* mice, the obese partner died of starvation. Coleman proposed that the mutant genes responsible for obesity in the two strains were probably involved in the same pathway. He made the prescient suggestion that the *ob* gene coded for a circulating satiety factor and that the *db* gene product was the receptor for that protein. In 1994, Friedman's group[22] reported the positional cloning of the mouse and human *obese* genes, and this initiated a rapid burst of activity in studies on the hormonal regulation of food intake and energy balance.

The mouse obese gene is localized on chromosome 6 in mice[22] and 7q31.3 in humans.[27] The coding region of the gene consists of three exons separated by a 2-kb intron in both mouse and human. The 5′ promoter region is complex and spans approximately 3 kb. It contains a TATA box and multiple CCAAT/enhancer binding protein (C/EBP) and Sp-1 binding sites, plus a glucocorticoid and several cAMP response element-binding sites.[27-29] The 4.5-kb *ob* mRNA codes for a 167 amino acid protein[22] which contains a signal sequence that is cleaved off to produce a 146 amino acid secreted protein, which has been named leptin (Greek: *leptos* = thin).[30] Human and rat leptins share 84% and 95 to 96% sequence identity with the mouse protein, respectively, indicating that leptin is highly conserved in mammals.[22,31] The leptin protein has been assigned, on structural grounds, to the hematopoietic cytokine family.

The *ob* allele contains a nonsense mutation (C → T substitution) that results in the introduction of a stop codon in place of an arginine at position 105. This leads to the production of a truncated, nonfunctional protein.[22] In the SM/Ckc-⁺ᴰᵃᶜ*ob²ʲ/ob²ʲ* strain no *ob* mRNA is transcribed due to a 5-kb insertion in the first *ob* intron.[22,32] Both strains lack circulating leptin, but there is a large increase in adipose *ob* mRNA levels.[22] No leptin mutations have been found in other animal obesity models. In human population studies, no deleterious mutations were found in American patients with NIDDM of various descent.[33-37] However, two severely obese children with congenital leptin deficiency were described recently.[20] These children were both members of a highly consanguinous ped-igree, and their serum leptin levels were undetectable, despite their markedly elevated fat mass. A homozygous frame-shift mutation was detected, resulting in the deletion of a single G in codon 133 of the leptin gene, and the resultant protein does not appear to be efficiently targeted to the secretory pathway. The children were normoglycemic, but basal insulin levels were elevated, suggestive of insulin resistance. Although the American population studies demonstrated that it is unlikely that defects in the *ob* gene are respon-sible for common forms of obesity and NIDDM, linkage studies have suggested that there may be an association between the leptin gene and extreme obesity in some families.[38]

14.4.1.2 Identification of the Diabetes Gene and the Leptin Receptor

A leptin receptor cDNA was isolated from a murine choroid plexus library using an expression cloning system.[39,40] Sequencing of the cDNA predicted that the receptor consisted of a single membrane-spanning protein and belonged to the class I cytokine receptor family, and was closely related to gp130 and the receptors for granulocyte stimulating factor and leukemia inhibitory factor. The predicted extracellular domain of the receptor was large, consisting of 816 amino acids, while the intracellular domain was predicted to consist of only 34 amino acids. This suggested a lack of signal-transducing ability.[40] Further screening led to the identification of multiple isoforms of the leptin receptor resulting from alternative RNA splicing,[41,42] one of which was a longer form with a 303 amino acid intracellular domain (OB-R_b; OB-$R_{l(long)}$). Numerous short forms (OB-R_s) of the leptin receptor (OB-R_a, OB-R_c, OB-R_d, and OB-R_f) have been described in both mouse and rat.[40-43] Sequences of the human and mouse receptor are highly homologous.[41] A soluble form of the mouse receptor (OB-R_e) has been identified that exhibits similar binding kinetics to OB-R_b,[44] and appears to circulate in the blood. This protein constitutes only a small fraction of leptin-binding proteins in plasma,[45] and they probably play an important role in modulating the biological activity of leptin.

When probes based on the extracellular domain of the leptin receptor are used to detect leptin receptor mRNA, a widespread tissue distribution is evident. In mouse, OB-R mRNA levels are most abundant in the choroid plexus of the lateral and third ventricles of the brain, kidney, and lung.[39] Lower levels are found in several other brain regions[46] and virtually all tissues, including stomach, pancreas, thymus, and kidney. The majority of ObR mRNA detected encodes for short receptor isoforms. Of particular importance is the presence of high levels of OB-R_b mRNA in the hypothalamus,[47] particularly in the arcuate (ARN), ventromedial (VMN), paraventricular (PVN), and dorsomedial (DMN) nuclei,[48,49] regions demonstrated to play important roles in the regulation of food intake.

The mouse leptin receptor gene has been mapped to Chromosome 4.[39] This is within the genetic region to which the *db* locus had been previously localized. Sequencing of the *db* mouse gene revealed a single nucleotide substitution (G → T transversion), within an exon containing the extreme C-terminus and 3' untranslated region.[41] The mutation results in the generation of a new splice donor site, producing an exon that is inappropriately spliced into the transcript coding for the long intracellular domain. The majority of the intracellular domain is truncated in the resultant receptor,[40-42] and is unable to initiate the normal signal-transduction pathway.[40,47] Mutations in the mouse *db* locus and the rat fatty locus (see later) have arisen many times,[50] and the defect in 129 *db³ʲ/db³ʲ* mice was identified by Lee et al.[50] as also resulting in a truncated receptor. The *db^{Pas}* mutation involves a partial duplication of the coding sequence for the extracellular domain.[51] A number of studies have been directed at determining whether humans carry similar mutations to the *db/db* mouse, but, although several sequence polymorphisms have been identified,[51-54] if important functional mutations occur, they are probably extremely rare.[51]

The mechanism by which the long form of the leptin receptor signals is an important active area of research, since it is possible that faulty signal transduction could be involved in obesity/NIDDM. After it was determined that OB-R_b shared homology with the class I cytokine family, it was concluded that the receptor must act primarily via the JAK/STAT (Janus Kinase/Signal Transducers and Activators of Transcription) system.[55] Transfection studies have shown that OB-R_b can activate both STAT3 and STAT5,[56] although there is disagreement about whether or not it interacts with STAT1 and STAT6,[40] and it is unclear which STAT is most important *in vivo*. Although there is now strong evidence supporting a role for the JAK/STAT system, there have been recent reports indicating alternative modes of action for leptin, involving insulin receptor substrate (IRS)-1 and mitogen-activating protein (MAP) kinase,[57] and hyperpolarization of hypothalamic neurons[58] and pancreatic β-cells[59] via inhibition of ATP-sensitive K^+ channels. The majority of studies have shown that short forms of the receptor lack the ability to activate the JAK/STAT pathway, but they may signal via alternative pathways.[60] The shorter forms of the receptor located in endothelial cells of the choroid plexus in the brain most likely act as saturable leptin transporters.[61,62] The cerebrospinal fluid (CSF) levels of leptin are extremely low, and the blood–CSF gradient may be maintained via regulated transport of leptin from the blood into the CSF, from whence it diffuses to various other brain regions.[61-64] There is a strong correlation between CSF and plasma leptin levels,[64] and the differences in circulating levels between obese and lean individuals are much greater than those in CSF levels, suggesting that uptake may be compromised in obese individuals. This would be expected to result in a syndrome resembling leptin resistance.

Since the effects of leptin on food intake and energy expenditure are of paramount importance for an understanding of obesity/NIDDM in both animal models and humans, a fairly comprehensive overview will be provided of the regulation of leptin production and secretion and of the functions of leptin.

14.4.1.3 *Ob Gene Expression and Leptin Secretion*

Circulating leptin and *ob* mRNA levels in white adipose tissue are elevated in all rodent models of genetic and diet-induced obesity that have been studied.[65-67] This suggests that the level of *ob* gene expression and leptin synthesis reflects the size of the adipose tissue mass.[66,67] In agreement with this proposal, there is a positive correlation between body mass index (BMI), body fat, *ob* mRNA levels, and circulating leptin levels in adult humans,[66-71] the strongest correlation being between circulating leptin and percentage body fat.[68,69] However, in children, plasma leptin levels correlate with total energy expenditure and the level of physical activity, independent of body weight, emphasizing the importance of a second role for leptin in the maintenance of energy balance.[72] The elevated levels of circulating leptin in human obesity have been suggested to reflect resistance to the action of leptin, as previously mentioned.[61-64] Although a body of literature supports this contention, Ravussin et al.[73] found lower mean circulating leptin levels in Pima Indians who subsequently became obese than in those who did not. This interesting finding suggests that an early leptin deficiency may contribute to obesity and NIDDM in some groups. Female humans have higher circulating levels than males,[74,75] probably due to both a greater percentage of body fat and the effects of steroid hormones.[75] There is a diurnal rhythm in both *ob* gene expression[67] and leptin secretion[76] that is entrained to meal pattern.[77,78] The nocturnal increase may be involved in suppression of appetite during sleeping. There is an inverse relationship between rapid fluctuations in plasma leptin and those of adrenocorticotropin (ACTH) and cortisol,[77] implying that there is interaction between leptin and the hypothalamo–pituitary–adrenocortical axis. This will be returned to later.

Ob gene expression is restricted mainly to mature adipocytes,[79] and all rat fat deposits have been reported to contain *ob* mRNA.[80,81] Low levels of leptin mRNA have also been detected in the placenta,[82] but it is not known if leptin serves a different function in this site. The complexity of the leptin gene promoter suggests that regulation of gene expression is probably multifactorial. Since the level of *ob* gene expression reflects the size of the adipose depot, the major determinants may be cell stretching and/or lipid content. If the latter is involved, elevations of lipid levels due to either increased transcription rate or decreased turnover of components of triacylglycerol metabolism could be involved. The adipocyte leptin levels are clearly related to nutrient intake. In rodents, a diet high in fat results in markedly increased *ob* mRNA levels[83] and circulating leptin.[84] In contrast, *ob* gene expression is decreased following fasting[67,85] and rapidly increases again following refeeding.[85] Flier[86] pointed out that the suppression of leptin gene expression in response to starvation is greater than one would expect from the degree of reduction in adipocyte energy stores. He suggested that a primary role for leptin could be in the neuroendocrine adaptation to starvation, and that a drop in insulin may provide the link. In support of this proposal, Ahima et al.[87] showed that prevention of starvation-induced reductions in leptin, by addition of exogenous leptin, blunted changes in the gonadal, adrenal, and thyroid axes. There is also considerable evidence supporting a key role for insulin in the regulation of leptin gene expression. Fat deposition is one of the major end points of the anabolic actions of insulin, and during differentiation of preadipocytes into adipocytes synthesis of leptin mRNA occurs concomitantly with expression of other insulin-responsive genes. Insulin administration in fasted animals increases ob mRNA levels to those of fed controls.[88] All obese rodent models are both hyperleptinemic and hyperinsulinemic, and there is a positive correlation between leptin and insulin levels in obese humans.[89] In humans, insulin has been reported to have no acute effect on *ob* gene expression[90] or circulating leptin levels,[91] but chronic insulin administration in humans increases levels of both,[67,90] suggesting that the major effect of insulin is likely to be long term, and through a trophic effect on fat cells. One intracellular pathway by which leptin gene expression is increased is via C/EBPα, a transcriptional activator that is important during adipocyte differentiation,[92] but a direct link between insulin action and such a pathway has not as yet been established. As discussed later, in addition to its effects on food intake, leptin also regulates energy expenditure via activation of efferent autonomic pathways, and there is a feedback inhibitory pathway for gene expression mediated via the sympathetic nervous system. For example, activation of sympathetic nervous activity through exposure of rats to cold,[93,94] or administration of β_3-adrenergic agonists,[95] reduces ob mRNA levels. Leptin may also reduce expression of its own gene.[96] Inhibition of *ob* gene expression appears to be regulated at least in part through the peroxisome proliferator-activated receptor for PPARγ.[97]

14.4.1.4 *Actions of Leptin, Obesity, and NIDDM*

Following the availability of recombinant protein, numerous studies were performed to determine whether or not exogenous leptin could correct the deficiencies in thermogenesis, fat metabolism, insulin secretion, and fertility in obese rodents. Intraperitoneal administration of leptin reduced food intake, percentage body fat, and body weight in *ob/ob* mice[30,98-102] and mice with diet-induced obesity.[98] Circulating glucose[30,99,100] and insulin[99,100] levels in *ob/ob* mice are also reduced by leptin, and the lower metabolic rate, oxygen consumption, and temperature found in these rodents can be normalized.[99] Normal mice were found to be less sensitive to leptin, although they ate less following its administration.[30,98] Treatment of *ob/ob* mice with a recombinant adenovirus expressing mouse leptin resulted in large reductions in food intake and body weight. Serum insulin levels and glucose tolerance were also normalized.[103] Since injection of leptin into the lateral ventricles of the brain also reduces food intake, the peptide acts at least partially via central effects.[98] The ARN is now thought to play a major role in the action of leptin, and monosodium glutamate-induced damage to this region attenuates leptin-induced reductions in feeding.[104]

As a result of the above studies, plus numerous others, leptin has now been established to play an important role in body weight homeostasis, and the regulation of energy balance, by signaling to the brain information regarding the size of energy stores and activating centers involved in regulating food intake and energy expenditure.[71,105,106] Considerable efforts have been directed at clarifying the complex circuitry involved in the central actions of leptin. Although these pathways have not been completely delineated, it appears that there may be both rapid and more long-term effects of leptin involving multiple neuropeptides. Leptin acts as a synaptic modulator on arcuate neurons,[107] and it has profound effects on hypothalamic neuropeptide Y (NPY) neuron function. NPY, acting via specific NPY$_5$ "feeding" receptors,[108] is a powerful central appetite stimulant (orexigenic peptide), selective for carbohydrate and fat. Repeated central NPY injections ultimately lead to obesity, whereas exogenous leptin blocks all feeding responses to NPY. NPY is synthesized in the ARN, and NPY-containing neurons project to the PVN, where the neuropeptide is released. There is coexpression of leptin receptor mRNA and NPY mRNA in the mouse ARN, and administration of leptin inhibits both NPY gene expression and NPY release in *ob/ob*[101,102,109-111] and normal[102] mice via an action on the ARN. Therefore, leptin acts both at the site of synthesis and secretion of NPY. As expected, *db/db* mice are resistant to leptin treatment.[101] Paraventricular NPY secretion has been shown to be elevated in both *ob/ob* mice and *fa/fa* Zucker rats,[111] presumably as a result of leptin or leptin receptor deficiency. A central role has therefore been proposed for NPY in the obesity of these animals, as a result of hypothalamic overexpression. In addition to stimulating food intake, NPY also reduces energy expenditure, by inhibiting activity of the sympathetic innervation of BAT, decreases thermogenesis, and increases plasma insulin and corticosterone levels.[109,113] NPY is not, however, the sole hypothalamic mediator of the actions of leptin. Erickson et al.[114] showed that NPY-deficient *ob/ob* mice (NPY$^{-/-}$) had normal food intake, increased metabolic rate, and weighed less than NPY-replete *ob/ob* mice. Both decrease in food intake and loss of weight in response to leptin were also more pronounced than in the controls. It was concluded that there were compensatory responses involving other neuropeptides. Leptin does exert other central effects dissociated from those on the NPY system, and this includes interaction with the hypothalamo–pituitary–adrenocortical axis involving proopiomelanocortin (POMC)-containing neurons.

With the available data, it is possible to speculate on the mode of development of obesity in the *ob/ob* mouse.[109] The major deficiency is a complete lack of feedback from leptin. Both hypothalamic NPY content and secretion are consequently elevated, and this results in hyperphagia and decreased energy utilization, obesity, and hyperinsulinemia. The hypothalamo–pituitary–adrenocortical axis and hypercorticosteronism are also involved.[109] In normal animals, leptin inhibits CRH release from the hypothalamus, resulting in reduced ACTH secretion, and decreased circulating glucocorticoids. All centrally mediated NPY effects on obesity require the presence of glucocorticoids,[109] although the mechanism of action is unknown. In the *ob/ob* mouse, the lack of leptin removes its inhibitory action on CRH secretion,[115] pituitary ACTH content is increased, the adrenal cortex is enlarged,[5] and circulating cortisol levels are elevated. Hypercorticosteronism contributes to a state of muscle insulin resistance,[109] and adrenalectomy of *ob/ob* mice lowers blood glucose and partially restores insulin sensitivity. Glucocorticoids also directly inhibit insulin secretion *in vivo*.[116] In the *db/db* mouse, lack of the leptin receptor results in similar NPY abnormalities to the *ob/ob* mouse, but leptin is still produced, and NPY-induced hyperinsulinemia plus hypercorticosteronism result in *ob* hyperexpression and hyperleptinemia.

Other leptin-related factors may also be involved in the development of obesity. The weight-reducing effects of leptin injection cannot be completely accounted for by decreased food intake,[30,117] and leptin also increases both thermogenesis and energy expenditure. In addition to reversing NPY-mediated actions on the sympathetic nervous system, leptin appears to increase energy expenditure directly via activation of the sympathetic nervous system,[118] resulting in increased noradrenaline turnover in BAT.[119] Leptin-induced increases in thermogenesis in normal rats is associated with elevations of uncoupling protein (UCP-1) mRNA levels.[120] Intravenous leptin increases sympathetic nervous activity to other organs, including the adrenal, kidney, and hind limb,[118] and uncoupling proteins have now been found in multiple tissues.[121] Additionally, leptin influences parasympathetic function peripherally. Local application of leptin to terminals of the rat vagus altered the firing patterns of two types of afferent fibers.[122] One of these was suggested to be involved in the regulation of body weight by sending information regarding circulating concentrations of leptin centrally, and the second to be involved in the regulation of food intake. Sensitivity of the latter to leptin was increased by prior treatment with cholecystokinin (CCK). Leptin also appears to have direct actions on adipocyte metabolism, in addition to those mediated via activation of the autonomic nervous system, resulting in increased glucose utilization and lipolysis.[123] Chen et al.[124] showed a remarkable disappearance of whole-body fat in normal rats treated with a recombinant adenovirus vector overexpressing leptin, and this was associated with decreased circulating triglycerides and insulin, suggestive of enhanced insulin sensitivity. These studies suggest that leptin may normally exert lipoatrophic activity and that leptin deficiency contributes to insulin resistance, through resultant increases in free fatty acids (FFAs; see Section 14.4.6). However, there is also evidence to suggest that leptin can directly antagonize insulin action.[125]

The finding that insulin regulates leptin gene expression led to studies directed at determining whether there was a reciprocal effect of leptin on the pancreatic islet and whether this could provide an important link between leptin and altered islet function in the *ob/ob* mouse. Islet β-cells and βTC-3 tumor cells were indeed shown to express leptin receptors,[126] including the full-length form, Ob-R$_b$,[59,126,127] and leptin inhibits insulin secretion from *ob/ob* mouse islets or the perfused pancreas *in vitro*.[126,127] Leptin was shown to decrease islet intracellular Ca^{2+} (iCa^{2+}) in mouse islets by membrane hyperpolarization via activation of ATP-dependent K$^+$ channels.[59] What is the relationship between the lack of leptin and β-cell abnormalities? Kieffer et al.[59] pointed out that islets from *ob/ob* mice are depolarized in the absence of glucose and that basal insulin release is elevated, with little response to increasing glucose. They attribute this to the lack of leptin-activated K$_{ATP}$ channels. Unger[128] has proposed an interesting hypothesis implicating a primary role for intraislet FFAs in the pathology of islet function in the Zucker Diabetic Fatty rat and this important suggestion will be returned to later (Section 14.4.6).

14.4.2 The Agouti Mouse

The agouti mouse is believed to have first appeared in China, where it was treated as a curiosity because of its brilliant yellow hair color. The *agouti* locus was identified as a result of studies on coat color pigments, and was named after the South American rodent *Dasyprocta aguti*, which has a banded pattern of hair color.[129,130]

The mouse *agouti* gene is localized on chromosome 2. More than 25 phenotypically distinguishable *agouti* alleles have been identified,[129,131,132] and there are several dominant alleles which increase the amount of yellow pigment in the coat, including lethal yellow (A^y), intermediate yellow (A^{iy}), sienna yellow (A^{sy}), viable yellow (A^{vy}), A^{hvy} (hypervariable yellow), and intracisternal A-particle yellow (A^{iapy}). All of these also result in obesity. Homozygosity for the A^y allele results in preimplantation lethality and termination of development by the blastocyst stage. In the heterozygous state, A^y and A^{vy}, maintained on the C57BL/6J strain, produce several dominant pleiotropic effects,[130] including increased body length, increased susceptibility to hepatic, pulmonary, bladder, and mammary tumors, and mild hyperphagia. Obesity in the *agouti* mouse is the result of both the hyperphagia and enhanced efficiency for utilization of calories,[132,133] and it results in marked hypertrophy of adipocytes in subcutaneous, gonadal, and retroperitoneal fat depots. Obesity begins at puberty, is maximal between 7 and 18 months of age,[132,134] and can be influenced by diet. Stored triglycerides increase greatly in adults and can reach 25% of total body weight. This is associated with reduced basal lipolysis.[132] Initially, blood glucose is moderately elevated in nonfasted obese A^{vy}/A males, but normal in fasted males and females. Obese A^{vy}/A mice develop hyperinsulinemia, hyperglycemia, insulin resistance, and NIDDM in males from around weeks 4 to 5.[135,136] The level of hyperinsulinemia is much milder than that found in *ob/ob* and *db/db* mice and is capable of maintaining normoglycemia.[137] Pancreatic islets become enlarged and the β-cells hyperplastic.[3,5] The onset of hyperplasia and hyperinsulinemia in A^vy mice may precede obesity.[137,138] As with the *ob* and *db* mice, there is an essential involvement of the adrenal, since hypertrophy and hyperplasia of the adrenal cortex increases with age in A^y mice, and adrenalectomy results in weight reduction.

14.4.2.1 Identification of the Agouti Gene and Protein

The *agouti* gene is approximately 18 kb in length.[139,140] It contains two identified promoters that utilize three common coding exons. This results in four types of mature 0.7- to 0.8-kb mRNA transcripts with identical coding regions. The 131 amino acid precursor agouti protein contains an N-terminal signal sequence, cleavage of which results in the production of an 108 amino acid–secreted protein. It has a very basic central region and cysteine-rich C-terminus. The *agouti* gene is normally expressed in cells just below the hair bulb, with minor levels of mRNA found in the epidermis.[132] Although humans do not appear to develop agouti-pigmented hair, there is a human version of the mouse *agouti* gene, which maps to chromosome 20q11.2,[141,142] and is 85% identical to the mouse gene. The 132 amino acid human agouti signaling protein (ASP)[142] is 80% identical to the mouse protein, and both proteins share similarities with toxins produced by snails and spiders: the ω-conotoxins and plectotoxins. The *agouti* gene is expressed more widely in humans, predominantly in adipose tissue, testis, ovary, and heart, but at lower levels in liver, kidney, and foreskin.[141,142] This suggests that it may play a broader regulatory role in humans.

The agouti and extension loci are responsible for the temporal and spatial distribution of granules containing phaeomelanin (yellow to red pigment) and eumelanin (black to brown pigment) by regulating a switch in pigment synthesis within each hair shaft. The coloration of the wild-type agouti (A^w) is a result of a pulse of agouti expression during the hair growth cycle in the dorsal region, which produces agouti-colored hairs, and continuous expression during the hair-growth cycle in the ventral region, producing yellow to white hairs.[130,143] Two agouti isoforms are expressed in dorsal and ventral skin, and two further isoforms in the ventral skin. The level of expression correlates with the synthesis of yellow pigment. Agouti produced in the hair follicles acts on follicular melanocytes. These are neural crest-derived cells lying around the base of the hair follicle that produce the pigment and deposit it via dendritic processes into the growing hair shaft. As discussed below, the agouti gene product inhibits α-melanocyte-stimulating hormone (α-MSH)-induced eumelanin production, resulting in a subterminal band of phaeomelanin. The α-MSH receptor, MC1-R, via which these effects are mediated is encoded by the extension locus.[144]

A^y, A^vy, A^hvy, A^iapy, A^iy, and A^sy are all mutations that result in the introduction of a new promoter upstream of the *agouti* gene, leading to ubiquitous expression. The first of the mutations characterized, the A^y mutation, is caused by a deletion that results in the replacement of the normal agouti gene promoter with that of a ubiquitously expressed gene, *Raly*, which is normally constitutively active in all tissues.[145-147] Other dominant alleles, including A^iapy, A^iy, and A^vy also result from insertions that result in inappropriate and ubiquitous expression. The insertion associated with A^sy is unknown at present, but those associated with A^iy, A^vy, A^sy, and A^iapy are intracisternal A-particles (IAPs).[148,149] The IAPs are defective retroviruses encoded by a family of endogenous proviral sequences present at about 1000 copies per haploid genome in *Mus musculus*.[143] They integrate upstream of the first coding exon of the *agouti* gene,[145-148] and probably act by initiating transcription from a cryptic promoter within the IAP long terminal repeat. A^hvy is unique because mice carrying the mutation can display a range of coat color from obese pure yellow to almost pure black and normal weight.[150] A[hvy] results from integration of an IAP in an antisense orientation within the 5′ untranslated agouti exon 1C.[151] Klebig et al.[152] tested the hypothesis that ectopic expression of the normal agouti protein in dominant obese yellow a-locus mutants was directly responsible for the pleiotropic phenotype by generating transgenic mice ectopically expressing the normal agouti protein. Transgenic mice of both sexes had yellow fur, became obese, and developed hyperinsulinemia. Males developed hyperglycemia by 12 to 20 weeks of age.

14.4.2.2   Mode of Action of Agouti and Its Role in Obesity and NIDDM

It is now clear that obesity in agouti mice involves a complex network of peptides and their receptors, with ligands derived from the POMC precursor, ACTH and MSH, a family of five melanocortin (MC) receptors, and two inhibitory peptides for these receptors, agouti and the agouti-related transcript (protein).[153] MC receptors are members of the seven-transmembrane G protein–coupled family, that includes MSH and ACTH receptors, now renamed MC1-R and MC2-R, plus MC3-R, MC4-R, and MC5-R (reviewed by Cone et al.[144]). The five receptors are 39 to 61% identical at the amino acid level,[144] and all couple to adenylate cyclase.

A local mode of action of agouti was first suggested by studies involving parabiosis between A[y] and nonagouti (a/a) littermates. Following identification of agouti protein, it was demonstrated that it acts on hair color via MCR-1. Normally, α-MSH activates adenylate cyclase in the melanocyte via MC1-R, and the cAMP produced stimulates production of eumalanin.[144] Agouti protein is a high-affinity antagonist of the MC1-receptor[154] and, when present within the hair follicle, it acts in a paracrine manner to block binding of α-MSH, thus causing a shift from eumalanin to phaeomelanin. Millar et al.[155] tested this proposed mode of action by creating transgenic animals in which agouti was expressed in basal cells of the epidermis. These animals displayed stripes of yellow hairs corresponding to regions of epidermal agouti expression, confirming that agouti signals melanocytes to synthesize yellow pigment and providing direct evidence that it functions in a paracrine manner. Although it is not clear whether or not human ASP plays a major role in the regulation of hair color, α-MSH does stimulate melanogenesis, specifically eumelanogenesis, in human epidermal melanocytes. Expression of ASP in transgenic mice produces a yellow coat, and expression in mouse cultured melanoma cells blocked α-MSH-stimulated accumulation of cAMP,[140] so it has the potential to play a physiological role.

In mice, MC1-R is restricted to melanocytes and MC2-R to adrenal cortex and adipocytes. In contrast, MC3-R, 4-R, and 5-R show a much broader distribution.[144] MC4-R is found in high concentrations in the hypothalamus, including the VM, lateral DMN, and the PVN, important regions for regulating feeding behavior.[156] Additionally, there are links between neurons in the ARC nucleus, a major site of production of POMC in the brain, and the VMH, DMH, and PVN.[156] Agouti is an antagonist of MC4-R, but not MC-3R or MC-5R, and it is now considered likely that the major pathway by which agouti results in obesity is via interacting with these receptors. Inactivation of MC4-R by gene targeting resulted in mice with NIDDM associated with hyperphagia, hyperinsulinemia, and hyperglycemia, which recapitulated several of the characteristic features of the agouti obesity syndrome.[136] The NPY system is also involved. Expression of NPY in A[y] and MC4R-deficient mice was found to be greatly increased in the DMH.[156] This indicated that MC4-R-containing neuron terminals in the DMH normally inhibit NPY gene expression in this nucleus, and, when the receptor is suppressed or absent, NPY expression is elevated. As mentioned in discussing the interaction between leptin and NPY, projections of these neurons to the PVN increase feeding. The endogenous ligand acting on MC4-R is thought to be des-acetyl-MSH. Fan et al.[157] provided further evidence for a tonic inhibitory role for MC4-R in feeding. Intracerebroventricular administration of a cyclic agonist of central MC-4 receptors inhibited feeding in several models of hyperphagia, and this effect was blocked by an MC-4 receptor antagonist. The same antagonist also inhibited nocturnal feeding and feeding stimulated by a prolonged fast. Leptin has also been implicated in this pathway. The POMC neurons responsible for inhibiting NPY secretion coexpress leptin receptors,[158] and, as previously discussed, normally NPY gene expression and secretion is inhibited by leptin. *Ob* mRNA levels are elevated in adipose tissue from obese yellow agouti mice, the degree of increase correlating with elevations in body weight,[159] and these mice do not respond to exogenous leptin with a reduction in food intake.[160] It is therefore likely that part of the neural network distal to that activated via the leptin receptor is inactive.

The magnitude of change in eating behavior and thermogenesis in A^{vy} mice attributable to central effects cannot completely account for the degree of obesity observed. Therefore, it has been suggested that, apart from its central action, agouti also exerts peripheral effects, either via MC4-R[154] or its own receptor. In a series of papers from Zemel's laboratory,[161-165] evidence has been presented suggesting that agouti increases intracellular free Ca^{2+} concentrations $[iCa^{2+}]$, in cells via a mechanism distinct from an antagonistic action at MC receptors. As pointed out earlier, the spacing of cysteines in agouti peptide is almost identical to that found in ω-conotoxins and plectotoxins. These toxins are agonists or antagonists of various ion channels, including Ca^{2+} channels. Zemel et al.[162,163] showed that in mice carrying the A^{vy} mutation, the $[iCa^{2+}]$ was elevated in skeletal muscle, and the degree of elevation closely correlated with the degree to which the mutant traits were expressed. Additionally, it was demonstrated that agouti protein increased $[iCa^{2+}]$ in skeletal muscle myocytes from wild-type mice, and in vascular smooth muscle cells and 3T3-L1 adipocytes *in vitro*.[164] These workers have therefore suggested that agouti protein promotes insulin resistance in mutant animals through its ability to increase $[iCa^{2+}]$.[163,164] Adipose and hepatic mRNA levels for fatty acid synthase (FAS) and stearoyl-CoA desaturase (SCD), two key enzymes in *de novo* fatty acid synthesis and desaturation, respectively, are greatly increased in obese (A^{vy}) mice. Agouti also increases FAS and SCD mRNA levels and FAS activity and triglyceride in 3T3-L1 adipocytes, suggesting a direct action.[165] These responses are blocked by the Ca^{2+}-channel blocker, nitrendipine. The $[iCa^{2+}]$ studies have been criticized on the basis that the homologous snail and spider toxins block calcium channels, and this would not be expected to result in increased $[iCa^{2+}]$,[136] and that the effect of agouti on iCa^{2+} is only transient. The story is as yet incomplete.

Are these peripheral effects of agouti protein of relevance to the development of diabetes in humans? Human agouti protein has been reported to decrease melanogenesis directly in cultured human epidermal melanocytes,[166] without significant effects on the ability of α-MSH to stimulate melanogenesis, indicating that it can act peripherally. Insulin resistance has been suggested to be characterized by abnormal iCa^{2+} homeostasis in several cell types, and increased iCa^{2+} inhibits insulin-stimulated glucose transport and may also affect the phosphorylation/dephosphorylation state of various enzymes. Therefore, agouti-induced increases in $[iCa^{2+}]$ could play a role. Additionally, since islet hyperplasia develops early in obese A^{vy} mice an interaction between agouti and insulin could be important for triggering the onset of obesity.[133] A recent study from Mynatt et al.[167] provides credence for this proposal. They generated transgenic mice expressing agouti in BAT and WAT. These mice did not normally become obese or diabetic, but daily insulin injections significantly increased weight gain in the transgenic lines expressing agouti in adipose tissue, but not in nontransgenic mice. Such a synergistic effect is interesting since both hormones are lipogenic,[165] and Mynatt et al.[167] have suggested a possible scenario for the development of diabetes in which agouti expression in the pancreatic β-cell stimulates insulin secretion, and the resulting hyperinsulinemia acts in concert with agouti to promote weight increase. The sustained hyperinsulinemia also results in insulin resistance and hyperglycemia, leading to NIDDM.

14.4.2.3 Agouti-Related Transcript (Protein)

Recently, a human gene, located on Chromosome 16q22, was identified and named agouti-related transcript (*Agrt; Art*)[153] or agouti-related protein (*Agrp*),[168] because of its similarity to *Agouti*. This gene encodes a 132 amino acid protein that is 25% identical to human agouti, the highest degree of identity residing within the C-terminus. The murine homologue is a 131 amino acid protein and 81% identical to the human version. The gene is expressed primarily in the adrenal (cortex and medulla), subthalamic nucleus, and hypothalamus in both human and mouse,[153,168] with low-level expression in the testis, lung, and kidney. Although the function of the gene product is at present unclear, it is a selective antagonist of MC-4R, is concentrated in the ARN and median eminence, and there is a tenfold upregulation in the hypothalamus of *ob* and *db* mice. This protein is therefore probably important in feeding, and may act via MC receptors. The fact that Bardet–Biedl syndrome maps near to this locus (16q21) may also be of significance.[153] Overexpression of Art protein in transgenic mice resulted in weight gain, increased circulating insulin, delayed hyperglycemia, but no change in coat color.[168,169] Hypertrophic adipose tissue and pancreatic islets were also evident.

14.4.3 The Tubby Mouse

The *tub* mutation arose spontaneously in a mouse colony at the Jackson Laboratory,[169] and the *tubby* colony was bred from a single C57BL/6J male. Tubby mice are characterized by slowly developing obesity. Although hyperinsulinemia, hyperactivity of the islet β-cells, and β-cell degranulation are conspicuous features of these animals, hyperglycemia is not observed, and the obesity syndrome does not normally progress to "severe" diabetes. Somewhat surprisingly, apart from Coleman and Eicher's[169] original description, there is little information regarding glucose metabolism in these mutants.

It was determined from breeding experiments that the mutation associated with obesity is autosomal recessive and located on Chromosome 7.[169] Increases in body weight are slower than with the *ob* and *db* mutations, and obesity is not apparent until 9 to 12 weeks of age.[169,170] Obese males at 24 weeks average ~46 g in weight.[169] Both females and males develop a mild hypoglycemia and hyperinsulinemia at 12 weeks, but then become euglycemic. The hyperinsulinemia persists, increasing in severity with age and, ultimately, is associated with insulin resistance. In contrast, in *ob*, *db*, and *fat* mice, hyperinsulinemia is not associated with hypoglycemia.[171] There is a marked sexual dimorphism in the development of pancreatic abnormalities. The pancreas is normal up to about 12 weeks of age, when hypertrophy develops in males, and by 1 year the pancreas is characterized by multiple large islets. Hypertrophy is delayed in onset, and is less severe, in females. It has been reported that obesity in tubby mice is not associated with hyperphagia,[171] although Noben-Trauth et al.[172] observed increased food intake over time. Sexual dimorphism has also been reported for triglyceride and cholesterol levels.[173] Male *tub/tub* mice have significantly greater triglyceride and cholesterol levels than control strains,[173] but reduced susceptibility to fatty streak lesions.[174] This suggests that there may also be dominant effects of the mutation.[175]

14.4.3.1 Identification of the Tub Gene and Tubby Protein

Two groups identified the mutated *tub* gene by positional cloning.[172,175] The wild-type transcript is localized predominantly in the brain, and *in situ* hybridization shows highest expression in the hippocampus, cortex, and in the PVN, VMN, and ARN neurons of the hypothalamus. Northern and RT-PCR analyses identified lower concentrations of transcript in eye, testis, small and large intestines, adipose tissue, liver, ovary, thymus and lung, indicating that the gene is widely expressed.

In mutant mice, a single mutation (GT $\rightarrow$ TT) abolishes a donor splice site in the 3' coding region. This results in incorrect retention of a single intron in the mature *tub* mRNA transcript, and replacement of the carboxy-terminal 44 amino acids with 20 to 24 intron-encoded amino acids.[172,175] A second, prematurely truncated transcript containing the unspliced intron is also found in testis.[172] A two- to threefold increase in brain *tub* mRNA is observed in tubby mice,[172] and there is variability in the relative abundance of alternatively spliced products between inbred mouse strains, which appears to correlate with intron length polymorphism.[175] A mouse cDNA probe was used to isolate the human homologue of *tub* (*TUB*), which maps to chromosome 11p15. Sequencing revealed 89% identity between the human and mouse species at the DNA level, and 94% at the protein level. The protein is predicted to be hydrophilic, lacks any known secretory component, and exhibits strong sequence similarity to a putative mouse testis-specific phosphodiesterase. Two related human proteins, tubby-like protein (TULP) 1 and 2, have been identified recently.[176]

The *tub* gene is closely linked to a gene causing loss of vision and hearing, and it is possible that they are the same gene. Tubby mice exhibit retinal degeneration, involving loss of photoreceptors, as shown by electroretinography and histopathology. They also have progressive hearing loss, which involves the cochlea.[177] There is pronounced degeneration of the organ of Corti and selective loss of afferent neurons, as seen in human Usher syndrome Type I, a disease associated with the *USH1c* locus.[177,178] Similarity to Alström and Bardet–Biedl syndromes has also been noted.[177] The chromosomal localization of *TUB* was originally described as 11p15.1, suggesting it might be *USH1c*.[178] However, this possibility was recently questioned, and an alternative locus suggested (11p15.4).[176]

14.4.3.2 Mode of Action of Tubby Protein and Its Role in Obesity

The phenotypic features of tubby mice have been suggested to result from cellular apoptosis triggered by expression of the mutated *tub* gene,[177,178] but whether or not this accounts for the observed pathology is unclear. Similarly, although regions of the hypothalamus associated with body weight regulation express the *tub* gene, uncertainty regarding its function has so far precluded the establishment of a link between the protein product and the development of obesity.

14.4.4 The Fat Mouse

The *fat* (CPE^{fat}) mutation was discovered in an HRS/J inbred mouse colony at the Jackson Laboratory, and it was mapped to mouse Chromosome 8.[169] Inheritance is autosomal recessive. Animals develop obesity at 6 to 8 weeks of age, slightly earlier than tubby mice,[169] but *fat/fat* mutants may not be distinguishable from their littermates until 8 to 12 weeks of age.[179] Mutants can weigh 60 to 70g by 24 weeks. Unlike *tubby* mice, there is no sexual dimorphism for development of adiposity. In Coleman and Eicher's study[169] transient hyperglycemia (~14 m*M*) was observed at 7 to 8 weeks of age in males, and glucose levels then returned to normal, whereas females remained normoglycemic throughout. Chronic hyperinsulinemia was present in both sexes from weaning, and this was associated with hypertrophic and hyperplastic pancreatic islets, although there were no signs of β-cell atrophy.

14.4.4.1   Identification of the Fat Mutation

The *fat* mutation was backcrossed onto C57BLKS/J mice.[169,179] C57BLKS/J-*fat/fat* mice have elevated circulating insulin levels but are extremely responsive to exogenous insulin, and hyperglycemia can be completely controlled. In an elegant combination of molecular biology and protein chemistry, Naggert and co-workers[179] demonstrated that the major component of the elevated circulating immunoreactive insulin was in fact partially processed proinsulin. They proceeded to identify *fat* as the carboxypeptidase E (CPE) gene (*Cpe*). This enzyme is normally found in high concentrations in secretory granules, and processes intermediates during the processing of prohormones such as proinsulin and POMC, by removal of C-terminal paired basic residues. It was demonstrated that there was a virtual absence of immunoreactive CPE in extracts of *fat/fat* pancreatic islets and pituitaries, and in islet extracts there were increased quantities of B-chain-extended (31,32) di-arginyl insulins. The gene mutation was identified as a T → C transition resulting in a single $Ser_{202}Pro$ substitution. Introduction of this mutation into the wild-type protein was later shown to result in a product that is either folded incorrectly or is unstable and degraded in the endoplasmic reticulum.[180]

The *fat* mutation involves an enzyme that is of widespread importance in the processing of prohormone-derived peptides. The pancreas, pituitary, and other neuroendocrine tissues, including the brain, adrenal, testis,[181] stomach, and colon[182] are all CPE-deficient in *fat/fat* mice. Inappropriate processing of several propeptides has been demonstrated, associated with elevated amounts of precursors and peptides with C-terminal mono- or di-basic amino acid extensions. This includes POMC,[183] proenkephalin,[181] proneurotensin,[184] promelanin-concentrating hormone (MCH),[184] progastrin,[182,185] and pro-CCK.[186] An alternative C-terminal processing pathway for CCK in the rat duodenum was demonstrated recently,[186] and in some tissues carboxypeptidase D can partially compensate for the loss of CPE in processing in the *fat/fat* mouse.[181] Therefore, levels of some peptides considered to be normally produced by CPE trimming may not be significantly altered.

Loh and co-workers[183,187,188] proposed an additional function for membrane-associated CPE: as a sorting receptor for trafficking to the secretory granule. This finding would be important, since this is a crucial component of the pathway for sorting secretory proteins into granules in preparation for release via the regulated secretory pathway, and it would imply general disruption of regulated secretion in the body. POMC contains an amino-terminal disulfide bonded loop, and Loh et al.[183,187,188] reported that this loop binds specifically to membrane-associated CPE. Evidence was presented from studies on CPE-transfected neuroendocrine cells and *fat/fat* mouse pituitary cells suggesting that POMC is missorted to the constitutive pathway and secreted in an unregulated manner. In isolated pituitary cells, POMC levels were increased 24-fold and this precursor was poorly processed to ACTH.[187] Intracellular routing of GH was also altered, and there were high levels of "constitutive" secretion of both POMC and growth hormone. Hence, the suggestion that CPE regulates sorting. Unfortunately, there are strong arguments against this conclusion.[189] These cannot be discussed in detail, but in essence they question whether the observed increase in secretion was truly constitutive, and not increased regulated release. Thiele et al.[189] point out that the neurointermediate lobe POMC secretory kinetics with tissues from control and *fat/fat* mice were extremely similar. Additionally, β-cells of *fat/fat* mice have normal numbers of secretory granules,[179] unimpaired targeting of proinsulin to the regulated pathway,[190] and normal regulated secretion.[191] Therefore, CPE is unlikely to be an obligatory sorting receptor.

14.4.4.2 Lack of Carboxypeptidase E and Obesity

It is clear that the absence of CPE results in multiple endocrine disorders in *fat/fat* mice, although the relationship between increases in prohormones and late-developing obesity is unclear. Since CCK, products of POMC processing, MCH, and insulin have all been implicated in the regulation of satiety, energy balance, and nutrient partitioning via central actions, aberrant processing of any of these peptide precursors could contribute to hyperphagia. The failure to develop a marked diabetic state may be related to the absence of hypercorticosteronism in the *fat/fat* mouse.[179]

Although mutations in CPE have not as yet been reported in humans, alterations in hormone precursor-processing enzymes have been shown to result in NIDDM. A woman with early-onset extreme obesity, abnormal glucose tolerance, and elevations in circulating proinsulin and POMC, but reduced insulin levels, was shown to be deficient in active prohormone convertase 1 (PC1).[192] It was shown that a $Gly_{483}Arg$ substitution was present that prevented processing of proPC1. Mice lacking PC2 have also been shown to have greatly impaired islet hormone processing, plus hyperplasia of α- and δ-cells and a reduction in β-cells.[193] It seems likely therefore that human forms of NIDDM will be found that are associated with other processing hormone mutations. This is clearly important since hyperproinsulinemia in human NIDDM results from incomplete processing of proinsulin.[194]

14.4.5 Zucker Fatty Rat

The fatty (*fa; Lepr^fa*) mutation in rats arose spontaneously in an outbred stock in the Zucker laboratory,[195] but the background strain genetics has been complicated by breeding in both outbred and inbred strains.[9] There is an extensive literature on the Zucker rat and there are several excellent reviews dedicated to this animal model.[15,196,197] Obese (*fa/fa*) Zucker rats are characterized by hyperphagia,[198] hyperlipidemia,[199] and mild glucose intolerance.[200] Obesity is accompanied by profound hyperinsulinemia detectable as early as 21 days of age.[201,202] Pancreatic islets are enlarged and yield an exaggerated response to a glucose stimulus.[203] In the nondiabetic Zucker fatty rat, hyperinsulinemia persists throughout life. Islets from *fa/fa* rats exhibit a left shift in glucose-concentration response curves,[202,204,205] and the increased sensitivity to low glucose levels undoubtedly contributes to fasting hyperinsulinemia. Additionally, neurotransmitters and hormones that normally exhibit a glucose threshold for the potentiation of insulin secretion (5 to 6 m*M*) stimulate insulin secretion at basal glucose levels.[204,205]

14.4.5.1 Identification of the Fa Gene

The *fa* gene is a homologue of the mouse *db* gene located on rat chromosome 5. A single point mutation (CAG → CCG) results in a $Gln_{269}Pro$ substitution in the extracellular domain of the leptin receptor (Ob-R).[206,207] Transient transfection studies with mouse Ob-R cDNA containing the $Gln_{269}Pro$ mutation demonstrated greatly reduced surface leptin binding,[208] and impaired signaling via pathways involving both early response genes (*c-fos, c-jun, jun-B*),[208] and STAT 5B.[209]

14.4.5.2   The Role of the Fa Mutation in Obesity and NIDDM

Hyperphagia in the *fa/fa* rat can now be explained on the same basis, of reduced leptin binding, as for the *db* mouse. This results in a reduction in production and secretion of satiety-promoting neuropeptides, such as CRH, and an increase in orexigenic peptides, such as NPY. Paraventricular NPY secretion has been shown to be increased,[111] and NPY also continues its effect on the pancreas, contributing to hyperinsulinemia and hypercorticosteronism. Jeanrenaud et al.[210] proposed that a defect in the central regulation of autonomic function is a major causative factor in the metabolic abnormalities observed in the *fa/fa* rat. This is characterized by increased parasympathetic input to the endocrine pancreas, resulting in hyperinsulinemia and hyperglucagonemia, and decreased sympathetic drive to the periphery, particularly to BAT, resulting in impaired temperature regulation. When studied at normal room temperature, basal glucose uptake of BAT is similar in lean and obese animals, but when animals are exposed to a cold environment, sympathetic activation leading to glucose uptake into BAT is markedly reduced in obese animals, indicating blunted sympathetic responses.[211,212] The similar phenotype to the diabetic mouse with regard to increased *ob* gene expression[213] and circulating leptin levels[214] is consistent with leptin resistance.

The question of how a proposed hypothalamic defect in Zucker rats results in hyperinsulinemia and insulin resistance is now being answered on the basis of a deficiency in leptin receptor signaling. Insulin resistance in muscle and liver of *fa/fa* rats affects both glucose utilization and hepatic glucose production.[215,216] This is exemplified by the finding that in clamp experiments, insulin sensitivity was shown to be three- to fourfold lower in lean vs. obese Zucker rats.[216] It appears that abnormal glucose tolerance is due to metabolic defects in the liver, since glucose clearance in the obese rat was normal,[217] but hepatic glucose production was not suppressed following a glucose meal.[200] Abnormal regulation of glucagon secretion could also be a contributing factor to the increased hepatic glucose production.[218] The binding of insulin to isolated hepatocytes from *fa/fa* animals was reported to be decreased,[219] but there are conflicting reports of the status of liver insulin receptor tyrosine kinase activity,[220,221] although insulin receptor tyrosine kinase activity in muscle appears to be reduced.[218] The presence of both insulin resistance and a β-cell secretory defect in the Zucker rat has generally been held responsible for the impaired glucose-stimulated insulin release and hyperglycemia[222] in *fa/fa* rats. Treatment of Zucker rats with the insulin-sensitizing drug, proglitazone, was shown to correct the insulin resistance and enhance glucose-stimulated insulin secretion,[223] demonstrating the close link between the two abnormalities. However, the nature of the islet defect and the origin of the resistance have been undefined. A possible scenario, suggested by Unger from an extensive series of studies in the Zucker Diabetic Fatty (ZDF) rat is discussed below.

14.4.6   Zucker Diabetic Fatty (ZDF) Rat

A great deal of interest has been generated by the development of the ZDF strain as a model of NIDDM. These rats arose from the inbreeding of a substrain of *fa/fa* rats that exhibited hyperglycemia.[224] In this strain all males develop obesity, insulin resistance and overt NIDDM between 7 and 10 weeks of age, by which time their average plasma glucose exceeds 22 mM. Female littermates are also obese and insulin resistant but do not become diabetic. Although pre-diabetic animals exhibit normal glucose tolerance, islets from prediabetic animals show impaired ability of the β-cell to respond to alterations in glucose.[225] This results in a leftward shift in the dose–response curve relating glucose to insulin (low-K_m glucose usage) and a greater than normal insulin response to glucose. The same group noted that the islets of prediabetic animals were larger and more irregular in shape, and that these differences became more pronounced at 12 weeks of age, when animals became overtly diabetic. As noted above, the Zucker fatty rat, from which the ZDF strain was derived, exhibits islet hyperplasia.[202]

Normally, insulin is secreted in a pulsatile fashion of a fixed periodicity in humans,[226,227] as well as in the perfused pancreas and perifused islets,[228,229] a pattern that is disturbed in patients with NIDDM.[230] Additionally, it has been shown that pulsatile insulin delivery has a greater hypoglycemic effect than constant delivery.[231] Pulsatile insulin secretion was found to be disrupted in pancreata from ZDF rats,[232] and it was hypothesized that this disruption may contribute to the impairment in glucose-stimulated insulin secretion observed in the ZDF strain. Diabetic (10-week-old) ZDF animals exhibit many of the characteristics of human NIDDM including hyperglycemia and lack of responsiveness of the pancreas to glucose, while retaining the ability to release insulin in response to arginine.[232] There is also marked underexpression of β-cell immunoreactive GLUT-2 glucose transporters and GLUT-2 messenger RNA.[233,234] These data were interpreted as indicating that a reduced capacity for high Km glucose transport is involved in the impairment of glucose-stimulated insulin secretion in the ZDF islet with attendant hyperglycemia. However, it is now considered unlikely to play a major role. In their study of the transition from the prediabetic to the diabetic state, Tokuyama et al.[225] found many other abnormalities in the ZDF islet in addition to a reduction in GLUT-2 expression. This included reductions in islet mRNA levels for glucokinase, voltage-dependent Ca^{2+} and K^+ channels, Ca^{2+}-ATPase, and increases in glucose-6-phosphatase and 12-lipoxygenase. Impaired insulin secretion in response to glucose was also accompanied by reduced insulin mRNA levels, pancreatic insulin content, and β-cell number. The underlying cause of this multiplicity of islet defects is unknown. Decreased glucose transport activity and decreased levels of the insulin-sensitive glucose transporter GLUT-4 in adipose tissue have been reported in obese diabetic and nondiabetic humans,[235] implicating this transporter in the insulin resistance observed in obesity irrespective of the diabetic state (see Section 14.8.1.3). Decreased GLUT-4 levels were found in the hearts of obese *fa/fa* Zucker rats,[236,237] and in adipose tissue, heart, and skeletal muscle of ZDF rats.[238]

There is an extensive literature that has considered the possibility that direct effects of FFAs on glucose metabolism in tissues such as skeletal muscle play an important role in the link between obesity and NIDDM.[128,239-241] Recently, Unger[128] has proposed a unifying hypothesis linking elevations in circulating and intracellular FFAs and leptin deficiency or leptin resistance, to insulin resistance and NIDDM. A central point to the proposal is that FFAs are taken up, converted to triglycerides (TG), and stored in many cell types in addition to adipose tissue, including pancreatic β-cells. Islet β-cells contain leptin receptors,[59,126,127] and leptin may normally be involved in restricting β-cell TG accumulation.[128,242] Unger's group demonstrated recently that obesity in the ZDF rat results in the accumulation of TGs in islet cells,[128] and that isolated islets from ZDF rats have increased lipogenic capacity, probably due to chronic exposure to high levels of FFA.[243] It was proposed by Unger[128] that the increased β-cell TG results from a lack of islet responsiveness to leptin, and that it leads to lipotoxic β-cell damage. In support of this hypothesis is the finding that experimentally lowering TG levels in ZDF rats prevents the diabetic syndrome from developing.[244] In an extension of his hypothesis[128,245] it was proposed that the mechanism by which TGs cause lipotoxicity is via increasing levels of inducible nitric oxide synthase (iNOS), resulting in cell damage by nitric oxide (NO). That increased NO could result in the β-cell destruction observed late in ZDF diabetes is suggested by findings that inhibitors of iNOS prevent hyperglycemia and β-cell death when administered to prediabetic ZDF rats.[128]

14.4.7   The Koletsky and JCR:LA-Corpulent Rats

The obese, spontaneously hypertensive, Koletsky rat strain develops obesity, hyperlipidemia, and proteinuria with kidney disease, due to a single recessive gene originally called *f*.[247] From breeding studies with Zucker rats it was suggested that alleles from the same locus may be responsible for the obese phenotype, and *f* was renamed *fa^k^*.[247] Several substrains have been developed from Koletsky rats, including the SHR/N-cp, LA/N-cp,[248] and JCR:LA-cp (*fa^cp^*)[249] strains. The JCR:LA-cp rat will be discussed in some detail, as an example of the corpulent rat phenotype. The *cp/cp* rat exhibits marked hyperphagia and increased body weight and is highly prone to cardiovascular disease. It is identifiable by its phenotype at weaning (3 weeks of age). Plasma insulin and TG concentrations are mildly elevated in *cp/cp* rats at weaning,[249] and TG concentrations subsequently begin to rise. Marked hyperinsulinemia develops between 5 and 6 weeks of age and insulin-mediated glucose uptake decreases.[249,250] The hyperinsulinemia is due to an extreme pancreatic hypersecretion of insulin,[251] accompanied by increased β-cell glucokinase activity.[252] The hyperinsulinemia effectively maintains virtual normoglycemia, but this results in marked islet hyperplasia, and islets occupy 15 to 20% of the total pancreatic volume in 9-month-old *cp/cp* male rats.[253]

14.4.7.1   Identification of the Fa(Cp) Mutation

The recessive mutation in the Koletsky obese and corpulent rats maps to the same genetic interval as *fa*.[254] The mutation has been identified in both the Koletsky (*fa^k^/fa^k^*)[247,254] strain and corpulent (*fa^cp^/fa^cp^*)[50] substrain of rats as a T → A transversion in the leptin-receptor gene that results in a $Tyr_{763}Stop$ nonsense mutation just before the transmembrane domain. There is therefore complete lack of synthesis of the external and transmembrane domains common to all forms of Ob-R, a null mutation. Both *ob* gene expression and circulating leptin levels are increased in Koletsky rats to a greater degree than in *fa/fa* rats,[255] consistent with the more extreme leptin receptor deficiency.

14.4.7.2   The Cp Mutation and Vasculopathy in NIDDM

Hypertriglyceridemia in the *cp/cp* rat is a consequence of increased hepatic uptake of diet-derived glucose and TG synthesis, in the absence of peripheral insulin-mediated uptake,[256] resulting in hepatic hypersecretion of very-low-density lipoprotein (VLDL).[257] Increased FFAs may result in insulin resistance and islet defects as described above. The *cp/cp* male rat develops a vasculopathy before 12 weeks of age.[258,259] Atherosclerotic lesions reach an incidence of 100% on the aortic arch of 9-month-old animals. The lesions contain foam cells and debris, and are similar to those seen in humans and other animal models of atherosclerosis. The JCR:LA-cp rat is a useful model of the vasculopathy associated with NIDDM.

14.5   Polygenic Models of Obesity and NIDDM

No single gene has been demonstrated to be involved in the majority of patients with obesity and/or NIDDM. The overall contribution of single gene defects to the total NIDDM population is small, and only ~10% of the genetic risk factors for NIDDM are known.[1] The more common forms of NIDDM probably result from interaction between the environment and several gene defects, each of which when expressed individually has little effect on glucose tolerance. Therefore, polygenic animal models represent the human condition more closely, although knowledge of the genetic basis is rudimentary.

14.5.1 Inbred Mice

The most extensively studied inbred strains of mice are the New Zealand Obese (NZO), Japanese KK and NSY (Nagoya-Shibata-Yasuda), and PBB/Ld (Paul Bailey Black) strains.

14.5.1.1 New Zealand Obese (NZO) Mouse

Several groups have bred NZO mice from the strain first described by Bielschowsky and Bielschowsky,[260,261] which was developed from a mixed colony by inbreeding for coat color, starting with a pair of agouti mice. Variability has been introduced into the strain by continued inbreeding in separate colonies.[134] The NZO mouse is hyperphagic, obese, hyperglycemic, hyperinsulinemic, insulin resistant, and mildly glucose intolerant.[262,263] The NZO mouse is related to the autoimmune NZB strain, and there is evidence that the development of diabetes in the NZO strain might also involve an autoimmune component. Harrison and Itin[262] reported the presence of autoantibodies in serum from NZO mice which inhibited ^{125}I-insulin binding to mouse liver membranes, and suggested they were low-titer IgM antibodies to the insulin receptor. Circulating antibodies to both native and denatured, single-stranded DNA have also been detected.[264] A number of other abnormalities in both the humoral and cell-mediated immune systems are indicative of a generalized autoimmune disorder.[265] NZO mice become clearly obese by 8 to 10 weeks of age[262] and reach their maximal weight (males) of ~70 g at 12 months. Insulin and glucose levels are normal in overnight-fasted animals, but both are elevated in unfasted animals.[266,267] Glucagon levels are also increased in fasted animals.[266] Hyperinsulinemia and hyperglycemia develop early (by 4 weeks),[263] and pancreatic insulin stores are increased at this time.[268] Glucose intolerance decreases continuously with age and body weight.

Obesity in NZO mice involves increased retroperitoneal adipose deposits and both hypertrophy and hyperplasia of adipocytes in subcutaneous and gonadal fat depots.[134] This is associated with marked increases in the expression of adipose tissue leptin mRNA, and of stored and circulating leptin.[269] NZO mice do not decrease food intake in response to exogenous leptin, suggesting that leptin resistance contributes to the obesity/NIDDM syndrome. Two conservative and one nonconservative amino acid substitution in the leptin receptor have been found, but these also exist in the lean NZ black strain.[269] Therefore, these substitutions are unlikely to be responsible for the apparent leptin resistance, and the deficiency is likely to be either distal to the receptor or in the CNS uptake system. A number of abnormalities of adipocyte function have been described, which reflect the insulin resistance, including slightly decreased insulin receptor binding,[270] increased lipogenesis,[270] insulin unresponsiveness of pyruvate dehydrogenase,[270] and decreased GLUT-4 levels.[271]

First-phase insulin responses to glucose are decreased *in vivo*,[267,272] whereas integrated responses to other stimuli are increased. This has been interpreted as indicating a general secretory abnormality .[267] However, several *in vitro* studies point to a selective defect in glucose-induced insulin secretion.[273] It is unclear if such defects are primary or secondary to chronic hyperinsulinemia and hyperglycemia. Insulin resistance occurs at 4 to 5 weeks in several tissues,[272] the origin of which has also been investigated in a number of studies.

At 4 to 6 weeks of age, glucose uptake and utilization in soleus muscle in the absence of insulin is reduced, but there is a normal response to insulin.[263] However, from 11 weeks, insulin responsiveness is markedly impaired. Na^+-K^+-pump activity is also reduced in soleus muscle from NZO mice.[274] Changes in the intrinsic metabolic rate of skeletal muscle probably play an important role in the control of overall energy balance, and may be partly responsible for the altered energetic efficiency in this strain of mice. The liver also demonstrates insulin resistance, and hepatic glucose production is increased at an early age.[272,275,276] There appears to be an abnormality in fructose-1,6-bisphosphatase activity[277] and a failure in the normal mechanisms that reduce levels of glycogen synthase following birth,[278] which may contribute to the increased hepatic glucose production.

14.5.1.2   The Japanese KK Mouse

The KK mouse belongs to the Kasukabe (K) group of mouse strains.[9] It was produced by selective inbreeding for large body size and appears to be a polygenic model of obesity and NIDDM.[9,134] KK mice are hyperphagic and develop a moderate obesity, which can be observed at 2 months of age and which is maximal by 4 to 5 months. Islets become hyperplastic with increased insulin content, and there is hyperinsulinemia, nonfasting hyperglycemia, and glucose intolerance. Insulin resistance precedes the onset of obesity.[279] Restriction of food intake prevents the obesity, and many of the abnormalities revert to normal with age. The original strain produced in Japan became normoglycemic in the 1970s,[9] but inbred mice (T-KK) resulting from a cross between the KK and C57B1/6J mice develop a similar syndrome to the KK mouse. Introduction of the lethal yellow (A^y) gene into KK mice resulted in a congenic lethal yellow obese KK strain, KKA^y, which has severe obesity and NIDDM.[280] The genetics of these various strains is unclear. *Ob* gene expression in the KKA^y, but not the KK strain, was found to be increased in mesenteric and subcutaneous WAT at 12 weeks of age, a time when the markedly greater obesity develops in the KKA^y mice.[280] A reduced hypothalamic GLP-1 content was also found in hyperinsulinemic hyperglycemic KKA^y mice when compared with KK mice,[281] but whether the hyperphagia is associated with this defect or not is unclear. Insulin resistance has been concluded to be due to defects in both the insulin receptor and postreceptor signal-transduction systems, including glucose uptake,[282] pentose pathways,[282] and impaired insulin-sensitive phosphodiesterase in fat cells.[283] This strain therefore appears to have a complex set of abnormalities, but the relationship of these to NIDDM is unknown.

14.5.1.3   The Nagoya-Shibata-Yasuda (NSY) Mouse

NSY mouse was established as an inbred strain from a Jcl:ICR mouse colony by selective breeding for glucose intolerance.[284] Spontaneous diabetes develops in ~98% of males and ~30% of females by 48 weeks of age.[285] NSY mice do not become obese, although epididymal fat pad size is increased. NSY mice exhibit fasting hyperinsulinemia, and pancreatic insulin content is elevated in male mice at 36 weeks of age, but there are no morphological abnormalities of the pancreas.[286] Fasting blood glucose is not significantly elevated,[286] but glucose and insulin responses to an OGTT are markedly reduced after 12 weeks of age. *In vitro* glucose-induced insulin secretion from isolated islets is also reduced.[286] Old NSY mice develop amyloidosis and die from renal failure. Amyloid deposits can also be observed in many other organs, including the stomach, small intestine, large intestine, lung, heart, and adrenals.[286] Diabetes in the NSY mouse results from both impaired glucose-induced insulin secretion and insulin resistance, but the genetic basis is not known.

14.5.1.4 The PBB/Ld Mouse

The PBB/Ld mouse originated from pet store stock, selected on the basis of black coat color, and further generations were produced by brother–sister mating.[134,287] PBB/Ld mice were hyperphagic, and obesity became apparent when they were 3 to 4 months old when fed a low-fat diet. Obesity was associated with hypertrophy of adipocytes in retroperitoneal and subcutaneous fat, and to both hypertrophy and hyperplasia in the epididymal fat pad.[287] Obese animals exhibited hyperlipidemia, hyperinsulinemia, mild hyperglycemia, and reduced tolerance to a glucose load. Pancreatic islets appeared normal histologically. The origin of the obesity in the PBB/Ld mouse is thought to be polygenic,[287] but there do not appear to have been any further detailed studies, and the origin of the hyperphagia is unknown.

14.5.2 Inbred Rats

The OLETF (Long-Evans Takushima Fatty) and GK (Goto-Kakisaki) rats are the inbred rat strains that have been most comprehensively studied.

14.5.2.1 The Otsuka-Long-Evans-Tokushima Fatty Rat

Kawano and co-workers[288] established the OLETF rat strain by selective inbreeding of members of a normal colony of Long-Evans rats which developed polyuria, polydypsia, hyperinsulinemia, persistent hyperglycemia, hypertriglyceridemia, and mild to moderate obesity.[288-290] Obesity is evident approximately 2 weeks after weaning. The various disorders develop in severity with age, and there is a late onset of hyperglycemia (after 18 weeks of age) associated with marked glucose intolerance. Diabetes has been shown to develop in 80 to 100% of males by 25 weeks of age;[8] females do not show any disability until 40 weeks of age. There is evidence for an immunological component in some colonies, but not all.[291] At an early stage (less than 9 weeks of age), islets have mild lymphocytic infiltration. Hyperplasia with fibrosis develops from 10 to 40 weeks of age, and islets become atrophic with animals becoming hypoinsulinemic. Insulin resistance appears to be associated with the development of obesity and with impaired insulin-mediated glucose uptake.[288,289]

Segregation studies comparing OLETF rats and a control strain, Long-Evans Tokushima (LETO), which appears to share some of the diabetogenic genes with OLETF rats,[289] led Hirashima et al.[292] to conclude that multiple recessive genes are involved in the development of diabetes in the OLETF strain. Linkage studies confirmed that one of the responsible genes is located on the X chromosome (*Odb-1*); however, testosterone is involved in the development of diabetes.[289] An increased incidence of diabetes was later found to be associated with a coat color gene, *h* (hooded),[293] which is located on Chromosome 14. Additionally, a high linkage of hyperglycemia with a microsatellite marker, D14Mit4, was shown and the gene designated *Odb-2*.[293] Both *Odb-1* and *Odb-2* were found to be required for development of elevated plasma glucose in OGTTs. One genetic defect in the OTSUKA rat is a deficiency in the CCK_A receptor.[294,295] CCK_A receptor mRNA was shown to be absent, and intracerebroventricular administration of CCK-8 had no satiety effect in OLETF rats, providing a possible explanation for the hyperphagia.[296] No CCK_A receptor gene expression was detected in the pancreas,[296] and ^{125}I-CCK binding to isolated pancreatic acini from OLETF rats was undetectable,[290] and pancreatic weight was also reduced.[295]

Up to around 3.5 weeks of age, body weight, glucose tolerance, and plasma insulin levels after a glucose load are all normal in OLETF rats, but *in vitro* islet glucose-stimulated insulin release is exaggerated.[291] Obesity and glucose intolerance subsequently develop. Treatment with diazoxide, a β-cell K^+_{ATP} channel opener, from 4 to 12 weeks of age, normalized the β-cell response, prevented the development of obesity and insulin resistance, and resulted in a marked improvement in glucose tolerance.[291] This suggests the existence of a primary β-cell hypersecretory defect. However, Ishida et al.[297] showed that reductions in insulin-mediated glucose uptake, observed at ~16 weeks of age, precede decreased plasma insulin responses to glucose, which are only evident at 40 weeks. Islet hyperplasia and fibrosis also develop late. Early insulin treatment protected animals from development of defective β-cell secretory dynamics and altered morphology.[298] These studies indicate that, since insulin resistance precedes impaired β-cell function, islet secretory abnormalities are partly compensatory responses to insulin resistance. Recently, Man et al.[299] provided further evidence in support of Unger's lipotoxic theory by showing accumulation of TG droplets in islets of OLETF rats and linked this to reduced glucokinase activity.

Despite the considerable evidence regarding a gene defect related to the CCK-A receptor, it is not clear as to how this deficiency relates to *Odb-1* or *Odb-2*. However, it is interesting that two missense variants of the human CCK receptor gene associated with obesity and NIDDM have been identified.[300] These mutations appear to be rare, and their functional importance needs to be determined.

14.5.2.2 Goto-Kakisaki Rat

The GK rat was developed by Goto and Kakisaki[301] through the selection of 18 rats from the local Wistar stock that were slightly glucose intolerant. These hyperglycemic animals were mated and interbred until, after 30 generations, the diabetic state became stable in subsequent generations. The GK rat is one of the best-characterized animal models of spontaneous *nonobese* NIDDM, since it exhibits similar metabolic, hormonal, and vascular disorders to the human disease. This includes mild fasting hyperglycemia, pronounced glucose intolerance, peripheral and hepatic insulin resistance, impaired glucose-induced insulin secretion, and late complications such as neuropathy and nephropathy.[8]

From the manner in which the GK rat developed, it was concluded that selective breeding concentrated specific genetic traits, and that the NIDDM in these rats was polygenic. A number of studies have been directed at dissecting out susceptibility loci. Two groups, using quantitative trait locus (QTL) analysis on matings between diabetic and control rats,[302,303] established conclusively that NIDDM is polygenic in the GK rat, and that fasting and postprandial hyperglycemia have different genetic bases. The two studies differed in the strains used for crossing, genetic markers, and mode of analysis,[304] but they arrived at similar conclusions. The strongest linkage in both studies was between postprandial, but not fasting, hyperglycemia and markers on chromosome 1.[302,303] This locus is believed to be associated with impaired insulin responses to glucose. Additional loci affecting glucose tolerance included regions of chromosomes 2, 5, 10, and 17. Those on chromosomes 2 and 10 affect both fasting and postprandial hyperglycemia. Loci on chromosomes 4 and 8 showed linkage to insulin secretion.[302,303] An important factor affecting body weight, but not glucose tolerance, was identified on chromosome 7,[302,303] and a further ten regions were suggestive of linkage.[302]

There has been considerable interest in determining the origin of the altered pancreatic β-cell response to glucose, which is observed both *in vivo* and *in vitro*.[303] Basal and glucose-stimulated insulin release from diabetic rat islets are both greatly decreased.[305,306] Glucose-induced insulin release was reported to be decreased in islets from 8-day-old rats,[307] and isolated pancreases from 2-month-old animals were almost completely unresponsive to high glucose.[306,308-310] Somatostatin secretory responses to glucose were also greatly reduced.[309] Interestingly, the glucose threshold for agents potentiating insulin secretion via increasing cAMP was reduced to 3.3 mM. This is similar to the Zucker *fa/fa* rat.[206] Additionally, proinsulin biosynthesis was doubled in islets from GK rats in the presence of low (2.8 mM) glucose; biosynthesis was stimulated normally by 16.7 mM glucose.[305] Although irregular-shaped and fibrotic islets have been described in 4-week-old islets, and their number increases with age,[301] islets from animals 2 to 4 months of age do not have a grossly abnormal density of β-cells,[307] and most,[305,306,309] but not all,[308] studies have shown little change from normal in insulin content. Altered secretory responses are unlikely to result from a reduction in islet hormone content, and defective stimulus-secretion coupling mechanisms are probably involved. However, Movasset et al.[311] have suggested that a reduced β-cell mass is a primary event.

Reduced islet levels of GLUT-2 are not considered to be important for reductions in glucose-induced insulin secretion.[312] Among the alterations in islet glucose metabolism that have been implicated in the decreased responsiveness are deficient oxidative metabolism of glucose in islet mitochondria,[305] increased glucose cycling,[306,312] and decreased activity of the glycerol phosphate shuttle ultimately resulting in insufficient closure of ATP-sensitive K^+ channels (K_{ATP} channels), decreased membrane depolarization, and reduced insulin release.[313,314] Such a scenario has been questioned by Hughes and co-workers,[315] and it seems likely that different colonies of GK rats exhibit different phenotypes. The following discussion may therefore not apply to all GK colonies.

The pancreatic β-cell ATP-sensitive K^+ channel consists of two subunits: the sulfonylurea receptor (SUR) and a member of the inwardly rectifying channel family, Kir6.2. The susceptibility locus identified on chromosome 1 of the GK rat,[302,303] is homologous with human chromosome 11p15, and SUR gene maps to 11p.15.1. The K^+ channel (BUR) lies within 5 kb of the SUR gene. Mutations in the SUR gene exon 22 were found to be more common in morbidly obese and NIDDM families,[316,317] and defects in function could be important contributors to NIDDM in Northern European populations. Several mutations were identified in the Kir6.2 gene, but there were no differences in allelic frequencies between NIDDM and normals, and it was considered unlikely that they played a role in altered β-cell function.[318,319] Defects in either of these genes would therefore appear to be potentially important,[304] and glucose inhibition of the K_{ATP} channel was shown to be impaired in the GK rat.[313] However, the channel itself is not abnormal since responses to ATP are intact.[313] In contrast, both inhibition of K_{ATP} channel activity and stimulation of insulin secretion in response to dihydroxyacetone (DHA) were severely impaired.[314] This metabolite is converted to DHA-phosphate, which preferentially enters the glycerol phosphate shuttle. Further metabolism of DHA-phosphate via the glycerol phosphate shuttle is therefore a possible site of metabolic block. One enzyme potentially involved is mitochondrial FAD-dependent glycerol-3-phosphate dehydrogenase (mGPD), since it is present at less than 50% of normal in the GK rat.[320] Additionally, mGPD was recently mapped[321] close to the susceptibility locus on rat chromosome 3,[302] suggesting a possible link between changes in its function and the diabetic state in the GK rat. However, it is unlikely to be a primary cause of diabetes since MacDonald et al.[320] showed that treatment of GK rats with insulin restored activities of mGPD, indicating that the reduction was secondary to diabetes, and mGPD mRNA levels in GK rats were found to be equivalent to those in Wistar rats, indicating that differences probably arise post-transcriptionally.[322] In a recent linkage study Warren-Perry et al.[323] concluded that mutations involving the human mGPD gene are unlikely to contribute to NIDDM in Caucasians.

What other sites could be involved in altered insulin secretion? There have been a number of suggestions. There is an overall decrease in islet mitochondrial DNA content, but no major deletions or restriction fragment polymorphisms,[324] and it was suggested that reduced levels may occur as a consequence of the disturbed metabolic environment. Roles for reductions in ADP-ribosyl cyclase activity and intracellular cyclic ADP-ribose levels,[325] and reduced expression of a Ca^{2+}-ATPase, SERCA-3, which is involved in the active uptake of cytosolic Ca^{2+} into the endoplasmic reticulum, have also been reported.[326] Additionally, Leckström et al.[327] showed that the plasma islet amyloid polypeptide (IAPP)/insulin ratio was higher in GK rats after glucose injection, equivalent to a relative hypersecretion of IAPP. Increased amounts of islet IGF II mRNA and a high-molecular-weight IGF II peptide were found in the 2- and 6-month-old GK rats compared with 1-month-old rats.[328] The authors suggested that it could have resulted in the development of fibrosis, and the Nidd/gk1 region of rat chromosome 1, identified by Gauguier et al.[303] as a susceptibility locus, contains the IGF II gene. The hyperglycemic–hyperinsulinemic pattern observed in GK rats is also associated with hepatic glucose overproduction, decreased responsiveness to insulin in the basal state, and moderate insulin resistance in muscles and adipose tissues, present by 8 weeks of age in GK females. The origin of insulin resistance has been associated with decreased receptor number.[329] However, there is probably also a deficiency in the signal-transduction pathways. Farese et al.[330] suggested that diabetic GK rats have a defect in synthesizing or releasing functional chiro-inositol-containing inositol phosphoglycan in adipocytes, and that defective IPG-regulated intracellular glucose metabolism contributes to insulin resistance.

14.5.3   Hamsters

14.5.3.1   The Chinese Hamster

A diabetic syndrome in the Chinese hamster (*Cricetulus griseus*) was first reported by Meier and Yerganian,[331] and several diabetic lines have subsequently been established with well-defined ages of onset.[7,134,332] Prediabetic Chinese hamsters are hyperphagic from birth and develop hyperglycemia, polydipsia, and glycosuria early, but they do not become obese. The diabetes, which may progress to ketosis in some genetic lines, is thought to be polygenic with one to four genes contributing, but little progress has been made in identifying the genes responsible. The quantity and quality of the diet affect the level of obesity, and dietary restriction delays the onset of glucosuria and reduces the diabetic severity. In diabetic animals, blood glucose levels range from 11 to 33 mM, but insulin levels are extremely variable depending on the diabetic line. β-cells appear degranulated and decrease in number,[7] and both plasma and tissue insulin levels decrease as the syndrome progresses. Insulin secretion in the perfused pancreas and isolated islets is severely depressed, and there is defective mobilization of Ca^{2+} from intracellular stores.[332] The overall syndrome is suggestive of excessive demand for insulin followed by functional islet exhaustion.

14.5.3.2   The Djungarian (Siberian) Hamster

An extremely high incidence of spontaneous diabetes has been reported in Djungarian (Siberian) hamsters (*Phodopus sungorus*). For example, Voss et al.[333] reported that 98% of their animals in a recently established colony showed ketoacidosis soon after birth, 10% of which later developed persistent hyperglycemia. Following the development of hyperglycemia, degranulation of β-cells, and deposition of glycogen occurred. However, there have not been any detailed reports, apart from limited metabolic studies, related to the disease. Siberian hamsters have naturally occurring seasonal cycles of food intake, triggered by changes in the photoperiod, and in studies on food intake responses vary during the day. This may be one reason for the paucity of the literature on this species. Nevertheless, they appear to have similar control systems to other small mammals since NPY is a very powerful stimulant of food intake, in a photoperiod independent manner,[334] and food deprivation was accompanied by increases in both hypothalamic NPY and prepro-NPY mRNA in the ARN.[335]

14.5.3.3 The South African Hamster

The South African hamster (*Mystromys albicaudatus*) also develops diabetes without obesity. The degree of hyperglycemia and glucose intolerance varies in age of onset, incidence, and degree of severity in different colonies. Diabetic animals are characterized by polydypsia, glucosuria, and ketonuria. A number of islet lesions have been described, including hyperplasia, cytoplasmic vacuolization, and glycogen infiltration.[6,7]

14.6 Animal Models of NIDDM with Unknown Heredity and an Environmental Component

A number of models of NIDDM have been developed as a result of the observation that animals taken from their natural environment developed diabetes mellitus when fed a laboratory diet. Among these are the sand rat (*Psammomys obesus*), the spiny mouse (*Acomys cahirinus*), and the tuco-tuco (*Ctenomys talaru*).

14.6.1 The Sand Rat

Psammomys obesus is a small rodent (gerbil), indigenous to desert regions of the Middle East where access to food and water is limited. They normally eat saltbush, a succulent halophilic plant with high salt and water content, and under these conditions they are lean and normoglycemic.[134] However, sand rats exhibit a genetic predisposition to the development of NIDDM and cataracts, when fed a standard high-calorie laboratory diet *ad libitum*.[336] The mode of inheritance is complex: some rats develop hyperinsulinemia but remain relatively normoglycemic, others develop NIDDM, whereas some remain normal.[337,338] In the hyperglycemic group, fatty acid oxidation has been shown to play an important role since administration of the oxidation inhibitor etomoxir reduced tissue uptake of glucose and circulating levels of glucose and insulin.[337]

A number of alterations in both structure and function of pancreatic islets of *P. obesus* have been reported. β-cells of diabetic animals contain very few granules, large deposits of glycogen, depleted stores of insulin, plus a marked increase in the proinsulin:insulin ratio.[339,340] This is accompanied by hyperproinsulinemia[341] and increased circulating proinsulin conversion intermediates. Insulin mRNA levels of *P. obesus* fed a high-energy diet (hyperglycemic, hyperinsulinemic) are increased, the rate of proinsulin biosynthesis is greatly increased, and electron micrographs reveal increased β-cell secretory activity.[339,340] The glucose threshold for insulin secretion is also found to be abnormal, with significant secretion in the absence of glucose. Using colloidal gold immunocytochemistry at the electron microscopic level to study the distribution of processing enzymes the labeling intensity of both PC1 and PC2 was shown to be weak compared with cells of normoglycemic rats. Abnormally high levels of PC2 were found in the Golgi apparatus rather than in the immature granules suggesting that the β-cells are in a chronic secretory state during which the impaired processing of proinsulin takes place.[340] The hyperglycemia-driven increase in secretory demand eventually cannot be met by increasing biosynthetic capacity and there can be up to a 90% reduction in insulin stores.[342] Following food deprivation, insulin depletion in diabetic *P. obesus* was partially corrected, and the proinsulin/insulin ratio normalized. Nondiabetic *P. obesus* showed only ~50% reduction in pancreatic insulin stores with no change in the proinsulin/insulin ratio. Cerasi and co-workers[342] suggest that in the diabetic *P. obesus*, the pancreatic capacity for biosynthesis and storage of insulin is restricted. The increased secretory requirement, which is secondary to insulin resistance, eventually overcomes this restricted capacity resulting in hyperglycemia. It was further suggested that diabetic *P. obesus* islets are more susceptible to glucose toxicity. The development of insulin resistance in *P. obesus* is associated with reduced insulin receptor number,[343] and multisite phosphorylation of the receptor, including serine and threonine residues of the receptor β-subunit,[344] which are inhibitory to tyrosine kinase activity.

14.6.2   Spiny Mice

The development of diabetes has been studied in two species of spiny mice, *Acomys russatus* and *A. cahirinus*. These are not truly mice, and *A. cahirinus* was recently shown to be closely related to the Mongolian gerbil *Meriones unguiculatus*.[345,346] This may be the reason a number of peculiarities set the spiny mouse apart from other rodent models of diabetes.[134] The gestation period is ~40 days, and the young are fairly mature at birth. Both males and females have congenital hyperplasia of pancreatic islets, with a high insulin content. When laboratory bred, *A. cahirinus* exhibits a moderate weight gain on a fat diet, accompanied by hyperglycemia but neither hyperlipidemia nor ketonuria.[347] *A. russatus* become obese on either a regular or fatty diet, but do not exhibit hyperglycemia or hyperlipidemia, although they have greatly increased hepatic TG content and circulating FFAs. Ketonuria develops in ~25% of animals.[347] *A. cahirinus* exhibits low insulin responses to glucose with a nearly absent first phase of release up to 35 weeks of age.[348,349] Responses to direct activation of the adenylate cyclase/cAMP system are relatively normal,[349] suggesting that there is a deficiency in the link between glucose metabolism and secretion. Animals older than 40 weeks have a restored biphasic insulin secretory profile.[348] Glucose utilization appears normal[350] in islets from *A. cahirinus* and Malaisse-Lagae et al.[351] suggested that there is a deficiency in the microtubule system that contributes to the overall reduction in insulin release.

Several metabolic abnormalities in spiny mice have been observed including fatty diet–associated increases in adipose tissue activities of lipoprotein lipase and gluconeogenic enzymes, and suppression of glycolytic and lipogenic enzymes.[347] Studies on perfused livers from *A. cahirinus* demonstrated an increased sensitivity of hepatic glucose output to insulin and decreased maximal stimulation by glucagon.[352] It was suggested that this may counteract, to some extent, the impaired insulin secretion and thereby reduce the severity of glucose intolerance. It is not clear why spiny mice do not develop insulin resistance, but it may be related to the fact they are low insulin secretors as discussed by Shafrir.[344]

14.6.3   The Tuco-Tuco

Specimens of the tuco-tuco (*Ctenomys talarum*), a burrowing rodent related to the guinea pig, were captured in Argentina and a colony established in captivity in England.[353-355] It was observed that at 3 months of age many of these animals developed cataracts,[353] and that those with cataracts were hyperglycemic and some were also mildly obese.[353] There was also a strong correlation between the level of glycemia in the mother and those of the litter, suggesting involvement of a genetic component.[354-356] Dietary restriction reduced the level of glycemia without loss in body weight. The rodents demonstrated variable pancreatic pathology, with islets ranging among normal, hypertrophic, and atrophic. Degranulation was also evident in some normal-sized islets. Responses to bovine insulin infusion were weak, but, since hystricomorph insulins differ significantly from other mammalian peptides, it is unclear whether this indicates a resistant state or not. The tuco-tuco is normally extremely active in its natural environment, and the relative inactivity and unrestricted access to food in captivity appear to have precipitated the hyperglycemia.[353,354] Many of the animals in captivity were infertile, compromising breeding programs and there has, unfortunately, not been further progress in studies on spontaneous diabetes in the tuco-tuco.

14.7 Polygenic Animal Models Produced by Hybrid Crosses

A few groups have undertaken the task of analyzing the complex genetics of obesity and diabetes in multigenic animal models, including the development of models that are dependent upon environmental factors. The methodology is based on the use of two inbred strains of an animal, a detailed genetic map of its genome, and the technique of QTL analysis. This is a statistical approach developed by Lander and co-workers[357,358] to facilitate mapping of genetic loci that control a quantitative phenotype. Coupled with the detection of sequence length polymorphisms, sophisticated mapping is possible. This approach has been applied to the identification of regions containing genes influencing body mass, fat content and distribution, glycemia, and insulin secretion.[6,21,359-361] The procedure involves crossing two inbred strains, of divergent phenotype for the specific trait under study, to produce F1 and F2 or backcross progeny.[21,359] The progeny are genotyped using markers spanning the complete genome, and phenotypes are assayed. Statistical associations of markers and phenotypes are then performed to identify specific loci underlying the traits. For further details, see Fisler and Warden.[359] Mice and rats are the preferred species at present because of the detail of their genetic maps. Chagon and Bouchard[21] and Bray and Bouchard[360] have summarized the QTLs identified and proposed human cytological locations based on synteny of flanking markers between rat or mouse and humans, as outlined in Table 14.2.

14.7.1 The BSB Model

A spontaneously obese strain (BSB) was developed by Warden et al.[362] from a backcross of the C57BL/6J strain and F1 females from a cross between C57BL/6J and *Mus spretus*. These animals exhibit basal hyperinsulinemia, glucose intolerance, and hyperlipidemia similar to many obese humans.[352] The individual body fat content in BSB mice varies between 1 and 50%.[10] Four loci located on different chromosomes have been identified, and termed multigenic obesity 1–4 (*Mob1–4*) which differ with respect to effects on fat distribution, percentage of body fat and plasma lipoprotein levels.[21] The gene on chromosome 6 lies near to the *ob* gene and that on chromosome 7 is proximal to the *tub* locus.[21,360,361] A cross between NZB and SM/J strains revealed two further loci contributing to fatness, one of which is in the same chromosomal region as the melanocortin receptor type-3 and adenosine deaminase (*Mob5*). This suggests that allelic variants that do not themselves cause major phenotypic effects may have some phenotypic effect.[361]

TABLE 14.2

Genes and Loci for Mouse and Rat Mendelian or Polygenic Models of Obesity

Crosses	Genes	Chromosome Location		Associations/Candidate Genes (Mice)
		Mouse	Human	
Mouse QTL, BSB	*Mob-1*	7	11pter-p14	*Tub/Igfrl*; *Ath3*, carcass fat
	Mob-2	6	7q22-q36	*Ob*; subcutaneous fat
	Mob-3	12	14q13-q32	*Tshr*; body fat
	Mob-4	15	5p15-p12	*Ghr*; mesenteric fat
Mouse QTL, NZB	*Mob-5*	2	20p11-q13	*Agouti (Mc3r)*; *Ada*
Mouse QTL,	*Do1*	4	1p35-p32	*Db/Glut1*, total adiposity
AKR × SWR	*Do2*	9	3p22-q21	Total adiposity
	Do3	15	5p14-p12	*Ghr*; total adiposity
Rat QTL,	*Nidd/gk1*	1	11p	*IgfII,Ins*; AI; BW; IS; G
GK × BN	*Nidd/gk5*	8	3p	AI; BW; IS; G
	Nidd/gk6	17	1q41-q44	AI; BW; IS; G
	bw/gk 1	7	8q	AI; BW
Rat QTL,	*Niddm 1*	1	10q24-q26	BW; IS; G
GK X F	*Niddm 3*	10	17pter-q32	BW; IS; G
	Weight 1	71	12q22-q23	*Igfl*
Mouse QTL, ASB, HSB	*BWl-3*	X	X	BW

Ath3 = susceptibility locus for atherosclerosis; *Ada* = adenosine deaminase; *Agouti (Mc3r)* = melanocortin receptor-3; *Db* = diabetes; *Glut1* = glucose transporter 1; *Ghr* = growth hormone receptor; *Igfl* = IGF (insulin-like growth factor)-I; *Igfrl* = IGF-I receptor; *IgfII* = IGF-II; *Ins* = insulin; *Ob* = obese; *Tshr* = thyroid-stimulating hormone receptor;*Tub* = tubby, carcass fat; AI = adiposity index; BW = body weight; IS = insulin secretion; G = glycemia.

Based on Bray, Chagnon, and Bouchard.[21,360,361]

14.7.2   AKR/J × SWR/J Model

West[361] and West and co-workers[363] noted that inbred SWR/J mice are much leaner than AKR/J mice, and that on a high-fat diet the AKR/J strain become approximately fivefold fatter than the SWR/J strain. From crosses, genetic loci called *Do 1–3*, for dietary obesity, have been mapped to chromosomes 4, 9, and 15.[361] These genes confer susceptibility to obesity when the animals are placed in an obesity-inducing environment, similar to humans. The QTL on chromosome 4 includes the *db* locus, but the sequence of this gene in the AKR/J × SWR/J cross is unknown.[361] Three loci linked to body weight (*Bw1–3*), located on the X chromosome were detected with HSM and ASB strains.

14.7.3   GK Crosses

These have already been discussed in Section 14.5.2.2. A cross between GK and the Fischer-344 strain resulted in the detection of seven loci (*Nidd/gk1–6, bw/gk1*), and one QTL related to body weight (*Weight1*) and two related to body weight and insulin secretion were detected in crosses between GK and the nondiabetic Brown-Norway rat.

14.8   Transgenic and Knockout Animals

The animal models used to date have provided a wealth of information regarding individual obesity genes, which can also result in NIDDM. It has only recently been possible to identify specific human gene mutations, which ultimately result in defined subtypes of diabetes. The earliest example of this was insulin itself. Families have been identified in several populations in which one or more members have single-point mutations in insulin genes resulting in amino acid substitutions in their proinsulin.[364] Some of these mutations result in the secretion of peptide with reduced biological activity due to functionally important changes in the A or B chain. Individuals in which insulin demonstrates reduced receptor binding are mildly diabetic or hyperglycemic, and hyperinsulinemic. Other mutations result in hyperproinsulinemia. The prevalence of such mutations is rare.[1] Two major approaches to the identification of further diabetogenic genes in humans have been taken. The first of these, the candidate gene approach,[2,12,14] involves the characterization of molecules involved in normal insulin secretion and action, and determining whether or not patients with inherited forms of diabetes have genetic defects in these molecules. Many of the studies discussed earlier involved this approach in the study of animal diabetes. The second approach, random gene searching,[12,14] is based on the identification of families with inherited forms of diabetes and mapping to the human genome. By using positional cloning, defective genes can then be identified. By using these two approaches, specific single-gene disorders have been identified (Table 14.3), and these have generally been associated with early-onset NIDDM or severe insulin resistance.[1]

TABLE 14.3
Identified Single Gene Disorders Resulting in Specific Subtypes of NIDDM

Gene	Mode of Inheritance	Basis for Hyperglycemia
Insulin	Dominant	Inactive insulin
Insulin receptor	Dominant or recessive	Insulin signaling impaired
Glucokinase	Dominant	Impaired insulin secretion
HNF1α	Dominant	Progressive impairment of insulin secretion
HNF4α	Dominant	Progressive impairment of insulin secretion
Mitrochondrial genome	Maternal	Impaired insulin secretion

Modified from O'Rahilly.[14]

A major effort is now under way to study the normal function of these and other candidate diabetogenic genes to determine how multiple interacting mutations can result in NIDDM. In some cases, this involves manipulation of the genetic makeup of animals by producing transgenics in which mutated forms of genes are introduced, and animals in which genes are deleted (knockouts), or normal or mutated proteins are overexpressed. In this section, such models are discussed.

14.8.1   Transgenic Models for Studying Genes Involved in Insulin Resistance

Impaired insulin-stimulated glucose disposal is a major characteristic of NIDDM. The offspring of two NIDDM parents from populations of Pima Indians, San Antonio Hispanics, and Utah caucasians were found to be insulin resistant several years before the development of NIDDM.[11,12] This observation led to the conclusion that insulin resistance is inherited autosomally and that a single gene may be involved.[11] However, the identity of such a gene has remained elusive, and the search for defects at all levels of the pathway of insulin action have been studied, many of which have been discussed. Transgenic animals expressing mutated genes or overexpressing genes for components of this pathway have been shown to develop insulin resistance.

14.8.1.1 The Insulin Receptor

Reduced numbers of insulin receptors have been found in subjects with impaired glucose tolerance and obesity, which in most cases is a secondary effect resulting from hyperinsulinemia. However, since there is a large excess of insulin receptors in most cells and since only 10 to 20% occupancy is required for maximal effects, such reductions have only minor effects on insulin responsiveness.[13] Both receptor knockout and overexpression mouse models have been used to study the effect of more dramatic changes in receptor number. Homozygous insulin receptor knockout mice die shortly following birth, due to severe hyperglycemia and ketosis, whereas mice that are heterozygous have compensated insulin resistance and normal glucose tolerance.[365] Overexpression of kinase-deficient insulin receptors results in only mild insulin resistance and no diabetes.[366] Receptor mutations are extremely uncommon in NIDDM, estimated at <1% of patients,[1,14] and abnormalities range from mild glucose intolerance to overt diabetes, suggesting that additional factors are involved. The most common mutation associated with NIDDM, a $Val_{973}Met$ substitution, was recently shown to have no effect on receptor function in transfected cells.[367] A number of receptor mutations have also been found in rare syndromes associated with insulin resistance, such as leprechaunism and type A insulin resistance with acanthosis nigricans.[368] These individuals do not develop severe diabetes or ketoacidosis, possibly due to compensatory mechanisms.[366] Reduced tyrosine kinase activity in isolated receptors from liver, adipocytes, and skeletal muscle has been found in individuals with NIDDM, but the underlying cause is unclear.[13]

14.8.1.2 Insulin Receptor Substrates 1 and 2

The insulin receptor substrate (IRS) proteins act as interfaces between activated receptors and signaling proteins with Src homology-2 (SH2) domains. Following insulin stimulation IRS-1, for example, associates with several proteins including phosphatidylinositol (PI) 3-kinase, Syp, Nck, Grb-2, and Fyn. Polymorphisms in the IRS-1 gene have been detected in both the normal population and patients with NIDDM.[13] However, the incidence of mutations in the diabetics is two to four times greater,[366] and two polymorphisms are slightly more common in NIDDM than the general population.[2] Homozygous mice with a null mutation in the IRS-1 gene exhibit intrauterine and postnatal growth retardation,[369] hyperinsulinemia, glucose intolerance, and resistance to both insulin and IGF-I, but they are not markedly diabetic.[370] This is presumed to be due to IRS-2 compensation for the loss in IRS-1.[366] Mice double homozygous for null alleles in the insulin receptor and IRS-1 genes died from diabetic ketoacidosis, whereas heterozygotes were found to be lean but very insulin resistant. Animals had the expected 50% reduction in the two proteins, but synergism was evident with respect to the insulin resistance, with islet insulin levels elevated 5- to 50-fold.[371] Islet hyperplasia was increased by a similar amount, and 40% of the double heterozygotes became diabetic at 4 to 6 months of age.[371] This important study clearly demonstrates that interaction between relatively minor defects can result in overt NIDDM.

14.8.1.3 Glucose Transporters

Since insulin stimulates glucose uptake via translocation of intracellular GLUT-4 transporters to the plasma membrane, defects in this system could have an effect on insulin responsiveness. Glucose uptake in skeletal muscle and adipocytes is impaired in NIDDM. Uptake of glucose into fat accounts for only 5 to 10% of total glucose uptake, but reductions of insulin-stimulated glucose uptake in adipocytes from patients with NIDDM correlates with the degree of insulin resistance measured by glucose clamp.[13] Adipocytes from obese subjects have reductions in both the intracellular pool and plasma membrane–associated protein, which some consider to be sufficient to explain the reduction in basal and insulin-stimulated glucose transport in NIDDM.[13] However, no significant mutations in genes encoding GLUT-4 or GLUT-1[2] have been detected, and GLUT-4 levels in skeletal muscle are normal in obesity. It has therefore been speculated that transporter translocation or phosphorylation are impaired.[2] In tissue from both NIDDM and obese subjects such deficient translocation has been demonstrated by laser scanning microscopy. A large number of transgenic studies have been performed on glucose transporters,[372,373] and only those related to GLUT-4 will be discussed. Overexpression of GLUT-4, under its own promoter, results in a general increase in insulin action, obesity when fed a high-fat diet, and increased whole-body glucose disposal rates.[369,372] Surprisingly, homozygous GLUT-4 (null) knockout mice were found to be only mildly insulin resistant, with postprandial hyperinsulinemia and a mild hyperglycemic response to oral glucose.[373] They did not become diabetic. It was speculated that the mice compensated by appropriate increases in insulin levels,[373] and overexpression of another glucose transporter.[366] Mice heterozygous for GLUT-4 deficiency (GLUT-4$^{+/-}$) become hyperinsulinemic and eventually hyperglycemic,[374] and therefore could prove useful as models of nonobese NIDDM.

14.8.1.4 Hexokinase II

Phosphorylation of glucose to glucose 6 phosphate by the low-K_m hexokinase II is an important step in the regulation of glucose metabolism. Despite the existence of hexokinase II polymorphisms, the majority of evidence favours the finding of reduced activity in NIDDM as being secondary to the insulin resistance.[2] Transgenic mice overexpressing human hexokinase II had relatively normal OGTTs, intravenous insulin tolerance, and insulin levels.[369]

14.8.1.5 Tumor Necrosis Factor-α (TNF-α)

It has been proposed that an insulin antagonist is secreted by adipocytes and thereby provides the link between adiposity and insulin resistance. Increased adipose tissue size in obesity would therefore result in increased levels of this factor. TNF-α, is a cytokine that has been found to be overexpressed in adipose tissue of obese humans and most animal models of obesity.[375-377] There is a positive correlation between the level of TNF-α mRNA in fat tissue and the prevailing level of hyperinsulinemia[2] and between plasma levels of TNF-α and the rate of insulin-stimulated glucose metabolism, in humans. Additionally, a sib-pair analysis study revealed linkage between obesity and a marker near the TNF-α locus in Pima Indians.[2] These studies provide strong support for a relationship between elevated TNF-α and obesity in humans, and animal studies have supported this contention. TNF-α can induce insulin resistance by inhibition of tyrosine phosphorylation of the insulin receptor β chain and IRS-1.[377,378] TNF-α induces serine phosphorylation of IRS-1 and this form of the protein acts as an inhibitor of the insulin receptor tyrosine kinase activity.[377,378] Neutralization of TNF-α in Zucker rats improved insulin sensitivity and the insulin receptor kinase defect in muscle and adipose tissue.[375] *Ob/Ob* mice and mice with diet-induced obesity, but with a targeted null mutation in the TNF-α gene, had greatly improved insulin sensitivity.[379] Circulating FFAs were also reduced. Knockout of one or both of the receptor types for TNF-α also results in significant improvements in insulin sensitivity.[379] TNF-α is therefore a strong candidate for involvement in the development of insulin resistance.

14.8.1.6 Fatty Acid–Binding Protein 2

Adipocyte fatty acid–binding protein 2 (FABP2) binds to fatty acids such as oleic acid and retinoic acid, although its function is not entirely clear. Linkage analysis indicated that a gene on human chromosome 4q(26) close to the FABP2 gene (*aP2*) is associated with NIDDM in Pima indians.[380] Mice with a null mutation in *aP2* were metabolically and developmentally normal.[381] However, the knockout (*aP2-–*) animals developed dietary obesity but, unlike *aP2+/+* mice, they did not become either insulin resistant or diabetic. Interestingly, obese *aP2-/-* mice did not express TNF-α in adipose tissue. These authors therefore speculated that FABP2 links obesity and insulin resistance by coupling fatty acid metabolism to TNF-α expression.

14.8.1.7 Ras Associated with Diabetes (Rad)

Reynet and Kahn.[382] identified a small GTP-binding protein (*rad*: Ras-related protein associated with diabetes), and reported that it was overexpressed in skeletal muscle of patients with NIDDM. Rad appears to play a role as a negative regulator of insulin-stimulated glucose transport,[384] and overexpression could therefore result in insulin resistance. A polymorphism in the *rad* gene was initially reported to be associated with NIDDM in American Caucasians, but subsequent studies have not confirmed this observation.[13,385] The status of rad is therefore unclear.

14.8.2   Transgenic Models for Studying Genes Involved in Defective Insulin Secretion

Insulin secretion in rodents and humans, and the ability to compensate for insulin resistance, are genetically determined.[366] Among the candidate genes associated with insulin secretion proposed to be defective in NIDDM are those for GLUT-2 and glucokinase.

14.8.2.1 GLUT-2

The GLUT-2 transporter in the rat β-cell has a high capacity, and it is believed to result in near equalization of extra- and intracellular glucose concentrations. Islet GLUT-2 has been proposed to interact with glucokinase,[386] resulting in phosphorylation of glucose at a rate that is sensitive to the concentration of glucose within the physiological range. The observation that loss of glucose-stimulated insulin secretion in several animal models of diabetes was associated with greatly reduced expression of GLUT-2[234,235] was initially interpreted as demonstrating a primary role in the development of NIDDM. However, it was subsequently shown that expression of oncogenic H-*ras*[387] in transgenic islets resulted in a 90% decrease in GLUT-2 without major effects on glucose-stimulated insulin secretion or glucose homeostasis *in vivo*.[388] One case of a mutation in the human GLUT-2 gene, which results in an inactive protein, has been found associated with NIDDM.[389] However, the role of GLUT-2 glucose sensing in humans is unclear because De Vos et al.[390] showed that the human β-cell contains very little GLUT-2, and GLUT-1 is the major species. Sweet and Matschinsky[391] concluded that since GLUT-2 is not an essential component of the glucose-sensing system,[388] GLUT-1 can perform the function of islet glucose transporter perfectly adequately.

14.8.2.2 Glucokinase

Three subtypes of maturity-onset diabetes of the young (MODY), which usually develops before 25 years of age, have been characterized in humans. The disease is inherited in an

TABLE 14.4

Subtypes of MODY

Type	Inheritance	Genetic/Molecular Defect	Function	Prevalence (% of total NIDDM)
MODY 1	Autosomal dominant	TCF14/HNF-4α	Transcription factor expressed in liver and β-cells	<0.0001
MODY 2	Autosomal dominant	GCK/glucokinase	β-cell glucose sensing	<0.2
MODY 3	Autosomal dominant	TCF1/HNF-1α	Transcription factor expressed in liver and β-cells	1–2

Modified from Yki-Järvinen.[392]

autosomal dominant fashion (Table 14.4). MODY Type 2, accounts for about 50% of French patients with MODY[393] and is caused by a mutation in the glucokinase gene that results in defective β-cell glucose sensing, hyperglycemia, and mild NIDDM. In all, 42 different mutations and two amino acid polymorphisms have been identified;[393] mutations in one allele are sufficient to cause diabetes. Several transgenic models have been produced.[366,369] In mice with only one functional allele, blood glucose levels are increased and insulin secretion reduced.[394] Ablation of β-cell glucokinase results in severe diabetes shortly following birth, and animals die of extreme hyperglycemia within 1 week of birth.[394,395] When both liver and β-cell glucokinase are disrupted, the phenotype is even more severe, and there is embryonic or early postnatal death.[394,395] Heterozygotes, with ~50% reductions in glucokinase in β-cells develop mild diabetes. Several other transgenic studies have confirmed that glucokinase is the most important component of the β-cell glucose sensor.[366,369] Since the relative contributions of β-cell and liver deficiencies of glucokinase to diabetes in MODY are still not clear, these models should prove extremely useful for future studies.

14.8.2.3 *Hepatic Nuclear Factors*

Genome scans and linkage analysis have identified MODY 3 as the most common form of MODY worldwide. The mutated gene was recently identified as the transcription factor hepatic nuclear factor (HNF)-1α,[396] which is involved in the regulation of several hepatic genes. In pancreatic cells, it is a weak transactivator of the insulin-I gene. The mutated gene in MODY 1 was identified as HNF-4α, a member of the steroid/thyroid hormone superfamily that regulates expression of HNF-1α.[397] Late-onset NIDDM appears in some family members who carry the mutation.[11] Homozygous transgenic mice lacking HNF-1α did not thrive and died around the time of weaning.[398] However, although they suffered from phenylketonurea and renal tubular dysfunction, they had normal blood glucose levels. The response to an intravenous glucose infusion appeared normal, but since there was a massive glycosuria any diabetic state may have been masked. It is not known how mutations in the HNF-1α and HNF-4α genes result in diabetes when present on a single allele. It was postulated that partial deficiency may lead to β-cell dysfunction and diabetes, or mutations may cause diabetes by acting in a dominant-negative fashion.[396] HNF-4α acts on regulatory elements and promoters of a number of genes the products of which are involved in cholesterol, fatty acid, amino acid, and glucose metabolism.[399] In transgenic studies, HNF-4α[+/-] mice did not have diabetes or abnormal glucose tolerance, however loss of both genes resulted in early embryonic death due to dysfunction of the visceral endoderm in which it is expressed,[399] preventing studies on these animals. *In vitro* studies by Stoffel and Duncan[399] showed that mutant ($Gln_{268}X$ (nonsense)) HNF-4α protein does not bind to DNA-binding site as a homodimer or heterodimer. Several genes involved in glucose uptake and glycolysis were shown to be dependent upon HNF-4α, including

GLUT-2, aldolase B, and glyceraldehyde-3-phosphate dehydrogenase. Deficient expression of these proteins in β–cells probably accounts for the altered insulin secretion in patients with MODY. It was also found that levels of HNF-1α mRNA were only slightly reduced by the complete absence of HNF-4α. Therefore, other pathways are presumably also involved in patients with MODY 1.

14.8.2.4 Islet Amyloid Polypeptide

Islet amyloid polypeptide (IAPP; amylin) is cosecreted with insulin by the normal β-cell,[400] and it has effect on both insulin secretion and action. The presence of amyloid deposits in islets of Langerhans is commonly associated with NIDDM in animals and humans, and they have been proposed to play a pathogenic role in β-cell destruction. A $Ser_{20}Gly$ mutation has been associated with a group of Japanese patients with early onset NIDDM.[401] Transgenic mice overexpressing human IAPP, and fed a normal diet, had increased circulating IAPP and increased insulin storage but no signs of amyloid deposits over a 19-month period.[400,402,403] These studies indicated that the mere overproduction of an amyloidogenic form of IAPP is not sufficient to produce amyloid deposits. Subsequently, it was found that feeding a high-fat diet resulted in the majority of males developing amyloid deposits,[404] and ~50% of these were hyperglycemic. An association between apolipoprotein E and amyloid deposition has been suggested to occur.[405] These interesting observations suggest that defects in IAPP may contribute to human NIDDM.

14.8.3   Transgenic Animals with Increased Body Fat

Examples of the use of transgenic animals in studying the physiology of leptin and the agouti protein have been discussed earlier. Identification of the genes involved in the rare, probably monogenic, obesity syndromes, such as Prader–Willi, Bardet–Biedl, Alström, and Cohen, is likely to provide interesting information regarding specific pathways involved in body weight control, and the introduction of equivalent mutations into animals should provide important information regarding their function. Apart from leptin, carboxypeptidase E, and agouti plus ART, a plethora of candidate obesity genes have been identified. For example, DNA polymorphism studies have provided evidence for linkage with uncoupling proteins, the $β_3$-adrenergic receptor, and TNF.[406] Evidence supporting or refuting a role for some of these genes has come from transgenic mouse models.

14.8.3.1 Knockout of Uncoupling Proteins

Several uncoupling proteins have now been identified. The original protein cloned (UCP1) was identified as a membrane proton transporter found in mitochondria, expressed specifically in brown adipose tissue. Activation of the protein results in dissipation of the proton gradient and heat production. DNA polymorphisms in human UCP1 were found to correlate with age-associated increases in body fat.[406] Mutations in the protein could lead to reduced energy expenditure and, thus, weight gain. UCP1 knockout mice were shown to consume less oxygen in response to a $β_3$-adrenergic receptor agonist and were more sensitive to cold.[407] However, neither obesity nor hyperphagia was observed. Since animals in which BAT had been completely ablated developed marked obesity with increasing age, hyperglycemia, marked hyperinsulinemia, and glucose intolerance,[408] the mild pathology of the UCP1 knockout was probably due to compensation by UCP2,[409,410] therefore, double knockouts are needed to determine the effect of overall UCP ablation. It is of interest that UCP2 is also found in pancreatic islet β-cells, where it is likely to play a role in insulin secretion, and overexpression of leptin resulted in tenfold increases in

UCP2 gene expression.[411] This suggests that altered UCP2 expression, resulting from loss of leptin responsiveness, could contribute to the development of obesity/NIDDM.

14.8.3.2 Knockout of β₃-Adrenergic Receptors

The β₃-adrenergic receptor (adrenoceptor) is expressed in the BAT of rodents and in human adipose tissue, and it is now considered to be of prime importance in thermogenesis. Low levels of β₃-adrenoceptor could promote obesity as a result of decreased thermogenesis and reduced lipolysis. A mutation in the first intracellular loop of the human receptor, in which there is a Trp₆₄Arg substitution, was first discovered in Pima Indians.[412] This mutation results in reduced maximal cAMP production when receptors are expressed in clonal cell lines.[413] The Trp₆₄Arg mutation has been found in all populations of the world, except people from Naurua.[414] Pima Indians and Japanese homozygous for the mutation have a lower metabolic rate, and it is associated with earlier onset of NIDDM.[414] The Trp₆₄Arg receptor form is not found at higher frequencies in obese individuals in Western societies, and there is only a weak association with obesity, but its presence is linked to a greater tendency to weight gain. Complete functional disruption of the β₃-adrenoceptor gene resulted in animals with increased body fat and a small increase in food intake, and these responses were potentiated by high-fat diet.[415] Overall, loss of the receptor leads to a propensity for a gradual increase in body fat. It has been shown that specific β₃-adrenoceptor agonists are potent antiobesity and antidiabetic agents in obese animals, probably at least partially acting through activation of thermogenesis in BAT and inducing uncoupling protein gene expression in WAT.[416] Studies on animals bearing mutant or altered amounts of β₃-adrenoceptor receptor is a promising system for defining the mechanisms involved.

14.9 The Future

The various animal models of obesity and NIDDM have allowed experimentation that would be impossible in humans. This has resulted in the identification of several new factors involved in the regulation of food intake and of a number of genes that might contribute to these conditions. Each of these will undoubtedly be studied in depth over the coming years. One should be encouraged by the spectacular advances that have been made since the isolation of leptin and by the fact that other peptides, which may play important roles in the regulation of food intake and energy balance, are still being identified. There is an extensive literature on the stimulation of food intake by NPY and inhibition of intake by serotonin and neuropeptides such as CCK, insulin, and CRF, and roles for new peptides are appearing almost weekly. For example, melanin-concentrating hormone,[417] glucagon-like peptide-1,[418] galanin,[419] urocortin,[420] and ciliary neurotrophic factor[421] have all been localized to brain regions involved in the regulation of food intake and have been shown to have potent effects on feeding behavior. Indications for the involvement of other neuropeptides in the regulation of energy balance have come from unlikely sources. For example, in knockout mice studies aimed at determining the role of bombesin-3 receptors, it was observed that such animals became spontaneously obese.[422] Clearly, there is still a tremendous amount to be learned regarding the complex neurotransmitter systems involved in the normal regulation of food intake and abnormalities resulting in obesity.

In contrast to the successes in understanding the monogenic rodent obesity syndromes, progress in identifying diabetogenic genes involved in insulin secretory defects and insulin resistance has been slow, and there are still no established genetic defects associated with the majority of patients with obesity and/or NIDDM. Three important factors have contributed to the difficulty in identifying sequence variations in specific human genes that predispose to diabetes:[14]

1. The ill-defined nature of the progressive decrease in glucose tolerance;
2. The presentation of NIDDM relatively late in life, making it difficult to study multigenerational families by linkage analysis; and
3. The genetic and clinical heterogeneity of the disease.

Nevertheless, the success of genetic screening approaches in identifying specific genes associated with MODY indicates that successful identification of further genes could occur in the near future. However, this will also provide new challenges since animal models appropriate for studying the pathophysiology will probably have to be developed. For example, the association of A to G mutation in the mitochondrial gene for tRNA[Leu] with the triad of diabetes, maternal inheritance, and deafness is intriguing, but also confusing. In some cases patients present as IDDM-like, while others are NIDDM-like.[423] In Japan and the Netherlands, this diabetic subtype may account for 1 to 1.5% of diabetic cases,[423] but it is not clear why this mutation is so common, nor why it causes diabetes. There is a suggestion that it results in the production of an abnormally processed protein, accumulation of which results in changes in glucose sensing and reduced oxygen consumption and β-cell mass.[424] At present, there are no animal models appropriate for studying such mitochondrial diseases. The final-level challenge will be to develop methods for the identification of the different gene variants that interact and result in the major forms of human NIDDM. Each of these defects may have only small individual effects on glucose tolerance, and the combinations of deleterious genes are probably different for lean- and obese-related diabetes. The following are some of the genes for which there is an indication of involvement in human NIDDM: glycogen synthase,[2,425] lipoprotein lipase,[406] Na+,K+-ATPase,[406] phosphoenolpyruvate carboxykinase,[426] the glucagon receptor,[427,428] and the glucose-dependent insulinotropic polypeptide receptor.[429] Studies on animal models may well provide important insights into their role.

Acknowledgments

We would like to thank the Canadian Medical Research Council, Canadian Diabetes Association, and British Columbia Health Research Foundation for supporting our research and Dr. J. C. Russell, University of Alberta, Edmonton, Alberta, for assistance with the section on the JCR:LA-cp rat.

References

1. Froguel, P. and Hager, J., Human diabetes and obesity: tracking down the genes, *TibTech*, 13, 52, 1995.
2. Groop, L. C. and Tuomi, T., Non-insulin-dependent diabetes mellitus — a collision between thrifty genes and an affluent society, *Ann. Med.*, 29, 37, 1997.

3. Bray, G. A. and York, D. A., Genetically transmitted obesity in rodents, *Physiol. Rev.*, 51, 598, 1971.

4. Bray, G. A. and York, D. A., Hypothalamic and genetic obesity in experimental animals: an autonomic and endocrine hypothesis, *Physiol. Rev.*, 59, 719, 1979.

5. Herberg, L. and Coleman, D. L., Laboratory animals exhibiting obesity and diabetes syndromes, *Metabolism*, 26, 59, 1977.

6. Mordes, J. P. and Rossini, A. A., Animal models of diabetes, *Am. J. Med.*, 70, 353, 1981.

7. Bell, R. H. and Hye, R. J., Animal models of diabetes mellitus: physiology and pathology, *J. Surg. Res.*, 35, 433, 1983.

8. Ktorza, A., Bernard, C., Parent, V., Penicaud, L., Froguel, P., Lathrop, M., and Gauguier, D., Are animal models of diabetes relevant to the study of the genetics of noninsulin-dependent diabetes in humans? *Diabetes Metab.*, 2, 38, 1997.

9. Fiedorek, F. T., Rodent genetic models for obesity and noninsulin-dependent diabetes mellitus, in *Diabetes Mellitus*, LeRoith, D., Taylor, S. I., and Olefsky, J. M., Eds., Lippincott-Raven, Philadelphia, 1996, 604.

10. York, D. A., Lessons from animal models of obesity, *Endocrinol. Metab. Clin. North Am.*, 25, 781, 1996.

11. Elbein, S. C., The genetics of human noninsulin-dependent (type 2) diabetes mellitus, *J. Nutr.*, 127, 1891S, 1997.

12. Groop, L. C., The molecular genetics of noninsulin-dependent diabetes mellitus, *J. Int. Med.*, 241, 95, 1997.

13. Kruszynska, Y.T. and Olefsky, J.M., Cellular and molecular mechanisms of noninsulin-dependent diabetes mellitus, *J. Invest. Med.*, 44, 413, 1996.

14. O'Rahilly, S., Non-insulin dependent diabetes mellitus: the gathering storm, *Br. Med. J.*, 314, 955, 1997.

15. Bray, G. A., York, D. A., and Fisler, J. S., Experimental obesity: a homeostatic failure due to defective nutrient stimulation of the sympathetic nervous system, *Vitam. Horm.*, 45, 1, 1989.

16. Bonner-Weir, S., Leahy, J. L., and Weir, G. C., Induced rat models of noninsulin-dependent diabetes, in *Frontiers in Diabetes Research. Lessons from Animal Models*, Vol. II, Shafrir, E. and Renold, A. E., Eds., John Libbey & Co., London, 1988, 295.

17. Blair, S. C., Caterson, I. D., and Cooney, G. J., Glucose and lipid metabolism in the gold thioglucose injected mouse model of diabesity, in *Lessons from Animal Diabetes VI*, Shafrir, E., Ed., Birkhäuser, Boston, 1996, 237.

18. Hansen, B., Primate animal models of noninsulin-dependent diabetes mellitus, in *Diabetes Mellitus*, LeRoith, D., Taylor, S. I., and Olefsky, J. M., Eds., Lippincott-Raven, Philadelphia, 1996, 595.

19. Leibel, R. L., Chung, W. K., and Chua, S. C., Jr., The molecular genetics of rodent single gene obesities, *J. Biol. Chem.*, 272, 31937, 1997.

20. Montague, C. T., Farooqi, I. S., Whitehead, J. P., Soos, M. A., Rau, H., Wareham, N. J., Sewter, C. P., Digby, J. E., Mohammed, S. N., Hurst, J. A., Cheetham, C. H., Earley, A. R., Barnett A. H., Prins, J. B., and O'Rahilly, S., Congenital leptin deficiency is associated with severe early-onset obesity in humans, *Nature*, 387, 903, 1997.

21. Chagnon, Y. C. and Bouchard, C., Genetics of obesity: advances from rodent studies, *Trends Genet.*, 12, 441, 1996.

22. Zhang, Y., Proenca, R., Maffei, M., Barone, M., Leopold, L., and Friedman, J.M., Positional cloning of the mouse *obese* gene and its human homologue, *Nature*, 372, 425, 1994.

23. Coleman, D. L., Effect of parabiosis of obese with diabetes and normal mice, *Diabetologia*, 9, 294, 1973.

24. Coleman, D. L., Obese and diabetes: two mutant genes causing diabetes-obesity syndromes in mice, *Diabetologia*, 14, 141, 1978.

25. Falconer, D. S. and Isaacson, J. H., Adipose, a new inherited obesity of the mouse, *J. Hered.*, 50, 290, 1959.

26. Chehab, F.F., Lim, M.E., and Lu, R., Correction of the sterility defect in homozygous obese female mice by treatment with the human recombinant leptin, *Nature Genet.*, 12, 318, 1996.

27. Isse, N., Ogawa, Y., Tamura, N., Masuzaki, H., Mori, K., Okazaki T, Satoh, N., Shigemoto, M., Yoshimasa, Y., Nishi, S., Hosoda, K., Inazawa, J., and Nakao, K., Structural organization and chromosomal assignment of the human *obese* gene, *J. Biol. Chem.*, 270, 27728, 1995.

28. Hwang, C. S., Mandrup, S., Macdougald, O. A., Geiman, D. E., and Lane, M. D., Transcriptional activation of the mouse *obese* (*ob*) gene by CCAAT enhancer binding protein α, *Proc. Natl. Acad. Sci. U.S.A.*, 93, 873, 1996.

29. He, Y., Chen, H., Quon, M. J., and Reitman, M., The mouse *obese* gene. Genomic organization, promoter activity, and activation by CCAAT/enhancer-binding protein α, *J. Biol. Chem.* 270, 28887, 1995.

30. Halaas, J. L., Gajiwala, K.S., Maffei, M., Cohen, S. L., Chait, B. T., Rabinowitz, D., Lallone, R. L., Burley, S. K., and Friedman, J. M., Weight-reducing effects of the plasma protein encoded by the *obese* gene, *Science*, 269, 543, 1995.

31 Murakami, T. and Shima. K., Cloning of rat obese cDNA and its expression in obese rats, *Biochem. Biophys. Res. Commun.*, 299, 944, 1995.

32. Moon, B. C. and Friedman, J. M., The molecular basis of the obese mutation in *ob²ʲ* mice, *Genomics*, 42, 152, 1997.

33. Tritos, N. A. and Mantzoros, C. S. Leptin: its role in obesity and beyond, *Diabetologia*, 40, 1371, 1997.

34. Maffei, M., Stoffel, M., Barone, M., Moon, B., Dammerman, M., Ravussin, E., Bogardus, C., Ludwig, D. S., Flier, J. S., Talley, M., Auerbach, S., and Friedman, J. M., Absence of mutations in the human *OB* gene in obese/diabetic subjects, *Diabetes*, 45, 679, 1996.

35. Considine, R. V., Considine, E. L., Williams, C. J., Nyce, M. R., Zhang, P., Opentanova, I., Ohannesian, J. P., Kolaczynski, J. W., Bauer, T. L., Moore J. H., and Caro, J. F., Mutation screening and identification of a sequence variation in the human *ob* gene coding region, *Biochem. Biophys. Res. Commun.*, 220, 735, 1996.

36. Niki, T., Mori, H., Tamori, Y., Kishimoto-Hashiramoto, M., Ueno, H., Araki, S., Masugi, J., Sawant, N., Majithia, H. R., Rais, N., Hashiramoto, M., Taniguchi, H., and Kasuga, M., Molecular screening in Japanese and Asian Indian NIDDM patients associated with obesity, *Diabetes*, 45, 675, 1996.

37. Stirling, B., Cox, N. J., Bell, G. I., Hanis, C.L., Spielman, R. S., and Concannon, P., Identification of microsatellite markers near the human *ob* gene and linkage studies in NIDDM-affected sib pairs, *Diabetes*, 44, 999, 1995.

38. Clement, K., Garner, C., Hager, J., Philippi, A., LeDuc, C., Carey, A., Harris, T. J., Jury, C., Cardon, L. R., Basdevant, A., Demenais, F., Guy-Grand, B., North, M., and Froguel, P., Indication for linkage of the human OB gene region with extreme obesity, *Diabetes*, 45, 687, 1996.

39. Tartaglia, L. A., Dembski, M., Weng, X., Deng, N. H., Culpepper, J., Devos, R., Richards, G. J., Campfield, L. A., Clark, F. T., Deeds, J., Muir, C., Sanker, S., Moriarty, A., Moore, K. J., Smutko, J. S., Mays, G. G., Woolf, E. A., Monroe, C. A., and Tepper, R. I., Identification and expression cloning of a leptin receptor, OB-R, *Cell*, 83, 1263, 1995.

40. Tartaglia, L. A., The leptin receptor, *J. Biol. Chem.*, 272, 6093, 1997.

41. Chen, H., Charlat, O., Tartaglia, L. A., Woolf, E. A., Weng, X., Ellis, S. J., Lakey, N. D., Culpepper, J., Moore, K. J., Breitbart, R. E., Duyk, G. M., Tepper, R. I., and Morgenstern, J. P., Evidence that the diabetes gene encodes the leptin receptor: identification of a mutation in the leptin receptor gene in *db/db* mice, *Cell*, 84, 491, 1996.

42. Lee, G. H., Proenca, R., Montez, J. M., Carroll, K. M., Darvishzadeh, J. G., Lee, J. I., and Friedman, J. M., Abnormal splicing of the leptin receptor in diabetic mice, *Nature*, 379, 632, 1996.

43. Wang, M.-Y., Zhou, Y. T., Newgard, C. B., and Unger, R. H., A novel leptin receptor isoform in rat, *FEBS Lett.*, 392, 87, 1996.

44. Liu, C., Liu, X. J., Barry, G., Ling, N., Maki, R. A., and De Souza, E.B., Expression and characterization of a putative high affinity human soluble leptin receptor, *Endocrinology*, 138, 3548, 1997.

45. Sinha, M. K., Opentanova, I., Ohannesian, J. P., Kolaczynski, J. W., Heiman, M. L., Hale, J., Becker, G. W., Bowsher, R. R., Stephens, T. W., and Caro, J. F., Evidence of free and bound leptin in human circulation. Studies in lean and obese subjects and during short-term fasting, *J. Clin. Invest.*, 98, 1277, 1996.

46. Huang, X. F., Koutcherov, I., Lin, S., Wang, H. Q., and Storlien, L., Localization of leptin receptor mRNA expression in mouse brain, *Neuroreport*, 7, 2635, 1996.
47. Baumann, H., Morella, K. K., White, D. W., Dembski, M., Bailon, P. S., Kim, H. K., Lai, C. F., and Tartaglia, L. A., The full-length leptin receptor has signaling capabilities of interleukin 6-type cytokine receptors, *Proc. Natl. Acad. Sci. U.S.A.*, 93, 8374, 1996.
48. Fei, H., Okano, H. J., Li, C., Lee, G-H, Zhao, C., Darnell, R., and Friedman, J. M., Anatomic localization of alternatively spliced leptin receptors (Ob-R) in mouse brain and other tissues, *Proc. Natl. Acad. Sci. U.S.A.*, 94, 7001, 1997.
49. Mercer, J. G., Hoggard, N., Williams, L. M., Lawrence, C. B., Hannah, L. T., and Trayhurn, P., Localization of leptin receptor mRNA and the long form splice variant (Ob-Rb) in mouse hypothalamus and adjacent brain regions by *in situ* hybridization, *FEBS Lett.*, 387, 113, 1996.
50. Lee, G.-H., Li, C., Montez, J., Halaas, J., Darvishzadeh, J., and Friedman, J. M. Leptin receptor mutations in 129 *db^{3J}/db^{3J}* mice and NIH *fa^{cp}/fa^{cp}* rats, *Mamm. Genome*, 8, 445, 1997.
51. Chua, S. C., Chung, W. K., Wu-Peng, S., Zhang, Y., Liu, S.-M., Tartaglia, L., and Leibel, R. L., Phenotypes of mouse *diabetes* and rat *fatty* due to mutations in the OB (leptin) receptor, *Science*, 271, 994, 1996.
52. Considine, R. V., Considine, E. L., Williams, C. J., Hyde, T. M., and Caro, J. F., The hypothalamic leptin receptor in humans: identification of incidental sequence polymorphisms, *Diabetes*, 45, 992, 1996.
53. Matsuoka, N., Ogawa, Y., Hosoda, K., Matsuda, J., Masuzaki, H., Miyawaki, T., Azuma, N., Natsui, K., Nishimura, H., Yoshimasa, Y., Nishi, S., Thompson, D. B., and Nakao, K., Human leptin receptor gene in obese Japanese subjects: evidence against either obesity-causing mutations or association of sequence variants with obesity, *Diabetologia*, 40, 1204, 1997.
54. Thompson, D. B., Ravussin, E., Bennett, P. H., and Bogardus, C., Structure and sequence variation at the human leptin receptor gene in lean and obese Pima Indians, *Human Mol. Gen.*, 6, 675, 1997.
55. Darnell, J. E., Jr., Reflections on STAT3, STAT5 and STAT 6 as fat STATs, *Proc. Natl. Acad. Sci. U.S.A.*, 93, 6221, 1996.
56. Vaisse, C., Halaas, J. L., Horvath, C. M., Darnell, J. E., Jr., Stoffel, M., and Friedman, J. M., Leptin activation of Stat3 in the hypothalamus of wildtype and *ob/ob* mice but not *db/db* mice, *Nature Genet.*, 14, 95, 1996.
57. Bjørbaek, C., Uotani, S., da Silva, B., and Flier, J. S. Divergent signaling capacities of the long and short isoforms of the leptin receptor, *J. Biol. Chem.*, 272, 32686, 1997.
58. Spanswick, D., Smith, M. A., Groppi, V. E., Logan, S. D., and Ashford, M. L. J., Leptin inhibits hypothalamic neurons by activation of ATP-sensitive potassium channels, *Nature*, 390, 521, 1997.
59. Kieffer, T. J., Heller, R. S., Leech, C. A., Holz, G. G., and Habener, J. F., Leptin suppression of insulin secretion by the activation of ATP-sensitive K+ channels in pancreatic beta-cells, *Diabetes*, 46, 1087, 1997.
60. Murakami, T., Yamashita, T., Iida, M., Kuwajima, M., and Shima, K., A short form of leptin receptor performs signal transduction, *Biochem. Biophys. Res. Commun.*, 231, 26, 1997.
61. Banks, W. A., Kastin, A. J., Huang, W. T., Jaspan, J. B., and Maness, L. M., Leptin enters the brain by a saturable system independent of insulin, *Peptides*, 17, 305, 1996.
62. Golden, P. L., Maccagnan, T. J., and Pardridge, W. M., Human blood-brain barrier leptin receptor. Binding and endocytosis in isolated human brain microvessels, *J. Clin. Invest.*, 99, 14, 1997.
63. Malik, K. F. and Young, W. S., Localization of binding sites in the central nervous system for leptin (OB protein) in normal, obese (*ob/ob*), and diabetic (*db/db*) C57BL/6J mice, *Endocrinology*, 137, 1497, 1996.
64. Schwartz, M. W., Peskind, E., Raskind, M., Boyko, E. J., and Porte, D., Jr., Cerebrospinal fluid leptin levels: relationship to plasma levels and to adiposity in humans, *Nature Med.*, 2, 589, 1996.
65. Weigle, D. S. and Kuijper, J. L. Obesity genes and the regulation of body fat content, Bioessays, 18, 867, 1996.
66. Campfield, L. A., Smith, F. J., and Burn, P., The OB protein (leptin) pathway — a link between adipose tissue mass and central neural networks, *Horm. Metab. Res.*, 28, 619, 1996.

67. Saladin, R., Staels, B., Auwerx, J., and Briggs, M., Regulation of *ob* gene expression in rodents and humans, *Horm. Metab. Res.*, 28, 638, 1996.
68. Considine, R. V., Sinha, M. K., Heiman, M. L., Kriauciunas, A., Stephens, T. W., Nyce, M R., Ohannesian, J. P., Marco, C. C., Mckee, L. J., Bauer, T. L., and Caro, J. F., Serum immunoreactive leptin concentrations in normal-weight and obese humans, *N. Engl. J. Med.*, 334, 292, 1996.
69. Considine, R. V. and Caro, J. F., Leptin in humans: current progress and future directions, *Clin. Chem.*, 42, 843, 1996.
70. Lönnqvist, F., Arner, P., Nordfors, L., and Schalling, M., Overexpression of the obese (*ob*) gene in adipose tissue of human obese subjects, *Nature Med.*, 1, 950, 1995.
71. Caro, J. F., Sinha, M. K., Kolaczynski, J. W., Zhang, P. L., and Considine, R. V, Leptin: the tale of an obesity gene, *Diabetes*, 45, 1455, 1996.
72. Salbe, A. D., Nicolson, M., and Ravussin, E., Total energy expenditure and the level of physical activity correlate with plasma leptin concentrations in five-year-old children, *J. Clin. Invest.*, 99, 592, 1997.
73. Ravussin, E., Pratley, R. E., Maffei, M., Wang, H., Friedman, J. M., Bennett, P. H., and Bogardus, C., Relatively low plasma leptin concentrations precede weight gain in Pima Indians, *Nature Med.*, 238, 1997.
74. Havel, P.J., Kasim-Karakas, S., Dubuc, G. R., Mueller, W., and Phinney, S. D., Gender differences in plasma leptin concentrations, *Nature Med.*, 2, 949–950, 1996.
75. Rosenbaum, M., Nicolson, M., Hirsch, J., Heymsfield, S.B., Gallagher, D., Chu, F., and Leibel, R. L., Effects of gender, body composition, and menopause on plasma concentrations of leptin, *J. Clin. Endocrinol. Metab.*, 81, 3424, 1996.
76. Sinha, M. K., Ohannesian, J. P., Heiman, M. L., Kriauciunas, A., Stephens, T. W., Magosin, S., Marco, C., and Caro, J. F., Nocturnal rise of leptin in lean, obese, and noninsulin-dependent diabetes mellitus subjects, *J. Clin. Invest.*, 97, 1344, 1996.
77. Licinio, J., Mantzoros, C., Negrao, A. B., Cizza, G., Wong, M. L., Bongiorno, P. B., Chrousos, G. P., Karp, B., Allen, C., Flier, J. S., and Gold, P. W., Human leptin levels are pulsatile and inversely related to pituitary-adrenal function, *Nature Med.*, 3, 575, 1997.
78. Schoeller, D. A., Cella, L. K., Sinha, M. K., and Caro, J. F., Entrainment of the diurnal rhythm of plasma leptin to meal timing, *J. Clin. Invest.*, 100, 1882, 1997.
79. Masuzaki, H., Ogawa, Y., Isse, N., Satoh, N., Okazaki, T., Shigemoto, M., Mori, K., Tamura, N., Hosoda, K., Yoshimasa, Y., Jingami, H., Kaeada, T., and Nakao, K., Human obese gene expression. Adipocyte-specific expression and regional differences in the adipose tissue, *Diabetes*, 44, 855, 1995.
80. Moinat, M., Deng, C. J., Muzzin, P., Assimacopoulos-Jeannet, F., Seydoux, J., Dulloo, A. G., and Giacobino, J. P., Modulation of obese gene expression in rat brown and white adipose tissues, *FEBS Lett.*, 373, 131, 1995.
81. Tsuruo, Y., Sato, I., Iida, M., Murakami, T., Ishimura, K., and Shima, K., Immunohistochemical detection of the *ob* gene product (leptin) in rat white and brown adipocytes, *Horm. Metab. Res.*, 28, 753, 1996.
82. Masuzaki, H., Ogawa, Y., Sagawa, N., Hosoda, K., Matsumoto, T., Mise, H., Nishimura, H., Yoshimasa, Y., Tanaka, I., Mori, T., and Nakao, K., Nonadipose tissue production of leptin — leptin as a novel placenta-derived hormone in humans, *Nature Med.*, 3, 1029, 1997.
83. Masuzaki, H., Hosoda, K., Ogawa, Y., Shigemoto, M., Satoh, N., Mori, K., Tamura, N., Nishi, S., Yoshimasa, Y., Yamori, Y., and Nakao, K., Augmented expression of obese (*ob*) gene during the process of obesity in genetically obese-hyperglycemic Wistar fatty (*fa/fa*) rats, *FEBS Lett*, 378, 267, 1996.
84. Frederich, R. C., Hamann, A., Anderson, S., Lollmann, B., Lowell, B. B., and Flier, J. S., Leptin levels reflect body lipid content in mice: evidence for diet-induced resistance to leptin action, *Nature Med.*, 1, 1311, 1995.
85. Becker, D. J., Ongemba, L. N., Brichard, V., Henquin, J.-C., and Brichard, S. M., Diet- and diabetes-induced changes of *ob* gene expression in rat adipose tissue, *FEBS Lett.*, 371, 324, 1995.
86. Flier, J. S., Leptin expression and action: new experimental paradigms, *Proc. Natl. Acad. Sci. U.S.A.*, 94, 4242, 1997.

87. Ahima, R. S., Prabakaran, D., Mantzoros, C., Qu, D., Lowell, B., Maratos-Flier, E., and Flier, J., Role of leptin in the neuroendocrine response to fasting, *Nature*, 382, 250, 1996.

88. Saladin, R., De Vos, P., Guerre-Millo, M., Leturque, A., Girard, J., Staels, B., and Auwerx, J., Transient increase in obese gene expression after food intake or insulin administration, *Nature*, 377, 527, 1995.

89. Zimmet, P., Hodge, A., Nicolson, M., Staten, M., Decourten, M., Moore, J., Morawiecki, A., Lubina, J., Collier, G., Alberti, G., and Dowse, G., Serum leptin concentration, obesity, and insulin resistance in Western Samoans: cross sectional study, *Br. Med. J.*, 313, 965, 1996.

90. Kolaczynski, J. W., Nyce, M. R., Considine, R. V., Boden, G., Nolan, J. J., Henry, R., Mudaliar, S. R., Olefsky, J., and Caro, J. F., Acute and chronic effect of insulin on leptin production in humans: studies *in vivo* and *in vitro*, *Diabetes*, 45, 699, 1996.

91. Dagogo-Jack, S., Fanelli, C., Paramore, D., Brothers, J., and Landt, M., Plasma leptin and insulin relationships in obese and nonobese humans, *Diabetes*, 45, 695, 1996.

92. Mandrup, S. and Lane, M. D., Regulating adipogenesis, *J. Biol. Chem.*, 272, 5367, 1997.

93. Hardie, L. J., Rayner, D. V., Holmes, S., and Trayhurn, P., Circulating leptin levels are modulated by fasting, cold exposure and insulin administration in lean but not Zucker (*fa/fa*) rats as measured by ELISA, *Biochem. Biophys. Res. Commun.*, 223, 660, 1996.

94. Trayhurn, P., Duncan, J. S., and Rayner, D. V., Acute cold-induced suppression of *ob* (obese) gene expression in white adipose tissue of mice: mediation by the sympathetic system, *Biochem. J.*, 311, 729, 1995.

95. Mantzoros, C. S., Qu, D. Q., Frederich, R. C., Susulic, V. S., Lowell, B. B., Maratos-Flier, E., and Flier, J. S., Activation of β_3-adrenergic receptors suppresses leptin expression and mediates a leptin-independent inhibition of food intake in mice, *Diabetes*, 45, 909, 1996.

96. Zhang, Y. Y., Olbort, M., Schwarzer, K., Nuesslein-Hildesheim, B., Nicolson, M., Murphy, E., Kowalski, T. J., Schmidt, I., and Leibel, R. L., The leptin receptor mediates apparent autocrine regulation of leptin gene expression, *Biochem. Biophys. Res. Commun.*, 240, 492, 1997.

97. Zhang, B., Graziano, M. P., Doebber, T. W., Leibowitz, M. D., White-Carrington, S., Szalkowski, D. M., Hey, P. J., Wu, M., Cullinan, C. A., Bailey, P., Lollmann, B., Frederich, R., Flier, J. S., Strader, C. D., and Smith, R. G., Down-regulation of the expression of the obese gene by an antidiabetic thiazolidinedione in Zucker diabetic fatty rats and *db/db* mice, *J. Biol. Chem.*, 271, 9455, 1996.

98. Campfield, L. A., Smith, F.J., Guisez, Y., Devos, R., and Burn, P., Recombinant mouse ob protein: evidence for a peripheral signal linking adiposity and central neural networks, *Science*, 269, 546, 1995.

99. Pellymounter, M., Cullen, M., Baker, M., Hecht, R., Winters, D., Boone, T., and Collins, F., Effects of the obese gene product on body weight regulation in *ob/ob* mice, *Science*, 269, 540, 1995.

100. Weigle, D. S., Bukowski, T. R., Foster, D. C., Holderman, S., Kramer, J. M., Lasser, G., Loftonday, C. E., Prunkard, D. E., Raymond, C., and Kuijper, J. L., Recombinant ob protein reduces feeding and body weight in the ob/ob mouse, *J. Clin. Invest.*, 96, 2065, 1995.

101. Schwartz, M. W., Baskin, D. G., Bukowski, T. R., Kuijper, J. L., Foster, D., Lasser, G., Prunkard, D. E., Porte, D., Woods, S. C., Seeley, R. J., and Weigle, D. S., Specificity of leptin action on elevated blood glucose levels and hypothalamic neuropeptide Y gene expression in ob/ob mice, *Diabetes*, 45, 531, 1996.

102. Stephens, T. W., Basinski, M., Bristow, P. K., Bue-Valleskey, J. M., Burgett, S. G., Craft, L., Hale, J., Hoffmann, J., Hsiung, H. M., Kriauciunas, A., MacKellar, W., Rosteck, P. R., Jr, Schoner, B., Smith, D., Tinsley, F. C., Zhang, X.-Y., and Heiman, M., The role of neuropeptide Y in the antiobesity action of the *obese* gene product, *Nature*, 377, 530-532, 1995.

103. Muzzin, P., Eisensmith, R. C., Copeland, K. C., and Woo, S. L., Correction of obesity and diabetes in genetically obese mice by leptin gene therapy, *Proc. Natl. Acad. Sci. U.S.A.*, 93, 14804, 1996.

104. Dawson, R., Pelleymounter, M. A., Millard, W. J., Liu, S., and Eppler, B., Attenuation of leptin-mediated effects by monosodium glutamate-induced arcuate nucleus damage, *Am. J. Physiol.*, 273, E202, 1997.

105. Spiegelman, B. M. and Flier, J. S., Adipogenesis and obesity: rounding out the big picture, *Cell*, 87, 377, 1996.

106. Flier, J. S., The adipocyte: storage depot or node on the energy information superhighway, *Cell*, 80, 15-18, 1995.

107. Glaum, S. R., Hara, M., Bindokas, V. P., Lee, C. C., Polonsky, K. S., Bell, G. I., and Miller, R. J., Leptin, the obese gene product, rapidly modulates synaptic transmission in the hypothalamus, *Mol. Pharmacol.*, 50, 230, 1996.

108. Gerald, C., Walker, M. W., Criscione, L., Gustafson, E. L., Batzl-Hartmann, C., Smith, K. E., Vaysse, P., Durkin, M. M., Laz, T. M., Linemeyer, D. L., Schaffhauser, A. O., Whitebread, S., Hofbauer, K. G., Taber, R. I., Branchek, T. A., and Weinshank, R. L., A receptor subtype involved in neuropeptide-Y-induced food intake, *Nature*, 382, 168, 1996.

109. Rohner-Jeanrenaud, F., Cusin, I., Sainsbury, A., Zakrzewska, K. E., and Jeanrenaud, B., The loop system between neuropeptide Y and leptin in normal and obese rodents, *Horm. Metab. Res.*, 28, 642, 1996.

110. Wang, Q., Bing, C., Al-Barazanji, K., Mossakowaska, D. E., Wang, X.-E., McBay, D. L., Neville, W. A., Taddayon, M., Pickavance, L., Dryden, S., Thomas, M. E. A., McHale, M. T., Gloyer, I. S., Wilson, S., Buckingham, R., Arch, J. R. S., Trayhurn, P., and Williams, G., Interactions between leptin and hypothalamic neuropeptide Y neurons in the control of food intake and energy homeostasis in the rat, *Diabetes*, 46, 335, 1997.

111. Schwartz, M. W., Seeley, R. J., Campfield, L. A., Burn, P., and Baskin, D. G., Identification of targets of leptin action in rat hypothalamus, *J. Clin. Invest.*, 98, 1101, 1996.

112. Dryden, S., Pickavance, L., Frankish, H. M., and Williams, G., Increased neuropeptide Y (NPY) secretion in the hypothalamic paraventricular nucleus of obese *(fa/fa)* Zucker rats, *Brain Res.*, 690, 185, 1995.

113. Sainsbury, A., Rohner-Jeanrenaud, F., Cusin, I., Zakrzewska, K. E., Halban, P. A., Gaillard, R. C., and Jeanrenaud, B., Chronic central neuropeptide Y infusion in normal rats: status of the hypothalamo-pituitary-adrenal axis, and vagal mediation of hyperinsulinemia, *Diabetologia*, 40, 1269, 1997.

114. Erickson, J. C., Clegg, K. E., and Palmiter, R. D., Sensitivity to leptin and susceptibility to seizures of mice lacking neuropeptide Y, *Nature*, 381, 415, 1996.

115. Heiman, M. L., Ahima, R. S., Craft, L. S., Schoner, B., Stephens, T. W., and Flier, J. S., Leptin inhibition of the hypothalamic-pituitary-adrenal axis in response to stress, *Endocrinology*, 138, 3859, 1997.

116. Delaunay, F., Khan, A., Cintra, A., Davani, B., Ling, Z.-C., Andersson, A., Östenson, C. G., Gustafsson, J.-Å., Efendic, S., and Okret, S., Pancreatic β-cells are important targets for the diabetogenic effects of glucocorticoids, *J. Clin. Invest.*, 100, 2094, 1997.

117. Levin, N., Nelson, C., Gurney, A., Vandlen, R., and Desauvage, F., Decreased food intake does not completely account for adiposity reduction after ob protein infusion, *Proc. Natl. Acad. Sci. U.S.A.*, 93, 1726, 1996.

118. Haynes, W. G., Morgan, D. A., Walsh, S. A., Mark, A. L., and Sivitz, W. I., Receptor-mediated regional sympathetic nerve activation by leptin, *J. Clin. Invest.*, 100, 270, 1997.

119. Collins, S., Kuhn, C. M., Petro, A. E., Swick, A. G., Chrunyk, B. A., and Surwit, R. S., Role of leptin in fat regulation, *Nature*, 380, 677, 1996.

120. Scarpace, P. J., Matheny, M., Pollock, B. H., and Tümer, N., Leptin increases uncoupling protein expression and energy expenditure, *Am. J. Physiol.*, 273, E226, 1997.

121. Solanes, G., Vidal-Puig, A., Grujic, D., Flier, J. S., and Lowell, B. B., The human uncoupling protein-3 gene, *J. Biol. Chem.*, 272, 25433, 1997.

122. Wang, Y. H., Tache, Y., Sheibel, A. B., Go, V. L., and Wei, J. Y., Two types of leptin-responsive gastric vagal afferent terminals: an *in vitro* single-unit study in rats, *Am. J. Physiol.*, 273, R833, 1997.

123. Siegrist-Kaiser, C. A., Pauli, V., Juge-Aubry, C. E., Boss, O., Pernin, A., Chin, W. W., Cusin, I., Rohner-Jeanrenaud, F., Burger, A. G., Zapf, J., and Meier, C. A., Direct effects of leptin on brown and white adipose tissue, *J. Clin. Invest.*, 100, 2858, 1997.

124. Chen, G., Koyama, K., Yuen, X., Lee, Y., Zhou, Y.-T., O'Doherty, R., Newgard, C. B., and Unger, R. H., Disappearance of body fat in normal rats induced by adenovirus-mediated leptin gene therapy, *Proc. Natl. Acad. Sci. U.S.A.*, 93, 14795, 1996.

125. Cohen, B., Novick, D., and Rubinstein, M., Modulation of insulin activities by leptin, *Science*, 274, 1185, 1996.
126. Kieffer, T. J., Heller, R. S., and Habener, J. F., Leptin receptors expressed on pancreatic β-cells, *Biochem. Biophys. Res. Commun.*, 224, 522, 1996.
127. Emilsson, V., Liu, Y.-L., Cawthorne, M. A., Morton, N. M., and Davenport, M., Expression of the functional leptin receptor mRNA in pancreatic islets and direct inhibitory action of leptin on insulin secretion, *Diabetes*, 46, 313, 1997.
128. Unger, R. H., How obesity causes diabetes in Zucker diabetic fatty rats, *Trends Endo. Metab.*, 8, 276, 1997.
129. Siracusa, L. D., The agouti gene: turned on to yellow, *Trends Genet.*, 10, 423, 1994.
130. Manne, J., Argeson, A. C., and Siracusa, L. D., Mechanisms for the pleiotropic effects of the agouti gene, *Proc. Natl. Acad. Sci. U.S.A.*, 92, 4721, 1995.
131. Kucera, G. T., Bortner, D. M., and Rosenberg, M. P., Overexpression of an *agouti* cDNA in the skin of transgenic mice recapitulates dominant coat color phenotypes of spontaneous mutants, *Dev. Biol.*, 173, 162, 1996.
132. Miltenberger, R. J., Mynatt, R. L., Wilkison, J. E., and Woychik, R. P., The role of the *agouti* gene in the yellow obese syndrome, *J. Nutr.*, 127, 1902S, 1997.
133. Yen, T. T., Gill, A. M., Frigeri, L. G., Barsh, G. S., and Wolff, G. L., Obesity, diabetes, and neoplasia in yellow A$^{vy/-}$ mice: ectopic expression of the agouti gene, *FASEB J.*, 8, 479, 1994.
134. Hunt, C. E., Lindsey, J. R., and Walkley, S. U., Animal models of diabetes and obesity, including the PBB/Ld mouse, *Fed. Proc.*, 35, 1206, 1976.
135. Frigeri, L. G., Teguh, C., Ling, N., Wolff, G. L., and Lewis, U. J., Increased sensitivity of adipose tissue to insulin after *in vivo* treatment of yellow A^{vy}/A obese mice with amino-terminal peptides of human growth hormone, *Endocrinology*, 122, 2940, 1988.
136. Huszar, D., Lynch, C. A., Fairchild-Huntress, V., Dunmore, J. H., Fang, Q., Berkemeier, L. R., Gu, W., Kesterson, R. A., Boston, B. A., Cone, R. D., Smith, F. J., Campfield, L. A., Burn, P., and Lee, F., Targeted disruption of the melanocortin-4 receptor results in obesity in mice, *Cell*, 88, 131, 1997.
137. Wolff, G. L., Greenman, D. L., Frigeri, L. G., Morrissey, R. L., Suber, R. L., and Felton, R. P., Diabetogenic response to streptozotocin varies among obese yellow and among lean agouti (BALB/c × VY)F1 hybrid mice, *Proc. Soc. Exp. Biol. Med.*, 193, 155, 1990.
138. Warbritton, A., Gill, A. M., Yen, T. T., Bucci, T., and Wolff, G. L., Pancreatic islet cells in preobese yellow A$^{vy/-}$ mice: relation to adult hyperinsulinemia and obesity, *Proc. Soc. Exp. Biol. Med.*, 206, 145, 1994.
139. Bultman, S. J., Michaud, E. J., and Woychik, R. P., Molecular characterization of the mouse agouti locus, *Cell*, 71, 1195, 1992.
140. Miller, M. W., Duhl, D. M., Vrieling, H., Cordes, S. P., Ollmann, M. M., Winkes, B. W., and Barsh, G. S., Cloning of the mouse *agouti* gene predicts a secreted protein ubiquitously expressed in mice carrying the *lethal yellow* mutation, *Genes Dev.*, 7, 454, 1993.
141. Kwon, H. Y., Bultman, S. J., Loffler, C., Chen, W.-J., Furdon, P. J., Powell, J. G., Usala, A. L., Wilkison, W., Hansmann, I., and Woychik, R. P., Molecular structure and chromosomal mapping of the human homolog of the agouti gene, *Proc. Natl. Acad. Sci. U.S.A.*, 91, 9760, 1994.
142. Wilson, B. D., Ollmann, M. M., Kang, L., Stoffel, M., Bell, G. I., and Barsh, G. S., Structure and function of ASP, the human homolog of the mouse *agouti* gene, *Hum. Mol. Gen.*, 4, 223, 1995.
143. Perry, W. L., Copeland, N. G., and Jenkins, N. A., The molecular basis for dominant yellow agouti coat color mutations, *Bioessays*, 16, 705, 1994.
144. Cone, R. D., Lu, D., Koppula, S., Vage, D. I., Klungland, H., Boston, B., Chen, W., Orth, D. N., Pouton, C., and Kesterson, R. A., The melanocortin receptors: agonists, antagonists, and the hormonal control of pigmentation, *Recent Prog. Horm. Res.*, 51, 287, 1996.
145. Duhl, D. M., Stevens, M. E., Vrieling, H., Saxon, P. J., Miller, M. W., Epstein, C. J., and Barsch, G. S., Pleiotropic effects of the mouse lethal yellow (A^y) mutation explained by deletion of a maternally expressed gene and the simultaneous production of *agouti* fusion RNAs, *Development*, 120, 1695, 1994.
146. Michaud, E. J., Bultman, S. J., Stubbs, L. J., and Woychik, R. P., The embryonic lethality of homozygous lethal yellow mice (A^y/A^y) is associated with the disruption of a novel RNA-binding protein, *Genes Dev.*, 7, 1203, 1993.

147. Michaud, E. J., Bultman, S. J., Klebig, M. L., Van Vugt, M. J., Stubbs, L. J., Russell, L. B., and Woychik, R. P., A molecular model for the genetic and phenotypic characteristics of the mouse lethal yellow (A^y) mutation, *Proc. Natl. Acad. Sci. U.S.A.*, 91, 2562, 1994.

148. Duhl, D. M. J., Vrieling, H., Miller, K. A., Wolff, G. L., and Barsh, G. S., Neomorphic *agouti* mutations in obese yellow mice, *Nature Genet.*, 8, 59, 1994.

149. Michaud, E. J., van Vugt, M. J., Bultman, S. J., Sweet, H. O., Davisson, M. T., and Woychik, R. P., Differential expression of a new dominant agouti allele (A^{iapy}) is correlated with methylation state and is influenced by parental lineage, *Genes Dev.*, 8, 1463, 1994.

150. Siracusa, L. D., Washburn, L. L., Swing, D. A., Argeson, A. C., Jenkins, N. A., and Copeland, N. G., Hypervariable yellow (A^{hvy}), a new murine agouti mutation: A^{hvy} displays the largest variation in coat color phenotypes of all known agouti alleles, *J. Hered.*, 86, 121, 1995.

151. Argeson, A. C., Nelson, K. K., and Siracusa, L. D., Molecular basis of the pleiotropic phenotype of mice carrying the hypervariable yellow (A^{hvy}) mutation at the agouti locus, *Genetics*, 142, 557, 1996.

152. Klebig, M. L., Wilkinson, J. E., Geisler, J. G., and Woychik, R. P., Ectopic expression of the agouti gene in transgenic mice causes obesity, features of Type II diabetes, and yellow fur, *Proc. Natl. Acad. Sci. U.S.A.*, 92, 4728, 1995.

153. Shutter, J. R., Graham, M., Kinsey, A. C., Scully, S., Lüthy, R., and Stark, K. L., Hypothalamic expression of *ART*, a novel gene related to *agouti*, is upregulated in *obese* and *diabetic* mutant mice, *Genes Dev.*, 11, 593, 1997.

154. Lu, D., Willard, D., Patel, I. R., Kadwell, S., Overton, L., Kost, T., Luther, M., Chen, W., Woychik, R. P., Wilkison, W. O., and Cone, R. D., Agouti protein is an antagonist of the melanocyte-stimulating-hormone receptor, *Nature*, 371, 799, 1994.

155. Millar, S. E., Miller, M. W., Stevens, M. E., and Barsh, G. S., Expression and transgenic studies of the mouse agouti gene provide insight into the mechanisms by which mammalian coat color patterns are generated, *Development*, 121, 3223, 1995.

156. Kesterson, R. A., Huszar, D., Lynch, C. A., Simerly, R. B., and Cone, R. D., Induction of neuropeptide Y gene expression in the dorsal medial hypothalamic nucleus in two models of the *Agouti* obesity syndrome, *Mol. Endocrinol.*, 11, 630, 1997.

157. Fan, W., Boston, B. A., Kesterson, R. A., Hruby, V. J., and Cone, R. D., Role of melanocortinergic neurons in feeding and the agouti obesity syndrome, *Nature*, 385, 165, 1997.

158. Cheung, C. C., Clifton, D. K., and Steiner, R. A., Proopiomelanocortin neurons are direct targets for leptin in the hypothalamus, Endocrinology, 138, 4489, 1997.

159. Mizuno, T. M., Bergen, H., Funabashi, T., Kleopoulos, S. P., Zhong, Y.-G., Bauman, W. A., and Mobbs, C. V., Obese gene expression: reduction by fasting and stimulation by insulin and glucose in lean mice, and persistent elevation in acquired (diet-induced) and genetic (yellow agouti) obesity, *Proc. Natl. Acad. Sci. U.S.A.*, 93, 3434, 1996.

160. Halaas, J. L., Boozer, C., Blair-West, J., Fidahusein, N., Denton, D. A. and Friedman, J. M., Physiological response to long-term peripheral and central leptin infusion in lean and obese mice, *Proc. Natl. Acad. Sci. U.S.A.*, 94. 8878, 1997.

161. Zemel, M. B., Insulin resistance vs. hyperinsulinemia in hypertension: insulin regulation of Ca^{2+} transport and Ca^{2+}-regulation of insulin sensitivity, *J. Nutr.*, 125, 1738S, 1995.

162. Zemel, M. B., Kim, J. H., Woychik, R. P., Michaud, E. J., Kadwell, S. H., Patel, I. R., and Wilkison, W. O., Agouti regulation of intracellular calcium: role in the insulin resistance of viable yellow mice, *Proc. Natl. Acad. Sci. U.S.A.*, 92, 4733, 1995.

163. Kim, J. H., Mynatt, R. L., Moore, J. W., Woychik, R. P., Moustaid, N., and Zemel, M. B., The effects of calcium channel blockade on *agouti*-induced obesity, *FASEB J.*, 10, 1646, 1996.

164. Kim, J. H., Kiefer, L. L., Woychik, R. P., Wilkison, W. O., Truesdale, A., Ittoop, O., Willard, D., Nichols, J., and Zemel, M. B., Agouti regulation of intracellular calcium: role of melanocortin receptors, *Am. J. Physiol.*, 272, E379, 1997.

165. Jones, B. H., Kim, J. H., Zemel, M. B, Woychik, R. P., Michaud, E. J., Wilkison, W. O., and Moustaid, N., Upregulation of adipocyte metabolism by agouti protein: possible paracrine actions in yellow mouse obesity, *Am. J. Physiol.*, 270, E192, 1996.

166. Hunt, G. and Thody, A. J., Agouti protein can act independently of melanocyte-stimulating hormone to inhibit melanogenesis, *J. Endocrinol.*, 147, R1, 1995.

167. Mynatt, R. L., Miltenberger, R. J., Klebig, M. L., Zemel., M. B., Wilkison, J. E., Wilkison, W. O., and Woychik, R. P., Combined effects of insulin treatment and adipose tissue-specific agouti expression on the development of obesity, *Proc. Natl. Acad. Sci. U.S.A.*, 94, 919, 1997.

168. Ollmann, M. A., Wilson, B. D., Yang, Y.-K., Kerns, J. A., Chen, Y., Gantz, I., and Barsh, G. S., Antagonism of central melanocortin receptors *in vitro* and *in vivo* by agouti-related protein, *Science*, 278, 135, 1997.

169. Coleman, D. L., and Eicher, E. M., Fat (*fat*) and tubby (*tub*): two autosomal recessive mutations causing obesity syndromes in the mouse, *J. Hered.*, 8, 424, 1990.

170. Naggert, J., Harris, T., and North, M., The genetics of obesity, *Curr. Opin. Gen. Dev.*, 7, 398, 1997.

171. Chung, W. K., Goldberg-Berman, J., Power-Kehoe, L., and Leibel, R. L., Molecular mapping of the tubby (*tub*) mutation on mouse Chromosome 7, *Genomics*, 32, 210, 1996.

172. Noben-Trauth, K., Naggert, J. K, North, M. A., and Nishina, P. M., A candidate gene for the mouse mutation tubby, *Nature*, 380, 534, 1996.

173. Nishina, P. M., Lowe, S., Wang, J., and Paigen, B., Characterization of plasma lipids in genetically obese mice: the mutants obese, diabetes, fat, tubby, and lethal yellow, *Metabolism*, 43, 549, 1994.

174. Nishina, P. M., Naggert, J. K., Verstuyft, J., and Paigen, B., Atherosclerosis in genetically obese mice: the mutants obese, diabetes, fat, tubby, and lethal yellow, *Metabolism*, 43, 554, 1994.

175. Kleyn, P. W., Fan, W., Kovats, S. G., Lee, J. J., Pulido, J. C., Wu, Y., Berkemeier, L. R., Misumi, D. J., Holmgren, L., Charlat, O., Woolf, E. A., Tayber, O., Brody, T., Shu, P., Hawkins, F., Kennedy, B., Baldini, L., Ebeling, C., Alperin, G. D., Deeds, J., Lakey, N. D., Culpepper, J., Chen, H., Glucksmann-Kuis, M. A., and Moore, K. J., Identification and characterization of the mouse obesity gene tubby: a member of a novel gene family, *Cell*, 85, 281, 1996.

176. North, M. A., Naggert, J. K., Yan, Y., Noben-Trauth, K., and Nishina, P. M., Molecular characterization of *TUB*, *TULP1*, and *TULP2*, members of the novel tubby gene family and their possible relation to ocular diseases, *Proc. Natl. Acad. Sci. U.S.A.*, 94, 3128, 1997.

177. Ohlemiller, K. K., Hughes, R. M., Mosinger-Ogilvie, J., Speck, J. D., Grosof, D. H., and Silverman, M. S., Cochlear and retinal degeneration in the tubby mouse, *Neuroreport*, 6, 845, 1995.

178. Heckinlively, J. R., Chang, B., Erway, L. C., Peng, C., Hawes, N. L., Hageman, G. S., and Roderick, T. H., Mouse model for Usher syndrome: linkage mapping suggests homology to Usher Type I reported at human chromosome 11p15, *Proc. Natl. Acad. Sci U.S.A.*, 92, 11100, 1995.

179. Naggert, J. K., Fricker, L. D., Varlamov, O., Nishina, P. M., Rouille, Y., Steiner, D. F., Carroll, R. J., Paigen, B. J., and Leiter, E. H., Hyperproinsulinemia in obese *fat/fat* mice associated with a carboxypeptidase E mutation which reduces enzyme activity, *Nature Genet.*, 10, 135, 1995.

180. Varlamov, O., Leiter, E. H., and Fricker, L., Induced and spontaneous mutations at Ser^{202} of carboxypeptidase E. Effect on enzyme expression, activity, and intracellular routing, *J. Biol. Chem.*, 271, 13981, 1996.

181. Fricker, L. D., Berman, Y. L., Leiter, E. H., and Devi, L. A., Carboxypeptidase E activity is deficient in mice with the fat mutation. Effect on peptide processing, *J. Biol. Chem.*, 271, 30619, 1996.

182. Udupi, V., Gomez, P., Song, L., Varlamov, O., Reed, J. T., Leiter, E. H., Fricker, L. D., and Greeley, G. H., Jr., Effect of carboxypeptidase E deficiency on progastrin processing and gastrin messenger ribonucleic acid expression in mice with the fat mutation, *Endocrinology*, 138, 1959, 1997.

183. Cool, D. R., Normant, E., Shen, F., Chen, H. C., Pannell, L., Zhang, Y., and Loh, Y. P., Carboxypeptidase E is a regulated secretory pathway sorting receptor: genetic obliteration leads to endocrine disorders in Cpe^{fat} mice, *Cell*, 88, 73, 1997.

184. Rovere, C., Viale, A., Nahon, J., and Kitabgi, P., Impaired processing of brain proneurotensin and promelanin-concentrating hormone in obese *fat/fat* mice, *Endocrinology*, 137, 2954, 1996.

185. Lacourse, K. A., Friis-Hansen, L., Rehfeld, J. F., and Samuelson, L. C., Disturbed progastrin processing in carboxypeptidase E-deficient *fat* mice, *FEBS Lett.*, 416, 45, 1997.

186. Cain, B. M., Wang, W. G., and Beinfeld, M. C., Cholecystokinin (CCK) levels are greatly reduced in the brains but not the duodenums of Cpe^{fat}/Cpe^{fat} mice: a regional difference in the involvement of carboxypeptidase E (Cpe) in pro-CCK processing, *Endocrinology*, 138, 4034, 1997.

187. Shen, F. S. and Loh, Y. P., Intracellular misrouting and abnormal secretion of adrenocorticotropin and growth hormone in Cpe^fat mice associated with a carboxypeptidase E mutation, *Proc. Natl. Acad. Sci. USA*, 94, 5314, 1997.

188. Loh, Y. P., Snell, C. R., and Cool, D. R., Receptor-mediated targeting of hormones to secretory granules — role of carboxypeptidase E, *Trends Endocrinol. Metab.*, 8, 130, 1997.

189. Thiele, C., Gerdes, H. H., and Huttner, W. B., Protein secretion: puzzling receptors, *Curr. Biol.*, 7, R496, 1997.

190. Irminger, J.-C., Verchere, C. B., Meyer, K., and Halban, P. A., Proinsulin targeting to the regulated pathway is not impaired in carboxypeptidase E-deficient Cpe^fat/Cpe^fat mice, *J. Biol. Chem.*, 272, 27532, 1997.

191. Varlamov, O., Fricker, L. D., Furukawa, H., Steiner, D. F., Langley, S. H., and Leiter, E. H., β-cell lines derived from transgenic Cpe^fat/Cpe^fat mice are defective in carboxypeptidase E and proinsulin processing, *Endocrinology*, 138, 4883, 1997.

192. Jackson, R. S., Creemers, J. W. M., Ohagi, S., Raffin-Sanson, M. L., Sanders, L., Montague, C. T., Hutton, J. C., and O'Rahilly, S., Obesity and impaired prohormone processing associated with mutations in the human prohormone convertase 1 gene, *Nature Genet.*, 16, 303, 1997.

193. Furuta, M., Yano, H., Zhou, A., Rouillé, Y., Holst, J. J., Carroll, R., Ravazzola, M., Orci, L., Furuta, H., and Steiner, D. F., Defective prohormone processing and altered pancreatic islet morphology in mice lacking active SPC2, *Proc. Natl. Acad. Sci. U.S.A.*, 94, 6646, 1997.

194. Kahn, S. E. and Halban, P. A., Release of incompletely processed proinsulin is the cause of the disproportionate proinsulinemia of NIDDM, *Diabetes*, 46, 1725, 1997.

195. Zucker, L. M. and Zucker, T. F., Fatty, a new mutation in the rat, *J. Hered.*, 52, 275, 1961.

196. Jeanrenaud, B., An hypothesis on aetiology of obesity: dysfunction of the central nervous system as a primary cause, *Diabetologia*, 28, 502, 1985.

197. Kava, R., Greenwood, M. R. C., and Johnson, P. R., Zucker (fa/fa) rat, *ILAR News*, 32, 4, 1990.

198. Bray, G. A and York, D. A., Studies on food intake of genetically obese rats, *Am. J. Physiol.*, 223, 176, 1972.

199. Zucker, T. F. and Zucker, L. M., Hereditary obesity in the rat associated with high serum fat and cholesterol, *Proc. Soc. Exp. Biol. Med.*, 110, 165, 1962.

200. Ionescu, E., Sauter, J. F., and Jeanrenaud, B., Abnormal oral glucose tolerance in genetically obese (fa/fa) rats, *Am. J. Physiol.*, 248, E500, 1985.

201. Zucker, O. M. and Antoniades, H. N., Insulin and obesity in the Zucker genetically obese rat "fatty," *Endocrinology*, 90, 1320, 1972.

202. Chan, C. B., Pederson, R. A., Buchan, A. M. J., Tubesing K. B., and Brown, J. C., Gastric inhibitory polypeptide and hyperinsulinemia in the Zucker (fa/fa) rat: a developmental study, *Int. J. Obesity*, 9, 137, 1985.

203. Shino, A., Matsuo, T., Iwatsuka, H., and Suzuoki, F., Structural changes of pancreatic islets in genetically obese rats, *Diabetologia*, 9, 413, 1973.

204. Chan, C. B., Pederson, R. A., Buchan, A. M. J., Tubesing, K. B., and Brown, J. C., Gastric inhibitory polypeptide (GIP) and insulin release in the obese Zucker rat, *Diabetes*, 33, 536, 1984.

205. Jia, X., Elliott, R., Kwok, Y. N., Pederson, R. A., and McIntosh, C. H. S., Altered glucose dependence of glucagon-like peptide I(7-36)-induced insulin secretion from the Zucker (fa/fa) rat pancreas, *Diabetes*, 44, 495, 1995.

206. Chua, S. C., Jr., White, D. W., Wu-Peng, X. S., Liu, S.-W., Okada, N., Kershaw, E. E., Chung, W. K., Power-Kehoe, L., Chua, M., Tartaglia, L., and Leibel, R. L., Phenotype of fatty due to Gln269Pro mutation in the leptin receptor (*Lepr*), *Diabetes*, 45, 1141, 1996.

207. Iida, M., Murukami, T., Ishida, K., Mizuno, A., Kuwajima, M., and Shima, K., Phenotype-linked amino acid alteration in leptin receptor cDNA from Zucker fatty (fa/fa) rat, *Biochem. Biophys. Res. Commun.*, 222, 19, 1996.

208. Yamashita, T., Murukami, T., Iida, M., Kuwajima, M., and Shima, K., Leptin receptor of Zucker fatty rat performs reduced signal transduction, *Diabetes*, 46, 1077, 1997.

209. White, D. W., Wang, Y., Chua, S. C., Jr., Morgenstern, J. P., Leibel, R. L., Baumann, H., and Tartaglia, L. A., Constitutive and impaired signaling of leptin receptors containing the Gln → Pro extracellular domain fatty mutation, *Proc. Natl. Acad. Sci. U.S.A.*, 94, 10657, 1997.

210. Jeanrenaud, B., Halimi, S., and van de Werve, G., Neuroendocrine disorders seen as triggers of the triad: obesity-insulin resistance-abnormal glucose tolerance, *Diabetes Metab. Rev.*, 1, 261, 1985.
211. Greco, R., Zaninetti, D., Assiimacopoulos-Jeannet, F., and Jeanrenaud, B., Stimulatory effect of cold adaptation on glucose utilization by brown adipose tissue: relationship with changes of the glucose transporter system, *J. Biol. Chem.*, 262, 7732, 1987.
212. Greco-Perotto, R., Bobbioni E., Assimacopoulos-Jeannet, F., and Jeanrenaud, B. Properties of glucose transporters after cold-adaptation or insulin in brown adipose tissue of normal and obese rats, in *Int. Workshop, Lesson Anim. Diabetes II*, Geneva, 1987, 250 (abstr.).
213. Ogawa, Y., Masuzaki, H., Isse, N., Okazaki, T., Mori, K., Shigemoto, M., Satoh, N., Tamura, N., Hosoda, K., Yoshimasa, Y., Jingami, H., Kawada, T., and Nakao, K., Molecular cloning of rat obese cDNA and augmented gene expression in genetically obese Zucker fatty (fa/fa) rats, *J. Clin. Invest.*, 96, 1647, 1995.
214. Pagano, C., Englaro, P., Granzotto, M., Blum, W. F., Sagrillo, E., Ferretti, E., Federspil, G., and Vettor, R., Insulin induces rapid changes of plasma leptin in lean but not in genetically obese (fa/fa) rats, *Int. J. Obesity Rel. Metab. Dis.*, 2, 614, 1997.
215. Ferré, P., Burnol, A. F., Leturque, A., Leturque, A., Terretaz, J., Penicaud, L., Jeanrenaud, B., and Girard, J., Glucose utilization *in vivo* and insulin-sensitivity of rat brown adipose tissue in various physiological and pathological conditions, *Biochem. J.*, 233, 249, 1986.
216. Terrettaz, J., Assimacopoulos-Jeannet, F., and Jeanrenaud, B., Severe hepatic and peripheral insulin resistance as evidenced by euglycemic clamps in genetically obese *fa/fa* rats, *Endocrinology*, 118, 674, 1986.
217. Rohner-Jeanrenaud, F. and Jeanrenaud, B., A role for the vagus nerve in the etiology and maintenance of the hyperinsulinemia of genetically obese *fa/fa* rats, *Int. J. Obesity*, 9, 71, 1985.
218. Slieker, L. J., Roberts, E. F., Shaw, W. N., and Johnson, W. T., Effect of streptozotocin-induced diabetes on insulin receptor tyrosine kinase activity in obese Zucker rats, *Diabetes*, 39, 619, 1990.
219. Czech, M. P., Richardson, D. K., Becker, S. G., Walters, C. G., Glitomer, W., and Heinrich, J., Insulin response in skeletal muscle and fat cells of the genetically obese Zucker rat, *Metabolism* 27, 1967, 1978.
220. Karakash, C. and Jeanrenaud, B., Insulin binding and removal by livers of genetically obese rats, *Diabetes* 32, 605, 1983.
221. Shemer, J., Ota, A., Adamo, M., and LeRoith, D., Insulin-sensitive tyrosine kinase is increased in livers of adult obese Zucker rats: correction with prolonged fasting, *Endocrinology*, 123, 140, 1987.
222. DeFronzo, R. A., Bonadonna, R. C., and Ferrannini, E., Pathogenesis of NIDDM: a balanced overview, *Diabetes Care*, 15, 318, 1992.
223. De Souza, C. J., Yu, J. H., Robinson, D. D., Ulrich, R. G., and Meglasson, M. D., Insulin secretory defect in Zucker *fa/fa* rats is improved by ameliorating insulin resistance, *Diabetes*, 44, 984, 1995.
224. Peterson, R. G., Shaw, W. N., Neel, M., Little, L. A., and Eichberg, J., Zucker diabetic fatty rat as a model for noninsulin-dependent diabetes mellitus, *ILAR News*, 32, 16, 1990.
225. Tokuyama, Y., Sturis, J., DePaoli, A. M., Takeda, J., Stoffel, M., Tang, J., Sun, X., Polonsky, K. S., and Bell, G. I., Evolution of β-cell dysfunction in the male Zucker diabetic fatty rat, *Diabetes*, 44, 1447, 1995.
226. Ahansen, B. C., Jen, K. C., Pek, S. B., and Wolfe, R. A., Rapid oscillations in plasma insulin, glucagon and glucose in obese and normal weight humans, *J. Clin. Endocrinol. Metab.*, 54, 785, 1982.
227. Lang, D. A., Matthews, J., and Turner, R. C., Cyclic oscillations of plasma glucose and insulin concentrations in human beings, *N. Engl. J. Med.*, 301, 1023, 1979.
228. Goodner, C. J., Koerker, J., Stagner, I., and Samols, E., *In vitro* pancreatic hormonal pulses are less regular and more frequent than *in vivo*, *Am. J. Physiol.*, 260, E422, 1991.
229. Bergsten, P. and Hellman, B., Glucose-induced amplitude regulation of pulsatile insulin secretion from individual pancreatic islets, *Diabetes*, 42, 670, 1993.
230. Lang, D. A., Matthews, D. R., Burness, M., and Turner, R. C., Brief, irregular oscillations of basal plasma insulin and glucose concentrations in diabetic man, *Diabetes*, 30, 435, 1981.

231. Matthews, D. R., Lang, D. A., Burnett, M. A., and Turner, R. C., Control of pulsatile insulin secretion in man, *Diabetologia*, 24, 231, 1983.

232. Sturis, J., Pugh, W. I., Tang, J., Ostrega, D., Polonski, J. S., and Polonski, K. S., Alterations in pulsatile secretion in the Zucker diabetic fatty rat, *Am. J. Physiol.*, 267, E250, 1994.

233. Johnson, J. H., Ogawa, A., Chen, L., Orci, L., Newgard, C. B., Alam, T., and Unger, R. H., Underexpression of β-cell high K_m glucose-transporters in noninsulin-dependent diabetes, *Science*, 250, 546, 1990.

234. Unger, R. H., Diabetic hyperglycemia: link to impaired glucose transport in pancreatic β-cells, *Science*, 251, 1200, 1991.

235. Sinha, M. K., Raineri-Maldonado, C., Buchanan, C., Pories, W. J., Carter-Su, C., Pilch, P. F., and Caro, J. F., Adipose tissue glucose transporters in NIDDM. Decreased levels of muscle/fat isoform, *Diabetes*, 40, 472, 1991.

236. Uphues, I., Kolter, T., Goud, B., and Eckel, J., Failure of insulin-regulated recruitment of the glucose transporter GLUT4 in cardiac muscle of obese Zucker rats is associated with alterations of small-molecular-mass GTP-binding proteins, *Biochem. J.*, 311, 161, 1995.

237. Zaninetti, D., Crettaz, M., and Jeanrenaud, B., Dysregulation of glucose transport in hearts of genetically obese (*fa/fa*) rats, *Diabetologia*, 25, 525, 1983.

238. Slieker, L. J., Sundell, K. L., Heath, W. F., Osborne, H. E., Bue, J., Manetta, J., and Sportsman, J. R., Glucose transporter levels in tissues of spontaneously diabetic Zucker *fa/fa* rat (ZDF/drt) and viable yellow mouse (A^{vy}/a), *Diabetes*, 41, 187, 1992.

239. Ferrannini, E., Barrett, E. J., Bovilacqua, S., and DeFronzo, R. A., Effect of fatty acids on glucose production and utilization in man, *J. Clin. Invest.*, 72, 1737, 1983.

240. DeFronzo, R. A., The triumvirate β-cell, muscle, liver: a collusion responsible for NIDDM, *Diabetes*, 37, 667, 1988.

241. Reaven, G. M., The fourth musketeer — from Alexandre Dumas to Claude Bernard, *Diabetologia*, 38, 8, 1995

242. Shimabukuro, M., Koyama, K., Chen, G., Wang, M.-Y., Trieu, F., Lee, Y., Newgard, C. B., and Unger, R. H., Direct antidiabetic effect of leptin through triglyceride depletion of tissues, *Proc. Natl. Acad. Sci. U.S.A.*, 94, 4637, 1997.

243. Lee, Y., Hirose, H., Zhou, Y.-T., Esser, V., McGarry, J. D., and Unger, R. H., Increased lipogenic capacity of the islets of obese rats, *Diabetes*, 46, 408, 1997.

244. Ohneda, M., Inman, L. R., and Unger, R. H., Caloric restriction in obese prediabetic rats prevents β-cell depletion, *Diabetologia*, 38, 173, 1995.

245. Shimabukuro, M., Koyama, K., Lee, Y., and Unger, R. H., Leptin- or troglitazone-induced lipopenia protects islets from interleukin 1β cytotoxicity, *J. Clin. Invest.*, 100, 1750, 1997.

246. Koletsky, S., Obese spontaneously hypertensive rats — a model for study of atherosclerosis, *Exp. Mol. Pathol.*, 19, 53, 1973.

247. Takaya, K., Ogawa, Y., Hiraoka, J., Hosoda, K., Yamori, Y., Nakao, K., and Koletsky, R. J., Nonsense mutation of leptin receptor in the obese spontaneously hypertensive Koletsky rat, *Nature Genet.*, 14, 130, 1996.

248. Michaelis, O. E., Ellwood, K. C., Hallfrisch, J., and Hansen, C. T., Effect of dietary sucrose and genotype on metabolic parameters of a new strain of genetically obese rat: LA/N corpulent, *Nutr. Res.*, 3, 217, 1983.

249. Russell, J. C., Bar-Tana, J., Shillabeer, G., Lau, D. C. W., Richardson, M., Wenzel, L. M., Graham, S. E., and Dolphin, P. J., Development of insulin resistance in the JCR:LA-cp rat: role of triacylglycerols and effects of MEDICA 16, *Diabetes*, 47, 770, 1998.

250. Russell, J. C., Graham, S., and Hameed, M., Abnormal insulin and glucose metabolism in the JCR:LA-corpulent rat, *Metabolism*, 43, 538, 1994.

251. Pederson, R. A., Campos, R. V., Buchan, A. M. J., Chisholm, C. B., Russell, J. C., and Brown, J. C., Comparison of the enteroinsular axis in two strains of obese rats: the fatty Zucker and the JCR:LA-corpulent, *Int. J. Obesity*, 15, 461, 1991.

252. Chan, C. B., MacPhail, R. M., Kibenge, M. T., and Russell, J. C., Increased glucose phosphorylating activity correlates with insulin secreting capacity of male JCR:LA-corpulent rat islets, *Can. J. Physiol. Pharmacol.*, 73, 501, 1995.

253. Ahuja, S., Manickavel, V., Amy, R. M., and Russell, J. C., Age-related qualitative and quantitative changes in the endocrine pancreas of the LA/N-corpulent rat, *Diabetes Res.*, 6, 137, 1987.

254. Wu-Peng, X. S., Chua, S. C., Okada, N., Liu, S.-M., Nicolson, M., Leibel, R. L., Phenotype of the obese Koletsky (*f*) rat due to Tyr763Stop mutation in the extracellular domain of the leptin receptor (Lepr), *Diabetes*, 46, 513, 1997.

255. Hiraoka, J., Hosoda, K., Ogawa, Y., Ikeda, K., Nara, Y., Masuzaki, H., Takaya, K., Nakagawa, K., Mashimo, T., Sawamura, M., Kolejsky, R. J., Yamori, Y., and Nakao, K., Augmentation of obese (*ob*) gene expression and leptin secretion in obese spontaneously hypertensive rats (obese SHR or Koletsky rats), *Biochem. Biophys. Res. Commun.*, 231, 582, 1997.

256. Russell, J. C., Graham, S. E., Dolphin, P. J., and Brindley, D. N., Effects of benfluorex on serum triacylglycerols and insulin sensitivity in the corpulent rat, *Can. J. Physiol. Pharmacol.*, 74, 879, 1996.

257. Vance, J. E. and Russell, J. C., Hypersecretion of VLDL, but not HDL, by hepatocytes from the JCR:LA-corpulent rat, *J. Lipid Res.*, 31, 1491, 1990.

258. O'Brien, S. F. and Russell, J. C., Insulin resistance and vascular wall function: lessons from animal models, *Endocrinol. Metab.*, 4 155, 1997.

259. Richardson, M., Schmidt, A. M., Graham, S. E., DeReske, M., Achen, B., and Russell, J. C., Vasculopathy in the insulin resistant JCR:LA-cp rat, *Atherosclerosis*, 138, 135, 1998.

260. Bielschowsky, M. and Bielschowsky, F., A new strain of mice with hereditary obesity, *Proc. Univ. Otago Med. Sch.*, 31, 29, 1953.

261. Bielschowsky, M. and Bielschowsky, F., The New Zealand strain of obese mice. Their response to stilboestrol and to insulin, *Aust. J. Exp. Biol. Med. Sci.*, 34, 181, 1956.

262. Harrison, L. C. and Itin, A., A possible mechanism for insulin resistance and hyperglycemia in NZO mice, *Nature*, 279, 334, 1979.

263. Veroni, M. C. and Larkins, R. G., Evolution of insulin resistance in isolated soleus muscle of the NZO mouse, *Horm. Metab. Res.*, 18, 299, 1986.

264. Melez, K. A., Harrison, L. C., Gilliam, J. N., and Steinberg, A. D., Diabetes is associated with autoimmunity in the New Zealand obese (NZO) mouse, *Diabetes*, 29, 835, 1980.

265. Melez, K. A., Attallah, A. M., Harrison, E. T., and Raveche, E. S., Immune abnormalities in the diabetic New Zealand obese (NZO) mouse: insulin treatment partially suppresses splenic hyperactivity measured by flow cytometric analysis, *Clin. Immunol. Immunopathol.*, 36, 110, 1985.

266. Upton, J. D., Sneyd, J. G., and Livesey, J., Blood glucose, plasma insulin and plasma glucagon in NZO mice, *Horm. Metab. Res.*, 12, 173, 1980.

267. Cameron, D. P., Opat, F., and Insch, S., Studies of immunoreactive insulin secretion in NZO mice *in vivo*, *Diabetologia*, 10, 649, 1974.

268. Sneyd, J. G. T., Pancreatic and serum insulin in the New Zealand strain of obese mice, *J. Endocrinol.*, 28, 163, 1964.

269. Igel, M., Becker, W., Herberg, L., and Joost, H. G., Hyperleptinemia, leptin resistance, and polymorphic leptin receptor in the New Zealand obese mouse, *Endocrinology*, 138, 4234, 1997.

270. Macaulay, S. L. and Larkins, R. G., Impaired insulin action in adipocytes of New Zealand obese mice: a role for postbinding defects in pyruvate dehydrogenase and insulin mediator activity, *Metabolism*, 37, 958, 1988.

271. Ferreras, L., Kelada, A. S., McCoy, M., and Proietto, J., Early decrease in GLUT4 protein levels in brown adipose tissue of New Zealand obese mice, *Int. J. Obesity Rel. Metab. Dis.*, 18, 760, 1994.

272. Veroni, M. C., Proietto, J., and Larkins, R. G., Evolution of insulin resistance in New Zealand obese mice, *Diabetes*, 40, 1480, 1991.

273. Larkins, R. G., Simeonova, L., and Veroni, M. C., Glucose utilization in relation to insulin secretion in NZO and C57Bl mouse islets, *Endocrinology*, 107, 1634, 1980.

274. De Luise, M. and Harker, M., Skeletal muscle metabolism: effect of age, obesity, thyroid and nutritional status, *Horm. Metab. Res.*, 21, 410, 1989.

275. Andrikopoulos, S., Rosella, G., Gaskin, E., Thorburn, A., Kaczmarczyk, S., Zajac, J. D., and Proietto, J., Impaired regulation of hepatic fructose-1,6-bisphosphatase in the New Zealand obese mouse model of NIDDM, *Diabetes*, 42, 1731, 1993.

276. Andrikopoulos, S. and Proietto, J., The biochemical basis of increased hepatic glucose production in a mouse model of type 2 (noninsulin-dependent) diabetes mellitus, *Diabetologia*, 38, 1389, 1995.

277. Andrikopoulos, S., Rosella, G., Kaczmarczyk, S. J., Zajac, J. D., and Proietto, J., Impaired regulation of hepatic fructose-1,6-biphosphatase in the New Zealand obese mouse: an acquired defect, *Metabolism*, 45, 622, 1996.

278. Thorburn, A., Andrikopoulos, S., and Proietto, J., Defects in liver and muscle glycogen metabolism in neonatal and adult New Zealand obese mice, *Metabolism*, 44, 1298, 1995.

279. Ikeda, H., KK mouse, *Diabetes Res. Clin. Pract.*, 24, Suppl., S313, 1994.

280. Hayase, M., Ogawa, Y., Katsuura, G., Shintaku, H., Hosoda, K., and Nakao, K., Regulation of obese gene expression in KK mice and congenic lethal yellow obese KKA^y mice, *Am. J. Physiol.*, 271, E333, 1996.

281. Kreymann, B., Ghatei, M. A., Burnet, P., Williams, G., Kanse, S., Diani, A. R., and Bloom, S. R., Characterization of glucagon-like peptide-1-(7-36)amide in the hypothalamus, *Brain Res.*, 502, 325, 1989.

282. Taketomi, S., Fujita, T., and Yokono, K., Insulin receptor and postbinding defects in KK mouse adipocytes and improvement by ciglitazone, *Diabetes Res. Clin. Pract.*, 5, 125, 1988.

283. Makino, H., Kanatsuka, A., Suzuki, T., Kuribayashi, S., Hashimoto, N., Yoshida, S., and Nishimura, M., Insulin resistance of fat cells from spontaneously diabetic KK mice. Analysis of insulin-sensitive phosphodiesterase, *Diabetes*, 34, 844, 1985.

284. Shibata, M. and Yasuda, B., New experimental congenital diabetic mice (N.S.Y. mice), *Tohoku J. Exp. Med.*, 130, 139, 1980.

285. Ueda, H., Ikegami, H., Yamato, E., Fu, J., Fukuda, M., Shen, G., Kawaguchi, Y., Takekawa, K., Fujioka, Y., and Fujisawa, T., The NSY mouse: a new animal model of spontaneous NIDDM with moderate obesity, *Diabetologia*, 38, 503, 1995.

286. Shimizu, K., Morita, H., Niwa, T., Maeda, K., Shibata, M., Higuchi, K., and Takeda, T., Spontaneous amyloidosis in senile NSY mice, *Acta Pathol. Japon.*, 43, 215, 1993.

287. Walkley, S. U., Hunt, C. E., Clements, R. S., and Lindsey, J. R., Description of obesity in the PBB/Ld mouse, *J. Lipid Res.*, 19, 335, 1978.

288. Kawano, K., Hirashima, T., Mori, S., Saitoh, Y., Kurosumi., M., and Natori, T., Spontaneous long-term hyperglycemic rat with diabetic complications. Otsuka Long-Evans Tokushima Fatty (OLETF) strain, *Diabetes*, 41, 1422, 1992.

289. Kawano, K., Hirashima, T., Mori, S., and Natori, T., Spontaneously diabetic rat "OLETF" as a model for NIDDM in humans, in *Lessons from Animal Diabetes VI*, Shafrir, E., Ed., Birkhäuser, Boston, 1996, 225.

290. Otsuki, M., Akiyama, T., Shirohara, H., Nakano, S., Furumi, K., and Tachibana, I., Loss of sensitivity to cholecystokinin stimulation of isolated pancreatic acini from genetically diabetic rats, *Am. J. Physiol.*, 268, E531, 1995.

291. Aizawa, T., Taguchi, N., Sato, Y., Nakabayashi, T., Kobuchi, H., Hidaka, H., Nagasawa, T., Ishihara, F., Itoh, N., and Hashizume, K., Prophylaxis of genetically determined diabetes by diazoxide: a study in a rat model of naturally occurring obese diabetes, *J. Pharmacol. Exp. Ther.*, 275, 194, 1995.

292. Hirashima, T., Kawano, K., Mori, S., Matsumoto, K., and Natori, T., A diabetogenic gene (ODB-1) assigned to the X-chromosome in OLETF rats, *Diabetes Res. Clin. Pract.*, 27, 91, 1995.

293. Hirashima, T., Kawano, K., Mori, S., and Natori, T., A diabetogenic gene, ODB2, identified on chromosome 14 of the OLETF rat and its synergistic action with ODB1, *Biochem. Biophys. Res. Commun.*, 224, 420, 1996.

294. Funakoshi, A., Miyasaka, K., Shinozaki, H., Masuda, M., Kawanami, T., Takata, Y., and Kono, A., An animal model of congenital defect of gene expression of cholecystokinin (CCK)-A receptor, *Biochem. Biophys. Res. Commun.*, 210, 787, 1995.

295. Funakoshi, A., Miyasaka, K., Kanai, S., Masuda, M., Yasunami, Y., Nagai, T., Ikeda, S., Jimi, A., Kawanami, T., and Kono, A., Pancreatic endocrine dysfunction in rats not expressing the cholecystokinin-A receptor, *Pancreas*, 12, 230, 1996.

296. Miyasaka, K., Kanai, S., Ohta, M., Kawanami, T., Kono, A., and Funakoshi, A., Lack of satiety effect of cholecystokinin (CCK) in a new rat model not expressing the CCK-A receptor gene, *Neurosci. Lett.*, 180, 143, 1994.

297. Ishida, K., Mizuno, A., Min, Z., Sano, T., and Shima, K., Which is the primary etiologic event in Otsuka Long-Evans Tokushima Fatty rats, a model of spontaneous noninsulin-dependent diabetes mellitus, insulin resistance, or impaired insulin secretion? *Metabolism*, 44, 940, 1995.

298. Ishida, K., Mizuno, A., Sano, T., Noma, Y., and Shima K., Effect of timely insulin administration on pancreatic B-cells of Otsuka-Long-Evans-Tokushima-Fatty (OLETF) strain rats. An animal model of noninsulin-dependent diabetes mellitus (NIDDM), *Horm. Metab. Res.*, 27, 398, 1995.

299. Man, Z.-W., Zhu, M., Noma, K., Toide, K., Sato, T., Asahi, Y., Hirashima, T., Mori, S., Kawano, K., Mizuno, A., Sano, Y., and Shima, K., Impaired β-cell function and deposition of fat droplets in the pancreas as a consequence of hypertriglyceridemia in OLETF rat, a model of spontaneous NIDDM, *Diabetes*, 46, 1718, 1997.

300. Inoue, H., Iannotti, C. A., Welling, C. M., Veile, R., Donis-Keller, H., and Permutt, M. A., Human cholecystokinin type A receptor gene: cytogenetic localization, physical mapping, and identification of two missense variants in patients with obesity and noninsulin-dependent diabetes mellitus (NIDDM), *Genomics*, 42, 331, 1997.

301. Goto, Y., Suzuki, K., Sasaki, M., Ono, T., and Abe, S., GK rat as a model of nonobese, noninsulin-dependent diabetes. selective breeding over 35 generations, in *Frontiers in Diabetes Research. Lessons from Animal Diabetes II*, Shafrir, E., and Renold, A. E., Eds., John Libby and Co., London, 1988, 301-303.

302. Galli, J., Li, L. S., Glaser, A., Ostenson, C. G., Jiao, H., Fakhrai-Rad, H., Jacob, H. J., Lander, E. S., and Luthman, H., Genetic analysis of noninsulin-dependent diabetes mellitus in the GK rat, *Nature Genet.*, 12, 31, 1996.

303. Gauguier, D., Froguel, P., Parent, V., Bernard, C., Bihoreau, M. T., Portha, B., James, M. R., Penicaud, L., Lathrop, M., and Ktorza, A., Chromosomal mapping of genetic loci associated with noninsulin-dependent diabetes in the GK rat, *Nature Genet.*, 12, 38, 1996.

304. Permutt, M. A. and Ghosh, S., Rat model contributes new loci for NIDDM susceptibility in man, *Nature Genet.*, 12, 4, 1996.

305. Giroix, M. H., Vesco, L., and Portha, B., Functional and metabolic perturbations in isolated pancreatic islets from the GK rat, a genetic model of noninsulin-dependent diabetes, *Endocrinology*, 132, 815, 1993.

306. Ostenson, C. G., Khan, A., Abdel-Halim, S. M., Guenifi, A., Suzuki, K., Goto, Y., and Efendic, S., Abnormal insulin secretion and glucose metabolism in pancreatic islets from the spontaneously diabetic GK rat, *Diabetologia*, 36, 1, 1993.

307. Guenifi, A., Abdel-Halim, S. M., Höög, A., Falkmer, S., and Ostenson, C. G., Preserved beta-cell density in the endocrine pancreas of young, spontaneously diabetic Goto-Kakizaki (GK) rats, *Pancreas*, 10, 148, 1995.

308. Portha, B., Serradas, P., Bailbe, D., Suzuki, K., Goto, Y., and Giroix, M. H., β-cell insensitivity to glucose in the GK rat, a spontaneous nonobese model for Type II diabetes, *Diabetes*, 40, 486, 1991.

309. Abdel-Halim, S. M., Guenifi, A., Efendic, S., and Ostenson, C. G., Both somatostatin and insulin responses to glucose are impaired in the perfused pancreas of the spontaneously noninsulin-dependent diabetic GK (Goto-Kakizaki) rats, *Acta Physiol. Scand.*, 148, 219, 1993.

310. Abdel-Halim, S. M., Guenifi, A., Khan, A., Larsson, O., Berggren, P. O., Ostenson, C. G., and Efendic, S., Impaired coupling of glucose signal to the exocytotic machinery in diabetic GK rats: a defect ameliorated by cAMP, *Diabetes*, 45, 934, 1996.

311. Movasset, J., Saulnier, C., Serradas, P., and Portha, B., Impaired development of pancreatic beta-cell mass is a primary event during the progression to diabetes in the GK rat, *Diabetologia*, 40, 916, 1997.

312. Ostenson, C.-G., Abdel-Halim, S. M., Andersson, A., and Efendic, S., Studies on the pathogenesis of NIDDM in the GK (Goto-Kakizaki) rat, in *Lessons from Animal Diabetes VI*, Shafrir, E., Ed., Birkhäuser, Boston, 1996, 299-315.

313. Tsuura, Y., Ishida, H., Okamoto, Y., Kato, S., Sakamoto, K., Horie, M., Ikeda, H., Okada, Y., and Seino, Y., Glucose sensitivity of ATP-sensitive K⁺ channels is impaired in β-cells of the GK rat, a new genetic model of NIDDM, *Diabetes*, 42, 1446, 1993.

314. Tsuura, Y., Ishida, H., Okamoto, Y., Kato, S., Horie, M., Ikeda, H., and Seino, Y., Reduced sensitivity of dihydroxyacetone on ATP-sensitive K⁺ channels of pancreatic beta cells in GK rats, *Diabetologia*, 37, 1082, 1994.

315. Hughes, S. J., Faehling, M., Thorneley, C. W., Proks, P., Ashcroft, F. M., and Smith, P. A., Electrophysiological and metabolic characterization of single β-cells and islets from diabetic GK rats, *Diabetes*, 47, 73, 1998.

316. Hani, E. H., Clément, K., Velho, G., Vionnet, N., Hager, J., Philippi, A., Dina, C., Inoue, H., Permutt, M. A., Basdevant, A., North, M., Demenais, F., Guy-Grand, B., and Froguel, P., Genetic studies of the sulfonylurea receptor gene locus in NIDDM and in morbid obesity among French Caucasians, *Diabetes*, 46, 688, 1997.

317. Inoue, H., Ferrer, J., Welling, C. M., Elbein, S. C., Hoffman, M., Mayorga, R., Warren-Perry, M., Zhang, Y., Millns, H., Turner, R., Province, M., Bryan, J., Permutt, M. A., and Aguilar-Bryan, L., Sequence variants in the sulfonylurea receptor (SUR) gene are associated with NIDDM in Caucasians, *Diabetes*, 45, 825, 1996.

318. Inoue, H., Ferrer, J., Warren-Perry, M., Zhang, Y., Millns, H., Turner, R. C., Elbein, S. C., Hempe, C. L., Suarez, B. K., Inagaki, N., Seino, S., and Permutt, M. A., Sequence variants in the pancreatic islet β-cell inwardly rectifying K⁺ channel Kir6.2 (Bir) gene, *Diabetes*, 46, 825, 1997.

319. Hansen, L., Echwald, S. M., Hansen, T., Urhammer, S. A., Clausen, J. O., and Pederson, O., Amino acid polymorphisms in the ATP-regulatable inward rectifier Kir6.2 and their relationships to glucose- and tolbutamide-induced insulin secretion, the insulin sensitivity index, and NIDDM, *Diabetes*, 46, 508, 1997.

320. MacDonald, M. J., Efendic, S., and Ostenson, C. G., Normalization by insulin treatment of low mitochondrial glycerol phosphate dehydrogenase and pyruvate carboxylase in pancreatic islets of the GK rat, *Diabetes*, 45, 886, 1996.

321. Koike, G., Van Vooren, P., Shiozawa, M., Galli, J., Li, L. S., Glaser, A., Balasubramanyam, A., Brown, L. J., Luthman, H., Szpirer, C., MacDonald, M. J., and Jacob, H. J., Genetic mapping and chromosome localization of the rat mitochondrial glycerol-3-phosphate dehydrogenase gene, a candidate for noninsulin-dependent diabetes mellitus, *Genomics*, 38, 96, 1996.

322. Matsuoka, T., Kajimoto, Y., Watada, H., Umayahara, Y., Kubota, M., Kawamori, R., Yamasaki, Y., and Kamada, T., Expression of CD38 gene, but not of mitochondrial glycerol-3-phosphate dehydrogenase gene, is impaired in pancreatic islets of GK rats, *Biochem. Biophys. Res. Commun.*, 214, 239, 1995.

323. Warren-Perry, M. G., Stoffel, M., Saker, P. J., Zhang, Y., Brown, L. J., MacDonald, M. J., and Turner, R. C., Mitochondrial FAD-glycerophosphate dehydrogenase and G-protein-coupled inwardly rectifying K⁺ channel. No evidence for linkage in maturity-onset diabetes of the young or NIDDM, *Diabetes*, 45, 639, 1996.

324. Serradas, P., Giroix, M. H., Saulnier, C., Gangnerau, M. N., Borg, L. A., Welsh, M., Portha, B., and Welsh, N., Mitochondrial deoxyribonucleic acid content is specifically decreased in adult, but not fetal, pancreatic islets of the Goto-Kakizaki rat, a genetic model of noninsulin-dependent diabetes, *Endocrinology*, 136, 5623, 1995.

325. Matsuoka, T., Kajimoto, Y., Watada, H., Umayahara, Y., Kubota, M., Kawamori, R., Yamasaki, Y., and Kamada, T., Expression of CD38 gene, but not of mitochondrial glycerol-3-phosphate dehydrogenase gene, is impaired in pancreatic islets of GK rats, *Biochem. Biophys. Res. Commun.*, 214, 239, 1995.

326. Varadi, A., Molnar, E., Ostenson, C. G., and Ashcroft, S. J., Isoforms of endoplasmic reticulum Ca²⁺-ATPase are differentially expressed in normal and diabetic islets of Langerhans, *Biochem. J.*, 319, 521, 1996.

327. Leckström, A., Ostenson, C. G., Efendic, S., Arnelo, U., Permert, J., Lundquist, I., and Westermark, P., Increased storage and secretion of islet amyloid polypeptide relative to insulin in the spontaneously diabetic GK rat, *Pancreas*, 13, 259, 1996.

328. Höög, A., Sandberg-Nordqvist, A. C., Abdel-Halim, S. M., Carlsson-Skwirut, C., Guenifi, A., Tally, M., Ostenson, C. G., Falkmer, S., Sara, V. R., Efendic, S., Schalling, M., and Grimelius, L., Increased amounts of a high molecular weight insulin-like growth factor II (IGF-II) peptide and IGF-II messenger ribonucleic acid in pancreatic islets of diabetic Goto-Kakizaki rats, *Endocrinology*, 137, 2415, 1996.
329. Bisbis, S., Bailbe, D., Tormo, M. A., Picarel-Blanchot, F., Derouet, M., Simon, J., and Portha, B., Insulin resistance in the GK rat: decreased receptor number but normal kinase activity in liver, *Am. J. Physiol.*, 265, E807, 1993.
330. Farese, R. V., Standaert, M. L., Yamada, K., Huang, L. C., Zhang, C., Cooper, D. R., Wang, Z., Yang, Y., Suzuki, S., Toyota, T., and Larner, J., Insulin-induced activation of glycerol-3-phosphate acyltransferase by a chiro-inositol-containing insulin mediator is defective in adipocytes of insulin-resistant, Type II diabetic, Goto-Kakizaki rats,*Proc. Natl. Acad. Sci. U.S.A.*, 91, 11040, 1994.
331. Meier, H., and Yerganian, G. A., Spontaneous hereditary diabetes mellitus in Chinese hamster (*Cricetulus griseus*). 1, Pathological findings, *Proc. Soc. Exp. Biol. Med.*, 100, 810, 1959.
332. Frankel, B. J., Diabetes in the Chinese hamster, in *Lessons from Animal Diabetes VI*, Shafrir, E., Ed., Birkhäuser, Boston, 1996, 267-298.
333. Voss, K. M., Herberg. L., and Kern, H. F., Fine structural studies of the islets of langerhans in the Djungarian hamster (*Phodopus sungorus*), *Cell Tissue Res.*, 191, 333, 1978.
334. Boss-Williams, K. A. and Bartness, T. J., NPY stimulation of food intake in Siberian hamsters is not photoperiod dependent, *Physiol. Behav.*, 59, 157, 1996.
335. Mercer, J. G., Lawrence, C. B., Beck, B., Burlet, A., Atkinson, T., and Barrett, P., Hypothalamic NPY and prepro-NPY mRNA in Djungarian hamsters: effects of food deprivation and photoperiod, *Am. J. Physiol.*, 269, R1099, 1995.
336. Schmidt-Nielsen, K. and Haines, K. K. B., Diabetes mellitus in the sand rat induced by standard laboratory diets, *Science*, 143, 689, 1964.
337. Barnett, M., Habito, R., Cameron-Smith, D., Yamamoto, A., and Collier, G. R., The effect of inhibiting fatty acid oxidation on basal glucose metabolism in *Psammomys obesus*, *Horm. Metab. Res.*, 28, 165, 1996.
338. Kalderon, B. A., Gutman, A., Levy, E., Shafrir, E., and Adler, J. H., Characterization of stages in development of obesity-diabetes syndrome in *Psammomys obesus*, *Diabetes*, 6, 717, 1986.
339. Bendayan, M., Malide, D., Ziv, E., Levy, E., Ben-Sasson, R., Kalman, R., Bar-On, H., Chrétien, M., and Seidah, N., Immunocytochemical investigation of insulin secretion by pancreaticβ-cells in control and diabetic *Psammomys obesus*, *J. Histochem. Cytochem.*, 43, 771, 1995.
340. Gadot, M., Ariav, Y., Cerasi, E., Kaiser, N., and Gross, D. J., Hyperproinsulinemia in the diabetic *Psammomys obesus* is a result of increased secretory demand on the β-cell, *Endocrinology*, 136, 4218, 1995.
341. Gadot, M., Leibowitz, G., Shafrir, E., Cerasi, E., Gross, D. J., and Kaiser, N., Hyperproinsuline-mia and insulin deficiency in the diabetic *Psammomys obesus*, *Endocrinol.*, 135, 610, 1994.
342. Cerasi, E., Kaiser, N., and Gross, D. J., Is noninsulin-dependent diabetes mellitus a disease of the β-cell? *Diabetes Metab.*, 23, 47, 1997.
343. Kanety, H., Moshe, S., Shafrir, E., Lunenfeld, B., and Karasik, A., Hyperinsulinemia induces a reversible impairment in insulin receptor function leading to diabetes in the sand rat model of noninsulin-dependent diabetes mellitus, *Proc. Natl. Acad. Sci. U.S.A.*, 91, 1853, 1994.
344. Shafrir, E., Development and consequences of insulin resistance: lessons from animals with hyperinsulinemia, *Diabetes Metab.*, 22, 122, 1996.
345. Agulnik, S. I. and Silver, L. M., The Cairo spiny mouse*Acomys cahirinus* shows a strong affinity to the Mongolian gerbil *Meriones unguiculatus*, *Mol. Biol. Evol.*, 13, 3, 1996.
346. Chevret, P., Denys, C., Jaeger, J. J., Michaux, J., and Catzeflis, F. M., Molecular evidence that the spiny mouse (*Acomys*) is more closely related to gerbils (Gerbillinae) than to true mice (Murinae), *Proc. Natl. Acad. Sci. U.S.A.*, 90, 3433, 1993.
347. Shafrir, E. and Adler, J. H., Enzymatic and metabolic responses to affluent diet of two diabetes-prone species of spiny mice: *Acomys cahirinus* and *Acomys russatus*, *Int. J. Biochem.*, 15, 1439, 1983.

348. Butter, R., Keilacker, H., Heinke, P., Kloting, I., and Hahn, H. J., Delayed or biphasic glucose-induced insulin secretion of pancreatic islets isolated from spiny mice (*Acomys cahirinus*): relation to age of animals, *Diabetes Metab.*, 6, 47, 1980.

349. Nesher, R., Abramovitch, E., and Cerasi, E., Reduced early and late phase insulin response to glucose in isolated spiny mouse (*Acomys cahirinus*) islets: a defective link between glycolysis and adenylate cyclase, *Diabetologia*, 32, 644, 1989.

350. Grill, V. and Cerasi, E., The metabolism of cyclic AMP and glucose in isolated islets from *Acomys cahirinus*, *Diabetologia*, 16, 47, 1979.

351. Malaisse-Lagae, F., Ravazzola, M., Amherdt, M., Gutzeit, A., Stauffacher, W., Malaisse, W. J., and Orci, L., An apparent abnormaltiy of the B-cell microtubular system in spiny mice (*Acomys cahirinus*), *Diabetologia*, 11, 71, 1975.

352. Cerasi, E. and Jeanrenaud, B., Glucose production by the perfused liver of the spiny mouse (*Acomys cahirinus*): sensitivity to glucagon and insulin, *Isr. J. Med. Sci.*, 15, 134, 1979.

353. Wise, P. H., Weir, B. J., Hime, J. M., and Forrest, E., Implications of hyperglycemia and cataract in a colony of tuco-tucos (*Ctenomys talarum*), *Nature*, 219, 1374, 1968.

354. Weir, B.J., The development of diabetes in the tuco-tuco (*Ctenomys talarum*), *Proc. R. Soc. Med.*, 67, 843, 1974.

355. Weir, B., Wise, P. H., Hime, J. M., and Forrest, E., Hyperglycemia and cataract in the tuco-tuco, *J. Endocrinol.*, 43, 7, 1969.

356. Wise, P.H., Weir, B. J., Hime, J. M., and Forrest, E., The diabetic syndrome in the tuco-tuco (*Ctenomys talarum*), *Diabetologia*, 8, 165, 1972.

357. Paterson, A. H., Lander, E. S., Peterson, S., Lincoln, S. E., and Tanksley, S. D., Resolution of quantitative traits into Mendelian factors by using a complete linkage map of restriction fragment length polymorphisms, *Nature*, 335, 721, 1988.

358. Lander, E. S. and Botstein, D., Mapping Mendelian factors underlying quantitative traits using RFLP linkage maps, *Genetics*, 121, 185, 1989.

359. Fisler, J. S., and Warden, C. H. Mapping of mouse genes: a generic approach to a complex trait, *J. Nutr.* 127, 1909S, 1997.

360. Bray, G. and Bouchard, C., Genetics of obesity: research directions, *FASEB J.*, 11, 937, 1997.

361. West, D. B., Genetics of obesity in human and animal models, *Endocrinol. Metab. Clin. North Am.*, 25, 801, 1996.

362. Warden, C. H., Fisler, J. S., Shoemaker, S. M., Wen, P.-Z., Svenson, K. L., Pace, M. J., and Lusis, A. J., Identification of four chromosomal loci determining obesity in a multifactorial mouse model, *J. Clin. Invest.*, 95, 1545, 1995.

363. West, S. B., Gouday-Lefevre, J., York, B., and Truett, G. E., Dietary obesity linked to genetic loci on chromosomes 9 and 15 in a polygenic mouse model, *J. Clin. Invest.*, 94, 1410, 1994.

364. Steiner, D. F., Tager, H. S., Chan, S. J., Nanjo, K., Sanke, T., and Rubenstein, A. H., Lessons learned from molecular biology of insulin-gene mutations, *Diabetes Care*, 13, 600, 1990.

365. Acilli, D., Insulin receptor knock-out mice, *Trends Endocrinol. Metab.*, 8, 101, 1997.

366. Patti, M.-E. and Kahn, C. R. Lessons from transgenic and knockout animals about noninsulin-dependent diabetes mellitus, *Trends Endocrinol. Metab.*, 7, 311, 1996.

367. Strack, V., Bossenmeier, B., Stoyanov, B., Mushack, J., and Häring, H. U., A 973 valine to methionine mutation of the human receptor: interaction with insulin-receptor substrate-1 and Shc in HEK 293 cells, *Diabetologia*, 40, 1135, 1997.

368. Kadowaki, H., Takahashi, Y., Ando, A., Momomura, K., Kaburagi, Y., Quin, J. D., MacCuish, A. C., Koda, N., Fukushima, Y., Taylor, S. I., Akanuma, Y., Yazaki, Y., and Kadowaki, T., Four mutant alleles of the insulin receptor gene associated with genetic syndromes of extreme insulin resistance, *Biochem. Biophys. Res. Commun.*, 237, 516, 1997.

369. Joshi, R. L., Lamothe, B., Bucchini, D., and Jami, J., Genetically engineered mice as animal models for NIDDM, *FEBS Lett.*, 401, 99, 1997.

370. Araki, E., Lipes, M. A., Patti, M. E., Brüning, J. C., Haag, B., III, Johnson, R. S., and Kahn, C. R., Alternative pathway of insulin signaling in mice with targeted disruption of the IRS-1 gene, *Nature*, 372, 186, 1994.

371. Brüning, J. C., Winnay, J., Bonner-Weir, S., Taylor, S. I., Accili, D., and Kahn, C R., Development of a novel polygenic model of NIDDM in mice heterozygous for IR and IRS-1 null alleles, *Cell*, 88, 561, 1997.

372. Mueckler, M. M., Glucose transport and glucose homeostasis: new insights from transgenic mice, *News Physiol. Sci.*, 10, 22, 1995.

373. Katz, E. B., Burcelin, R., Tsao, T.-S., Stenbit, A. E., and Charron, M. J., The metabolic consequences of altered glucose transporter expression in transgenic mice, *J. Mol. Med.*, 74, 639, 1996.

374. Stenbit, A. E., Tsao, T.-U., Li, J., Burcelin, R., Geenen, D. L., Factor, S. M., Houseknecht, K., Katz, E. B., and Charon, M. J., *GLUT4* heterozygous knockout mice develop muscle insulin resistance and diabetes, *Nature Med.*, 3, 1096, 1997.

375. Hotamisligil, G. and Spiegelman, B. M., Tumor necrosis factor α: A key component of the obesity-diabetes link, *Diabetes*, 43, 1271, 1994.

376. Hotamisligil, G. S., Shargill, N. S., and Spiegelman, B. M., Adipose expression of tumor necrosis factor-α: Direct role in obesity-linked insulin resistance, *Science*, 259, 87, 1994.

377. Peraldi, P. and Spiegelman, B. M., Studies of the mechanism of inhibition of insulin signaling by tumor necrosis-α, *J. Endocrinol.*, 155, 219, 1997.

378. Hotamisligil, G. S., Peraldi, P., Budavari, A., Ellis, White, M. F., and Spiegelman, B. M., IRS-1-mediated inhibition of insulin receptor tyrosine kinase activity in TNF-α- and obesity-induced insulin resistance, *Science*, 271, 665, 1996.

379. Uysal, K. T., Wiesbrock, S. M., Marino, M. W., and Hotamisligill, G. S., Protection from obesity-induced insulin resistance in mice lacking TNF-α function, *Nature*, 389, 610, 1997.

380. Prochazka, M., Lillioja, S., Tait, J. F., Knowler, W. C., Mott, D. M., Spraul, M., Bennett, P. H., and Bogardus, C., Linkage of chromosomal markers on 4q with a putative gene determining maximal insulin action in Pima Indians, *Diabetes*, 42, 514, 1993.

381. Hotamisligil, G., Johnson, R. S., Distel, R. J., Ellis, R., Papaioannou, V. E., and Spiegelman, B. M., Uncoupling of obesity from insulin resistance through a targeted mutation in *aP2*, the adipocyte fatty acid binding protein, *Science*, 274, 1377, 1996.

382. Reynet, C. and Kahn, C. R., Rad: a member of the *ras* family overexpressed in muscle of Type II diabetic humans, *Science*, 262, 1441, 1993.

383. Kahn, C. R., Insulin action, diabetogenes, and the cause of Type II diabetes, *Diabetes*, 43, 1066, 1994.

384. Moyers, J. S., Reynet, C., Zhu, J., Bilan, P. J., and Kahn, C. R., A role for rad as an inhibitor of insulin-stimulate glucose transport, Diabetes, 44 (Suppl. 1), 302, 1995.

385. Orho, M., Carlsson, M., Kanninen, T., and Groop, L., Polymorphism at the rad locus is not associated with NIDDM in Finns, *Diabetes*, 45, 429, 1996.

386. Newgard, C. B., Ferber, S., Quaade C., Johnson, J. H., and Hughes, S. D., Molecular engineering of glucose-regulated insulin secretion, in *Molecular Biology of Diabetes*, Part 1. Draznin, B., and LeRoith, D., Eds., Humana Press, Totowa, NJ., 1994, 119-154.

387. Tal, M., Wu, Y.-J., Lweiser, M., Surana, M., Lodish, H., Fleischer, N., Weir, G., and Efrat, S., [Val12]Hras down regulates GLUT2 in beta cells of transgenic mice without affecting glucose homeostasis, *Proc. Natl. Acad. Sci. U.S.A.*, 89, 5744, 1992.

388. Efrat, S., Tal, M., and Lodish, H. F., The pancreatic β-cell sensor, *Trends Biochem. Sci.*, 19, 535, 1995.

389. Mueckler, M., Kruse, M., Strube, M., Riggs, A.C., Chiu, K. C., and Permutt, M. A., A mutation in the Glut2 glucose transporter gene of a diabetic patient abolishes transport activity, *J. Biol. Chem.*, 269, 765, 1994.

390. De Vos, A., Heimberg, H., Quartier, E., Huypens, P., Bouwens, L., Pipileers, D., and Schuit, F., Human and rat beta cells differ in glucose transporter but not in glucokinase gene expression, *J. Clin. Invest.*, 96, 2489, 1995.

391. Sweet, I. R. and Matschinsky, F. M. Are there kinetic advantages of GLUT2 in pancreatic glucose sensing? *Diabetologia*, 30, 112, 1997.

392. Yki-Järvinen, H., MODY genes and mutations in hepatocyte nuclear factors, *Lancet*, 349, 516, 1997.

393. Velho, G., Blanche, H., Vaxillaire, M., Bellanné-Chantelot, C., Pardini, V. C., Timsit, J., Passa, P. H., Deschamps, I., Robert, J.-J., Weber, I. T., Marotta, D., Pilkis, S. J., Lipkind, G. M., Bell, G. I., and Froguel, P. H., Identification of 14 new glucokinase mutations and description of the clinical profile of 42 MODY-2 families, *Diabetologia*, 40, 217, 1997.

394. Grupe, A., Hultgren, B., Ryan, A., Ma, Y. H., Bauer, M., and Stewart, T. A., Transgenic knockouts reveal a critical requirement for pancreatic β-cell glucokinase in maintaining glucose homeostasis, *Cell*, 83, 69, 1995.

395. Terauchi, Y., Sakura, H., Yasuda, K., Iwamoto, K., Takahashi, N., Ito, K., Kasai, H., Suzuki, H., Ueda, O., Kamada, N., Jishage, K., Komeda, K., Noda, M., Kanazawa, Y., Taniguchi, S., Miwa, I., Akanuma, Y., Kodama, T., Yazaki, Y., and Kadowaki, T., Pancreatic β-cell-specific targeted disruption of glucokinase gene, *J. Biol. Chem.*, 270, 30253, 1995.

396. Yamagata, K., Oda, N., Kaisaki, P. J., Menzel, S., Furuta, H., Vaxillaire, M., Southam, L., Cox, R. D., Lathrop, G. M., Boriraj, V. V., Chen, X., Cox, N. J., Oda, Y., Yano, H., Le Beau, M. M., Yamada, S., Nishigori, H., Takeda, J., Fajans, S. S., Hattersley, A. T., Iwasaki, N., Hansen, T., Pedersen, O., Polonsky, K. S., Turner, R. C., Velho, G., Chevre, J.-C., Froguel, P., and Bell, G. I., Mutations in the hepatocyte nuclear factor-1α gene in maturity-onset diabetes of the young (MODY3), *Nature*, 384, 455, 1996.

397. Yamagata, K., Furuta, H., Oda, N., Kaisaki, P. J., Menzel, S., Cox, N. J., Fajans, S. S., Signori, S., Stoffel, M., and Bell, G. I., Mutations in the hepatocyte nuclear factor-4α gene in maturity-onset diabetes of the young (MODY1), *Nature*, 384, 458, 1996.

398. Pontoglio, M., Barra, J., Hadchouel, M., Doyen, A., Kress, C., Bach, J. P., Babinet, C., and Yaniv, M., Hepatocyte nuclear factor 1 inactivation results in hepatic dysfunction, phenylkenonuria, and renal fanconi syndrome, *Cell*, 84, 575, 1996.

399. Stoffel, M., and Duncan, S. A., The maturity-onset diabetes of the young (MODY1) transcription factor HNF4α regulates expression of genes required for glucose transport and metabolism, *Proc. Natl. Acad. Sci. U.S.A.*, 94, 13209, 1997.

400. Verchere, C. B., D'Alessio, D. A., and Kahn, S. E., Consequences of human IAPP expression in transgenic mice, in *Lessons from Animal Diabetes VI*, Shafrir, E., Ed., Birkhäuser, Boston, 1996, 131.

401. Sakagashira, S., Sanke, T., Hanabusa, T., Shimomura, H., Ohagi, S., Kumagaye, K. Y., Nakajima, K., and Nanjo, K., Missense mutation of amylin gene (S20G) in Japanese NIDDM patients, *Diabetes*, 45, 1279, 1996.

402. D'Alessio, D. A., Verchere, C. B., Kahn, S. E., Hoagland, V., Baskin, D. G., Palmiter, R. D., and Ensinck, J. W., Pancreatic expression and secretion of human islet amyloid polypeptide in a transgenic mouse, *Diabetes*, 43, 1457, 1994.

403. Verchere, C. B., D'Alessio, D. A., Palmiter, R. D., and Kahn, S. E., Transgenic mice overproducing islet amyloid polypeptide have increased insulin storage and secretion *in vitro*, *Diabetologia*, 37, 725, 1994.

404. Verchere, C. B., D'Alessio, D. A., Palmiter, R. D., Weir, G. C., Bonner-Weir, S., Baskin, D. G., and Kahn, S. E., Islet amyloid formation with hyperglycemia in transgenic mice with beta cell expression of human islet amyloid polypeptide, *Proc. Natl. Acad. Sci. U.S.A.*, 93, 3942, 1996.

405. Charge, S. B. P., Esiri, M. M., Bethune, C. A., Hansen, B. C., and Clark, A., Apolipoprotein E is associated with islet amyloid and other amyloidoses-implications for Alzheimers disease, *J. Pathol.*, 179, 443, 1996.

406. Roberts, S. B. and Greenberg, A. S., The new obesity genes, *Nutr. Rev.*, 54, 41, 1996.

407. Enerbäck, S., Jacobsson, A., Simpson, E. M., Guerra, C., Yamashita, H., Harper, M.-E., and Kozak, L. P., Mice lacking mitochondrial uncoupling protein are cold-sensitive but not obese, *Nature*, 387, 90, 1997.

408. Lowell, B. B., Susulic, V. S., Hamann, A., Lawitts, J. A., Himms-Hagen, J., Boyer, B. B., Kozak, L. P., and Flier, J. S., Development of obesity in transgenic mice after genetic ablation of brown adipoase tissue, *Nature*, 366, 740, 1993.

409. Fleury, C., Neverova, M., Collins, S., Raimbault, S., Champigny, O., Levi-Meyrueis, C., Bouillaud, F., Seldin, M. F., Surwit, R. S., Ricquier, D., and Warden, C. H, Uncoupling protein-2: a novel gene linked to obesity and hyperinsulinemia, *Nature Genet.*, 15, 269, 1997.

410. Gimeno, R. E., Dembski, M., Weng, X., Deng, N., Shyjan, A. W., Gimeno C. J., Irir, F., Ellis, S. J., Woolf, E. A., and Tartaglia, L. A., Cloning and characterization of an uncoupling protein homolog, *Diabetes*, 46, 900, 1997.

411. Zhou, Y.-T., Shimabukuro, M., Koyama, K., Lee, Y., Wang, M.-Y., Trieu, F., Newgard, C. B., and Unger, R. H., Induction by leptin of uncoupling protein-2 and enzymes of fatty acid oxidation, *Proc. Natl. Acad. Sci. U.S.A.*, 94, 6386, 1997

412. Walston, J., Silver, K., Bogardus, C., Knowler, W. C., Celi, P. H. F. S., Austin, S., Manning, B., Strosberg, A. D., Stern, M. P., Raben, N., Sorkin, J. D., Roth, J., and Shuldiner, A. R., Time of onset of noninsulin-dependent diabetes and genetic variation in the β_3-adrenergic-receptor gene, *New Engl. J. Med.*, 333, 343, 1995.

413. Piétri-Rouxel, F., St. John Manning, B., Gros, J., and Strosberg, A. D., The biochemical effect of the naturally occurring Trp64 → Arg mutation on human $\beta3$-adrenoceptor activity, *Eur. J. Biochem.*, 247, 1174, 1997.

414. Strosberg, A. D., Association of β-3-adenoceptor polymorphism with obesity and diabetes: current status, *Trends Pharmacol. Sci.*, 18, 449, 1997.

415. Revelli, J.-P., Preitner, F., Samec, S., Muniesa, P., Kuehne, F., Boss, O., Vassalli, J.-D., Dulloo, A., Seydoux, J., Giacobino, J.-P., Huarte, J., and Ody, C., Targeted gene disruption reveals a leptin-independent role for the mouse β_3-adrenoceptor in the regulation of body composition, *J. Clin. Invest.*, 100, 1098, 1997.

416. Umekawa, T., Yoshida, T., Sakane, N., Saito, M., Kumamoto, K., and Kondo, M., Anti-obesity and anti-diabetic effects of CL316,243, a highly specific β_3-adrenoceptor agonist in Otsuka Long-Evans Tokushima fatty rats: induction of uncoupling protein and activation of glucose transporter 4 in white fat, *Eur. J. Endocrinol.*, 136, 429, 1997.

417. Qu, D., Ludwig, D. S., Gammeltoft, S., Piper, M., Pelleymounter, M. A., Cullen, M. J., Mathes, W. F., Przypek, J., Kanarek, R., and Maratos-Flier, E., A role for melanin-concentrating hormone in the central regulation of feeding behaviour, *Nature*, 380, 243, 1996.

418. Turton, M. D., O'Shea, D., Gunn, I., Beak, S. A., Edwards, C. M. B., Meeran, K., Choi, S. J., Taylor, G. M., Heath, M. M., Lambert, P. D., Wilding, P. H., Smith, D. M., Ghatei, M. A., Herbert, J., and Bloom, S. R., A role for glucagon-like peptide-1 in the central regulation of feeding, *Nature*, 379, 69, 1996.

419. Tang, C., Akabayashi, A., Manitiu, A., and Leibowitz, S. F., Hypothalamic galanin gene expression and peptide levels in relation to circulating insulin: possible role in energy balance, *Neuroendocrinology*, 65, 265, 1996.

420. Spina, M., Merlo-Pich, E., Chan, R. K. W., Basso, A. M., Rivier, J., Vale, W., and Koob, G. F., Appetite-suppressing effects of urocortin, a CRF-related neuropeptide, *Science*, 273, 1561, 1996.

421. Gloaguen, I., Costa, P., Demartis, A., Lazzaro, D., Di Marco, A., Graziani, R., Paonessa, G., Chen, F., Rosenblum, C. I., Van der Ploeg, L. H. T., Cortese, R., Ciliberto, G., and Laufer, R., Ciliary neurotrophic factor corrects obesity and diabetes associated with leptin deficiency and resistance, *Proc. Natl. Acad. Sci. U.S.A.*, 94, 6456, 1997.

422. Ohki-Hamazaki, H., Watase, K., Yamamoto, K., Ogura, H., Yamano, M., Yamada, K., Maeno, H., Imaki, J., Kikuyama, S., Wada E., and Wada, K., Mice lacking bombesin receptor subtype-3 develop metabolic defects and obesity, *Nature*, 390, 165, 1997.

423. Maassen, J. A., van den Ouweland, J. M. V., 't Hart, L. M., and Lemkes, H. H. P. J., Maternally inherited diabetes and deafness: a diabetic subtype associated with a mutation in mitochondrial DNA, *Horm. Metab. Res.*, 29, 50, 1997.

424. Gerbitz, K.-D., Gempel, K., and Brdiczka, D., Genetic, biochemical, and clinical implications of the cellular energy circuit, *Diabetes*, 45, 113, 1996.

425. Seldin, M., Mott, D., Bhat, D., Petro, A., Kuhn, C., Kingsmore, S. et al., Glycogen synthase: a putative locus for diet-induced hyperglycemia, *J. Clin. Invest.*, 94, 1, 1994.

426. Zouali, H., Hani, E. H., Philippi, A., Vionnet, N., Beckmann, J. S., Demenais, F., and Froguel, P., A susceptibility locus for early-onset noninsulin dependent (type 2) diabetes mellitus maps to chromosome 20q, proximal to the phosphoenolpyruvate carboxykinase gene., *Hum Mol. Gen*, 6, 1401-1408, 1997.

427. Hager, J., Hansen, L., Vaisse, C., Vionnet, N., Philippi, A., Poller, W., Velho, G., Carcassi, C., Contu, L., Julier, C., Cambien, F., Passa, P., Lathrop, M., Kindsvogel, W., Demenais, F., Nishimura, E., and Froguel, P., A missense mutation in the glucagon receptor gene is associated with noninsulin-dependent diabetes mellitus, *Nature Genet.*, 9, 299, 1995.
428. Burcelin, R., Katz, E. B., and Charron, M. J., Molecular and cellular aspects of the glucagon receptor: role in diabetes and metabolism, *Diabetes Metab.*, 22, 373, 1996.
429. Holst, J. J., Gromada, J., and Nauck, M. A., The pathogenesis of NIDDM involves a defective expression of the GIP receptor, *Diabetologia*, 40, 984, 1997.

Index

Index

A

differential inbred strain susceptibility, 278–280
HIV, 282
mechanism of differential strain sensitivity, 279–280
retroviruses and retroviral particles, 267, 274,
   281–282, 312, 349
triggers of diabetes in BB rat, 311–312
Vitamin C (ascorbic acid), 201–203
Vitamin E, 53, 203–204
V1-receptor, 182
V2-receptor, 182

W

Wallerian degeneration, 120
Warfarin, 90, 91
Water balance, 181
Weight change, *See also* Obesity
  BB diabetic rat, 297
  indicator of diabetes severity, 8
  obese phenotype, 342
  STZ-induced effects
    dose response, 8
    sex differences, 10
Wild rodents (captive) models, 365–367
Wistar rat, 9–12, 49, 53, 154, 160, 180, 183, 201, 207,
  233, 236–239, 249, 313, *See also* BB rat
Wistar-Kyoto (WKY) rat, 12, 154, 200, 245, 247, 250
Wistar-Lewis rat, 180
Worchester colony, 296, 317

X

Xenobiotic metabolism, 79–109
  acetylation, 93, 107
  activation and deactivation, 81–87
  cytochrome P450 enzymes, 87–91, 97–102, *See*
    Cytochrome P450-dependent oxidases
  epoxide hydration, 92, 107
  FAD monooxygenases, 91
  fate of reactive intermediates, 87
  glucuronide conjugation, 94, 106
  glutathione conjugation, 92–93, 107
  human diabetes, 108
  insulin-dependent diabetes mellitus and, 94–107
  insulin therapy and, 108
  noninsulin-dependent diabetes mellitus and, 108
  peroxidases, 91
  reactive intermediates, 87
  reductases, 91–92
  sensitization, 87
  sulfate conjugation, 93–94, 107

Z

Zinc, 199, 206, 206
Zizyphus spina-christi, 208
Zucker rat, 43, 250, 371
  diabetic fatty rat, 348, 356–357
  fatty rat, 355–356

T - #1068 - 101024 - C0 - 254/178/20 [22] - CB - 9780849316678 - Gloss Lamination